INTENSIVE CARE

A concise textbook

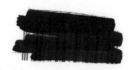

INTENSIVE CARE

A concise textbook

Second edition

C J Hinds FRCP FRCA
Senior Lecturer in Intensive Care and Anaesthesia,
The Medical College of St Bartholomew's Hospital
Director of Intensive Care, St Bartholomew's,
The Royal London and The London Chest Hospitals NHS Trust,
London UK

D Watson BSc (Hons) FRCA
Senior Lecturer in Intensive Care and Anaesthesia,
The Medical College of St Bartholomew's Hospital
Consultant, St Bartholomew's,
The Royal London and The London Chest Hospitals NHS Trust
and the Homerton Hospital, London UK

WB Saunders Company Ltd
London Philadelphia Toronto Sydney Tokyo

WB Saunders   24-28 Oval Road
Company Limited   London NW1 7DX, UK

The Curtis Center
Independence Square West
Philadelphia, PA 19106-3399, USA

Harcourt Brace & Company
55 Horner Avenue
Toronto, Ontario M8Z 4X6, Canada

Harcourt Brace & Company, Australia
30-52 Smidmore Street
Marrickville, NSW 2204, Australia

Harcourt Brace & Company, Japan
Ichibancho Central Building
22-1 Ichibancho
Chiyoda-ku, Tokyo 102, Japan

A catalogue record for this book is available from the
British Library

First edition published 1987

ISBN 0-7020-1541-5

This book is printed on acid-free paper

Typeset by Photo-graphics, Honiton, Devon, England
Printed and bound in Great Britain by The Bath Press, Bath

CONTENTS

FOREWORD

Intensive care medicine is a broad specialty covering a wide spectrum of potentially life-threatening illnesses and injuries in patients with various underlying conditions. Few medical specialties have evolved and grown as rapidly as intensive care medicine during the past few decades. Intensive clinical and fundamental research have resulted in a clearer understanding of the complex pathophysiology of the host's response to acute disease, whilst new methods of medical and surgical treatment, as well as new technologies to support vital organ functions, have been introduced. Decision-making in critically ill patients with complex pathophysiology and multisystem involvement requires the ability to assign priorities to diagnostic procedures and to tailor treatment to the needs of individual patients. Appropriate interpretation of information obtained from clinical examination, investigations, and monitoring forms the basis of a logical and comprehensive approach to the management of critical illness. The intensivist needs, therefore, theoretical knowledge and practical skills not included in training in the traditional specialties, in order to offer the best possible care to the critically ill.

In the rapidly evolving field of intensive care medicine trainees have to place scientific knowledge, as well as new treatment and monitoring techniques into a meaningful context. This requires a framework that includes an understanding of global pathophysiology, specific organ dysfunction, the systemic effects of the host's response, the technical aspects of patient monitoring and vital organ support, and the ability to interpret monitored data, as well as a knowledge of treatment modalities and the acquisition of practical skills. Doctors Hinds and Watson are to be congratulated on successfully producing such a framework in this concise textbook covering the main issues of intensive care medicine. The two authors from the same institution have achieved a uniformity of style and design, together with a balance between the various topics. In addition, overlap and repetition have been avoided, and recommendations are clear and nonconflicting. The intensive care trainee will find that information is easily accessible in this clearly written textbook and that by using the key references cited in each chapter particular subjects can be explored in greater depth.

This concise textbook is an excellent introductory text for those embarking on a career in intensive care medicine and should also prove useful to trainees in other specialties, medical students and intensive care nurses.

Lambert G. Thijs
Professor of Medicine, Director Medical Intensive Care Unit,
Free University Hospital, Amsterdam

PREFACE

To produce a second edition of *Intensive Care: A Concise Textbook* was a daunting task which was only feasible because of the contribution of my colleague, David Watson. Together we have been able to considerably expand and update the original text whilst avoiding, we hope, the difficulties and deficiencies associated with a multi-contributed work.

As before, this book is intended primarily as an introduction to intensive care medicine for doctors in training. It is aimed not only at those embarking on specialist training in intensive care but also at trainees in other acute specialties who may become involved in the management of critically ill patients. The book also targets those undertaking the various postgraduate examinations, which now include aspects of intensive care medicine. We anticipate that nurses specializing in intensive care, as well as some medical students and physiotherapists will find this book useful.

With these objectives in mind, we have attempted to produce a book which is sufficiently comprehensive to provide a sound working knowledge of the discipline and yet concise enough to be read in its entirety. This new edition includes additional chapters on some important aspects of intensive care practice which were not included in the first edition and the original chapters have been considerably expanded and updated. We have also attempted to provide clearer guidelines for management whilst continuing to discuss important theoretical principles of intensive care and provide a balanced view of current controversies. As before, key references are included for those who wish to pursue further a particular topic. Finally, it will be immediately obvious to the reader that the format has been radically altered with the intention of making the text more readable and the information more readily accessible.

We have been privileged to receive help and advice from friends and colleagues at St Bartholomew's Hospital and from elsewhere in the United Kingdom. In particular, we would like to acknowledge Dr DS Dymond (Consultant Cardiologist, St Bartholomew's Hospital), Professor MJG Farthing (Professor of Gastroenterology, St Bartholomew's Hospital), Professor AJ Pinching (Professor of Immunology, St Bartholomew's Hospital), Professor AEG Raine (Professor of Renal Medicine, St Bartholomew's Hospital), Dr HKF Van Saene (Consultant in Medical Microbiology, Alder Hey Children's Hospital) and Professor JAH Wass (Professor in Endocrinology, St Bartholomew's Hospital).

We would like to thank the publishers and especially Margaret Macdonald for her patience and good humour. Finally, we would like to express our gratitude to Miss Sandra Sims, Academic Secretary, for tirelessly typing the manuscript and to our consultant colleagues for their unstinting support.

CJ Hinds
D Watson

Glossary of Physiological Terms

C_aO_2	Arterial oxygen content
$C_{a-v}O_2$	Arteriovenous oxygen content difference
$C_{a-J}O_2$	Cerebral arteriovenous oxygen difference (also commonly abbreviated $AJDO_2$)
$C_{\bar{v}}O_2$	Mixed venous oxygen content
DO_2	Oxygen delivery
F_AO_2	Fractional concentration of oxygen in alveolar gas
F_IO_2	Fractional concentration of oxygen in inspired air
$M\dot{V}O_2$	Myocardial oxygen consumption
PO_2	Partial pressure of oxygen
P_aO_2	Arterial oxygen tension
P_AO_2	Alveolar oxygen tension
P_aCO_2	Arterial carbon dioxide tension
P_ACO_2	Alveolar carbon dioxide tension
$P_{A-a}O_2$	Alveolar-arterial oxygen difference
$P_{\bar{v}}CO_2$	Mixed venous carbon dioxide tension
$P_{\bar{v}}O_2$	Mixed venous oxygen tension
$\dot{Q}$	Perfusion per unit time
$\dot{Q}_t$	Cardiac output
SO_2	Oxygen saturation
S_aO_2	Arterial oxygen saturation
S_JO_2	Jugular bulb oxygen saturation
$S_{\bar{v}}O_2$	Mixed venous oxygen saturation
$\dot{V}$	Ventilation per unit time
$\dot{V}_A$	Effective alveolar ventilation per unit time
$\dot{V}_{CO_2}$	Amount of carbon dioxide excreted per unit time
V_D	Dead space
$\dot{V}_E$	Expired minute volume
$\dot{V}_{O_2}$	Oxygen consumption
V_T	Tidal volume

Dedication

To our wives and families without whose support this book could never have been completed. Also to the nurses, medical students and doctors in training who stimulated us to undertake this task and, through their encouragement, persuaded us to persevere to its completion.

CJH
DW

To Michael White, Professor of Medicine, University of Hull, a dear friend who died on Sunday 13th August 1995.

CJH

1 Planning, Organization and Management

INTRODUCTION

Intensive care medicine (or 'critical care medicine') is predominantly concerned with the management of patients with acute life-threatening conditions ('the critically ill') within the specialized environment of an intensive care unit. It also encompasses the resuscitation and transport of those who become acutely ill or are injured, either elsewhere in the hospital or in the community. Intensive care has been defined as *'a service for patients with potentially recoverable diseases who can benefit from more detailed observation and treatment than is generally available in the standard wards and departments'* (Spiby, 1989).

The creation of intensive care units and the subsequent development of intensive care medicine owes much to the introduction of intermittent positive pressure ventilation (IPPV) for the treatment of patients with respiratory failure. The therapeutic potential of this technique was first recognized during the 1950s when it was used to support patients with respiratory failure due to neuromuscular disorders, such as poliomyelitis, or acute exacerbations of chronic obstructive pulmonary disease (COPD) (see Chapter 7), and occasionally those with postoperative respiratory insufficiency. The more widespread adoption of therapeutic IPPV (as opposed to its established role in anaesthesia) during the early 1960s prompted many institutions to create 'respiratory care units' to facilitate the management of patients requiring mechanical ventilation. At the same time, it was appreciated that patients who had undergone cardiac surgery, which was then associated with an appreciable mortality, could benefit from intensive postoperative care, and that the complications of myocardial infarction could be detected and treated more effectively within specialized 'coronary care units.' It soon became apparent that other critically ill patients could be better managed within purpose-built units fully equipped with monitoring and technical facilities in which they could receive expert nursing care and the constant attention of appropriately trained medical staff. It also seemed likely that this concentration of special facilities and expertise would improve patient outcome and reduce costs.

The scope of intensive care medicine has since developed and expanded to include the management of patients with a wide variety of underlying medical and surgical disorders. In addition, patients with acute cardiorespiratory disturbances frequently develop failure of other organs or systems and, once the initial objective of sustaining life has been achieved, the primary disease must be diagnosed and appropriately treated. Although intensive care medicine therefore remains a discipline primarily concerned with the management of acute major disturbances of cardiovascular and respiratory function, a coordinated, multidisciplinary approach is essential for optimal patient care.

PLANNING, DESIGN AND ORGANIZATION OF INTENSIVE CARE UNITS (Intensive Care Society—Standards for Intensive Care Units)

Definitions

Intensive care units are usually reserved for patients with potential or established organ failure and must therefore provide the facilities for the diagnosis, prevention and treatment of multiple organ failure.

High dependency units offer a standard of care intermediate between that available on the general ward and that in the intensive care unit. They provide monitoring and support for patients at risk of developing organ failure, including facilities for short-term ventilatory support and immediate resuscitation (Intensive Care Society, 1990). They can also provide a 'step-down' facility for patients being discharged from intensive care (*progressive care unit*). It is important to establish clear lines of communication between the intensive care unit and the high dependency/ progressive care units.

In Australia three levels of intensive care provision have been defined.

- *Level 1 (small district hospital)* provides close nursing observation, basic monitoring, immediate resuscitation, and short-term (24 hours or less) ventilation.

These units are equivalent to 'high dependency units'.

- *Level 2 (larger general hospital)* provides more prolonged ventilation, a resident doctor, and access to pathology, radiology and physiotherapy at all times. These units are equivalent to the intensive care units found in some smaller district general hospitals in the UK. They do not provide more complex organ support (e.g. haemofiltration) and more complex invasive monitoring (e.g. intracranial pressure monitoring, pulmonary artery catheterization).

- *Level 3 (tertiary referral hospital)* provides all aspects of intensive care and is staffed by specialists in intensive care with trainees, specialist nurses and allied health professionals, and clinical and scientific staff. These units have access to complex investigations, complex imaging techniques and specialists from all disciplines. In the UK such units have been referred to as regional intensive care units.

The recent trend to stratify intensive care units in this way has the advantage of avoiding unnecessary duplication of expensive intensive care facilities, but it does mean that the transfer of critically ill patients between hospitals will probably become increasingly common. It has been suggested that early referral to a regional (Level 3) unit may decrease mortality in patients with complex critical illness and that sicker patients benefit from early referral. Mortality is, however, likely to be extremely high in those patients transferred after more than ten days of intensive care (Purdie *et al.*, 1990).

Planning

The type and size of intensive care unit suitable for a particular hospital depends on several factors including the number of acute beds and the type of cases being treated. The need for flexibility and for local, rather than national, planning has been emphasized (The Association of Anaesthetists of Great Britain and Ireland, 1988), although adherence to national and international standards and guidelines is clearly essential. Many years ago the Department of Health and Social Security recommended that approximately 1–2% of the acute beds of a general hospital should be allocated to intensive care, and suggested that bed numbers should be increased if there are special units within the hospital for cardiac, major vascular and neurosurgery (Department of Health and Social Security, 1970, revised 1974). Since then, however, there has been a progressive increase in the demand for intensive care, largely because, despite the recent decrease in the number of long-stay acute hospital beds (a trend that is likely to continue) the proportion of seriously ill patients has steadily increased (see also Chapter 4). As a result the proportion of hospital beds that should be allocated to intensive care is now

considerably greater than previously suggested; in one recent study involving 40 intensive care units in North America, the average number of beds in each hospital was 359 and the average number of intensive care beds in each institution was 21 (Knaus *et al.*, 1991). Overall in the USA, intensive care beds account for about 6–11% of all hospital beds and an expenditure of as much as 1% of gross national product (Osborne & Evans, 1994; Spivack, 1987). By contrast, in New Zealand about 1.7% of total beds are designated for intensive care (Zimmerman *et al.*, 1988) and, in the UK, the percentage of intensive care beds is around 1–2% (Spiby, 1989).

The size of a unit should also be governed by the fact that those with fewer than four beds and less than 200 admissions a year, or a bed occupancy less than 60%, are unlikely to acquire and retain the necessary expertise, and are probably uneconomic (The Association of Anaesthetists of Great Britain and Ireland, 1988), while units with more than 12–16 beds become increasingly difficult to manage. Although the average district general hospital is likely to have around 6–8 beds, units with 20–25 beds, or even more, may be appropriate in larger institutions, and can operate effectively, provided they are adequately staffed and working practices are adapted to cope with the increased workload.

In the UK and Australasia there has been a preference for developing general intensive care units, managed wherever possible by intensive care specialists, and for providing separate units only for neonatal, paediatric, post-cardiac surgery and, sometimes, neurosurgical intensive care. Coronary care units are usually separated from the other intensive care areas. In some large North American hospitals, however, units may be further subdivided (e.g. into medical, respiratory, surgical and trauma). Whatever the arrangements, the various units, including high-dependency and progressive care facilities, should be close to each other to make optimal use of pooled medical, nursing and technical staff, and equipment. They should also be adjacent to other acute areas such as the accident and emergency department, the operating theatres and the labour ward, and imaging facilities. The intensive care areas must also be easily accessible via capacious lifts, wide corridors and large doors.

Design

Intensive care units must be spacious to allow easy access to the patient; 20 m² per bed is recommended and ideally single rooms should be larger (e.g. 25.5 m²) (**Fig. 1.1**) (Intensive Care Society—Standards for Intensive Care Units, Health Building Note 27, 1992). The overall floor plan should minimize unnecessary through traffic (Aitkenhead *et al.*, 1993). The patient areas should consist of a large open-plan area containing

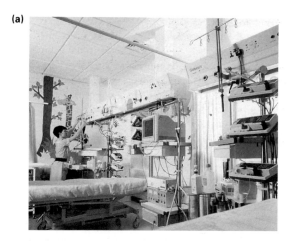

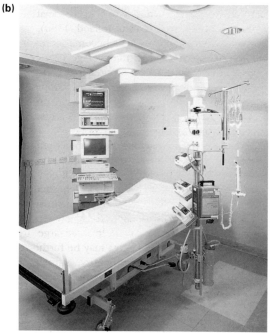

Fig. 1.1 Access to intensive care patients must be un-restricted. This is achieved by allowing adequate floor space for each bed area. The available space can be optimized by using (a) an overhead rail or (b) a 'pendant' system.

several beds, with some adjacent single-bedded cubicles, the exact proportion being determined by the types of patient being treated. Open-plan areas make the most efficient use of nursing staff, while single cubicles may be used to minimize the risks of cross-infection by isolating patients with impaired immune responses or those harbouring dangerous microorganisms, and to provide privacy for mentally alert, long-stay patients. It is recommended that not more than two or possibly three single rooms should be provided for every ten beds.

Positive/negative pressure air conditioning systems for single isolation rooms are expensive and of un-proven efficacy. Air conditioning is, however, rec-ommended to ensure a reasonable working environ-ment.

Each bed space must be equipped with monitors, suc-tion apparatus, piped oxygen and air, and a vacuum sup-ply. Three oxygen, two air and four suction outlets have been recommended. Low-pressure suction should be available. There should also be a bedside light. A plenti-ful supply of mains sockets (e.g. 20–24 per bed) is essen-tial, as are power points for mobile X-ray equipment. There must be emergency back-up supplies of air, oxy-gen, suction and power that are immediately available in the event of failure (Aitkenhead et al., 1993). Facil-ities for haemodialysis may be provided at selected bed areas. To avoid restricting access to the patient, services are normally delivered via 'trunking' and equipment is usually mounted on a rail system, both being located behind the bed. Less frequently, services and some equipment are ceiling-mounted or delivered via an 'over-head rail' (see **Fig. 1.1**) or a free-standing bollard (Kerr et al., 1985).

Bed dividers can be used not only to provide a degree of privacy for the patients, but also as storage space. By keeping all essential equipment at the bedside, staff movement can be reduced. A chart table and writing surface are also required at the bedside. There should be a central nursing station from which it is possible to see all patients and their bedside monitors. Central monitoring is not, however, as important as in a coron-ary care unit. It is essential to provide adequate radio-graph viewing facilities and a good communication network using telephones and an intercom system.

There should be separate 'clean' and 'dirty' utility rooms, with adequate facilities for the disposal of soiled linen and waste. Surfaces should be easily cleaned and there should be a good supply of wash-basins, with one in each single room (Aitkenhead et al., 1993).

As well as plenty of storage space (20–25% of the pa-tient and central nursing station areas is recommended), it is important to provide a doctor's on-call room, adequate office accommodation, a staff rest room, a waiting area, overnight accommodation for relatives and an interview room. Other facilities may include a library and a tutorial room. In most units there is also an on-site 'stat' laboratory allowing immediate blood gas ana-lysis and determination of plasma electrolytes, blood sugar levels, haemoglobin concentration and packed cell volume. In some units this laboratory will also be equipped with devices for measuring haemoglobin sat-uration with oxygen, blood lactate levels and plasma osmolality. Overall more than 50% of the total floor space of the unit should be for non-patient areas.

Finally, it is important for the psychological well-being of both patients and staff that all bed areas are well illuminated with natural daylight (Wilson, 1972) (see also Chapter 10). Ideally patients should be positioned facing a window with a view of the outside world.

Equipment

Clearly the quantity and level of sophistication of the equipment and monitoring required will be influenced by the size and role of the intensive care unit (**Table 1.1**). Monitoring equipment should preferably have the capacity for data storage and retrieval. The equipment for the following therapeutic interventions should be immediately available (Aitkenhead et al., 1993):

- tracheal intubation;
- DC cardioversion;
- bronchoscopy;
- insertion of chest drains;
- cardiac pacing;
- intra-aortic balloon pumping;
- invasive haemodynamic monitoring;
- establishing extracorporeal renal support.

STAFFING INTENSIVE CARE UNITS

Medical staff

It is essential that a suitably trained resident doctor is immediately available throughout the day and night to deal with emergencies occurring on the unit. Often this doctor is an anaesthetist, but if not they must be capable

Table 1.1 Some of the equipment required in a regional (Level 3) intensive care unit.

Monitoring and Investigations	
- Bedside monitors - Central monitors (optional) - Portable monitors - Facilities for: ● monitoring intravascular pressure ● intracranial pressure monitoring ● cerebral function monitoring ● cardiac output determination ● pulse oximetry ● capnography ● temperature monitoring	- Equipment for ● blood gas/acid–base analysis ● determination of electrolytes/blood sugar ● measurement of haemoglobin/packed cell volume ● measurement of blood lactate ● measurement of oxygen content ● bedside blood sugar measurements ● 12-lead electrocardiogram ● monitoring lung function ● weighing patients

Respiratory therapy	Renal support
- Ventilators (bedside and portable) - Humidifiers - Oxygen masks - Circuits - Self-inflating bags for manual ventilation - Fibre-optic bronchoscope - Anaesthetic machine	- Equipment for peritoneal dialysis - Equipment for continuous arteriovenous haemodiafiltration - Equipment for continuous veno–venous haemodiafiltration - Access to haemodialysis machine

Cardiovascular therapy	Other
- Defibrillators (including portable devices) - Intra-aortic balloon pump - Infusion pumps and syringe pumps - Pacemakers	- Pressure-relieving beds and mattresses - Heating/cooling blankets/devices - Drip stands - Dressing trolleys - Mobile curtains
Radiology	
- Portable X-ray machine - Image intensifier	

of emergency intubation and have a thorough knowledge of the techniques of ventilatory support and their complications. Resident medical staff must be closely supervised at all times by a consultant or an experienced senior registrar and a consultant intensive care specialist should always be immediately available for advice and be ready to attend the unit at short notice. In many larger units trainees in intensive care and research fellows will be important members of the medical team.

Each intensive care unit should have a nominated 'director' who should be an intensive care specialist. There is now a measure of agreement among those closely involved in intensive care that the 'base specialty' of the consultant in charge is largely irrelevant, provided that he or she is motivated and appropriately trained. The proportion of the consultant's time allocated to intensive care will depend largely on the size and type of hospital. In a large teaching hospital, most or all of their sessions may be devoted to intensive care so that additional teaching, training and research commitments can be fulfilled, while in some district general hospitals it may be appropriate to appoint consultants 'with an interest in intensive care' who will also have an appreciable number of sessions in their base specialty.

The on-call commitment will necessarily be shared between a number of suitably trained consultants. In many hospitals in the UK, the intensive care unit is run by a group of consultant anaesthetists specializing in intensive care, while in others the team consists of both anaesthetists and physicians. Only a few units are managed exclusively by physicians. In North America, surgeons also specialize in intensive care and are particularly involved in the management of critically ill trauma patients. These intensive care specialists should control and coordinate patient care in conjunction with the primary clinician; they should also, when appropriate, be guided by advice obtained from other specialists. Clear lines of responsibility must be established between the medical staff, and all those involved in the patients' care, including nurses and physiotherapists must be in constant communication.

Nursing staff

An adequate complement of suitably trained nurses is crucial to the success of an intensive care unit. Ideally there should be one nurse for each patient, a 'runner' and a senior nurse in charge on any one shift. Allowing for holidays, off-duty and sickness, this requires a total of at least 5-6 nurses per bed as well as several senior nurses and a 'nurse manager,' who assumes overall administrative responsibility. A clinical teacher who can develop the skills of the less experienced staff is an invaluable addition to the team.

In practice, because of economic constraints and a shortage of suitably qualified personnel, this ideal can be difficult to achieve. Further problems are posed by the inevitable fluctuations in both patient numbers and the level of nursing care that each requires. Although the optimum bed occupancy is said to be approximately 80%, in many units this figure is closer to 60%, while in others it approaches 100%. Furthermore, some units deal almost exclusively with seriously ill, ventilated patients, while others admit a larger proportion of relatively stable cases, mainly for observation. Units that are adequately staffed when full of highly dependent patients will therefore have an excess of nurses at other times. The alternative is a relatively understaffed unit, unable to cope during periods of peak demand. In an attempt to solve this problem and to achieve a balance between these two extremes, more exact methods of assessing the overall nursing requirements of a particular unit have been developed (Intensive Care Society—Standards for Intensive Care Units). Some of the difficulties can be minimized by managing the less-demanding patients in high-dependency or progressive care units where a 1 : 2 nurse : patient ratio is acceptable.

Recruitment and retention of nursing staff can be improved by attention to the designing and planning of units, as well as to the organizational and stress management aspects of intensive care discussed elsewhere in this chapter.

Administrative and ancillary staff

A *receptionist/ward clerk* who can answer the telephone, attend to relatives and perform clerical duties is a valuable addition to the team and can relieve the nurses' work load. *Secretarial assistance* will also be required.

Other health care professionals

Physiotherapists who are experienced in dealing with critically ill, ventilated patients have a vital role in successful intensive care (see later chapters) and must be integrated into the 'team'.

Adequate *technical support* for repair and maintenance of equipment is also essential. It is particularly important that on-site laboratory equipment such as automated blood gas analysers, are subjected to a strict quality control programme performed by experienced laboratory staff (see Chapter 5). These members of the team will also be involved in selecting and buying equipment.

Expert imaging (e.g. chest radiography, ultrasound, computerized tomographic (CT) scanning) is an important aspect of intensive care and requires the services of expert radiographers and close liaison with radiologists.

A *pharmacist* should be identified as having responsibility for the intensive care unit and should be available for advice. It is also important to be able to consult suitably experienced *dietitians*. Specialized '*respiratory therapists*' are important members of the team in North America, but have not established a role in the UK, Europe or Australasia.

Finally access to *social workers, counselling services* and *ministers of religion* is essential.

Work-related stress

The psychological pressures on those who work in intensive care units, particularly the nursing staff, are considerable. As well as the usual signs and symptoms of stress (**Table 1.2**), the syndrome of 'burnout' (**Table 1.3**) has been described in intensive care staff (Roberts, 1986). This is a process in which high and sustained levels of job stress produce feelings of tension, irritability and fatigue ending with a defensive reaction of detachment, apathy, cynicism or rigidity. Such work-related stress disorders are more likely to occur in the most dedicated, enthusiastic and idealistic members of staff.

Because of the sustained intimate contact between intensive care nurses and their patients a close relationship is inevitably established, particularly with those whose stay in the unit is prolonged. This exposes the nurse to considerable emotional pressures, which are

often exacerbated by frequent close contact with the patient's anxious and distressed relatives. The work of an intensive care nurse is both physically and mentally demanding, involving the ability to use complex equipment and to diagnose acute life-threatening events and administer appropriate emergency treatment. Moreover, many are reluctant to seek advice, fearing that this might be interpreted as incompetence. Medical staff are also subjected to stress (Lask, 1987) and it has been suggested that their frustration at being unable to help an

Table 1.2 Some effects of stress.

Physiological

Fatigue

Headache

Sexual difficulties

? Hypertension

? Peptic ulceration

? Coronary artery disease

Psychological

Anxiety

Depression

Irritability

Drug or alcohol abuse

Poor work performance

Relationship problems

Table 1.3 Signs and symptoms of 'burn-out' (Roberts, 1986).

Emotional

Loss of humour: 'Gallows humour'

Persistent sense of failure, guilt, blame

Cynical, blaming attitude towards patients

Frequent anger, resentment and bitterness

Increasing irritability, family and marital conflict

Feelings of discouragement and indifference

Eventual resignation to lack of power

Preoccupation with own needs and personal survival

Behavioural

Frequent clock watching

Increasing resistance to go to work each day

Postpone patient contacts, resist calls and visits

Increasingly go by the book, loss of creative problem solving

Work harder to achieve less

Avoid discussing work with colleagues

Increasing social isolation

Increasing use of mood-altering drugs

Physical

Feel tired and exhausted all day

Sleep disorders

Frequent and long-lasting minor ailments

Increasing use of sick leave, high absenteeism

Prone to accidents

Cognitive

Increasing thoughts of leaving job

Inability to concentrate on or listen to what patient is saying

Rigid thinking, resist all change

Increasing suspiciousness and distrust

See patients as objects rather than people

Stereotype patients

individual patient may precipitate excessive criticism of colleagues, overzealous treatment or even avoidance of the unit altogether.

Maintenance of staff morale is therefore crucial. Important aspects to be considered include the provision of adequate numbers of appropriately qualified personnel, close cooperation and discussion of management decisions among all members of staff, consistent unit policies, and comprehensive teaching in all aspects of intensive care. Unit design may also be important; for example it is now recognized that working in an environment devoid of natural light increases stress (Wilson, 1972).

Finally, faulty job design is an important cause of burn-out. Confusion about the exact nature and extent of one's responsibilities can lead to exhaustion, while overlapping responsibilities may precipitate competition and conflict with colleagues. These factors will be exacerbated by lack of meaningful support, 'negative' feedback and teaching that creates false expectations. Measures that may reduce the incidence of burn-out include:

- teaching stress awareness and personal stress management;
- improved management and organizational changes;
- adequate leave of absence;
- access to further education;
- adequate support;
- team approach;
- personal changes (e.g. exercise, relaxation).

Education and research

Staff morale and job satisfaction and the quality of patient care can be substantially enhanced by providing structured introductory training, offering specific opportunities for career development, and encouraging participation in continuing education, including attendance at national and international meetings. Larger units may also offer approved courses in intensive care nursing and more specialist training in intensive care medicine. An active research programme can also have a beneficial influence on *esprit de corps* by stimulating enquiry, discussion and enthusiasm for the specialty.

Audit

A system of continuing audit is essential to document activity, identify deficiencies and suggest ways of improving patient care. Audit should involve regular objective assessments of structure, processes and outcome (Aitkenhead *et al.*, 1993). It is important to 'close the loop' by auditing the impact of any changes that are made on the chosen outcome measures.

Incidents that either could, or did, reduce the margin of safety for a patient or staff member must be documented in a structured report so that measures can be taken to minimize the risk of a similar event in the future.

Policies and protocols

Intensive care and high-dependency units must have agreed, written policies for the admission and discharge of patients and for dealing with patient referrals. Management responsibilities and the clinical chains of command must also be clearly defined. Written protocols for all the common intensive care activities and procedures must be produced and adhered to, and should be regularly reviewed. Safe practice demands that protocols for all procedures should stipulate that (Aitkenhead *et al.*, 1993):

- the availability, correct functioning and calibration of all equipment should be checked in advance;
- the operator should be appropriately experienced or supervised;
- competent assistance should be available;
- the expected benefits should outweigh the anticipated risks.

Examples of activities for which protocols should be established include:

- vascular cannulation, including pulmonary artery catheterization;
- tracheal intubation and extubation;
- mechanical ventilation;
- antimicrobial policies and prevention of infection.

Written guidelines for the management of specific conditions, especially those that are encountered less frequently, are also valuable.

Documentation

Regular systematic clinical assessments of the patient should be recorded in the progress notes, including comments on vital signs, the function of each organ or system, and the results of haematological, biochemical and microbiological investigations. The treatment plan for the day and any alterations or additions to the drug regimen must be recorded. Interviews with relatives should also be documented, as should decisions to limit or withdraw treatment. Physiological measurements, clinical signs and blood results should be recorded on flow charts or in a computer that can produce 'trend' displays. This allows large amounts of data to be assimilated. Accurate fluid balance charts are essential.

OUTCOME AND COSTS

For many critically ill patients, intensive care is undoubtedly life-saving and resumption of a normal lifestyle is expected. In certain patients (e.g. those requiring mechanical ventilation for Guillain–Barré syndrome or drug overdose and those recovering from cardiac surgery), mortality rates should be very low and the majority should make a complete recovery. It also seems likely that the elective admission of selected high-risk patients into an intensive care or high-dependency unit, particularly in the immediate postoperative period, can minimize morbidity and mortality and possibly reduce costs (Teplick et al., 1983), as well as reduce the demands on medical and nursing personnel on the general wards.

Mortality

In the more seriously ill patients immediate mortality rates are high, while a significant number succumb soon after discharge from the intensive care unit and the quality of life for some of those who do survive may be poor. In one study from North America, for example, the mortality rate of a group of unstable patients who required continuous medical and nursing care with frequent changes of orders and therapy, was 57% at one month, rising to 69% at one year. By comparison in the less seriously ill patients, one-year mortality was 15–21% (Cullen et al., 1984). In a more recent evaluation of outcome in a heterogeneous group of critically ill patients admitted to a typical general intensive care unit in the UK, 24% died in the unit and a further 24% died within two years of discharge (Ridley et al., 1990). Long-term survival was related to age and severity of illness, but mortality was also influenced by the diagnosis: 71% of trauma patients survived to one year compared with only 41% of those admitted with gastrointestinal pathology (Ridley et al., 1990). Similar results have been reported from a European intensive care unit where the in-unit mortality was 18%, the hospital mortality was 29%, and a further 13% died after discharge from hospital within 12 months of admission to the intensive care unit (Dragsted et al., 1989; Dragsted & Qvist, 1989).

Quality of life

Although some investigators have concluded that quality of life after intensive care is good, and is generally determined by premorbid health (Sage et al., 1986), others have detected significant decreases in quality of life in some subgroups including younger patients, trauma patients, patients admitted with respiratory problems and those who previously had a good quality of life (Ridley & Wallace, 1990; Ridley et al., 1994). It has been shown that the patients perceived quality of life may be reduced by a decreased ability to think and remember, limitations on their contact with other family members, a perceived decrease in their contribution to society, a reduction in activities outside work and a fall in income (Ridley et al., 1994). In young trauma patients the reduction in quality of life after intensive care is associated with significant psychological difficulties as well as concerns about employment and leisure activities, and it has been suggested that rehabilitation programmes should concentrate on these areas (Thiagarajan et al., 1994).

Costs

The cost of intensive care, which is thought to be around 3–4 times more expensive than routine ward care, is also a cause for concern.

In some hospitals in the USA, 15–20% of all costs are attributable to intensive care (Spivack, 1987; Thibault et al., 1980), accounting for an annual expenditure estimated in 1987 as approximately 13–15 billion dollars; and it is likely that as new therapeutic techniques and agents become available these costs will continue to escalate. In 1984 the total charges for patients with adult respiratory distress syndrome admitted to a medical intensive care unit in the USA ranged from US$9263 to US$1,873,893 with a median cost of US$523,894; median daily charges were US$2430 (Bellamy & Oye, 1984). Since then these costs are likely to have increased significantly. In this and other studies the nonsurvivors cost considerably more than the survivors (approx- imately twice as much), partly because of the large quantities of blood and blood products usually required by the most seriously ill patients.

In the UK, it has been calculated that the costs of intensive care for a patient surviving for one year after an episode of acute cardiovascular or respiratory disease is approximately £2600, while the total hospital cost per quality adjusted life year was estimated at £7500 (Ridley et al., 1994). These estimates place intensive care at the higher end of health care expenditure, equivalent to heart transplantation, but cheaper than haemodialysis, and the costs increase considerably if expenditure of non-survivors is included in the calculation.

PATIENT SELECTION AND LIMITING TREATMENT

Apart from considerations of cost, inappropriate use of intensive care facilities has other implications (Jennett, 1984). The patient may experience unnecessary suffering and loss of dignity, while relatives may also have to endure considerable emotional pressures. In some cases, treatment may simply prolong the process of dying or sustain life of dubious quality, and in others the risks of interventions may outweigh the potential benefits. Finally, skilled medical and nursing staff may be diverted from caring for patients elsewhere in the hospital, and the ability of staff on general wards to manage seriously ill patients is diminished. Jennett (1984) has summarized the circumstances in which intensive care may be harmful as:

- unnecessary, because routine care would have achieved the same result;
- unsuccessful, because the patient is too ill to recover;
- unsafe, because the risks of complications exceed the potential benefits;
- unkind, because the subsequent quality of life is unacceptable;
- unwise, because of the diversion of limited resources.

To ensure a humane approach to the management of the critically ill and that limited resources are used appropriately it is important to identify those patients who are most likely to benefit from intensive care (who ideally should never be denied admission), and to withhold, limit or withdraw treatment when there is no prospect of recovery. It is also important to avoid admitting those who will make a good recovery without intensive care; an event which, for a variety of reasons including the availability of beds and the threat of litigation is more common in North America than in the UK. In one medical intensive care unit in the USA, for example, approximately 75% of patients were admitted solely for non-invasive monitoring and of those only 10% subsequently required major interventions (Thibault *et al.*, 1980).

As high mortality rates in the intensive care unit and soon after discharge contribute significantly to the high costs of intensive care, it has been suggested that efforts to contain costs should concentrate on selecting patients with a 'reasonable' prospect of survival (Ridley *et al.*, 1994). In practice, however, it is not usually acceptable to deny critically ill patients admission to intensive care, even when the chances of recovery from the acute illness seem to be remote. The long-term prognosis is usually uncertain, except in patients with disseminated, incurable malignancy or terminal chronic respiratory failure, and those in a persistent vegetative state, and it is often difficult to make a precise diagnosis on initial referral. In addition, the patient's response to treatment can rarely be anticipated with any degree of certainty. Decisions to deny patients access to intensive care may also be tempered by the knowledge that the prognosis of individual disorders frequently changes as standards of care improve or new treatments are introduced.

In the early days of intensive care some considered it reasonable to deny admission simply on the grounds of old age, but it was soon recognized that this approach could not be justified. Although it is clear that some elderly patients may have little or no chance of returning to an independent existence and there is evidence that age can affect long-term survival (Ridley *et al.*, 1990), it has been shown that old age alone does not influence either the cost or the outcome of intensive care (Fedullo & Swinburne, 1983). There is also evidence to suggest that age should not be a consideration when allocating intensive care beds to patients with malignancy (Chalfin & Carlon, 1990). It would seem that physiological age is more important than chronological age in determining survival and that a careful assessment of the patient's previous health, physical independence and social circumstances provides a better indication of the likely benefits of intensive care (Editorial, 1991).

Because it is rarely possible, or acceptable to discriminate between critically ill patients before admission the humanitarian and cost-effective practice of intensive care largely depends on a willingness to make decisions about withholding, withdrawing or limiting treatment once it becomes clear that the prognosis is hopeless. To persist with futile treatment is undignified and sometimes distressing for the patient, as well as upsetting and disruptive for the relatives, demoralizing for the staff and wasteful of limited resources. It is therefore now generally accepted that physicians are not obliged to administer '*extraordinary care*'. This has been defined (Schneiderman & Spragg, 1988) as care that is not morally obligatory because:

- it is medically impossible or futile;
- it provides no benefits in terms of prolonging life or alleviating suffering;
- the resulting burdens on the patient are excessive in relation to the benefits.

Ethically, withdrawing life support, including mechanical ventilation, is considered to be no different from discontinuing any other inappropriate medical intervention (Schneiderman & Spragg, 1988).

When making decisions to forego life-sustaining treatment clinicians may be helped by some of the statements that have appeared in landmark court decisions in the USA relating to patients in a persistent vegetative state (Schneiderman & Spragg, 1988). These have included the contention that '*prolongation of life does not mean a mere suspension of the act of dying, but contemplates at the very least a remission of symptoms enabling return towards a normal, functioning, integrated existence*' and the recommendation that '*the focal point of decision should be the prognosis as to the reasonable possibility of return to cognitive and sapient life, as distinguished from the forced continuance of that biological vegetative existence . . .*'. In another case it was stated that life-sustaining treatment can be withdrawn when it is clear that the patient will never '*regain cognitive behaviour, the ability to com-*

municate, or the capability of interacting purposefully with their environment' (Ruark & Raffin, 1988). Most would agree that these decisions should not be influenced by *'assessments of the personal worth, or social utility of another's life, or of that life to others'* (Schneiderman & Spragg, 1988). Finally, as in all branches of medicine, decision-making in intensive care should be based on generally accepted ethical principles (Ruark & Raffin, 1988) including:

- the primary objective is to preserve life, but this should be tempered by the need to alleviate suffering;
- first do no harm (*'primum non nocere'*);
- respect the autonomy of the patient;
- allocate medical resources fairly;
- tell the truth.

These judgements can be difficult and onerous, not least because there is often a degree of prognostic uncertainty. They should therefore always be taken by senior staff who are regularly present on the unit and continuously involved in patient care. Decisions should be reached in consultation with other intensive care clinicians, the primary physician or surgeon and the nurses, and, whenever possible, the patient's family.

It is important to appreciate that patients or their legal surrogates have the right to control what happens to them. Informed, rational and competent patients (e.g. those with incurable, but not immediately terminal illnesses), therefore have the right to refuse life-sustaining treatment. Not only do clinicians not have the right to force treatment on competent, unwilling patients, but if a competent patient requests that an intervention such as mechanical ventilation be discontinued, the wish should be honoured. Patients do not, however, have the right to demand life-sustaining treatment when the clinician considers it is inappropriate (Ruark & Raffin, 1988; Schneiderman & Spragg, 1988); neither is there any legal or moral obligation to provide treatment on request when there appears to be no possibility of benefit (Spiby, 1989). Clinicians should not, therefore, feel obligated to intervene with mechanical ventilation if it will not contribute to preserving life or alleviating suffering.

Finally, the patient's refusal, request or consent can only be truly informed when the clinician has communicated *all* the information the patient needs to make a knowledgeable decision, including any uncertainties.

Most critically ill patients, however, are either not competent or are unable to participate in decisions regarding their treatment. Under these circumstances, decisions must rest with the doctor, but always in close consultation with the family. The clinician must make a judgement in the patient's 'best interests', based not only on the expected duration, but also the anticipated quality of life, bearing in mind that a presumption in

favour of preserving life must always predominate (Spiby, 1989). Clearly, effective communication with the family or the patient's representative is essential, and they should whenever possible be included in discussions involving the initiation or withdrawal of life-sustaining treatment. Their views of the best interests of the patient are often invaluable. Such discussions are easier when the family has been kept fully informed during all stages of the patient's illness with regular updates on progress and when they have been prepared for the possibility that the patient may not survive.

In North America it is possible for patients to anticipate some of these decisions while still capable and rational and to make a formal statement about how they want to be treated should they become incompetent. These declarations are known as *'advanced directives'* or *'living wills'* (Higgs, 1987) and may take a form such as: 'If I should have an incurable or irreversible condition that will cause my death within a relatively short time and am no longer able to make decisions regarding my medical treatment I direct my attending physician . . . to withhold or withdraw treatment that only prolongs the process of dying and is not necessary to my comfort or to alleviate pain.'

Although these living wills have no binding force in some states in the USA and they currently have no legal status in the UK they are at least a clear expression of the patient's wishes. They are not, of course, a substitute for effective communication between staff, patients and relatives. Some have expressed concern that patients might be (or feel themselves to be) under pressure from friends, relatives or health workers, to indicate their willingness to have treatment discontinued because they think of themselves as a burden that nobody wishes (or can afford) to support. Others worry that living wills may compromise the autonomy of the profession (Higgs, 1987). In California it is possible to designate an 'attorney in fact' who is empowered to make medical decisions should the patient become incompetent. Occasionally the likely progression of an illness may have been explained to the patient who may then have indicated the choices he or she would wish to make at each stage.

Medical and nursing staff involved in making these decisions should be aware that their assessment of the usefulness of intensive care for an individual patient may differ substantially from that of patients or their relatives. In one study, for example, nurses significantly underestimated the usefulness of intensive care in comparison to the evaluation of patients or their families, and patients believed that quality of life was a less important consideration than their nurses did (Danis *et al.*, 1987). Moreover, the demand and expectations of patients and their families may conflict with efforts to ration intensive care on the basis of age, function or quality of life. Danis *et al.* (1988) found that 70% of a group of medical intensive care patients or their families were 100% willing to undergo intensive care again to achieve even just one month of survival, while only 8% were completely unwilling to undergo intensive care to achieve any prolongation of life. In the majority of cases, preferences did not seem to be closely related to functional status or quality of life and were not altered by life expectancy. The willingness to undergo intensive care again was not influenced by age, severity of the acute illness, length of stay or the cost of intensive care (Danis et al., 1988).

Once the decision to withdraw life-sustaining treatment has been made, the responsible clinicians, in consultation with the nurses and sometimes the patient's family, must decide which interventions should be discontinued. Such choices are important because they can influence the rapidity, the degree of discomfort and the dignity of the patient's death. Discussions with family and friends should stress the alleviation of suffering and emphasize that priority will be given to the comfort and dignity of the patient. On the rare occasions when mechanical ventilation is to be discontinued, for example, the patient must be given narcotics and sedatives to eliminate the discomfort of agonal efforts to breathe.

The feelings of family and friends may influence the manner in which treatment is withdrawn. In some cases it may therefore be appropriate to delay withdrawing treatment to allow them to cope with grief or to assimilate and come to terms with their loss. In one North American survey the order of physicians' preferences for treatments to be withdrawn was blood products, haemodialysis, intravenous vasopressors, total parenteral nutrition, antibiotics, mechanical ventilation, tube feeding and intravenous fluids. They preferred to withdraw:

- therapy supporting organs that failed for natural rather than iatrogenic reasons;
- recently instituted rather than long-standing interventions;
- treatment that would lead to rapid rather than delayed death;
- therapy resulting in delayed death when faced with diagnostic uncertainty.

Under some circumstances these biases could unnecessarily prolong the process of dying, increase the suffering of patients and their families, and waste resources. They also raise concerns about patient autonomy and might impede rational and compassionate decision-making (Christakis & Asch, 1993).

SEVERITY SCORING SYSTEMS

The outcome of critical illness is determined by:

- the severity of the acute illness;
- the patient's previous state of health;
- the nature of the underlying disease;
- the treatment given;
- the patient's response to treatment.

Early attempts to quantify the relationship between severity of illness and outcome were based on disease-specific indices such as the Glasgow Coma Score (GCS) for patients with acute brain injury (see Chapter 14) and the Ranson criteria for acute pancreatitis (see Chapter 15). Although these systems do accurately stratify patients according to risk they are limited by their disease specificity; a variety of more generally applicable methods for assessing illness severity, and thereby risk of death, have therefore been developed. These have included:

- assessments of the severity of the acute disturbance of physiological function—acute physiology and chronic health evaluation (APACHE) and the simplified acute physiology score (SAPS) (Knaus et al., 1981, 1985, 1991; Le Gall et al., 1984);
- a measure of the therapeutic effort expended on a patient—therapeutic intervention scoring system (TISS) (Cullen et al., 1974; Keene & Cullen, 1983);
- a mortality prediction model (MPM) (Lemeshow et al., 1988).

Other systems have been devised for particular categories of patients such as the combined trauma and injury severity scoring system (TRISS) (Boyd et al., 1987), which consists of calculations based on the injury severity score (ISS) and the revised trauma score (RTS).

The acute physiology, age, chronic health evaluation (APACHE) system

The APACHE scoring system is a widely applicable method for assessing severity of illness in the critically ill and has been extensively validated. It was originally designed as a classification system (Knaus et al., 1981), which would:

- control for case mix (that is the characteristics of the patient population in terms of diagnosis, age, sex, severity of illness and available treatment);
- allow meaningful comparisons of outcomes;
- assist in the evaluation of new therapies;
- be used to study the use of intensive care.

The original score consisted of two parts: the acute physiology score (APS) based on 34 physiological variables, and an assessment of the patient's previous state of health. Scores were assigned to each physiological variable depending on the extent to which they deviated from normal and their relative importance in determining outcome. There was a direct relationship between the calculated APS and the relative risk of death, although the chronic health indicators were associated with an increased risk of death only in patients with very poor and failing health before admission.

APACHE II

Largely because a number of the 34 physiological variables are not routinely measured in all patients the relatively complex APACHE system was simplified, refined and improved to produce the clinically more practical and now extensively used APACHE II score (Knaus *et al.*, 1985) (**Table 1.4**). The number of physiological variables was reduced to 12 easily measured values, the assessment of chronic health was changed to a system in which points were assigned for long-standing organ dysfunction and increasing age attracted additional risk points. The impact of emergency surgery on outcome was also incorporated into the risk assessment. The final APACHE II score is the sum of the acute physiology, age and chronic health points, calculated from the worst values during the first 24 hours of intensive care.

It is important to appreciate that the relationship between this score and outcome is crucially dependent on the underlying disease. For example for a given score the prognosis for a patient with septic shock is considerably worse than that for a patient with asthma or diabetic ketoacidosis. To provide an accurate assessment of illness severity and risk of death it is therefore essen-

Table 1.4 Assignment of points to derive APACHE II

	Assignment of points in acute physiology score								
	4	3	2	1	0	1	2	3	4
Rectal temperature (°C)	≥ 41.0	39.0–40.9		38.5–38.9	36.0–38.4	34.0–35.9	32.0–33.9	30.0–31.9	≤ 29.9
Mean blood pressure (mm Hg)	≥ 160	130–159	110–129		70–109		50–69		≤ 49
Heart rate (ventricular response/min)	≥ 180	140–179	110–139		70–109		55–69	40–54	≤ 39
Respiratory rate (breaths/min, spontaneous or mechanical)	≥ 50	35–49		25–34	12–24	10–11	6–9		≤ 5
Oxygenation (mm Hg):									
I (≥ 50%)	≥ 500	350–499	200–349		< 200				
II (< 50%)					> 70	61–70		55–60	< 55
Arterial pH	≥ 7.70	7.60–7.69		7.50–7.59	7.33–7.49		7.25–7.32	7.15–7.24	< 7.15
Serum sodium (mmol/l)	≥ 180	160–179	155–159	150–154	130–149		120–129	111–119	≤ 110
Serum potassium (mmol/l)	≥ 7.0	6.0–6.9		5.5–5.9	3.5–5.4	3.0–3.4	2.5–2.9		< 2.5
Serum creatinine (mg/100 ml)	≥ 3.5	2.0–3.4	1.5–1.9		0.6–1.4		< 0.6		
Haematocrit	≥ 60		50–59.9	46–49.9	30–45.9		20–29.9		< 20
White blood cell count (× 10³/ml³)	≥ 40		20–39.9	15–19.9	3–14.9		1–2.9		< 1

Glasgow coma score (GCS): subtract GCS from 15 to obtain points assigned

Points assigned to age and chronic disease as part of the APACHE II score

Age (years):	Score
< 45	0
45–54	2
55–64	3
65–74	5
≥ 75	6
History of chronic conditions	
None	0
Present:	
Elective surgical patient:	2
Emergency surgical or non-surgical patient	5

tial to weight the score using coefficients assigned to specific diagnostic categories (**Table 1.5**). When this is done there is a consistent relationship between APACHE II mortality predictions and observed hospital death rates throughout the spectrum from low to high risk of death.

Since APACHE II can accurately quantify the severity of illness and predict overall mortality for large groups of acutely ill patients it may be useful for auditing a unit's clinical activity, for evaluating the use of resources, and for characterizing groups of patients in clinical studies. Many believe that despite its limitations (see below), APACHE II mortality predictions can also be used to compare the efficacy of intensive care between different units and over time in the same unit. This involves calculating the expected mortality rate by dividing the sum of the predicted risks of death for all patients by the total number of patients. It is suggested that by relating the actual to the predicted mortality—the *standardized mortality ratio* (SMR)—the performance of individual units is adjusted for case mix and can be assessed and compared with other units. When this technique was used to compare outcome in 13 major medical centres in the USA results were significantly better than average in one hospital, while in another, outcome was significantly worse than predicted. These differences were thought to be related more to the interaction and coordination of each intensive care unit's staff than the administrative structure, amount of specialized treatment used or the hospital's teaching status (Knaus *et al.*, 1986). The calculation of SMRs is, however, a fairly blunt instrument for between-unit comparisons. Only extreme differences in SMR (0.59 and 1.58 respectively in the study just mentioned) can be considered to be significant and then only when based on large numbers. In addition, serious errors can be introduced, for example by overscoring on the GCS or the chronic health evaluation, or by misclassifying the diagnostic category. When using the APACHE II methodology it is important to appreciate that:

- it must not be used without taking into account the underlying disease;
- it cannot be used on samples of patients selected according to different criteria;
- it cannot be applied at times other than the first 24 hours of intensive care;
- the risk of death may not be accurately assessed in patients with rare conditions or in those with unusual presentations of common conditions.

The international applicability of the American-derived APACHE II equation has been assessed in a number of studies (Zimmerman *et al.*, 1988; Sirio *et al.*, 1992; Rowan *et al.*, 1993). When APACHE II was used in two hospitals in New Zealand (Zimmerman *et al.*, 1988) and in intensive care units in six hospitals in

Japan (Sirio *et al.*, 1992), the observed mortality did not differ significantly from that predicted by the American equation. In the UK and Ireland, however, it has been shown that although the overall predictive ability is good, the observed mortality is rather higher than predicted in two of the lower-risk groups and lower than expected in some of the highest-risk patients. Moreover, the equation did not adjust uniformly across some of the subgroups defined according to factors such as age and diagnosis. For example, deaths were underpredicted in patients over 76 years of age and mortality rates were less than predicted for surgical patients with respiratory disease. There are a number of possible explanations for these disparities including systematic differences in medical definitions and diagnostic labelling between the two countries, systematic variations in the effectiveness of treatment and the possibility that there are age-specific differences in health status between countries. These findings highlight some of the complexities of severity scoring and suggest that the uniformity of fit of the American APACHE II equation for UK and Irish patients needs to be improved (Rowan *et al.*, 1993).

APACHE III

Recently Knaus *et al.* (1991) have attempted to improve on the risk prediction derived from APACHE II by re-evaluating the selection and weighting of physiological variables, as well as examining the influence of differences in patient selection and timing of admission to intensive care on outcome. The improved explanatory power of this APACHE III score can be combined with major disease category and previous patient location to produce an estimated risk of death for each patient. This calculation can be performed at various times during the patient's intensive care unit stay. It is suggested that, provided patient selection and disease classification are precisely defined, this system can be used to improve the statistical power and precision of randomized clinical trials, and to identify patients with an intermediate risk of death who are most likely to benefit from new treatments. As with APACHE II the difference between predicted and actual death rates can be used to compare mortalities between units and to provide a quantitative assessment of quality of care. Finally, it might also be used to improve intensive care unit discharge decisions, thereby enhancing patient safety and improving the use of resources (Zimmerman *et al.*, 1994).

The improvements in predictive power achieved with APACHE III are, however, relatively modest and the coefficients and equation for calculation of risk are not in the public domain (Bion, 1993); most units therefore continue to use the APACHE II methodology for clinical audit and research.

Table 1.5 Diagnostic categories used to provide an accurate assessment of illness severity and risk of death from the APACHE II score.

Primary system
R, respiratory; C, cardiovascular; N, neurological; G, gastrointestinal; K, renal; M, metabolic; H, haematological

Precipitating factor
01   Infection
02   Neoplasm
03   Trauma
04   Self intoxication (overdose)
05   Intracerebral haemorrhage
06   Cranial haemorrhage
07   Seizures
08   Neuromuscular failure
09   Coronary artery disease
10   Myocardial infarction
11   Valvar heart disease
12   Peripheral vascular disease
13   Embolus
14   Congenital anomaly/anatomical defect
15   Congestive heart failure/pulmonary oedema
16   Hypertension
17   Rhythm disturbance
18   Pericardial disease
19   Cardiogenic shock/cardiomyopathy
20   Septic shock/sepsis
21   Anaphylactic/drug-induced shock
22   Haemorrhagic shock/hypovolaemic shock
23   Bleeding (significant but not shock)
24   Cardiac/respiratory arrest
25   Allergic reaction
26   Obstruction/perforation
27   Coma/mental derangement
28   Electrolyte imbalance/acid–base disturbance
29   Diabetic ketoacidosis
30   Endocrine emergency
31   Hypothermia/hyperthermia
32   Haematological insufficiency/crisis
33   Transplant surgery
34   Postoperative ventilation or respiratory support (unplanned)
35   Acute exacerbation of chronic end-stage disease
36   Toxic/chemical poisoning

Other scoring systems

SIMPLIFIED ACUTE PHYSIOLOGY SCORE (SAPS)

This arose from an independent attempt to simplify the APACHE system by reducing the original 34 variables to 13. The weights assigned to each physiological variable were nearly equivalent to those used in APACHE and the accuracy of predictions was comparable to that obtained using the original APACHE system.

MORTALITY PREDICTION MODELS (MPMs)

Lemeshow *et al.* (1988) devised MPMs based on step-wise linear discriminant function and multiple logistic regression analysis of data from a large cohort of adult general intensive care patients in a single hospital. A series of questions with predominantly yes or no answers relating to 11 admission variables are answered and these are weighted according to their individual contribution to mortality. Serial observations of the changing probability of mortality are then used to anticipate the likely outcome. More recently it has been shown that APACHE II is superior to the MPM as a means of predicting outcome in groups of adult intensive care patients from Britain and Ireland (Rowan *et al.*, 1994) although later developments of the MPM (MPM II at 24, 48 and 72 hours) may provide more accurate estimates of the probability of hospital mortality (Lemeshow *et al.*, 1994).

THERAPEUTIC INTERVENTION SCORING SYSTEM (TISS)

The TISS was originally designed to classify the severity of illness by quantitating the therapeutic interventions (Cullen *et al.*, 1974). Because TISS points are physician-dependent, the score cannot be used to compare the efficacy of intensive care in different units and is not an ideal method for assessing the relationship between severity of illness and outcome. It does, however, provide an accurate assessment of the level of care and monitoring and is therefore a valuable administrative tool. It can, for example, be used to assess the workload required by each patient, to establish nurse : patient ratios and to calculate costs.

INJURY SEVERITY SCORE (ISS) AND COMBINED TRAUMA AND INJURY SEVERITY SCORE (TRISS)

The ISS and TRISS system was developed to provide a standard approach for the evaluation of trauma care (Boyd *et al.*, 1987). Mortality following traumatic injury depends on the degree of physiological derangement, the extent of the anatomical injury, the age of the patient and whether the trauma was blunt or penetrating. The TRISS methodology combines these factors—the revised trauma score, the injury severity score, age, blunt or penetrating injury—to provide a measure of the probability of survival.

Predicting death in individual patients

Although the APACHE methodology and other severity scoring systems can be used to estimate individual risks of mortality, they clearly cannot predict with certainty the outcome in an individual patient, and were not designed to do so. Objective probabilities should not therefore be used in isolation as a basis for limiting or discontinuing treatment and should not be used as a substitute for clinical decision-making as outlined earlier in this chapter. It is, however, possible that reliable, well-calibrated prognostic scoring systems may be useful aids to such subjective assessments. Certainly objective outcome predictions do have a number of potential advantages compared with clinical judgement (Knaus *et al.*, 1991) including the following:

- Past experiences are taken into account in an unbiased manner, whereas with human decisions, recent experience has a disproportionate influence.
- Objective outcome predictions should be more reliable because they are based on reproducible data.
- The database supporting the risk estimate is substantially larger than any one clinician's experience.
- The risk estimates are based solely on the patient's response to treatment.

In practice APACHE III outcome predictions compare favourably with clinicians' assessments; indeed, the objective system is better calibrated, and there is evidence that daily prognostic estimates are sufficiently accurate to be used to assist clinical decision-making (Wagner *et al.*, 1994). Usually, however, daily risk assessments only serve to confirm prognostic uncertainty, albeit with a reduced chance of error, and most difficult clinical problems are unlikely to be resolved solely by objective probability estimates.

Chang *et al.* (1988) have taken risk prediction one step further and have designed algorithms to predict death in individual patients. They suggest that a decision to withdraw treatment might be more acceptable to clinicians, patients and their relatives when supported by an accurate prediction of death after a trial period of treatment. Potential advantages of such a system include reduced suffering of those for whom treatment is futile and more effective use of limited resources. Clearly these benefits will be offset by false predictions of death.

The 'Riyadh Intensive Care Program' uses computerized trend analysis of a daily organ failure score (OFS), which is derived from the APACHE II score weighted according to the number and duration of organ failures. Both the absolute value of the score and its rate of change relative to the previous day's score are taken into consideration. Unfortunately when the value of this system as an aid to clinical decision-making has been tested in different patient populations its predictive ability has not been impressive. In one study the sensitivity of the prediction of death was only 14.8% and the number of bed days that would have been saved expressed as a percentage of the proportion of total intensive care unit bed days occupied by non-survivors was only 2.8%. Moreover, three patients (all post-cardiac surgery, see below) were falsely predicted to die by the computer, but not by the treating physician (Jacobs et al., 1992). These authors stressed that the program had never been intended for general use in its present form and advocated extreme caution in the use of computer systems to predict death. More recently Atkinson et al. (1994) used the same system and found that although predictions of death were very specific, sensitivity was again poor (23.4%). Their results also suggested that the use of this system in isolation to determine when treatment should be withdrawn might cost the lives of 1 in 20 patients who would otherwise survive with a reasonable quality of life.

Criticisms of severity scoring

The introduction of prognostic scoring systems has been accompanied by considerable debate and controversy. While some have been concerned with practical difficulties related to data collection and consistency of scoring methods, others have questioned their accuracy and their use for audit, evaluating a unit's performance,

between unit comparisons and patient selection (Civetta, 1990; Boyd & Grounds, 1993). Some have gone so far as to suggest that it is virtually impossible to develop a useful scoring system (Civetta, 1990). Certain limitations of prognostic scoring systems such as their inability to predict either the sudden unexpected complications that often affect outcome or the subsequent development of multiple organ dysfunction are intuitively obvious.

Of more concern is the suggestion that scores based on physiological data that can be influenced by medical and nursing interventions, such as APACHE, cannot be used to compare unit performances and are not suitable for audit (Boyd & Grounds, 1993). It is claimed that the accuracy of such systems is compromised by 'lead time bias'; that is, they fail to take into account the effect that management before the initiation of intensive care (e.g. stabilization in the operating theatre or prompt retrieval and resuscitation of trauma patients) may have on physiological variables. This issue was, however, addressed in the development of APACHE III (see earlier in this chapter). Conversely the use of intentional hypotension, hypothermia, muscle relaxation and mechanical ventilation can result in a high APACHE score, despite a very low risk of death (Civetta, 1990). It is probably for this reason that APACHE II predictions cannot be applied to post-cardiac surgery patients.

There is also concern that inter-observer variations may have a profound effect on calculated probabilities of survival. With the TRISS system, for example, it has been shown that individual predictions of survival are potentially inaccurate, except at the extremes of probabilities (Zoltie & De Dombal, 1993).

Finally, some have contended that exclusion of patients from intensive care on the basis of APACHE II scores will not result in significant savings, but will instead create risks of increased morbidity, mortality and costs (Civetta, 1990).

REFERENCES

Aitkenhead AR, Booij LH, Dhainaut JF et al. (1993) International standards for safety in the intensive care unit. *Intensive Care Medicine* **19**: 178–181.

Atkinson S, Bihari D, Smithies M et al. (1994) Identification of futility in intensive care. *Lancet* **344**: 1203–1206.

Bellamy PE & Oye RK (1984) Adult respiratory distress syndrome: hospital charges and outcome according to underlying disease. *Critical Care Medicine* **12**: 622–625.

Bion J (1993) Outcomes in intensive care. *British Medical Journal* **307**: 953–954.

Boyd O & Grounds RM (1993) Physiological scoring systems and audit. *Lancet* **341**: 1573–1574.

Boyd CR, Tolson MA & Copes WS (1987) Evaluating trauma care: the TRISS method. *Journal of Trauma* **27**: 370–378.

Chalfin DB & Carlon GC (1990) Age and utilization of intensive

care unit resources of critically ill cancer patients. *Critical Care Medicine* **18**: 694–698.

Chang RWS, Jacobs S, Lee B & Pace N (1988) Predicting deaths among intensive care unit patients. *Critical Care Medicine* **16**: 34–42.

Christakis NA & Asch DA (1993) Biases in how physicians choose to withdraw life support. *Lancet* **342**: 642–646.

Civetta JM (1990) 'New and improved' scoring systems. *Critical Care Medicine* **18**: 1487–1490.

Cullen DJ, Civetta JM, Briggs BA & Ferrera LC (1974) Therapeutic intervention scoring system: a method for quantitative comparison of patient care. *Critical Care Medicine* **2**: 57–60.

Cullen DJ, Keene R, Waternaux C & Peterson H (1984) Objective, quantitative measurement of severity of illness in critically ill patients. *Critical Care Medicine* **12**: 155–160.

Danis M, Jarr SL, Southerland LI, Nocella RS & Patrick DL (1987) A comparison of patient, family, and nurse evaluations of the usefulness of intensive care. *Critical Care Medicine* **15**: 138-143.

Danis M, Patrick DL, Southerland LI & Green ML (1988) Patients' and families' preferences for medical intensive care. *JAMA* **260**: 797-802.

Department of Health and Social Security (1970) Intensive Therapy Unit. Hospital Building Note (HBN) 27. Revised 1974.

Dragstead L & Qvist J (1989) Outcome from intensive care. III. A 5-year study of 1308 patients: activity levels. *European Journal of Anaesthesiology* **6**: 385-396.

Dragsted L, Qvist J & Madsen M (1989) Outcome from intensive care II. A 5-year study of 1308 patients: short-term outcome. *European Journal of Anaesthesiology* **6**: 131-144.

Editorial (1991) Intensive care for the elderly. *Lancet* **337**: 209-210.

Fedullo AJ & Swinburne AJ (1983) Relationship of patient age to cost and survival in a medical ICU. *Critical Care Medicine* **11**: 155-159.

Health Building Note 27. London, HMSO, 1992.

Higgs R (1987) Living wills and treatment refusal. *British Medical Journal* **295**: 1221-1222.

Intensive Care Society Standards for Intensive Care Units. London, Biomedica. Available from the Intensive Care Society.

Intensive Care Society (1990) *The Intensive Care Service in the UK*. London, HMSO. Available from the Intensive Care Society.

Jacobs S, Arnold A, Clyburn PA & Willis BA (1992) The Riyadh Intensive Care Program applied to a mortality analysis of a teaching hospital intensive care unit. *Anaesthesia* **47**: 775-780.

Jennett B (1984) Inappropriate use of intensive care. *British Medical Journal* **289**: 1709-1711.

Keene AR & Cullen DJ (1983) Therapeutic intervention scoring system: update 1983. *Critical Care Medicine* **11**: 1-3.

Kerr JH, Coates DP & Gale LB (1985) Use of 'bollards' to improve patient access during intensive care. *Intensive Care Medicine* **11**: 33-38.

Knaus WA, Zimmerman JE, Wagner DP, Draper EA & Laurence DE (1981) APACHE—acute physiology and chronic health evaluation: a physiologically based classification system. *Critical Care Medicine* **9**: 591-597.

Knaus WA, Draper EA, Wagner DP & Zimmerman JE (1985) APACHE II: a severity of disease classification system. *Critical Care Medicine* **13**: 818-829.

Knaus WA, Draper EA, Wagner DP & Zimmerman JE (1986) An evaluation of outcome from intensive care in major medical centers. *Annals of Internal Medicine* **104**: 410-418.

Knaus WA, Wagner DP, Draper EA, *et al.* (1991) The APACHE III prognostic system: risk prediction of hospital mortality for critically ill hospitalised adults. *Chest* **100**: 1619-1636.

Lask B (1987) Forget the stiff upper lip. *British Medical Journal* **295**: 1584-1585.

Le Gall JR, Loirat P, Alperossteh A, *et al.* (1984) A simplified acute physiology score for ICU patients. *Critical Care Medicine* **12**: 975-977.

Lemeshow S, Teres D, Aurinin JS & Gage RW (1988) Refining intensive care unit outcome prediction by using changing probabilities of mortality. *Critical Care Medicine* **16**: 470-477.

Lemeshow S, Klar J, Teres D, *et al.* (1994) Mortality probability models for patients in the intensive care unit for 48 or 72 hours: a prospective, multicenter study. *Critical Care Medicine* **22**: 1351-1358.

Osborne M & Evans TW (1994) Allocation of resources in intensive care: a transatlantic perspective. *Lancet* **343**: 778-780.

Purdie JAM, Ridley SA & Wallace PGM (1990) Effective use of regional intensive therapy units. *British Medical Journal* **300**: 79-81.

Ridley SA & Wallace PGM (1990) Quality of life after intensive care. *Anaesthesia* **45**: 808-813.

Ridley S, Jackson R, Findlay J & Wallace P (1990) Long term survival after intensive care. *British Medical Journal* **301**: 1127-1130.

Ridley S, Biggam M & Stone P (1994) A cost-utility analysis of intensive therapy. II. quality of life in survivors. *Anaesthesia* **49**: 192-196.

Roberts GA (1986) Burnout: psycho babble or valuable concept? *British Journal of Hospital Medicine* **36**: 194-197.

Rowan KM, Kerr JH, Major E, McPherson K, Short A & Vessey MP (1993) Intensive Care Society's APACHE II study in Britain and Ireland. II. Outcome comparisons of intensive care units after adjustment for case mix by the American APACHE II method. *British Medical Journal* **307**: 977-981.

Rowan KM, Kerr JH, Major E, McPherson K, Short A & Vessey MP (1994) Intensive Care Society's acute physiology and chronic health evaluation (APACHE II) study in Britain and Ireland: a prospective, multicenter, cohort study comparing two methods for predicting outcome for adult intensive care patients. *Critical Care Medicine* **22**: 1392-1401.

Ruark JE & Raffin TA (1988) Initiating and withdrawing life support. Principles and practice in adult medicine. *New England Journal of Medicine* **318**: 25-30.

Sage WM, Rosenthal MH & Silverman JF (1986) Is intensive care worth it? An assessment of input and outcome for the critically ill. *Critical Care Medicine* **14**: 777-782.

Schneiderman LJ & Spragg RG (1988) Ethical decisions in discontinuing mechanical ventilation. *New England Journal of Medicine* **318**: 984-988.

Sirio CA, Tajimi K, Tase C, Knaus WA, Wagner DP, Hirasawa H, Sakanishi N, Katsuya H & Taenaka N (1992) An initial comparison of intensive care in Japan and the United States. *Critical Care Medicine* **20**: 1207-1215.

Spiby J (1989) Intensive care in the United Kingdom: report from the King's Fund panel. *Anaesthesia* **44**: 428-431.

Spivack D (1987) The high cost of acute health care: a review of escalating costs and limitations of such exposure in intensive care units. *American Review of Respiratory Diseases* **136**: 1007-1011.

Teplick R, Caldera DL, Gilbert JP & Cullen DJ (1983) Benefit of elective intensive care admission after certain operations. *Anesthesia and Analgesia* **62**: 572-577.

Thiagarajan J, Taylor P, Hogbin E & Ridley S (1994) Quality of life after multiple trauma requiring intensive care. *Anaesthesia* **49**: 211-218.

The Association of Anaesthetists of Great Britain and Ireland (1988) *Intensive Care Services—Provision for the Future*. Available from the Association of Anaesthetists.

Thibault GE, Mulley AG, Barnett GO *et al.* (1980) Medical intensive care: indications, interventions and outcomes. *New England Journal of Medicine* **302**: 938-942.

Wagner DP, Knaus WA, Harrell FE, Zimmerman JE & Watts C (1994) Daily prognostic estimates for critically ill adults in intensive care units: results from a prospective, multicenter, inception cohort analysis. *Critical Care Medicine* **22**: 1359-1372.

Wilson LM (1972) Intensive care delirium. The effect of outside deprivation in a windowless unit. *Archives of Internal Medicine* **130**: 225-226.

Zimmerman JE, Knaus WA, Judson JA *et al.* (1988) Patient selection for intensive care: a comparison of New Zealand and United States hospitals. *Critical Care Medicine* **16**: 318-326.

Zimmerman JE, Wagner DP, Draper EA & Knaus WA (1994) Improving intensive care unit discharge decisions: supplementing physician judgement with predictions of next day risk for life support. *Critical Care Medicine* **22**: 1373-1384.

Zoltie N & De Dombal FT on behalf of the Yorkshire Trauma Audit Group (1993) The hit and miss of ISS and TRISS. *British Medical Journal* **307**: 906-909.

2 Applied Cardiovascular and Respiratory Physiology

In all critically ill patients the immediate priority must be to preserve life and prevent, reverse or minimize damage to vital organs such as the brain, gut and kidneys. This is achieved by optimizing cardiovascular and respiratory function in order to *maximize delivery of oxygen* to the tissues. Subsequently, it is hoped that the underlying abnormality will resolve either spontaneously (e.g. postoperatively and in some viral illnesses such as Guillain–Barré syndrome) or as a result of specific treatment aimed at the underlying disease, such as the administration of antibiotics to a patient with pneumonia or surgery to control a source of infection. Occasionally, when the aetiology of the acute illness is unknown, successful resuscitation and stabilization provides a 'breathing space' during which the diagnosis can be made and specific therapy started.

OXYGEN DELIVERY

Oxygen delivery (D_O_2) is defined as the total amount of oxygen delivered to the tissues per unit time. It is dependent on:

- the volume of blood flowing through the microcirculation per unit time (i.e. the cardiac output, $\dot{Q}_t$);
- the amount of oxygen contained in that blood (i.e. the arterial oxygen content, C_aO_2) (**Table 2.1**).

Oxygen is transported in combination with haemoglobin (Hb) and dissolved in plasma, the amount combined with haemoglobin being determined by its oxygen capacity (usually taken as being 1.34 ml O_2/g Hb) and its percentage saturation with oxygen (S_O_2), while the volume in solution depends on the partial pressure of oxygen (P_O_2) (see **Table 2.1**).

For most practical purposes, except when hyperbaric oxygen is administered, the amount of dissolved oxygen is sufficiently small to be ignored.

In the normal, healthy adult approximately 1000 ml (550 ml/min/m²) of oxygen is delivered to the tissues each minute (see **Table 2.1**) and since the normal oxygen consumption ($\dot{V}_O_2$) is 250 ml/min (140 ml/min/m²), only about 25% of the available oxygen is used. Normal arterial blood, in which the Hb is fully saturated, con-

Table 2.1 Determinants of oxygen delivery. (S_aO_2, saturation of haemoglobin with oxygen in arterial blood; P_aO_2, partial pressure of oxygen in arterial blood; Hb, haemoglobin.)

Oxygen delivery = cardiac output × arterial oxygen content

Oxygen delivery = cardiac output × [(Hb × S_aO_2 × 1.34) + (P_aO_2 × 0.003)]

For representative values in a normal adult, and ignoring the small amount of dissolved oxygen

$$1000 \text{ ml/min} \simeq 5000 \text{ ml} \times \frac{15}{100} \text{ g/ml} \times \frac{99}{100} \times 1.34$$

Since oxygen consumption is normally approximately 250 ml/min there is an excess of supply over demand which provides a margin of safety if oxygen consumption increases or oxygen delivery falls.

tains 20 vol% of oxygen, and since 25% (or 5 vol%) is extracted by the tissues, this leaves 15 vol% in mixed venous blood, which is, therefore, 75% saturated with oxygen. The normal arteriovenous oxygen content difference is therefore 5 ml/100 ml of blood (**Fig. 2.1**) (Appendices 1 and 2).

There are, however, some important limitations to the application of the concept of oxygen flux in clinical practice.

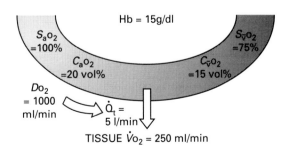

Fig. 2.1 Tissue oxygen delivery and consumption. S_aO_2, arterial oxygen saturation; C_aO_2, arterial oxygen content; D_O_2, oxygen delivery; $\dot{Q}_t$, cardiac output; $\dot{V}_O_2$, oxygen consumption; $C_{\bar{v}}O_2$, mixed venous oxygen content; $S_{\bar{v}}O_2$, mixed venous oxygen saturation.

- Some organs, notably the heart, have a very high oxygen requirement relative to their blood flow and may, therefore, receive insufficient supplies of oxygen even when overall oxygen delivery (D_{O_2}) is apparently adequate.
- It does not consider relative differences in blood flow to individual organs.
- It does not take into account maldistribution of flow in the microcirculation.
- Microcirculatory flow can be influenced by viscosity.

CARDIAC OUTPUT

The factors that determine the volume of blood delivered to the tissues (i.e. the cardiac output) will be considered first. It is useful to index the cardiac output and other haemodynamic and oxygen transport variables, per square metre of body surface area. In this way, comparisons can be made between patients, and the normal limits can be more closely defined (see Appendices 1 and 2).

Maintenance of an adequate cardiac output is obviously crucial to the survival of the critically ill and both the heart rate and the determinants of the stroke volume need to be considered (**Fig. 2.2**).

Heart rate and rhythm

The heart rate is largely dependent on the balance of sympathetic and parasympathetic nervous activity and, in health, is directly related to the metabolic rate. At rest, vagal tone predominates and maintains the heart rate at about 70 beats/min. If both the sympathetic and parasympathetic supply to the heart are interrupted, a rate of approximately 100 beats/min results.

Extreme bradycardias and tachycardias can cause cardiac output to fall.

- *As heart rate increases*, the duration of systole remains essentially unchanged, whereas diastole and therefore the time available for ventricular filling, becomes progressively shorter, and stroke volume eventually falls. In the normal heart this occurs at rates greater than about 160 beats/min, but in those

with cardiac pathology, especially when this restricts ventricular filling (e.g. in mitral stenosis), stroke volume may fall at much lower heart rates. Furthermore, tachycardias cause marked increases in myocardial oxygen consumption ($M_{V_{O_2}}$) and this may precipitate ischaemia in areas of myocardium with restricted coronary perfusion. It is therefore most important to control tachyarrhythmias; but it must be recognized that the majority have an underlying cause such as hypokalaemia, which should be diagnosed and treated before instituting specific therapy (see Chapter 8).

- *When heart rate falls*, on the other hand, a point is reached at which the increase in stroke volume is insufficient to compensate for the bradycardia and again cardiac output falls. Under these circumstances overdistension of the ventricles may impair myocardial performance and jeopardize subendocardial perfusion.

Alterations in heart rate are often caused by disturbances of rhythm in which atrial transport is lost (e.g. atrial fibrillation, complete heart block or nodal rhythm), thereby further reducing ventricular filling and stroke volume. In this situation, catastrophic reductions in cardiac output may occur and urgent treatment is then required (see also Chapter 8).

Stroke volume

The volume of blood ejected by the ventricle in a single contraction is the difference between the ventricular end-diastolic volume (VEDV) and end-systolic volume (VESV) (i.e. stroke volume = VEDV – VESV).

The *ejection fraction* describes the stroke volume as a percentage of VEDV

(i.e. ejection fraction = $\dfrac{VEDV - VESV}{VEDV} \times 100\%$)

and is an indication of myocardial performance.

Three interdependent factors determine the stroke volume: pre-load, myocardial contractility and after-load.

PRE-LOAD

Pre-load is defined as the tension of the myocardial fibres at end-diastole, just before the onset of ventricular contraction, and is therefore related to their degree of stretch (**Fig. 2.3**). The main factor influencing pre-load is the venous return. *Starling's law of the heart* states that 'the force of myocardial contraction is directly proportional to the initial fibre length.' Therefore, as the filling pressure, and consequently the VEDV increases, stroke volume rises (**Fig. 2.4**). If, however, the ventricle is overstretched, excessive dilatation and thinning of the myocardium may cause stroke volume to fall (**Fig. 2.5**). There is also a risk of pulmonary oedema.

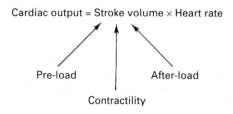

Cardiac output = Stroke volume × Heart rate

Pre-load   After-load

Contractility

Fig. 2.2 The determinants of cardiac output.

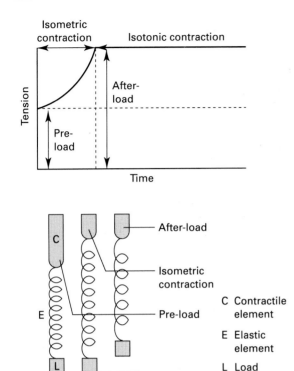

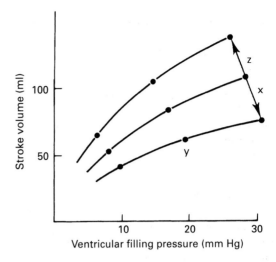

Fig. 2.5 Starling curve: as pre-load is increased, stroke volume rises. If the ventricle is overstretched, stroke volume will fall (x). In myocardial failure, the curve is depressed and flattened (y). Increasing contractility shifts the curve upwards and to the left (z).

Achieving the optimal pre-load improves cardiac output by increasing stroke volume without affecting the main determinants of myocardial oxygen requirements (i.e. heart rate and after-load, **Table 2.2**). Consequently, myocardial oxygen consumption (MVo_2) increases only slightly and manipulation of pre-load is therefore the most efficient way of improving cardiac output.

Fig. 2.3 The relationship between myocardial tension and contraction. 'Pre-load' is the tension of the myocardial fibres prior to the onset of systole and depends on the degree to which they are passively stretched. During isometric contraction, the tension in the contractile elements increases; the tension required to open the aortic valve and eject blood from the ventricle is the 'after-load'.

MYOCARDIAL CONTRACTILITY

Myocardial contractility refers to the ability of the heart to perform work independently of changes in pre-load and after-load. The state of myocardial contractility therefore determines the response of the ventricles to changes in pre-load and after-load. Unfortunately, contractility is often reduced in intensive care patients as a result of either pre-existing myocardial damage (e.g. due to ischaemic heart disease) or the acute disease process

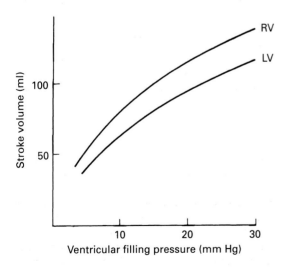

Fig. 2.4 In normal subjects the left ventricular function curve (LV) is displaced downwards because the left ventricle is less compliant and is working against a higher after-load than the right ventricle (RV).

Table 2.2 The determinants of myocardial oxygen consumption.	
Major effect	Heart rate
	After-load
Intermediate effect	Ventricular wall tension
	Contractility
Least effect	Pre-load
	Stroke volume

itself. Changes in myocardial contractility alter the slope and position of the ventricular function curve; worsening ventricular performance is manifested as a depressed, flat curve (see **Fig. 2.5**). Therefore, for a given pre-load, stroke volume is less and increasing the filling pressures leads to only limited improvement. Under these circumstances, cardiac output can be maintained only by increasing heart rate with an associated rise in MV_{O_2}.

AFTER-LOAD

After-load is defined as the myocardial wall tension developed during systolic ejection (see **Fig. 2.3**) and is a significant determinant of left ventricular performance. From *Laplace's law* the ventricular wall tension (T) is given by:

$$T = \frac{P_{tM} \times R}{2H},$$

where P_{tM} is the transmural pressure, R is the ventricular radius, and H is the ventricular wall thickness.

Left ventricular after-load will therefore be increased by

- ventricular dilatation;
- an increase in intraventricular pressure;
- a negative intrathoracic pressure.

Conversely after-load will be reduced by:

- a positive intrathoracic pressure;
- decreased intraventricular pressure;
- increased ventricular wall thickness.

Other important determinants of left ventricular after-load are:

- the resistance imposed by the aortic valve and the peripheral vasculature;
- the elasticity of major blood vessels.

Decreasing after-load can increase the stroke volume achieved at a given pre-load (**Fig. 2.6**), while at the same time ventricular wall tension and MV_{O_2} are reduced. The reduction in wall tension may produce an increase in coronary blood flow, thereby improving the myocardial oxygen supply : demand ratio. An increase in after-load, on the other hand, can cause a fall in stroke volume, particularly in those with myocardial dysfunction, and is a potent cause of increased MV_{O_2}.

Right ventricular after-load is normally negligible since the resistance of the pulmonary circulation is very low. In patients with stenosis of the pulmonary valve or pulmonary hypertension, however, right ventricular after-load may become the dominant influence on overall cardiac performance.

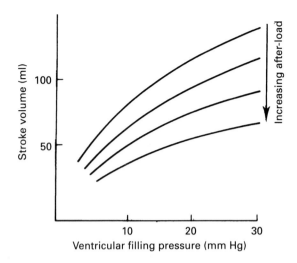

Fig. 2.6 The effect of changes in after-load on the ventricular function curve.

OXYGEN CONTENT

The oxygen content of arterial blood (C_aO_2) depends on the amount of Hb present per unit volume of blood, its oxygen capacity and its percentage saturation with oxygen (see **Table 2.1**). Maintenance of an 'adequate' Hb concentration is therefore essential in critically ill patients. Tissue oxygenation is, however, also dependent on blood flow. This in turn is determined not only by the cardiac output and its distribution, but also by the viscosity of the blood, which depends largely on the packed cell volume (PCV). It has been shown in dogs with haemorrhage that oxygen transport through the coronary circulation is maximal at a haematocrit of approximately 25%, whereas for the systemic circulation the optimal value is 45% (Jan *et al.*, 1980).

Oxyhaemoglobin dissociation curve

The saturation of Hb with oxygen is determined by the P_{O_2} in the blood, the relationship between the two being described by the *oxyhaemoglobin dissociation curve* (**Fig. 2.7**). The sigmoid shape of this curve is clinically important for a number of reasons.

- Falls in P_aO_2 may be tolerated provided percentage saturation remains above 90%.
- Increasing P_aO_2 to above normal has only a minimal effect on oxygen content unless hyperbaric oxygen is administered, when the amount of oxygen in solution in plasma becomes significant.
- Once on the steep portion of the curve (the 'slippery slope'), a small decrease in P_aO_2 can cause large falls in oxygen content, conversely increasing P_aO_2 only

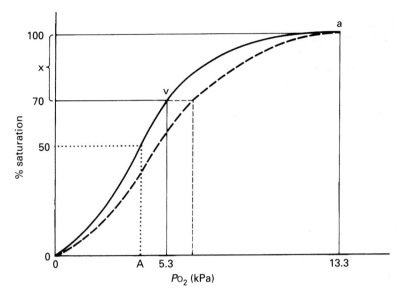

Fig. 2.7 The oxyhaemoglobin dissociation curve: this curve will move to the right (—−−) in the presence of an acidosis (metabolic or respiratory), pyrexia or an increased red cell 2,3-diphosphoglycerate (DPG) concentration. For a given arterio-venous oxygen content difference the mixed venous Po_2 will then be higher. Furthermore if the mixed venous Po_2 is unchanged, the arteriovenous oxygen content difference increases and more oxygen is off-loaded to the tissues (a, arterial point; v, venous point; x, arteriovenous oxygen content difference; A, P_{50}, which is normally 3.6 kPa (27 mm Hg).

slightly can lead to useful increases in oxygen saturation.

In contrast, *the carbon dioxide dissociation curve* is virtually linear over the range normally encountered in clinical practice so that alterations in Pco_2 cause proportional changes in carbon dioxide content (**Fig. 2.8**).

The arterial oxygen tension is influenced by the efficiency of pulmonary gas exchange and the mixed venous Po_2 ($P_{\bar{v}}O_2$).

PULMONARY VENTILATION AND GAS EXCHANGE

Alveolar ventilation and dead space

The volume of effective alveolar ventilation per unit time ($\dot{V}_A$) is determined by the expired minute volume ($\dot{V}_E$), reduced by the amount 'wasted' in terms of gas exchange (the *physiological, or total, dead space, V_D*).

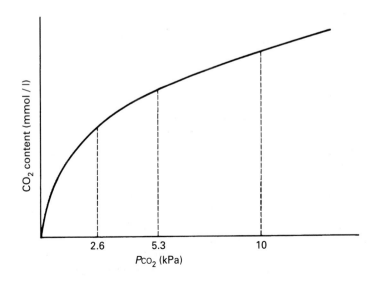

Fig. 2.8 The carbon dioxide dissociation curve: note that in the physiological range this is essentially linear.

The latter consists of 'anatomical' dead space (the conducting airways) and alveolar dead space (ventilated alveoli, which are either not perfused or relatively underperfused; see below under ventilation/perfusion inequalities), i.e:

$$\dot{V}_A = \dot{V}_E - V_D \qquad \textbf{2.1}$$

For a single breath, this can be rewritten as:

$$\dot{V}_A = V_T - V_D \qquad \textbf{2.2}$$

(where V_T is the tidal volume).

In practice, however, V_D varies in proportion to the tidal volume. This is due to the 'cone front effect' (**Fig. 2.9**). Because gas flow in the large airways is laminar, the leading front is conical, with the gas in the centre moving more rapidly than that towards the periphery; indeed, gas close to the walls of the conducting airways may be stationary. This reduces the effective volume of the dead space. As V_T falls, the amount of stationary gas increases and V_D is reduced (Briscoe *et al.*, 1954). In clinical practice it is therefore preferable to refer to the V_D/V_T ratio.

CALCULATION OF V_D/V_T

Since no gas exchange takes place in the conducting airways and there is essentially no carbon dioxide in inspired air, all the carbon dioxide in the mixed expired gas must originate from gas exchanging areas of the lung. Therefore:

$$\dot{V}_E \times F_E CO_2 = \dot{V}_A \times F_A CO_2 \qquad \textbf{2.3}$$

(where $F_E CO_2$ and $F_A CO_2$ are the fractional concentrations of carbon dioxide in mixed expired and alveolar gas respectively).

Then, substituting from equation **2.1** for V_A:

$$\dot{V}_E \times F_E CO_2 = (\dot{V}_E - V_D) \times F_A CO_2 \qquad \textbf{2.4}$$

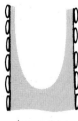 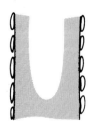

Large tidal volumes   Small tidal volumes

Fig. 2.9 The 'cone front effect': as tidal volume falls the volume of stationary gas increases, thereby reducing the effective dead space.

Substituting partial pressures for fractional concentrations and V_T for $\dot{V}_E$:

$$V_T \times P_E CO_2 = (V_T - V_D) \times P_A CO_2 \qquad \textbf{2.5}$$

Finally, in an 'ideal' alveolus, $P_A CO_2$ can be assumed to be identical to $P_a CO_2$, and rearranging the equation:

$$V_D/V_T = \frac{P_a CO_2 - P_E CO_2}{P_a CO_2} \qquad \textbf{2.6}$$

This is the *Bohr equation*. In normal subjects the V_D/V_T ratio is less than 0.3.

RELATIONSHIP BETWEEN ALVEOLAR VENTILATION AND ARTERIAL CARBON DIOXIDE TENSION

The amount of carbon dioxide excreted per unit time ($\dot{V}CO_2$) is clearly determined by the volume of the expired gas and the concentration of carbon dioxide in that gas, that is:

$$\dot{V}CO_2 = \dot{V}_E \times F_E CO_2 \qquad \textbf{2.7}$$

Substituting from equation **2.3**:

$$\dot{V}CO_2 = \dot{V}_A \times F_A CO_2 \qquad \textbf{2.8}$$

Substituting partial pressure for fractional concentration and rearranging:

$$\dot{V}_A = K \times \frac{\dot{V}CO_2}{P_A CO_2} \qquad \textbf{2.9}$$

(where K is a constant).

As before, $P_a CO_2$ can be substituted for $P_A CO_2$ and therefore rearranging gives:

$$P_a CO_2 \propto \frac{\dot{V}CO_2}{\dot{V}_A} \qquad \textbf{2.10}$$

If $\dot{V}CO_2$ remains constant, $P_a CO_2$ is determined solely by alveolar ventilation (i.e. V_T and V_D), while for a given level of alveolar ventilation, $P_a CO_2$ is proportional to carbon dioxide production.

THE ALVEOLAR AIR EQUATION

Derivation

The amount of oxygen taken up through the lungs per unit time (the oxygen consumption, $\dot{V}O_2$ must be given by the difference between the volume of oxygen breathed in and the volume breathed out. Therefore:

$$\dot{V}O_2 = (\dot{V}_A \times F_I O_2) - (\dot{V}_A \times F_A O_2) \qquad \textbf{2.11}$$

(where $F_I O_2$ and $F_A O_2$ are the fractional concentrations of oxygen in inspired air and expired alveolar gas respectively).

Rearranging gives:

$$F_AO_2 = F_IO_2 - \frac{\dot{V}O_2}{\dot{V}_A} \qquad \textbf{2.12}$$

Substituting for $\dot{V}_A$ from equation **2.8**:

$$F_AO_2 = F_IO_2 - (F_ACO_2 \times \frac{\dot{V}O_2}{\dot{V}CO_2}) \qquad \textbf{2.13}$$

$\dfrac{\dot{V}O_2}{\dot{V}CO_2}$ is, of course, the inverse respiratory exchange ratio R, and therefore:

$$F_AO_2 = F_IO_2 - \frac{F_ACO_2}{R} \qquad \textbf{2.14}$$

Fractional concentrations can be converted to partial pressures:

$$P_AO_2 = P_IO_2 - \frac{P_ACO_2}{R} \qquad \textbf{2.15}$$

In clinical practice it is usual to measure F_IO_2 and multiply this by the barometric pressure to obtain P_IO_2. Furthermore, P_ACO_2 is considered to be identical to P_aCO_2 and R is usually assumed to be 0.8. Therefore:

$$P_AO_2 = (F_IO_2 \times PB) - \frac{P_aCO_2}{0.8} \qquad \textbf{2.16}$$

(where PB = barometric pressure)

Composition of alveolar gas

Room air contains 20.93% oxygen so that the F_IO_2 is 0.21 and, for a normal barometric pressure of 101 kPa (760 mm Hg), the P_IO_2 is 21.2 kPa (159 mm Hg) (**Fig. 2.10**). There is virtually no carbon dioxide in inspired air, and the amount of water vapour is relatively small, so the remainder is largely nitrogen. However, by the time the inspired gases reach the alveoli they are fully saturated with water vapour at body temperature (37°C), which has a partial pressure of 6.3 kPa (47 mm Hg), and carbon dioxide has been added at a partial pressure of approximately 5.3 kPa (40 mm Hg). The P_AO_2 is thereby reduced to approximately 13.4 kPa (100 mm Hg).

The clinician can therefore influence P_AO_2 by altering the F_IO_2, the barometric pressure (i.e. administering hyperbaric oxygen) or the P_aCO_2.

The alveolar–capillary barrier

STRUCTURE

Alveolar gas is separated from blood in the pulmonary capillaries by the alveolar–capillary barrier, the detailed

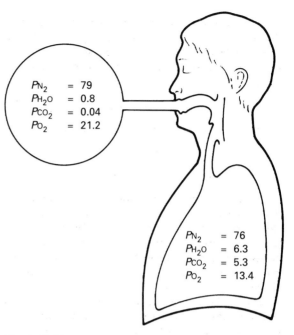

Fig. 2.10 The composition of inspired and alveolar gas (partial pressures in kPa).

structure of which has been demonstrated by Weibel (1984) and others using electron microscopy (**Fig. 2.11**). The pulmonary capillaries lie asymmetrically within the walls of the alveoli so that on one side where there is a single basement membrane the alveolar–capillary membrane is extremely thin (i.e. < 0.5 μm in cross-section), allowing rapid gas transfer,

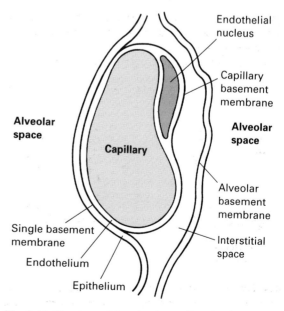

Fig. 2.11 Structure of the alveolar–capillary barrier.

while on the opposite 'thick' side, there is an interstitial space lying between the basement membranes of the capillary endothelium and the alveolar epithelium. This is the major site for fluid and solute exchange in the lungs and extends to surround the smaller blood vessels and airways from where fluid is drained by the terminal branches of the lymphatics.

SURFACTANT

Conventionally it is believed that the alveoli are lined by a continuous film of fluid, or 'aqueous hypophase' and that they therefore behave as one-sided bubbles, having an inherent tendency to collapse until the internal pressure exceeds the external by a difference, which can be quantified by the Laplace equation:

$$\Delta P = 2T/r$$

(where r is the radius of curvature of the bubble, and T is the surface tension).

In order to minimize the tendency for alveoli to collapse a monomolecular layer of a surface active phospholipid (predominantly dipalmitoyl phosphatidylcholine), secreted as *lamellar bodies* by the type II alveolar cells, is located at the liquid–air interface. This 'surfactant', it is suggested, acts as a detergent to lower surface tension, thereby stabilizing the alveoli and reducing the pressure differential required to inflate the lung. Nevertheless in this model the interconnecting fluid-lined alveoli remain inherently unstable since the smaller 'bubbles' will always have a tendency to empty into their larger neighbours. Indeed this would be an accelerating process because the pressure differences would increase progressively as one alveolus collapses into another.

Considerable controversy has surrounded the role of surfactant in excluding fluid from the alveoli. In the conventional model outlined above it is claimed that surfactant reduces the negative pressure in the aqueous lining, thereby minimizing the tendency for fluid to be sucked directly into the alveolus. This reduction in negative pressure would also reduce the chances of neighbouring alveoli collapsing and drawing fluid into the adjacent interstitial space.

An alternative proposal is that surfactant is directly adsorbed onto the epithelium, with no intervening aqueous layer, rendering the epithelial surface hydrophobic (Hills, 1990). It is suggested that the surfactant acts as a water repellent layer capable of impeding the penetration of water from the pulmonary capillary into the alveolus with a force well in excess of normal capillary hydrostatic pressure. Surface tension forces water to collect as convex droplets at the angles of the alveoli where they act as self-regulating 'corner pumps', which force fluid back into the pulmonary capillaries and interstitial spaces. This model of a 'dry' alveolus overcomes the problems associated with inherently unstable fluid-lined alveoli.

Surfactant may also be important in determining solute transport across the alveolar–capillary barrier. Depletion of surfactant is therefore associated not only with alveolar instability, but also with an increase in solute and water permeability of the alveolar–capillary barrier (Evander *et al.*, 1987).

STARLING FORCES

The factors governing fluid flux (Q_f) across a semipermeable membrane such as the pulmonary capillary endothelium can be described by the modified Starling equation (**Fig. 2.12**):

$$Q_f = K_f \left([P_{mv} - P_{pmv}] - \sigma \left[\pi_{mv} - \pi_{pmv} \right] \right)$$

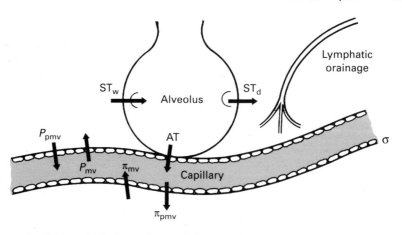

Fig. 2.12 Factors governing fluid flux in the lungs. P_{pmv}, perimicrovascular hydrostatic pressure; P_{mv}, microvascular hydrostatic pressure; π_{pmv}, perivascular colloid osmotic pressure; π_{mv}, microvascular colloid osmotic pressure; σ, reflection coefficient; ST_w, surface tension. (wet): ST_d, surface tension (dry); AT, active transport.

The membrane filtration coefficient (K_f) describes the permeability of the membrane to water. The direction and rate of fluid flux depends on the balance between the hydrostatic pressure gradient (i.e. the difference between microvascular and perimicrovascular pressures or $P_{mv} - P_{pmv}$) and the colloid osmotic pressure (COP) gradient (i.e. the difference between the COP in capillary blood and that in the interstitial space or $\pi_{mv} - \pi_{pmv}$), modified by the permeability of the membrane to protein—the reflection coefficient σ. When $\sigma = 1$ the membrane is perfectly semipermeable, when $\sigma = 0$ it is completely permeable. For albumin, the reflection coefficient of the pulmonary endothelium is normally about 0.6. These 'Starling forces' do not take into account the influence on overall lung fluid balance of lymphatic drainage or the surface area over which filtration takes place.

The Starling equation predicts a constant flow of protein and water across the capillary endothelium and into the interstitial space.

It has been estimated that in normal lungs the hydrostatic pressure falls from approximately 14 mm Hg in the pulmonary artery to about 8 mm Hg in the pulmonary capillary and 5 mm Hg in the pulmonary vein. Since the hydrostatic pressure in the interstitial space is thought to be slightly subatmospheric (i.e. − 2 mm Hg) there is a net transendothelial hydrostatic pressure gradient of the order of 10 mm Hg. This is counterbalanced by the difference between the COP in capillary blood (about 25 mm Hg) and the interstitial COP, which has been estimated to be approximately 19 mm Hg. There is therefore a transmural gradient of about 4 mm Hg, which produces about 10-20 ml of fluid per hour. There is also a pressure gradient between the perimicrovascular interstitial space (− 2 mm Hg) and the peribronchovascular interstitium (− 8 mm Hg), which promotes movement of fluid towards the lymphatics.

Oedema formation

If capillary hydrostatic pressure rises (e.g. in cardiac failure), there is a proportional increase in fluid flux across the endothelial membrane. Accumulation of extravascular lung water (EVLW) is, however, limited by:

- increased lymphatic drainage, which has a reserve capacity of approximately ten times basal flow;
- a dilutional reduction in the perimicrovascular COP (the capillary endothelium retains its 'barrier' function);
- a rise in hydrostatic pressure as fluid accumulates in the extravascular space.

Moreover, the interstitial compartment can accommodate a moderate increase in lung water (up to about 7 ml/kg), which does not directly interfere with gas exchange because the 'thin' side of the alveolar–capillary barrier remains dry.

In normal lungs these compensatory mechanisms are overwhelmed at hydrostatic pressures above about 18 mm Hg and interstitial oedema begins to form at pressures of around 20 mm Hg; marked increases in EVLW are seen when pressures exceed 25 mm Hg. The intercellular junctions between the alveolar epithelial cells are, however, approximately ten times 'tighter' (less permeable) than those of the endothelium, and the alveoli are therefore protected until the late stages of oedema formation. Eventually the mechanical stress of fluid distension causes a sudden disruption of the epithelial barrier and the alveoli are flooded. This occurs in an 'all or none' fashion—either an alveolus is flooded or it is completely dry.

A fall in COP (e.g. due to a reduction in serum albumin levels) rarely in itself precipitates pulmonary oedema because of a concomitant fall in interstitial COP and increased lymphatic drainage. Nevertheless both reductions in plasma COP and falls in the reflection coefficient, as occurs in the adult respiratory distress syndrome (see Chapter 6) will reduce the threshold hydrostatic pressure for oedema formation.

Active transport of sodium across the alveolar barrier accompanied by the passive movement of chloride and water also plays an important role in the clearance of fluid from the lungs. The ability of the epithelium to transport sodium actively, combined with its low permeability explains the large osmotic gradients that can be sustained across this membrane.

ELECTROSTATIC CHARGE

The distribution of electrostatic charges within the alveolar–capillary membrane (see **Fig. 2.11**) also has an important influence on the movement of fluid and solutes. The epithelial basement membrane has approximately five times more fixed, negative electrostatic charge than the capillary basement membrane; in fact it has been suggested that the latter is predominantly positively charged. This distribution of charge ensures that diffusion of anionic molecules such as albumin into the alveolar space is inhibited, while movement into the interstitial spaces and thence into the lymphatics is relatively unimpeded. In addition the charges are predominantly negative within the interstitial space so that negatively charged proteins are likely to be repelled from interstitial structures, enhancing their movement into the lymphatics.

Pulmonary gas exchange (Appendix 3)

If lung function was perfect, alveolar gas would equilibrate completely with arterial blood and P_aO_2 would equal P_AO_2. Even in normal individuals, however, a small pressure gradient exists between the oxygen in the alveoli and that in the arterial blood (the *alveolar–arterial oxygen difference*, $P_{A-a}O_2$) and this difference increases with age. Any disease of the lung parenchyma will interfere with oxygen transfer and cause an abnormal increase in $P_{A-a}O_2$. Three causes of the $P_{A-a}O_2$ can be identified: diffusion defects, right-to-left shunts and ventilation/perfusion mismatch.

DIFFUSION DEFECTS

A very small pressure gradient (0.133 kPa or 1 mm Hg) probably exists between oxygen in the alveoli and that in end-pulmonary capillary blood. This is probably not an important cause of hypoxaemia even in diseases such as fibrosing alveolitis in which the alveolar–capillary membrane is considerably thickened, except possibly during exercise when pulmonary capillary transit time is markedly reduced or when P_AO_2 is very low (e.g. at altitude). Because carbon dioxide is so much more soluble than oxygen its excretion is not influenced by diffusion defects.

RIGHT-TO-LEFT SHUNTS

Normally, a small amount of venous blood bypasses the lungs via the bronchial and Thebesian veins. Although this amounts to only 2% of the total cardiac output it is one cause of the normal $P_{A-a}O_2$. In some diseases of the lung, such as lobar pneumonia, and with certain cardiac lesions, such as Fallot's tetralogy, a much larger proportion of the cardiac output passes to the left side of the heart without taking part in gas exchange, thereby causing significant arterial hypoxaemia. This hypoxaemia cannot be corrected by administering oxygen to increase P_AO_2, because blood leaving normal alveoli is already fully saturated and further increases in P_AO_2 will not significantly affect its oxygen content. When this fully saturated blood is mixed with the shunted blood, arterial oxygen content, and therefore P_aO_2, falls proportionately. On the other hand, because of the shape of the carbon dioxide dissociation curve (see **Fig. 2.8**), the high P_{CO_2} of the shunted blood can be compensated by overventilating patent alveoli and thereby lowering the carbon dioxide content of the effluent blood. Indeed, in many patients with acute right-to-left shunts, hyperventilation reduces P_aCO_2.

VENTILATION/PERFUSION MISMATCH (West, 1977)

In a perfect lung each alveolus would be perfused with a quantity of blood exactly equal to its volume of ventila-

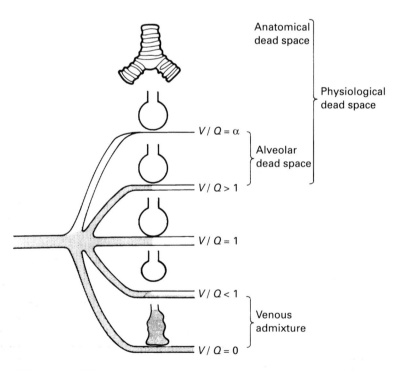

Fig. 2.13 Ventilation (*V*)/perfusion (*Q*) relationships.

tion (i.e. the ventilation (*V*)/perfusion (*Q*) ratio would be unity ($V/Q = 1$, **Fig. 2.13**). If alveoli are ventilated, but not perfused ($V/Q = \alpha$), or if ventilation is excessive relative to their perfusion ($V/Q > 1$), then a proportion of this ventilation is wasted, and behaves as alveolar 'dead space'. On the other hand, if an alveolus is well-perfused, but poorly ventilated ($V/Q < 1$), complete oxygenation of the blood in contact with that alveolus is impossible. Finally, alveoli that are perfused, but not ventilated ($V/Q = 0$) behave as true shunts.

Distribution of ventilation

Even in normal subjects, inspired gas is not evenly distributed throughout the lungs. Studies using inhaled radioactive xenon have demonstrated that ventilation increases from the upper to the lower regions of the lungs. The explanation is illustrated in **Fig. 2.14**. Furthermore, especially in diseased lungs, ventilation may be unevenly distributed due to variations in the time constants of individual respiratory units (**Fig. 2.15**). Finally, although air is moved through the conducting airways by convection, gas transfer in distal lung segments occurs by molecular diffusion. This diffusion may be incomplete, particularly in abnormal lungs, and may further contribute to an uneven distribution of ventilation.

Distribution of perfusion (West *et al.*, 1964)

In the normal lung, blood flow also increases downwards, but does so to a rather greater extent than ventilation (**Fig. 2.16**). Normally, the overall *V/Q* ratio is approximately 0.8. This has an effect equivalent to a right-to-left shunt of less than 3% of the cardiac output and causes a $P_{A-a}O_2$ of no more than 0.7 kPa (5 mm Hg).

Diseases of the lung parenchyma interfere with the distribution of both ventilation and perfusion, causing an increased 'scatter' of *V/Q* ratios. This produces an increase in alveolar V_D and hypoxaemia. As discussed above, the former can be compensated by increasing overall ventilation. *In contrast to the hypoxia resulting from a true right-to-left shunt, that due to areas of low V/Q can be partially corrected by administering oxygen and thereby increasing P_AO_2, even in poorly ventilated areas of lung.*

HYPOXIC PULMONARY VASOCONSTRICTION

The degree of hypoxaemia produced by *V/Q* mismatch or a right-to-left shunt is limited by the direct vasconstrictor effect of alveolar hypoxia on the pulmonary vasculature. In acute lung injury with increased capillary permeability (see Chapter 6) this response may also limit oedema formation. The constriction occurs in the small arteries and arterioles (< 200 μm in diameter) when the alveolar PO_2 decreases to below about 8 kPa

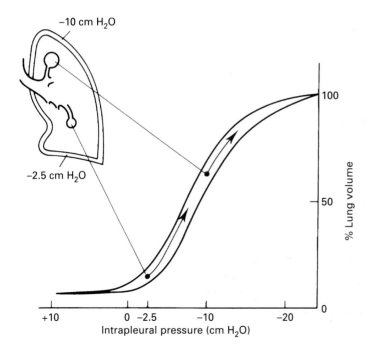

Fig. 2.14 Distribution of ventilation. Redrawn from West (1990), p. 99, with permission. Because of the weight of the lungs, intrapleural pressure is less negative at the base than at the apex. Consequently, there is less expansion of basal alveoli, which are on the steep portion of their compliance curve. For the same change in intrapleural pressure, therefore these alveoli expand more than those at the apex. Alveolar ventilation therefore increases from the apex to the base of the lungs. © 1990, The Williams & Wilkins Co., Baltimore.

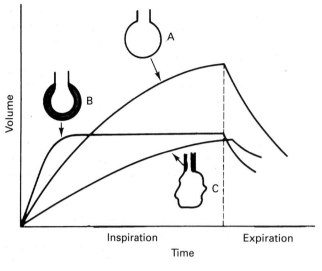

Fig. 2.15 Time constants. Redrawn from West (1990), p. 113, with permission. One time constant = compliance × resistance. For a normal alveolus (A): 0.6 sec = 0.2 l/cm H_2O × 3 cm H_2O/l/sec and by definition an alveolus is 95% filled in three time constants (i.e. 1.8 sec). A non-compliant alveolus (B) will have a short time constant, whereas the time constant will be prolonged in those with airway narrowing (C). © 1990, The Williams & Wilkins Co., Baltimore.

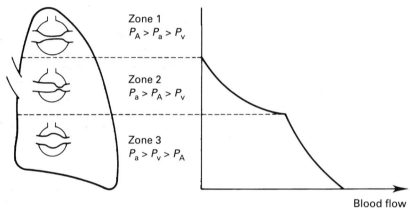

Fig. 2.16 Distribution of blood flow. Redrawn from West (1990), p. 41, with permission. Because of a hydrostatic effect the pressure in the pulmonary vessels increases from the apex to the base of the lungs. Consequently, in zone 1, alveolar pressure P_A exceeds both pulmonary arterial P_a and venous P_v pressures; the vessels are therefore collapsed and there is no blood flow (in fact, zone 1 does not exist in normal subjects). In zone 2, P_a exceeds P_A, which in turn is greater than P_v. Flow is therefore determined by the difference between P_A and P_a; since the former remains constant, flow increases progressively from the top to the bottom of this zone. In zone 3, both P_a and P_v exceed P_A. Flow therefore depends on the difference between these two pressures. Because of distension of the capillaries, blood flow increases slightly down this zone. A further zone, zone 4, may exist at the bases in which blood flow falls again due to compression of extra-alveolar vessels by poorly inflated lung tissue. © 1990, The Williams & Wilkins Co., Baltimore.

(60 mm Hg). The exact mechanism is unclear, but may be a direct effect on the vascular smooth muscle or an indirect effect via the release of vasoactive mediators from lung parenchyma. This response occurs in only about two-thirds of healthy people and is much more pronounced in the young.

THE THREE-COMPARTMENT MODEL OF PULMONARY GAS EXCHANGE (Riley & Cournand, 1949)

In clinical practice it is often convenient to consider the lungs as if they consisted of three compartments:

- physiological dead space;
- perfectly matched V/Q;
- venous admixture (**Fig. 2.17**).

The *dead space compartment* (wasted ventilation) therefore includes both the anatomical and the alveolar dead space, the latter consisting of 'true' dead space and lung units with V/Q ratios > 1 (see **Fig. 2.13**).

Venous admixture combines all sources of 'wasted blood flow' (i.e. diffusion defects, right-to-left shunts and V/Q ratios < 1 (see **Fig. 2.13**) and treats them as if a given proportion of the cardiac output bypassed the lungs altogether. *Venous admixture* is then expressed

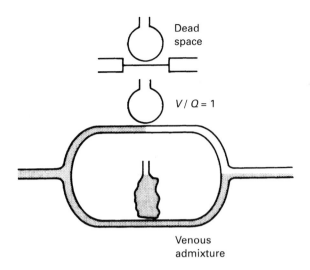

Fig. 2.17 The three-compartment model of pulmonary gas exchange.

as a percentage of the cardiac output—$\dot{Q}_s/\dot{Q}_t\%$, where $\dot{Q}_s$ is the flow per unit time through the shunt and $\dot{Q}_t$ is the total flow (i.e. the cardiac output). Both total dead space and venous admixture can be calculated relatively easily in clinical practice and, by administering 100% oxygen to correct any hypoxaemia due to V/Q inequalities, the relative contribution of true right-to-left shunt and V/Q inequalities to the total venous admixture can be determined. This information is, however, of limited clinical relevance and administration of high concentrations of oxygen, even for short periods, may adversely affect lung function. This is because alveolar nitrogen, which is not absorbed, is replaced by oxygen, which is rapidly taken up by pulmonary capillary blood, thereby rendering alveoli unstable and liable to collapse.

$\dot{Q}_s/\dot{Q}_t\%$ can be calculated from the shunt equation (**Fig. 2.18**).

Oxygen content can be derived from oxygen saturation and the Hb concentration (see **Table 2.1**). In the case of arterial and mixed venous blood, oxygen saturation can be derived from the P_{O_2} using a standard equation. Many automated blood gas analysers will perform this calculation, usually assuming that the oxyhaemoglobin dissociation curve is normally positioned. Some will then proceed to calculate oxygen content, either assuming a normal Hb or using a value entered by the operator. There are significant errors involved in obtaining oxygen content in this way and it is preferable to use a direct method such as spectrophotometry (see Chapter 5).

If a pulmonary artery catheter is not in place, true mixed venous blood cannot be obtained, but some authorities suggest that since in general only changes in venous admixture are of interest, central venous blood is adequate. Of course it is not possible to obtain end-pulmonary capillary blood; it is usual, therefore, to calculate $P_{A_{O_2}}$ from the alveolar air equation (see equation 2.16) and assume that equilibration in the ideal alveolus is complete so that $P_{c'O_2} = P_{A_{O_2}}$. Percentage saturation of Hb with oxygen is then calculated using a standard formula to represent the dissociation curve. Lastly, $C_{c'O_2}$ is derived from the Hb concentration. The V_D/V_T ratio can be calculated from the Bohr equation (2.6). This requires measurement of $P_{a_{CO_2}}$ and determination of the concentration of carbon dioxide in expired gas ($F_{E_{CO_2}}$).

MIXED VENOUS OXYGEN TENSION

If mixed venous oxygen tension ($P_{\bar{v}O_2}$) and therefore mixed venous oxygen content falls, the effect of a given degree of venous admixture on arterial oxygenation will be exacerbated (Kelman et al., 1967). If cardiac output, and therefore oxygen delivery, falls and/or oxygen

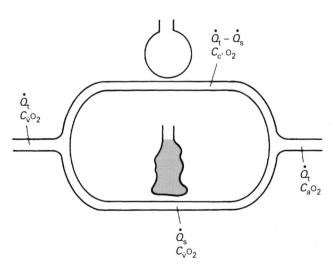

Fig. 2.18 Derivation of the shunt equation. The total amount of oxygen entering the systemic circulation per unit time must be equal to the sum of the amount leaving the ideal alveolus and the amount in the shunted blood. Therefore:

$$\dot{Q}_t \times C_{a_{O_2}} = [(\dot{Q}_t - \dot{Q}_s) \times C_{c'O_2}] + [\dot{Q}_s \times C_{\bar{v}O_2}].$$

This can be rearranged to give:

$$\frac{\dot{Q}_s}{\dot{Q}_t} = \frac{C_{c'O_2} - C_{a_{O_2}}}{C_{c'O_2} - C_{\bar{v}O_2}}$$

($\dot{Q}_t$, total flow (i.e. the cardiac output); $\dot{Q}_s$, flow through the shunt; ($\dot{Q}_t - \dot{Q}_s$), flow through ideal alveolus; $C_{a_{O_2}}$, arterial oxygen content; $C_{\bar{v}O_2}$, mixed venous oxygen content; $C_{c'O_2}$, end-capillary oxygen content in the ideal alveolus.)

requirements increase, more oxygen has to be extracted from each unit volume of blood arriving at the tissues and $P_{\bar{v}}O_2$ falls. Worsening arterial hypoxaemia therefore does not necessarily indicate a deterioration in pulmonary function, but may instead reflect a fall in cardiac output and/or a rise in oxygen consumption. Similarly, an increase in carbon dioxide production, if not compensated by greater alveolar ventilation, will cause P_aCO_2 to rise (see equation 2.10).

The extent to which $P_{c'}O_2$ is altered by a reduction in $P_{\bar{v}}O_2$ depends on the V/Q ratio of the lung unit in question. The effect will be most marked when there is a right-to-left shunt, while for ventilated units the impact of falls in $P_{\bar{v}}O_2$ will be greatest when the V/Q ratio is low. Overall the reduction in P_aO_2, which follows a fall in $P_{\bar{v}}O_2$ will depend on the V/Q distribution of the whole lung (i.e. the greater the V/Q mismatch the larger the fall in P_aO_2).

The $P_{\bar{v}}O_2$ is also influenced by the position of the oxy-haemoglobin dissociation curve (see **Fig. 2.7**). Therefore, if the arteriovenous oxygen content difference remains constant, a shift of the curve to the right, which occurs with acidosis, hypercarbia, pyrexia and a rise in red cell 2,3-DPG levels, may cause $P_{\bar{v}}O_2$ to rise. In addition, if $P_{\bar{v}}O_2$ remains unchanged, more oxygen will be unloaded at tissue level. A shift of the curve to the left, on the other hand, will cause a fall in $P_{\bar{v}}O_2$. It might be argued then that under certain circumstances an acidosis may be beneficial in terms of tissue oxygenation, provided that it is not sufficiently severe to interfere with cardiac function. It is probable though that shifts of the dissociation curve are of limited clinical significance. The position of the curve is conventionally described by specifying the P_{O_2} at which Hb is 50% saturated with oxygen (the P_{50}) (see **Fig. 2.7**).

LUNG VOLUMES (see Appendix 3)

Normally one breathes in and out from the resting end-expiratory position with a *tidal volume* V_T of approximately 500 ml. A maximal inspiration, followed by a maximal expiration, is the *vital capacity* (VC) and comprises the V_T, the *inspiratory reserve volume* (IRV) and the *expiratory reserve volume* (ERV) (**Fig. 2.19**).

At the end of a forced expiration, intrapleural pressure becomes positive, overcoming the elastic forces that normally keep the distal airways patent so that the terminal airways collapse. The amount of gas thereby trapped in the lungs is called the *residual volume* (RV). The volume of gas remaining in the lungs at the end of a normal quiet expiration is the *functional residual capacity* (FRC) and consists of the ERV plus the RV. The *closing volume* (CV) is defined as the lung volume at which airway closure first begins.

LUNG MECHANICS AND WORK OF BREATHING (see Appendix 3)

To achieve normal ventilation the respiratory muscles have to perform work against the *elastic* and *resistive forces* of the lungs and chest wall (**Fig. 2.20**); *viscoelastic* and *plastoelastic* forces must also be overcome. A negligible amount of work is expended in combating *inertial forces* (which depend on the mass of gases and tissues), *gravitational forces*, and the *compressibility of intrathoracic gases*, as well as in *distorting the chest wall* from its relaxed configuration. *Hyperventilation* is associated with an additional workload due to asynchronous or paradoxical motion of the rib cage and abdomen, particularly in those with pulmonary disease.

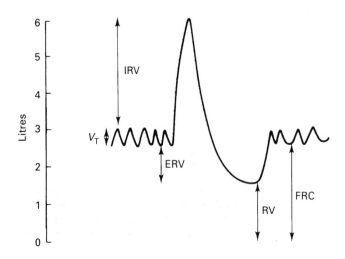

Fig. 2.19 Lung volumes. (V_T, tidal volume; IRV, inspiratory reserve volume; ERV, expiratory reserve volume; RV, residual volume; FRC, functional residual capacity.)

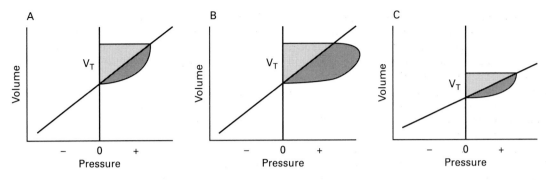

Fig. 2.20 Pressure volume curves illustrating the work performed in order to overcome the elastic (▨) and resistive (■) forces in the lungs. (A, normal lung mechanics; B, increased airway resistance; C, decreased compliance.)

In the presence of *airway obstruction and hyperinflation* further work is expended in compressing gas within the lungs and airways.

Since work = force × distance moved, the amount of work performed by the respiratory system per breath is determined by the transpulmonary pressure gradient and V_T. At rest the metabolic cost of the work of breathing is small and constitutes only 1–3% of total oxygen consumption. In respiratory disease, however, there is an increase in the elastic and resistive forces, a larger transpulmonary gradient has to be generated to achieve the same V_T and the work of breathing increases. Under these circumstances respiratory effort may account for as much as 25–30% of total body oxygen consumption.

Compliance

Compliance (elastic opposing forces) is defined as the change in lung volume produced by a given change in airway pressure ($\Delta V/\Delta P$). It is possible to determine the compliance of the lungs and chest wall separately by measuring intrapleural pressure changes (approximated by oesophageal pressure), but in clinical practice it is more usual to consider both together. Normal lung compliance is approximately 200 ml/cm H_2O whereas total thoracic compliance is around 70–100 ml/cm H_2O. Reductions in total thoracic compliance may be caused by disorders affecting the thoracic cage or by reductions in the number of functioning lung units (e.g. due to lung

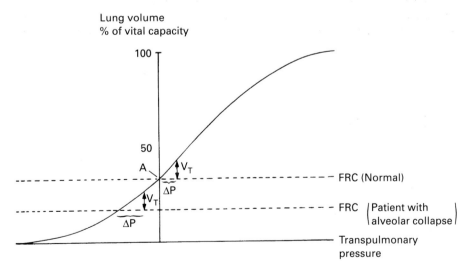

Fig. 2.21 Compliance curve for lung and chest wall combined. Tidal exchange takes place from the resting end-expiratory position (A), at which the tendency for the lungs to collapse is exactly counterbalanced by the tendency for the chest wall to expand. It can be seen that this is also the steepest part of the curve, where small changes in pressure produce large changes in volume (i.e. compliance is greatest). However, as FRC falls the curve becomes flatter (i.e. the lungs become stiffer and compliance falls).

resection, pneumothorax, pneumonia, or pulmonary oedema). An overall reduction in lung volume, reflected by a fall in FRC, is also associated with a decreased compliance (**Fig. 2.21**).

Effective dynamic compliance includes the influence of inspiratory airways resistance and is calculated as the ratio between the V_T delivered and the change in airway pressure (peak inspiratory pressure – end expiratory pressure, **Fig. 2.22**).

Static compliance is calculated from the change in volume produced by a given change in pressure *at a time of zero flow*. In practice if the inspiratory pause is sufficiently prolonged the dynamic component is eliminated and the 'quasi-static' compliance is obtained (see **Fig. 2.22**). Alternatively the expiratory tubing can be briefly occluded.

In general dynamic compliance is about 10–20% lower than compliance measured at plateau pressure. If dynamic compliance falls to a greater extent than total thoracic compliance it suggests an increase in airway resistance. This approach, however, only measures compliance within the range of tidal volumes employed and the value obtained may therefore alter depending on V_T and the level of positive end-expiratory pressure (see Chapter 7). An alternative is to perform a prolonged stepwise inspiratory-expiratory manoeuvre to obtain a true static pressure-volume loop. Frequently this pressure-volume curve is found to be non-linear and points can be identified on both the inspiratory and expiratory curves at which the slope suddenly changes (**Fig. 2.23**). During inflation this 'elbow', where compliance suddenly increases, may be caused by re-expansion of a large number of previously collapsed alveoli as a *'critical opening pressure'* is reached. During deflation, at a pressure generally lower than the opening pressure, these same alveoli collapse with a reduction in compliance. It has been suggested that this phenomenon of 'recruitment' should be used as a basis for

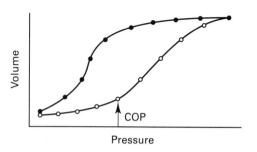

Fig. 2.23 Static pressure–volume curve illustrating a critical opening pressure (COP) during lung inflation (○) and a similar 'elbow' at a lower pressure in the deflationary curve (●).

selecting the optimal level of positive end-expiratory pressure (see Chapter 7).

Resistance

Airway resistance is expressed as the airway pressure required to generate a given gas flow rate (cm $H_2O/l/sec$). The relationship between the flow-resistance of the total respiratory system (R_{rs}) and flow at a fixed lung volume is given by:

$$R_{rs} = R_t + K_1 + K_2 V$$

(where R_t is the flow resistance of the thoracic tissues and K_1 and K_2 are empirical constants that describe the relationship between airway resistance (R_{aw}) and flow-$R_{aw} = K_1 + K_2 V$.)

At a given lung volume therefore, R_{rs} will rise as flow increases. Moreover, at a given flow, R_{rs} will fall as lung volume rises because of a decrease in both R_{aw} and R_t. The former reflects airway dilatation, while the latter is a result of a decrease in the linear velocity of thoracic tissues and therefore a reduction in flow-dependent pressure losses.

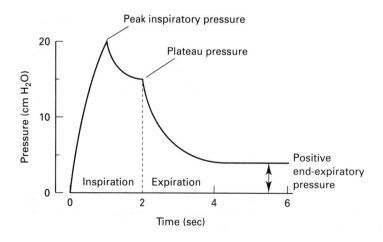

Fig. 2.22 Changes in airway pressure during mechanical ventilation. Effective dynamic compliance is calculated using peak inspiratory pressure–end expiratory pressure. Quasi-state compliance is calculated at time of zero flow (i.e. using plateau pressure – end expiratory pressure).

An increase in airway resistance will require greater transpulmonary pressures to achieve the same V_T and will increase the work of breathing (see **Fig. 2.20**).

CONTROL OF BREATHING

Breathing is normally precisely controlled by a tightly integrated feedback loop with three components:

- the respiratory control centres;
- the respiratory sensors;
- the respiratory effectors.

By balancing V_T and respiratory frequency to achieve the desired minute ventilation, this complex system maintains blood gas tensions within narrow limits despite marked fluctuations in V_{O_2} and V_{CO_2}, while at the same time minimizing the work of breathing. The body's capacity to store carbon dioxide far exceeds its ability to store oxygen and therefore changes in ventilation produce greater and more rapid changes in P_{O_2} than in P_{CO_2} or pH.

Respiratory control centres

The traditional concept of a single 'respiratory centre' has been superseded. It is now appreciated that there are several localized regions of respiratory regulation, which although situated at different levels within the brain stem, are highly interrelated by multilevel feedback connections. Functionally it is useful to consider two major centres of respiratory regulation, the *medullary centres* and the *groups of pontine neurones*, both of which can be overriden during wakefulness by projections from the *cerebral cortex*.

MEDULLARY CENTRES

Respiratory rhythm originates in the medulla, possibly due to the interactive function of individual inspiratory and expiratory neurones, although separate respiratory pacemaker cells may also exist. In isolation the respiratory rhythm generated by this centre is not necessarily regular. There are two major groups of respiratory neurones in the medullary region: *the dorsal respiratory group* (DRG) and the *ventral respiratory group* (VRG).

Dorsal respiratory group

The DRG is situated in the dorsomedial region of the medulla and is primarily composed of inspiratory neurones, which connect to the spinal inspiratory motor neurones of the phrenic and intercostal nerves. It seems likely that the DRG is the source of rhythmic respiratory drive, which is then transmitted to other regions, including the ventral respiratory group, for modulation.

Ventral respiratory group

The VRG is located ventrolaterally in the medulla and contains both inspiratory and expiratory neurones, which project to intercostal, abdominal and phrenic motor neurones, as well as to branches of the vagus, which supply the accessory muscles of respiration.

Other participating neurones

In addition there are other neurones in the vicinity of the DRG and VRG that may participate in some other aspects of inspiration, expiration and generation of respiratory rhythm.

PONTINE NEURONES

Pontine neurones may be responsible for 'fine tuning' respiratory adjustments. There are two major centres in this region:

- the *apneustic centre* in the lower pons;
- the *pneumotactic centre* in the upper pons.

Midpontine transection disinhibits the apneustic centre and produces a sustained inspiratory spasm, called *'apneusis'*. The pneumotactic centre regulates the relative duration of inspiration and expiration, although it is not essential for respiratory rhythmicity.

CORTICAL MODULATION

Cortical neurones project via corticobulbar and corticospinal pathways allowing conscious modulation of the respiratory neurones during activities such as speech and eating. In sleep the cortical drive to respiration is diminished and ventilation becomes more closely linked to the afferent input from chemoreceptors and vagal intrapulmonary receptors (see Chapter 6, Sleep related respiratory disturbances).

Respiratory sensors

Respiratory sensors consist of the *chemoreceptors*, which are sensitive to changes in blood gas tensions and acid–base status, and sensory *mechanoreceptors,* within the lung and chest wall.

CENTRAL CHEMORECEPTORS

The central chemoreceptors are located on the ventral surface of the medulla oblongata. They respond rapidly to an increase in the H^+ ion concentration $[H^+]$ within the cerebrospinal fluid (CSF) by a linear increase in ventilation. Because carbon dioxide diffuses rapidly into the CSF, increasing its $[H^+]$, increases in P_aCO_2 produce an immediate ventilatory response. Changes in systemic pH, on the other hand produce a delayed response because H^+ ions and HCO_3^- diffuse more slowly into the CSF. The central chemoreceptors are depressed by hypoxia.

PERIPHERAL CHEMORECEPTORS

The peripheral chemoreceptors are located at the bifurcation of the carotid arteries and along the aortic arch where they are exposed to a very high blood flow. They respond mainly to hypoxaemia and are activated to a much lesser extent by increases in PCO_2 and $[H^+]$, although the effects of combined hypoxaemia and hypercarbia are synergistic. The response to hypoxia is non-linear; as P_aO_2 falls below about 10 kPa (75 mm Hg) there is an exponential increase in respiratory stimulation.

Under normal circumstances, therefore, carbon dioxide has a greater influence on the control of ventilation than oxygen. The peripheral chemoreceptors respond to changes in partial pressure, not oxygen content, and in carbon monoxide poisoning, for example, there is therefore no increase in ventilation. They are also sensitive to reductions in blood pressure, and this may partly account for the hyperventilation often seen in the early stages of shock.

CHEST WALL MECHANORECEPTORS

Chest wall mechanoreceptors measure and modulate the forces generated by inspiratory effort. They respond to stretch of the respiratory muscles and reflexly modify the rate and depth of breathing. The *tendon receptors* within the intercostal muscles and diaphragm inhibit motor activity when the force of contraction is excessive. The *muscle spindles*, which are abundant in the intercostals, but more sparsely distributed in the diaphragm, may help to maintain V_T when chest wall movement is impeded (e.g. by changes in posture).

PULMONARY MECHANORECEPTORS

The V_T and respiratory rate may also be influenced by stimuli arising in pulmonary receptors. *Irritant receptors*, which are located within the epithelium of the airways, respond to chemical or physical stimuli (e.g. mechanical deformation) to produce an increase in ventilation and bronchoconstriction. They are also involved in coughing.

The *pulmonary stretch receptors* are located in the smooth muscle of the airways and respond to changes in lung volume. The *Hering–Breuer reflex*, for example, is a vagally-mediated reflex that normally terminates inspiration once a certain volume threshold has been reached. It is inoperative during quiet breathing, but is activated when V_T increases to about twice normal.

The *juxtacapillary (J) receptors* are found in the interstitium of the alveolar wall and are stimulated by distortion of the interstitial space as may occur with vascular engorgement, congestion or fibrosis. Stimulation of these receptors may explain the rapid shallow breathing seen in many patients with parenchymal lung disease.

Respiratory effectors

SPINAL PATHWAYS

The cortical pathways descend separately from the involuntary neuronal projections; there may also be spatial separation between the descending inspiratory and expiratory pathways.

RESPIRATORY MUSCLES

There are three major groups of respiratory muscles:

- the intercostal and accessory muscles;
- the diaphragm;
- the abdominal musculature.

The contractile properties of the respiratory muscles are governed by the same factors as those that control all striated muscles and their force of contraction is therefore influenced by force–length, force–velocity and force–frequency relationships. The greatest tension is generated when the muscle is at its resting 'optimal' length when there is maximum overlap of the cross-bridges between the thick and thin filaments. An increase in lung volume will therefore lead to shortening of the respiratory muscles and a marked reduction in the tension generated (see Chapter 6). As the frequency of contraction increases there is a steep rise in the force of contraction, which plateaus at a rate of about 60 cycles/s, while increasing velocity of contraction is associated with a reduction in force.

There are three types of respiratory muscle fibre:

- Slow-twitch type I fibres have the highest resistance to fatigue with a low glycolytic and high oxidative capacity. These fibres are best suited to sustained tonic activity and constitute about 50% of the diaphragm.

- Type II A fast-twitch red fibres are very resistant to fatigue and are suitable for sustained phasic activity.
- Type II B fast-twitch white fibres have a poor oxidative capacity and the least resistance to fatigue. They are used for fast and powerful, but short-term activity.

Diaphragm

The diaphragm is the major inspiratory muscle. It consists of a costal portion arising from the inner aspect of the lower six ribs and a crural portion originating from the upper lumbar vertebrae. In general, diaphragmatic contraction pushes down against the abdominal contents, leading to a rise in intra-abdominal pressure, and uses the resisting abdomen as a fulcrum to elevate the chest wall. The costal portion is capable of performing both these functions, while the major role of the crural portion is to increase intra-abdominal pressure. Diaphragmatic contraction therefore produces an outward movement of the anterior abdominal wall.

The efficiency with which the diaphragm translates its contraction into lung inflation depends on the ability of the abdominal wall to resist outward motion and create a positive pressure within the abdomen. Paradoxical inward movement of the abdomen during inspiration is a sign of diaphragmatic paralysis. Increases in lung volume will decrease the resting length of the diaphragm, thereby reducing its ability to develop tension. Moreover, the diaphragmatic fibres may come to lie at right angles to the chest wall and in this situation contraction may serve only to decrease the diameter of the inferior margin of the thoracic cage (see also Chapter 6). Nevertheless contraction of the diaphragm continues to fulfil a useful function because it fixes the lower boundary of the thorax.

Intercostals

Intercostals fulfil both an inspiratory and an expiratory function with the external intercostals being predominantly active during inspiration.

Abdominal muscles

The abdominal muscles are the major muscles of expiration and generate the increased intrathoracic pressures needed for coughing. They also act to facilitate inspiration as described above.

Muscle weakness

Muscle weakness can be defined as an impaired ability of a rested muscle to generate force.

Muscle fatigue

Muscle fatigue can be defined as a situation in which muscle loses its ability to generate and sustain a required force or velocity of contraction. It is the result of muscle activity under load and is reversible by rest. It is likely to be due to depletion of energy stores, but recovery is slow and may take as long as 24 hours. The long-lasting component of fatigue is thought to be the result of impaired excitation–contraction coupling. Fatigue is generally a relatively acute phenomenon; little is known about chronic fatigue in which muscle has not recovered from previous activity and there is a failure to generate a force, as opposed to sustaining a force. Central fatigue is considered to be present when a voluntary effort generates less force than electrical stimulation.

The respiratory muscles are relatively resistant to fatigue because they are continually active but, under extreme circumstances, they will eventually fail. Normal subjects are able to sustain minute ventilations less then 50–60% of maximum indefinitely. As the demand exceeds 60%, however, endurance times rapidly fall. Inspiratory resistive loads of less than 40% of maximum can be sustained indefinitely, but at higher loads the diaphragm fails as a pressure generator (Roussos & Macklem, 1977).

The bronchial circulation (Deffebach et al., 1987)

The lung is perfused by two circulations.

The *pulmonary circulation* receives the entire venous return and is the major site for gas exchange. The much smaller *bronchial circulation* fulfils an important role in sustaining vital airway defences, fluid balance and metabolic activity in the lungs. It is the 'systemic blood supply to the lungs,' supplying not only the bronchi, but also the trachea, the distal airways, the bronchoalveolar bundles, nerves, supporting structures, regional lymph nodes and visceral pleura. It also supplies, as the vasa vasorum, the walls of the pulmonary arteries and veins.

The bronchial veins draining the upper airways join the systemic veins to the right heart via the azygous and hemiazygous veins, while blood from the lower airways and lung parenchyma drains via the pulmonary veins into the left heart. This latter portion of the bronchial circulation is known as the 'pulmonary collateral', 'bronchopulmonary anastamotic' or 'bronchial systemic to pulmonary' flow. Branches from medium-sized bronchial arteries anastomose with the pulmonary alveolar microvasculature and with the pulmonary veins.

Bronchial blood flow is reduced by:

- systemic hypotension;
- raised intrathoracic pressure;
- increased lung volume;
- increases in pulmonary vascular pressures.

Systemic hypoxaemia increases both anastomotic and total bronchial blood flow. Although alveolar hypoxia may increase bronchial blood flow, in some situations simultaneous hypoxic pulmonary vasoconstriction may elevate downstream pressures and reduce flow. Systemic hypercarbia increases bronchial blood flow.

The bronchial circulation enlarges in response to lung injury and may provide the blood supply necessary for inflammation and subsequent healing in circumstances when pulmonary blood flow is often reduced. More-over, significant gas exchange may be possible (e.g. during pulmonary artery occlusion) via the bronchial circulation, across either the bronchial or the alveolar epithelium, downstream of its anastomosis with the pulmonary circulation. The volume of gas exchange via the first route is likely to be small, but overall the bronchial circulation can contribute as much as 37% of total carbon dioxide output, and oxygen uptake may also occur in the presence of systemic hypoxia.

REFERENCES

Briscoe WA, Forster RE & Comroe JH, Jr (1954) Alveolar ventilation at very low tidal volumes. *Journal of Applied Physiology* **7**: 27–30.

Deffebach ME, Charan NB, Lakshminarayan S & Butler J (1987) The bronchial circulation. Small, but a vital attribute of the lung. *American Review of Respiratory Diseases* **135**: 463–481.

Evander E, Wollmer P, Jonson B & Lachmann B (1987) Pulmonary clearance of inhaled 99m Tc-DTPA: effects of surfactant depletion by lung lavage. *Journal of Applied Physiology* **62**: 1611–1614.

Jan K-M, Heldman J & Chien S (1980) Coronary haemodynamics and oxygen utilization after hematocrit variations in hemorrhage. *American Journal of Physiology* **239**: H326–H332.

Hills BA (1990) The role of lung surfactant. *British Journal of Anaesthesia* **65**: 13–29.

Kelman GR, Nunn JF, Prys-Roberts C & Greenbaum R (1967) The influence of cardiac output on arterial oxygenation: a theoretical study. *British Journal of Anaesthesia* **39**: 450–458.

Riley RL & Cournand A (1949) 'Ideal' alveolar air and the analysis of ventilation–perfusion relationships in the lungs. *Journal of Applied Physiology* **1**: 825–847.

Roussos C & Macklem PT (1977) Diaphragmatic fatigue in man. *Journal of Applied Physiology* **43**: 189–197.

Weibel ER (1984) *The Pathway of Oxygen: Structure and Function in the Mammalian Respiratory System.* Cambridge, Massachusetts, Harvard University Press.

West JB (1977) State of the art: ventilation–perfusion relationships. *American Review of Respiratory Disease* **116**: 919–943.

West JB (1990) *Respiratory Physiology*, 5th edn. Baltimore, Williams & Wilkins.

West JB, Dollery CT & Naimark A (1964) Distribution of blood flow in isolated lung; relation to vascular and alveolar pressures. *Journal of Applied Physiology* **19**: 713–724.

APPENDICES

Appendix I Normal haemodynamic values.	
Mean arterial pressure (MAP)	70–100 mm Hg
Central venous pressure (CVP)	2–8 mm Hg
Right ventricular pressures	14–30/0–7 mm Hg
Pulmonary artery pressures	16–24/5–12 mm Hg
Mean pulmonary artery pressure	9–16 mm Hg
Pulmonary artery occlusion pressure (PAOP)	5–12 mm Hg
Left ventricular end-diastolic pressure (LVEDP)	4–10 mm Hg
Cardiac output ($\dot{Q}_T$)	4–6 l/min
Cardiac index (CI)	2.8–3.5 l/min/m²
Stroke volume (SV)	50–100 ml
Stroke volume index (SVI)	30–50 ml/m²
Right ventricular stroke work index (RVSWI)	4–12 g/m/m²
Left ventricular stroke work index (LVSWI)	44–68 g/m/m²

Appendix 1 continued.

Systemic vascular resistance (SVR)	900–1200 dyne.s/cm^5
Systemic vascular resistance index (SVRI)	1700–2600 dyne.s/cm^5/m^2
Pulmonary vascular resistance (PVR)	120–200 dyne.s/cm^5
Pulmonary vascular resistance index (PVRI)	210–360 dyne.s/cm^5/m^2
Ejection fraction	50–60%

Appendix 2 Normal oxygen transport values.

Oxygen delivery index (DO_2)	520–720 ml/min/m^2
Oxygen consumption index (VO_2)	100–180 ml/min/m^2
Arterial oxygen content (C_aO_2)	18–21 vol%
Mixed venous oxygen content ($C_{\bar{v}}O_2$)	13–16 vol%
Arteriovenous oxygen content difference ($C_{a-v}O_2$)	4–5 vol%
Oxygen extraction ratio (OER)	0.22–0.30

Appendix 3 Normal respiratory values.

Dead space fraction (V_D/V_T)	< 0.35
Alveolar–arterial oxygen difference ($P_{A-a}O_2$)	
$\quad F_IO_2 = 0.21$	5–25 mm Hg
$\quad F_IO_2 = 1.0$	< 150 mm Hg
Percentage venous admixture ($\dot{Q}_s/\dot{Q}_t$%) (shunt fraction)	3–8%
Static total thoracic compliance	70–100 ml/cm H$_2$O
Airflow resistance	< 3 cm H$_2$O/L/s

	Male	Female
FEV$_1$ (l)	2.2–4.7	1.3–3.6
FVC (l)	3.2–4.7	1.8–4.5
FEV$_1$/FVC (%)	66–83	71–81
PEFR (l/min)	460–680	280–490

Normal lung volumes in 60 kg male

Tidal volume (V_T)	400–600 ml
Inspiratory reserve volume (IRV)	3330–3740 ml
Expiratory reserve volume (ERV)	950–1200 ml
Functional residual capacity (FRC)	2300–2600 ml
Residual volume (RV)	1200–1700 ml
Vital capacity (VC)	3800–5000 ml

3 Assessment and Monitoring of Cardiovascular Function

Continuous monitoring allows rapid recognition of changes in the patient's condition and an accurate assessment of progress and response to therapy. In many cases invasive monitoring will be required to establish the precise diagnosis although, because these techniques incur a significant risk of complications (see below), they should be used selectively and non-invasive methods should be chosen whenever possible.

HEART RATE

As discussed in Chapter 2, heart rate is an important determinant of cardiac output and almost all intensive care patients require *continuous electrocardiographic (ECG) monitoring*. Not only can changes in heart rate be observed immediately, but arrhythmias may be detected, diagnosed and treated. Moreover, changes in the ECG pattern may suggest the presence of electrolyte disturbances such as hypo- or hyperkalaemia and hypo- or hypercalcaemia (see Chapter 10) and allow the detection of episodes of myocardial ischaemia (ST segment/T wave changes).

BLOOD PRESSURE

Alterations in blood pressure are often interpreted as reflecting changes in cardiac output. However, if the patient is vasoconstricted, with a high peripheral resistance, blood pressure may be normal, or occasionally high, even when cardiac output is low. Conversely the vasodilated patient may be hypotensive despite a very high cardiac output.

As well as its value as a guide to cardiac output, the absolute level of blood pressure is important since hypotension may jeopardize perfusion of vital organs, while excessively high pressure increases myocardial work and can cause bleeding from arterial suture lines or precipitate cerebrovascular accidents. *The adequacy of blood pressure in an individual patient must always be assessed in relation to their premorbid value.*

Measuring blood pressure

Traditionally, blood pressure is measured intermittently using a sphygmomanometer cuff and auscultation. Automated instruments are now available, which use a microphone to detect Korotkoff sounds. These automatically record and digitally display blood pressure and heart rate at intervals of 1–15 minutes. Although expensive, they are reliable and accurate and have the advantage of being non-invasive.

INTRA-ARTERIAL CANNULATION

If rapid alterations in blood pressure are anticipated (e.g. when administering vasoactive or inotropic agents), continuous monitoring using an *intra-arterial cannula* is essential. An additional advantage of an indwelling arterial cannula is that repeated sampling for blood gas analysis can be performed without repeated puncture of the artery, which may well be more traumatic than prolonged cannulation.

Approaches

Percutaneous puncture of the radial artery (**Fig. 3.1**) is usually preferred because this superficial vessel is readily accessible, sterility of the insertion site is easily maintained, pressure can be applied to control bleeding and there is minimal restriction of patient mobility. Moreover, there is usually an adequate collateral circulation.

Some feel that cannulation of a larger vessel such as the femoral artery carries less risk of occlusive complications since good blood flow continues around the cannula. Femoral artery cannulation has been recommended as a safer alternative to difficult percutaneous radial artery cannulation or a surgical cut-down, both of which carry an increased risk of complications (Russell *et al.*, 1983). Certainly, cannulation of the femoral artery is relatively easy and is a useful approach in an emergency, particularly if the patient is hypotensive and other pulses are difficult to palpate.

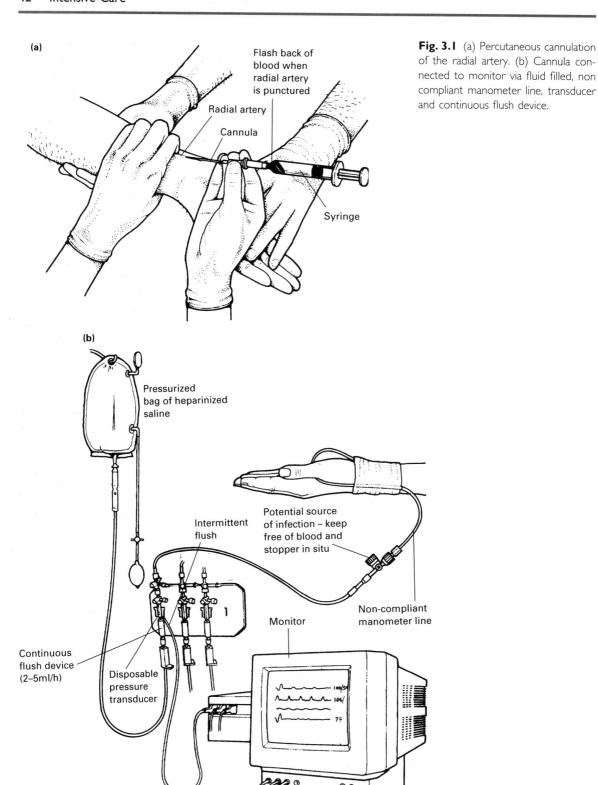

(a)

Flash back of blood when radial artery is punctured

Radial artery

Cannula

Syringe

(b)

Pressurized bag of heparinized saline

Intermittent flush

Potential source of infection – keep free of blood and stopper in situ

Non-compliant manometer line

Monitor

Continuous flush device (2–5ml/h)

Disposable pressure transducer

Fig. 3.1 (a) Percutaneous cannulation of the radial artery. (b) Cannula connected to monitor via fluid filled, non compliant manometer line, transducer and continuous flush device.

In difficult cases the brachial or dorsalis pedis arteries may be cannulated, while in children the axillary artery can be used.

Cannulae

Relatively small (20 gauge for adults, 22 gauge for children) short parallel-sided cannulae allow blood flow to continue past the cannula, and those made of Teflon are less irritant than, for example, those made of polypropylene or PVC; the use of such cannulae is therefore considered to minimize the risk of thrombosis.

Sources of error

It is important that the clinician is aware of some common sources of error in intra-arterial pressure measurement. If the arterial trace is 'over-damped', the recorded systolic pressure will be less than the actual systolic pressure (**Fig. 3.2**). This can occur if the cannula is kinked or partially obstructed by blood clot, if its tip is against the vessel wall or if there are air bubbles in the manometer line or transducer. Soft manometer lines can also produce a damped signal. Conversely, an 'under-damped' trace will 'over-read', particularly at high pressures (see **Fig. 3.2**). Long manometer lines (more than 3–4 feet) can also introduce inaccuracies since the natural resonant frequency of the system is decreased until it approaches the harmonics of the input signal, accentuating the recorded pressure. The mean arterial pressure is not influenced by either damping or resonance.

It should be appreciated that in peripheral vessels the systolic pressure is 1.1–1.3 times higher than in the ascending aorta (probably because of resonance in the arterial system) and that the diastolic pressure is lower by up to 5 mm Hg. Conversely vasoconstriction may cause damping of pressures recorded from peripheral vessels. *Catheter tip transducers* have a number of advantages:

- artefacts due to catheter movement are avoided;
- there is no fluid-filled tubing;
- the frequency response is improved;
- correct positioning of the transducer is simplified.

Technique

- The arm should be supported, with the wrist extended, by an assistant (see **Fig. 3.1a**).
- Assessment of the ulnar collateral circulation using Allen's test is no longer recommended since a normal result does not preclude ischaemia neither does an abnormal result reliably predict this complication. Regular inspection of the cannulated hand is more likely to prevent ischaemic damage.
- Gloves should be worn.
- Palpate the radial artery where it arches over the head of the radius and make a small skin incision over the proposed puncture site. In conscious patients, raise a wheal of local anaesthetic, taking care not to puncture the vessel or obscure its pulsation.
- Insert the cannula over the point of maximal pulsation and advance in line with the direction of the vessel, at an angle of approximately 30°. 'Flash back' of blood indicates that the radial artery has been punctured.

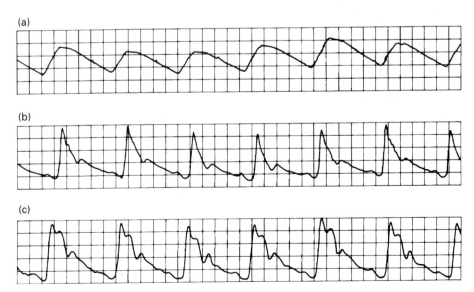

Fig. 3.2 Intra-arterial pressure recordings: (a) excessively damped; (b) critically damped to provide accurate readings; (c) under-damped.

- To ensure that the shoulder of the cannula enters the vessel, lower the needle and cannula and advance a few mm into the vessel and then thread the cannula off the needle into the vessel.
- Following withdrawal of the needle connect the cannula to a non-compliant manometer line filled with heparinized saline. This is then connected via a transducer and continuous flush device to an oscilloscope (see **Fig. 3.1b**). The transducer should be zeroed.
- Spray the puncture site with povidone iodine and cover with a transparent dressing.
- The manometer line should be changed every 48 hrs and the cannulation site every 4-5 days.

Some prefer to transfix the artery and when there is difficulty advancing the cannula into the vessel a guide wire may prove useful. If cannulation fails, digital compression should be applied to the vessel for three minutes. In some cases this may result in vasospasm, in which case the return of a good volume pulse should be awaited (usually 15 minutes) or cannulation should be attempted at another site.

Complications

Loss of arterial pulsation occurs in a significant proportion of patients and *digital ischaemia* is the most common complication of arterial cannulation. However, the much feared complication of necrosis of one or more digits is fortunately rare, provided ischaemia is recognized early and the cannula is then removed promptly (Russell *et al.*, 1983). Risk factors for ischaemia include:

- prolonged cannulation;
- low cardiac output;
- administration of vasoconstrictors;
- pre-existing peripheral vascular disease.

Ischaemia is commoner:

- in females;
- following multiple attempts at cannulation;
- if a haematoma develops.

Transfixation of the artery does not increase the incidence of ischaemia. Persistent ischaemia may require aggressive management (e.g. brachial plexus or stellate ganglion block or even surgical exploration).

Some consider that there is an increased risk of *infection* with the femoral approach (Band & Maki, 1979), others feel this is insignificant (Thomas *et al.*, 1983); the overall complication rate is similar for both radial and femoral artery cannulation (7.5% and 6.9%, respectively) (Russell *et al.*, 1983).

Two other important complications associated with intra-arterial cannulation include:

- *accidental injection of drugs*, which can cause widespread vascular occlusion with the development of gangrene distally;
- *disconnection*, which, if unnoticed, can rapidly produce serious hypovolaemia, particularly in children.

The risk of these complications can be minimized by clearly labelling the arterial line, using Luer locks for all connections and leaving the site exposed at all times so that disconnection is immediately recognized.

The development of an *arteriovenous fistula* and formation of an *aneurysm* or *pseudoaneurysm* are unusual, while *bruising* and *haematomas* are common (**Table 3.1**).

PRE-LOAD

As discussed in the preceding chapter, the force with which myocardial fibres contract is dependent on the degree to which they are stretched prior to the onset of systole. This is in turn dependent on the ventricular end-diastolic volume (VEDV), which is directly related to the ventricular end-diastolic pressure (VEDP). The latter can, of course, be measured by direct catheterization of the ventricle, but in clinical practice it is more usual to measure the pressure in the relevant atrium as this is nearly always closely related to VEDP. The relationship between VEDV and VEDP depends on ventricular compliance, so a stiff ventricle will need a higher EDP to achieve an adequate VEDV—a situation frequently encountered in the critically ill. Also, atrial pressure will not equal VEDP when there is an obstruction, such as a stenosed valve, between the two chambers.

Central venous pressure

In the case of the right ventricle the pressure within one of the large veins in the thorax is usually measured—the 'filling pressure' of the right ventricle. This provides a

---

Table 3.1 Complications of intra-arterial cannulation.

Bruising and haematoma

Occlusive complications (loss of arterial pulsation, digital ischaemia, digital necrosis)

Infection

Accidental injection of drugs

Disconnection

Arteriovenous fistula

Aneurysm/Pseudo-aneurysm

fairly simple method of assessing the adequacy of a patient's circulating volume and the contractile state of the myocardium. It is important to realize, however, that the absolute value of the central venous pressure (CVP) is not as important as its response to a fluid challenge (**Fig. 3.3**) (Sykes, 1963); it should always be interpreted in conjunction with other monitored variables (e.g. heart rate, blood pressure, urine flow and cardiac output) and with clinical assessment (e.g. skin colour, peripheral temperature and perfusion). The hypovolaemic patient will initially respond to transfusion with little or no change in CVP, together with some cardiovascular improvement (falling heart rate, rising blood pressure and increased peripheral temperature). As the normovolaemic state is approached, the CVP usually rises slightly and stabilizes, while other cardiovascular values normalize. At this stage transfusion should be slowed, or even stopped, to avoid overloading the patient, which results in an abrupt and sustained rise in CVP, usually accompanied by some deterioration in the patient's condition.

The CVP may be read:

- intermittently using a manometer system, which is only used when facilities for transducing the pressure are not available (e.g. on a general ward);
- continuously using a transducer connected to an oscilloscope (see **Fig. 3.1b** for intra-arterial pressure monitoring).

Whichever method is used, there are several common pitfalls when interpreting CVP measurements, many of which also apply to interpretation of other intravascular pressure measurements. These are:

- catheter obstruction;
- failure to refer the recorded pressure to the level of the right atrium;

- incorrect calibration;
- measuring the CVP while an infusion is in progress through the CVP catheter;
- taking a measurement when the cather tip is in the right ventricle;
- effect of respiratory oscillations.

Catheter obstruction

Catheter obstruction will result in a sustained high reading with a damped trace, which often does not correlate with the patient's overall clinical state. Check that a venous waveform and respiratory oscillations are present and that venous blood can be easily aspirated. A chest radiograph may be taken to confirm satisfactory positioning of the catheter.

Pressure recording not referred to level of the right atrium

The recorded pressure is a combination of the pressure within the right atrium and a hydrostatic pressure caused by any difference in vertical height between the right atrium and the point of measurement. To allow meaningful comparisons between patients and between repeated readings obtained in the same patient, it is essential that the pressure recorded is always related to the level of the right atrium. Failure to adjust the level of the manometer or transducer after changing the patient's position is therefore a common cause of erroneous readings. Various landmarks are advocated to indicate the level of the right atrium, but it is largely immaterial which is chosen as long as it is used consistently and the readings are obtained with the patient in

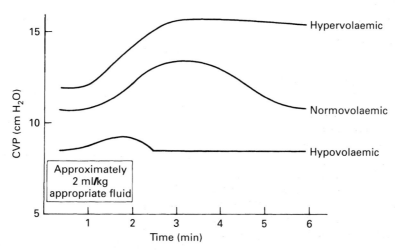

Fig. 3.3 The effects of rapid administration of a 'fluid challenge' to patients with a central venous pressure (CVP) within the normal range. From Sykes (1963), with permission.

the appropriate position, i.e. sternal notch when the patient is supine or sternal angle when the patient is at 45°; the axillary fold or the midpoint between the antero-posterior diameter of the thorax above the level of the fourth intercostal space can be used in either position.

Incorrect calibration

If an electronic transducer and oscilloscope is used, it is important that the system is carefully zeroed and calibrated against a mercury column before use and that the calibration and zero are checked if clinically doubtful values are obtained.

Infusion(s) in progress

If access to central veins proves difficult, the CVP catheter may be used for other infusions and the pressure measured intermittently. If these infusions continue to be administered by an infusion pump via a Y-piece or three-way tap while the pressure is read, a falsely high reading will result. Moreover, if the infusions contain inotropic or vasodilator agents, these may be 'flushed' into the patient when the CVP is measured. This can cause sudden episodes of cardiovascular instability.

Catheter tip in right ventricle

If the catheter is advanced too far it may enter the right ventricle. This should be suspected when an unexpectedly high pressure is recorded, particularly if oscillations are pronounced, and is easily recognized when the waveform is displayed.

Influence of respiratory oscillations

Respiratory oscillations may be particularly pronounced when patients are in respiratory distress and during mechanical ventilation. Pressures should be taken at end-expiration (i.e. when intrathoracic pressure is close to ambient pressure) in both spontaneously breathing and mechanically ventilated patients.

CENTRAL VENOUS CANNULATION

Indications

The indications for central venous cannulation are:

● to monitor right ventricular filling pressure;

● to administer drugs (e.g. inotropes, concentrated potassium);
● to administer parenteral nutrition;
● for cardiac pacing;
● to allow rapid fluid administration;
● difficult peripheral venous access.

Approaches

The aim is to position a catheter with its tip in the superior vena cava or the right atrium (high up to avoid damage to the tricuspid valve). Failing this, any large intrathoracic vein is generally satisfactory. This is usually achieved by percutaneous puncture of a central vein such as the *internal jugular* or *subclavian*. An advantage of the internal jugular approach is that pressure can be applied in the event of haemorrhage or inadvertent carotid artery puncture. The infraclavicular approach to the subclavian vein is also popular. It is ideal for long-term cannulation and is preferred for the administration of parenteral nutrition, but probably carries a higher risk of complications (particularly pneumothorax). A long line may be inserted via an *antecubital vein*, but frequently it proves impossible to advance the catheter into a satisfactory position. This approach is useful in those with a coagulopathy and when a head down tilt is contraindicated. Less commonly, the *femoral* or *external jugular* veins may be used. A few clinicians still prefer to 'cut down' on an arm vein while, if the chest is open, a cannula may be inserted *directly into the innominate vein*.

Cannulae

The relatively short and rigid *catheter-over-needle* devices, which are merely long intravenous cannulae, are easy to use and are particularly useful in an emergency. They have the disadvantage that the needle protrudes beyond the end of the catheter, making it possible to aspirate blood even when the catheter itself is outside the vein. Furthermore, the catheter needs to be fairly sharp and rigid, since it has to be pushed through the skin and subcutaneous tissues. Consequently, it can damage the vein when advanced and may gradually erode through the vessel wall once in position. These devices are therefore only safe when inserted via the right internal jugular vein so that the catheter lies in a straight line with its tip in the superior vena cava or high right atrium.

Long *catheter-through-cannula* devices are particularly useful when using the basilic vein in the antecubital fossa. With these, venepuncture is first performed using a standard intravenous cannula. The needle is then withdrawn and a soft, flexible catheter is advanced through the cannula into the vein. The cannula is then removed. The main disadvantage of this technique is that the hole in the vein is larger than the catheter so there is a risk of bleeding around the puncture site.

Techniques using a *guide wire* (**Fig. 3.4a**) are generally safer and less traumatic. They are particularly useful in difficult cases and can be used in conjunction with a vein dilator for inserting introducers for *pulmonary artery catheters* (see below) and *triple-lumen catheters*. The latter are now used extensively in intensive care units, almost to the exclusion of other devices, because they allow CVP monitoring and the safe administration of multiple infusions through the various separate lumens of a single central venous catheter.

The procedure

The general principles of a safe technique are common to all the approaches to central venous cannulation and should be learnt from instruction and demonstration in patients by an expert. The low anterior approach to the internal jugular vein will be described (**Fig. 3.4b**), since this is probably the safest and most consistently successful route to use in an emergency. Recently a technique in which the head is maintained in the neutral position has been proposed for internal jugular venous cannulation in trauma patients with suspected cervical instability (Willeford & Reitan, 1994).

- If the patient is conscious the procedure must be fully explained and should be carried out with the best sterile precautions allowed by the urgency of the situation. Generally the operator should 'scrub up' and wear a sterile gown and gloves, but in extremely urgent cases (e.g. cardiac arrest), a 'no touch' technique can be acceptable, although gloves should always be worn for protection.
- Place the patient in the head-down position so that the central veins are distended; this makes can-

(a)

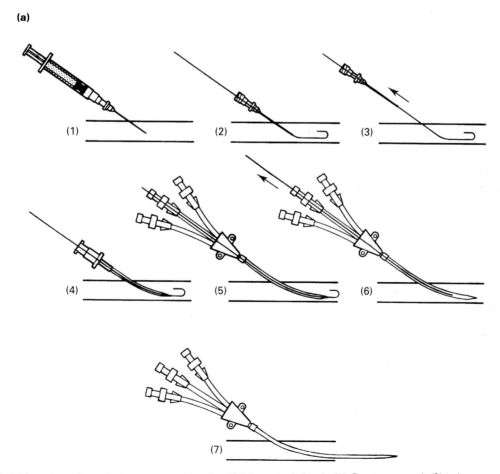

Fig. 3.4 (a) Insertion of a catheter over a guide wire (Seldinger technique). (1) Puncture vessel, (2) advance guard wire, (3) remove needle, (4) dilate vessel, (5) advance catheter over guide wire, (6) remove guide wire, (7) catheter *in situ.*

(b)

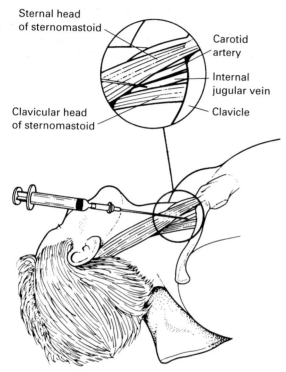

Sternal head of sternomastoid

Carotid artery

Internal jugular vein

Clavicular head of sternomastoid

Clavicle

Fig. 3.4 (b) Cannulation of the right internal jugular vein (see text).

nulation easier and minimizes the risk of air embolism. This position will, however, exacerbate any respiratory difficulty, particularly if due to cardiac failure. The head-down position is also dangerous in patients with raised intracranial pressure.

- Clean the skin over the proposed puncture site with an antiseptic solution, such as iodine tincture, and place sterile towels in position.
- Turn the patient's head away from the proposed site of entry. Usually, the right side is chosen because this is technically easier for a right-handed operator and on the left there is a danger of damaging the thoracic duct.
- Palpate the apex of the triangle formed by the two heads of sternomastoid, with the clavicle as its base and raise a wheal of 2% plain lignocaine over this point.
- Determine the position of the carotid artery to avoid the risk of accidental arterial puncture.
- Make a small incision in the anaesthetized skin and insert the cannula or introducing needle through this, directed laterally downwards and backwards so that the vein is punctured just beneath the skin, deep to the lateral head of sternomastoid. If the vein is not encountered, the needle must not be advanced more than a few cm because of the risk of a pneumothorax.

Failure suggests that either the vein is not sufficiently distended or the cannula is incorrectly positioned. The anatomical landmarks should be checked and the patient can be placed more steeply head-down before the attempt is repeated.

- Once the catheter has been inserted and is thought to be correctly positioned, venous blood should be easily aspirated; then, the CVP manometer line can be connected. There is always a risk of air embolism whenever the catheter is open to air, so necessary periods of disconnection should be as short as possible and Luer locks must be used on all connections. The CVP can then be measured.
- It is important to check that the fluid level in the manometer falls rapidly and fluctuates with respiration because this indicates that the tip of the catheter is in an intrathoracic vein. Similarly, when transduced, there should be a clear venous wave-form with respiratory oscillations.
- Obtain a chest radiograph as soon as possible to verify that the tip of the catheter is centrally placed and not too low in the atrium, and to exclude the presence of a pneumothorax (**Fig. 3.5**). This is particularly important before infusing large volumes of fluid, especially hypertonic solutions such as those that might be used for intravenous feeding (**Fig. 3.6**).

Complications

The complications of central venous cannulation include:

- pneumothorax (see **Fig. 3.5**);
- vascular perforation;
- thrombosis (particularly with the femoral approach);
- catheter-related sepsis;
- air embolism.

Less common complications include:

- pericardial tamponade;
- hydrothorax (see **Fig. 3.6**);
- haemothorax;
- injury to the brachial plexus;
- damage to the thoracic duct.

Cardiac arrhythmias and endocardial damage may occur, but are more commonly associated with pulmonary artery catheterization (see below) (Editorial, 1986). It has been shown that the overall incidence of failed cannulation and complications is related not to the approach used (internal jugular or subclavian), but to operator experience (Sznajder *et al.*, 1986). The failure rate was 10.1% for experienced and 19.4% for inexperienced operators, while the incidence of complications was 5.4% and 11% respectively. The incidence of failed attempts is higher in the obese and those who have undergone major surgery in the region of cannulation

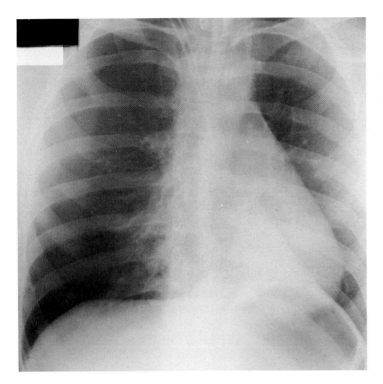

Fig. 3.5 Pneumothorax following insertion of two central venous cannulae via the internal jugular vein. Note also the collapsed left lower lobe (sail-shaped shadow behind the heart obscuring the outline of the elevated left hemidiaphragm; the mediastinum is deviated to the left).

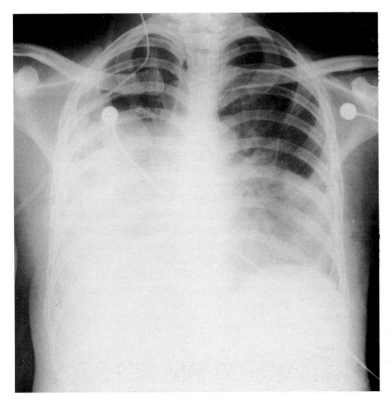

Fig. 3.6 Fluid has been infused into the right pleural space via an incorrectly positioned catheter. There is also bilateral consolidation in the mid and lower zones.

or in whom the vein has been previously cannulated. Moreover, complications are strongly associated with failed attempts (Mansfield *et al.*, 1994). *Ultrasound-guided puncture* has been recommended for difficult cases and to reduce the incidence of complications, particularly for cannulation of the subclavian vein. In a recent study, however, the use of ultrasound did not appear to influence the incidence of complications (Mansfield *et al.*, 1994).

Left atrial pressure

In uncomplicated cases careful interpretation of the CVP provides a reasonable guide to the 'filling pressures' of both sides of the heart. In many critically ill patients, however, this is not the case and there is a *'disparity in ventricular function'*. Most commonly, left ventricular performance is more impaired so that the left ventricular function curve is displaced downward and to the right (**Fig. 3.7**). This situation is encountered in many patients with clinically significant ischaemic heart disease and has also been reported in multisystem trauma, sepsis, peritonitis, hepatic failure, valvular heart disease and after cardiac surgery. High right ventricular filling pressure with normal or low left atrial pressure (LAP), is less common, but may occur in situations in which pulmonary vascular resistance (i.e. right ventricular after-load) is raised, such as acute respiratory failure, as well as in those with right ventricular ischaemia. These discrepancies between right and left ventricular performance can be exacerbated by the use

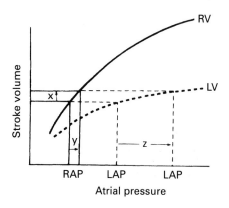

Fig. 3.7 Left (LV) and right (RV) ventricular function curves in a patient with left ventricular dysfunction. Since the stroke volume of the two ventricles must be the same (except perhaps for a few beats during a period of circulatory adjustment), left atrial pressure (LAP) must be higher than right atrial pressure (RAP). Moreover, an increase in stroke volume (x) produced by intravascular volume expansion will be associated with a small rise in RAP (y), but a marked increase in LAP (z).

of inotropic and vasoactive drugs. If there is a disparity in ventricular function after cardiac surgery the left atrium can be cannulated directly, but if the thorax is not open, some other means of determining left ventricular filling pressure must be devised.

Pulmonary artery pressure (Expert Panel (ESICM) 1991)

In 1970, Swan *et al.* described a modified cardiac catheter that incorporated an inflatable balloon at its tip (Swan *et al.*, 1970). This *'balloon flotation catheter'* allowed prompt and reliable catheterization of the pulmonary artery without the need for screening, and minimized the incidence of arrhythmias. Later, a catheter with a slightly increased diameter, a larger balloon, a proximal lumen for CVP measurement and a thermistor located near the tip was introduced, the thermistor allowing determination of cardiac output by the thermodilution technique (see below) (Forrester *et al.*, 1972). Balloon flotation catheters have also been modified for other purposes, including cardiac pacing, pulmonary angiography, continuous monitoring of venous oxygen saturation (see Chapter 5) and determination of right ventricular ejection fraction. Recently techniques have been developed for the continuous measurement of cardiac output (see later).

Approaches

Swan–Ganz catheters can be inserted centrally, through the femoral vein or via a vein in the antecubital fossa. The latter route is perhaps the most comfortable, but it may be difficult to advance the catheter beyond the shoulder region. Furthermore secure fixation is not easily achieved and involves some degree of immobilization of the arm. On the other hand, the complication rate, particularly the risk of pneumothorax, is less. The left infraclavicular approach to the subclavian vein conforms most closely to the natural curvature of the catheter, and secure fixation is most easily achieved at this site. Catheterization of the right internal jugular vein, however, provides the shortest and most direct route to the right side of the heart.

The procedure

Gaining vascular access. Because pulmonary artery catheters have to be introduced through a wide-bore cannula, a guide wire technique is used (see **Fig. 3.4a**).

● First an incision is made in the anaesthetized skin and

the vein punctured with a standard intravenous cannula.

- A guide wire with a very flexible, blunt-ended or preferably J-shaped tip is then introduced and the cannula removed.
- A tapered vein dilator carrying a wide-bore cannula is inserted over the guide wire, which is then withdrawn. (If the original skin incision is not sufficiently large and deep, pushing the dilator and cannula through the skin and subcutaneous tissues may prove difficult.)
- The dilator is then removed and the Swan–Ganz catheter passed through the introducer into the vein. The latter incorporates a valve mechanism, which prevents air embolism and spillage of blood after the dilator is removed and during insertion of the catheter. This introducer cannula should be left *in situ* and provides an extra central venous access point. A plastic sleeve is provided with some introducer kits, which protects a length of catheter, thereby maintaining its sterility. This can subsequently be manipulated without risking contamination if the catheter becomes misplaced.

Precautions

Before the Swan–Ganz catheter is inserted:

- The balloon should be inflated with the recommended volume of air to check for leaks and to ensure that inflation is symmetrical.
- It should be confirmed that the thermistor is functioning.
- The various lumens should be flushed with heparinized saline.

The technique must be learnt under supervision because complications are inversely related to operator experience.

Introducing the catheter

- Passage of the catheter from the major veins, through the chambers of the heart into the pulmonary artery and the 'wedge' position is monitored and guided by the pressure wave-forms recorded from the distal lumen (**Fig. 3.8**).
- The catheter should not be advanced too rapidly since redundant loops may form in the right atrium or ventricle, with a risk of knotting.

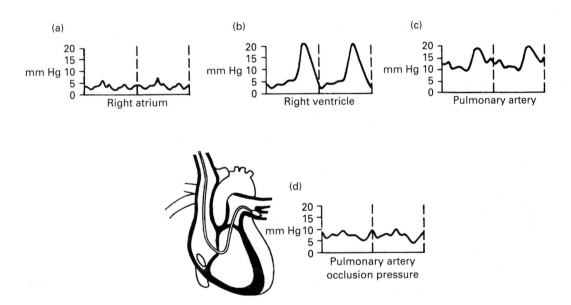

Fig. 3.8 Pressure wave-forms as a Swan–Ganz catheter is passed through the chambers of the heart into the 'wedge' position. (a) Once in the thorax, marked respiratory oscillations are seen. The catheter should be advanced further towards the lower superior vena cava/right atrium when oscillations become more pronounced (15–20 cm of catheter inserted). The balloon should then be inflated and the catheter advanced. (b) In the right ventricle (25–35 cm) there is no dicrotic notch and the diastolic pressure is close to zero. *The patient should be returned to the horizontal, or slight head-up, position before advancing the catheter further.* (c) In the pulmonary artery (35–50 cm) a dicrotic notch appears and there is elevation of the diastolic pressure. The catheter should be advanced further with the balloon inflated. (d) Reappearance of a venous wave-form indicates that the catheter is 'wedged'. Stop advancing. The balloon should be deflated to obtain pulmonary artery pressure, and then inflated intermittently to obtain pulmonary artery 'wedge' or occlusion pressure.

- Radiographic control must be used if any difficulty is encountered and is most often required in those with a low cardiac output.
- A chest radiograph should always be obtained to check the position of the catheter; the tip should be within 2 cm of the cardiac silhouette (**Fig. 3.9**). Some recommend a lateral chest radiograph in a supine patient to ensure that the tip of the catheter is posterior.

Pressure measurements

Once in position, the balloon is deflated and pulmonary artery systolic pressure, end-diastolic pressure (PAEDP) and mean pulmonary artery pressure (PAP) can be obtained. The balloon is then inflated intermittently with the recommended volume of air (0.8–1.5 ml), thereby propelling the catheter distally where it will impact in a medium-sized pulmonary artery and record pulmonary artery occlusion pressure (PAOP) (see **Fig. 3.9**). If a PAOP is obtained when the balloon is inflated with less than 0.8 ml of air the catheter should be withdrawn a few cm to reduce the risk of pulmonary artery rupture or infarction (see later).

All intravascular pressures should be measured relative to atmospheric pressure and should therefore be obtained at end-expiration. The digital pressure display does not provide an accurate end-expiratory value, and so pressures should be determined from a paper chart recording or using algorithms within the monitor designed specifically for this purpose. In patients receiving a positive end-expiratory pressure (PEEP) (see Chapter 7), the recorded pressure will be incremented by an amount proportional to the level of PEEP. This effect is, however, difficult to quantify in the individual patient and depends on a number of factors, including lung compliance. PEEP should not be discontinued while obtaining pressure measurements because this unpredictably alters the haemodynamic conditions, there may be a sudden increase in venous return and it is usually associated with a significant fall in P_aO_2. It is important to remember that in obstructive airways disease there may be an 'intrinsic PEEP' (see Chapter 6).

Interpretation

When the pulmonary artery catheter is in the wedge position, there is a continuous column of fluid between its distal lumen and the left atrium (**Fig. 3.10**). PAOP is therefore usually closely related to LAP. The measurement of PAOP is, however, prone to errors and misinterpretation. It is clearly essential to *establish that a genuine PAOP reading has been obtained*. When the catheter 'wedges':

- a damped venous wave-form should appear;

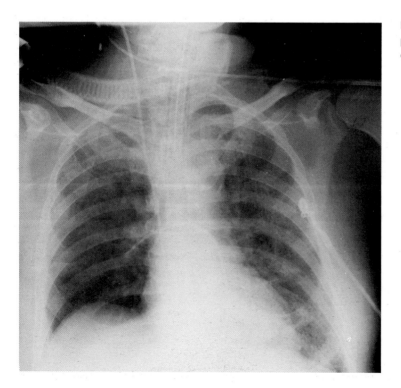

Fig. 3.9 Swan–Ganz catheter correctly positioned in a patient with adult respiratory distress syndrome (ARDS).

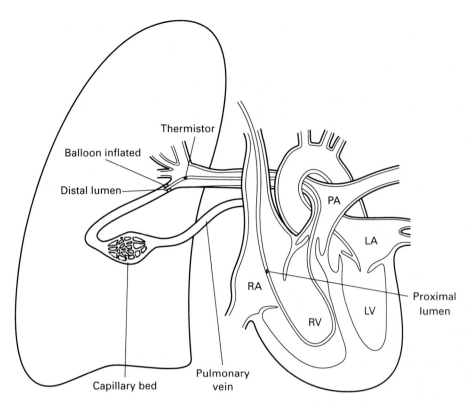

Fig. 3.10 Balloon flotation pulmonary artery catheter in the 'wedged' position. There is now a continuous column of blood between the tip of the catheter and the left atrium; pulmonary artery occlusion pressure (PAOP) is therefore usually closely related to left atrial pressure.

- respiratory oscillations should be apparent;
- the PAOP should be a few mm Hg less than PAEDP;
- some check that it is possible to withdraw 'arterialized' blood, although as much as 20–40 ml of blood may have to be aspirated to obtain a fully oxygenated sample.

Occasionally, when the balloon is inflated, a PAOP trace is obtained only intermittently. This *'transitional wave-form'* can occur when the fluctuations in PAP cause the catheter to 'wedge and unwedge' in a branch of the pulmonary artery. The recorded PAOP may be higher than PAEDP if:

- the balloon is overinflated;
- the balloon inflates eccentrically;
- the wave-form is abnormal (e.g. large V waves in mitral regurgitation or cannon waves in complete heart block).

Once a genuine PAOP has been obtained, a number of *potential causes of misinterpretation* remain. The assumption is that:

$$PAOP = LAP = LVEDP = LVEDV.$$

As discussed above, the relationship between LVEDP and LVEDV depends on the compliance of the vent-

ricles, which is altered in many critically ill patients, and some have found PAOP to be a poor predictor of left ventricular pre-load (Calvin *et al.*, 1981). Furthermore, LAP may not accurately reflect LVEDP in the presence of mitral valve disease, left atrial myxoma or severe left ventricular dysfunction. Finally, PAOP will only be equivalent to LAP when there is a continuous column of blood between the catheter tip and the left atrium (i.e. West's zone 3 conditions prevail, see Chapter 2). This will not be the case when the intervening pulmonary vessels are collapsed by intra-alveolar pressures that are higher than pulmonary venous pressure. This can occur in ventilated patients requiring high inflation pressures or PEEP, and in those with airway obstruction, particularly if they are hypovolaemic and/or the catheter is in the upper zones of the lungs (West's zones 1 and 2, see Chapter 2) (Lozman *et al.*, 1974; Kane *et al.*, 1978). Non-zone 3 conditions are suggested:

- by the absence of normal cardiac oscillations in the PAOP trace;
- when PAOP exceeds PAEDP;
- if, during the application of increasing levels of PEEP, PAOP is incremented by a similar amount.

In the supine patient a lateral chest radiograph taken

with the catheter wedged can determine whether the tip is correctly positioned at or below left atrial level. Fortunately, because the catheter enters the right ventricle anteriorly through the tricuspid valve and leaves it to enter the pulmonary artery in a posterior direction, the curve on the catheter usually causes it to enter a posterior branch of the pulmonary artery, which supplies the right lower lobe. Also blood flow is greatest in zone 3, increasing the likelihood of the catheter 'floating' into this region of the lung.

The PAOP may overestimate LVEDP if there is a tachycardia because premature closure of the mitral valve will increase the atrioventricular pressure gradient and there is limited time for equilibration between PAOP and LAP.

If it proves impossible to obtain a satisfactory PAOP (e.g. if the balloon ruptures), it has been suggested that PAEDP can provide a reasonable guide to LAP. There is, however, normally a gradient of 1-3 mm Hg between PAEDP and PAOP, and this is increased in the presence of pulmonary hypertension, in those with tachycardias and during rapid transfusion (Lappas et al., 1973). In general, PAEDP is an unreliable index of left ventricular filling pressures in the critically ill. It must be emphasized, however, that, as with CVP measurement, the response of PAEDP and PAOP to a fluid challenge is often of more significance than the absolute value.

Complications

There are a large number of complications associated with the use of Swan-Ganz catheters (Pace, 1977), some of which may be very serious and even fatal (**Table 3.2**).

Table 3.2 Complications of pulmonary artery catheters.
Haemorrhage
Pneumothorax
Arrhythmias (during passage of catheter through the right ventricle, usually benign, can often be prevented with lignocaine)
Sepsis (at insertion site, bacteraemia)
Endocarditis (seldom recognized clinically)
Knotting (catheter coils in right ventricle)
Valve trauma (catheter withdrawn with balloon inflated, valves repeatedly closing on catheter)
Thrombosis/embolism
Pulmonary infarction (catheter remains in 'wedge' position)
Pulmonary artery rupture (frequently fatal)
Balloon rupture/leak/embolism

Arrhythmias are more common when the larger thermodilution catheters are used and there is a higher incidence in patients with electrolyte disorders, acidosis or myocardial ischaemia. It is important to inflate the balloon to the recommended volume to conceal the tip of the catheter and prevent it irritating the endocardium during its passage through the right ventricle. Although fatal ventricular tachycardia has been reported (Sise et al., 1981), these arrhythmias are usually transient and consist of a few benign ventricular premature contractions, which stop as soon as the catheter enters the pulmonary artery. If troublesome, they can usually be suppressed with intravenous lignocaine, although in some very unstable patients it may be safer to abandon the procedure. Transient right bundle branch block occurs in up to 5% of patients, but usually resolves within 24 hrs. In the presence of pre-existing left bundle branch block this may precipitate complete atrioventricular block or asystole.

Knotting. To avoid *knotting*, which is more common in those with enlarged cardiac cavities and in low-flow states, the catheter should not be advanced by more than 30 cm without observing a change in wave-form (see **Fig. 3.8**).

Heart valve damage. Heart valves can be severely damaged if the operator withdraws the catheter without deflating the balloon while, in the longer term, valve cusps can be progressively traumatized by repeated closure against the catheter.

Pulmonary infarction. This may be related to thrombus formation in and around the catheter, but will also occur if the catheter 'wedges' for any length of time. The latter can be avoided by continuously displaying the pulmonary artery pressure so that the spontaneous appearance of a 'wedge' pressure (caused by softening and migration of the catheter) can be detected and remedied immediately. It is important to minimize the length of time for which the catheter is wedged.

Pulmonary artery rupture. Although rare, pulmonary artery rupture may be fatal due to intractable haemorrhage. This complication appears to be commoner in the elderly, particularly in those with pulmonary hypertension, and is due either to continuous impaction of the catheter with erosion of the vessel wall, or rapid inflation of a distally placed balloon. It may also occur if the catheter is advanced with the balloon deflated or if a wedged catheter is flushed by hand.

Overview of the complications. Despite the rather formidable list of potential hazards, in practice haemodynamic monitoring using the Swan-Ganz catheter has an acceptably low morbidity and mortality (Sise et al.,

1981). The majority of complications are closely related to user inexperience and their incidence is falling as world-wide expertise grows. Pulmonary artery catheters should preferably be removed within 72 hours because the incidence of infective complications increases (Sise et al., 1981).

CARDIAC OUTPUT AND MYOCARDIAL FUNCTION

As discussed in Chapter 2, cardiac output is a major determinant of oxygen delivery and is therefore one of the most clinically relevant haemodynamic variables.

Non-invasive techniques for assessing cardiac function (Parker et al., 1985)

Over the years, there have been many attempts to develop clinically viable, non-invasive techniques for determining cardiac output and myocardial function when pulmonary artery catheterization is either unavailable or considered unwarranted. These have included impedance cardiography, Doppler ultrasound, echocardiography and various radioisotope techniques. The value of these non-invasive methods in the more seriously ill patients is, however, limited because they do not allow sampling of mixed venous blood or the measurement of pulmonary artery pressures (PAPs).

IMPEDANCE CARDIOGRAPHY

Electrical conductors are placed around the patient's neck and thorax. Some of the electrodes are supplied with a current, while others detect voltage changes produced by the alterations in thoracic bioimpedance caused by ventricular ejection. Stroke volume can then be calculated from the magnitude of the voltage fluctuations. This method tends to overestimate low cardiac outputs and underestimate high cardiac outputs. Fur-

thermore, other factors such as sweating, lung volume and oedema fluid influence thoracic bioimpedance, and limit the accuracy of the technique, particularly in the critically ill. In patients with sepsis, for example, the bioimpedence method overestimated low cardiac outputs, markedly underestimated high cardiac outputs and was too insensitive for clinical monitoring of changes in cardiac output in individual patients (Young & McQuillan, 1993).

AORTIC DOPPLER ULTRASOUND (Singer & Bennett, 1991; Singer et al., 1991)

When transmitted sound waves are reflected from a moving object their frequency is shifted by an amount proportional to the relative velocity between object and observer. This effect, originally described by Doppler, can be described by the equation:

$$V = \frac{C\,fd}{2\,f_T\,\cos}$$

(where V is flow velocity, C is speed of sound, fd is the frequency shift, f_T is the frequency of transmitted sound, and cos is the cosine of the angle between the sound beam axis and the velocity).

Therefore, provided the frequency of the transmitted sound and the angle of interrogation remain constant, the flow velocity will be proportional to the shift in frequency. The Doppler effect is greater the smaller the angle between the beam and the velocity vector; when the beam is perpendicular to the direction of flow no shift can be detected whereas maximal shift is seen with a parallel beam. Best results are obtained when the angle of interrogation is less than 20°.

The *Doppler ultrasound technique* uses an acoustic wave with a frequency exceeding the upper range of human audibility, which may be transmitted continuously or in pulses *(pulse wave Doppler)*. Back-scattered Doppler signals can be processed to produce velocity–time wave-forms, which are visually displayed (**Fig. 3.11**).

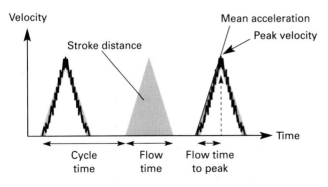

Fig. 3.11 Stylized velocity wave-form traces obtained using oesophageal Doppler (reproduced from Singer et al., 1991, Critical Care Medicine 19: 1184, with permission © 1991 The Williams & Wilkins Co. Baltimore).

So that changes in the velocity wave-form can be used as an estimate of proportional changes in stroke volume, the velocity profile must be flat, flow should be laminar and it has to be assumed that the aortic cross-sectional area remains constant throughout systole. Although the aortic diameter increases slightly in early systole, these conditions are largely fulfilled over a wide range of flow, pressure and temperature. The angle of interrogation must also be known and remain constant.

Aortic blood flow can be determined at a number of sites including suprasternal and oesophageal sites.

Suprasternal site

This site has the advantage of being entirely non-invasive, but it is often difficult to achieve an interrogation angle of less than 20° and good signals cannot be obtained in about 5% of patients (e.g. after cardiac surgery and in those with emphysema). It is also difficult to achieve secure fixation of the probe for continuous beat to beat monitoring and there may be interference from breathing or patient movement. Finally, turbulence makes quantification of the signal impossible in patients with aortic valve disease.

Oesophageal site

A Doppler probe is passed into the oesophagus until it lies approximately 35–40 cm from the mouth. In this position velocity wave-forms from descending aortic blood flow can be continuously monitored. The sensor is securely positioned and high-quality signals with minimal artefact are easily obtained. Measurements are unaffected by mediastinal air and the technique can be used during and after cardiac surgery. Oesophageal Dopplers can be left in place for up to three days but, because of discomfort, are only suitable for use in patients who are sedated and mechanically ventilated. Because of the risk of oesophageal perforation or haemorrhage they should not be used in patients with known pharyngo-oesophagogastric pathology or a bleeding diathesis.

When using the oesophageal approach it has to be assumed that blood flow in the descending aorta remains a fixed proportion of total left ventricular output over a wide range of flows and pressures. Approximately 75% of the total cardiac output passes through the descending aorta and this proportion is little changed in high output states; in those with low cardiac outputs, however, it falls by about 10%.

The interobserver variability with oesophageal Doppler is less than 2% and there is a reasonable correlation between Doppler and thermodilution determinations of cardiac output, although absolute values are generally underestimated.

Derived and measured variables

A number of derived or measured variables can be obtained from the velocity wave-form (see **Fig. 3.11**).

Stroke distance. The distance a column of blood travels along the aorta with each ventricular contraction can be calculated by integrating the velocity–time wave-form. Assuming that the cross-sectional area of the aorta changes little during systole the product of stroke distance and cross-sectional area gives the volume of blood passing along the aorta with each ventricular ejection. In the case of the ascending aorta this is the left ventricular stroke volume.

Minute distance. Multiplying stroke distance in the ascending aorta by heart rate provides an estimate of cardiac output.

The rate of change of velocity during systole (acceleration) and *peak velocity*. These provide some indication of left ventricular function.

Aortic Doppler ultrasound is a safe, non-invasive and reliable means of continuous haemodynamic monitoring. Although reasonable estimates of stroke volume and cardiac output can be obtained, the technique is best used for trend analysis rather than for making absolute volumetric measurements.

ECHOCARDIOGRAPHY

Echocardiography is a non-invasive technique in which the ultrasound beam is transmitted via a transducer placed on the chest wall. It allows intermittent real-time imaging of the heart at the patient's bedside and provides immediate diagnostic information about cardiac structure and function.

In *two-dimensional (2D) echocardiography* the beam is moving continuously to produce a cross-sectional slice through the heart and great vessels; this image is displayed 'real-time'. Usually an *M-mode examination* is also performed in which the heart is examined by a single beam of ultrasound to obtain measurements of ventricular wall thickness, size of the ventricular cavities and valve leaflet excursions. M mode echocardiography is better than 2D for detecting rapid intravascular movements and for quantitation of temporal relationships. Additional information can be derived using *Doppler echocardiography*, which allows determination of the direction and velocity of blood flow. This can be combined with *colour flow mapping* in which normal and abnormal flows are colour-coded and shown as real-time 2D images.

The quality of information obtained with echocardiography depends on the skill and experience of the operator. To locate a suitable *'acoustic window'* through which to image the heart the examination is best performed in the left recumbent position; this may be difficult in some critically ill patients. In others access to the precordium may be obscured (e.g. by dressings or chest wounds). The beam may also be interrupted by overexpanded lungs, and this can lead to particular difficulties in those receiving mechanical ventilation, especially when levels of PEEP in excess of 10 cm H_2O are used.

Indications for echocardiography in the critically ill

Indications for echocardiography in the critically ill include the following.

- Assessment of ventricular function. Echocardiography can be used to determine left ventricular end-diastolic and end-systolic diameters from which a reasonable estimation of ejection fraction can be derived. Visualization of the right ventricle may reveal anterior wall hypokinesia or akinesia, cavity enlargement or paradoxical septal motion.
- Assessment of myocardial ischaemia and infarction. Echocardiography can be used to diagnose and assess the extent of myocardial ischaemia or infarction and to detect complications of ischaemia such as left ventricular aneurysm, mitral regurgitation or ventricular septal defect. Right ventricular infarction may also be diagnosed.
- Diagnosis of valvular heart disease and malfunction of prosthetic valves.
- Confirmation of infective endocarditis. Vegetations may be visualized, thereby confirming the diagnosis, although a negative echocardiogram does not exclude endocarditis. Complications of endocarditis such as valvular incompetence may be detected.
- Diagnosis of congenital heart disease.
- Distinction between hypertrophic, congestive and restrictive cardiomyopathies.
- Detection and location of pericardial effusions. Compression of the right atrium or ventricle is indicative of cardiac tamponade. Echocardiography can be used to guide pericardiocentesis.
- Diagnosis of diseases of the aorta (e.g. aortic dissection).

NUCLEAR CARDIAC IMAGING

Radionuclide techniques can also be performed at the bedside using a portable gamma camera to detect intravenously administered radioisotopes.

First pass technique

A high-speed scintillation camera follows the transit of a bolus of radionuclide (e.g. technetium-99m), as it passes through the chambers of the heart.

Equilibrium technique

Human serum albumin or red blood cells are labelled with technetium-99m and allowed to equilibrate in the blood pool for 8–10 min. The detection of the emitted radiation is timed, or 'gated', to end-systole and end-diastole using the ECG and performed repeatedly (*multi-gated technique* or 'Muga' scan). Counts can then be averaged over several cardiac cycles. Ejection fraction is calculated as:

$$\frac{\text{end-diastolic counts} - \text{end-systolic counts}}{\text{end-diastolic counts}},$$

and corrected for background activity.

For accurate results, heart rhythm and function must be relatively stable. By using multiple projections, regional wall motion abnormalities (hypokinesia or akinesia) can be detected.

Perfusion imaging

By using an isotope such as thallium-20, which is concentrated in viable myocardium by active transport via Na^+/K^+/ATPase the ventricular muscle can be directly visualized. Ischaemia or infarction will appear as areas of low uptake.

Although non-invasive, these techniques do expose the patient to radioactivity, therefore limiting the number of occasions on which the investigation can be performed, and cannot be used for continuous monitoring. Moreover, portable gamma cameras are extremely expensive.

NON-IMAGING RADIONUCLIDE DETECTORS

An alternative radionuclide technique involves the use of a non-imaging detector (or *'nuclear stethoscope'*) to provide continuous on-line monitoring of ejection fraction derived from end-diastolic and end-systolic counts. This technique seems to be a practical, relatively low-cost, bedside method for reliably estimating ejection fraction in critically ill, patients. It may prove to be particularly useful for continuously monitoring changes in left ventricular function in response to therapeutic interventions (Timmins *et al.*, 1994).

Invasive techniques

DIRECT FICK METHOD

Fick's principle states that if an indicator is added to a column of flowing liquid at a constant rate, then the flow of that liquid is equal to the amount of substance entering the stream divided by the difference between the concentration of the indicator either side of the entry point. The principle is also valid for the removal of a substance and can therefore be applied to the consumption of oxygen by the body ($\dot{V}O_2$). Thus:

$$Q_t = \frac{\dot{V}O_2}{C_aO_2 - C_vO_2}, \qquad \textbf{3.1}$$

where $\dot{Q}_t$ is cardiac output, C_aO_2 is arterial oxygen content, and C_vO_2 is mixed venous oxygen content.

Conceptually, it may be easier to appreciate that the amount of oxygen consumed by the body can be calculated from the product of the flow of blood to the tissues and the amount of oxygen extracted from each unit of blood. Thus:

$$\dot{V}O_2 = \dot{Q}_T \times (C_aO_2 - C_vO_2) \qquad \textbf{3.2}$$

and this can be rearranged in order to derive $\dot{Q}_T$ as above. This formula is commonly used clinically to calculate $\dot{V}O_2$.

To obtain cardiac output by the direct Fick method arterial and mixed venous oxygen contents and $\dot{V}O_2$ have to be measured directly as described in Chapter 5. In practice, however, a number of difficulties limit the clinical application of this method (see Chapter 5) and it is in fact rarely used in intensive care units.

INDICATOR DILUTION TECHNIQUES

Indicator dilution techniques are based on a modification of the Fick principle in which a substance is added to the central circulation as a bolus, rather than continuously. The appearance and disappearance of this substance is then recorded at a distal site. The cardiac output is calculated from the total amount of indicator injected divided by its average concentration and the time taken to pass the recording site.

Dye dilution

In this technique a bolus of dye (usually indocyanine green) is injected into the pulmonary artery. Its subsequent passage through the systemic circulation is recorded at a downstream site (usually the radial artery) by continuously aspirating blood through a densitometer. This records the changing concentration of dye, thereby describing an 'indicator dilution curve' as shown in **Fig. 3.12**. (It is essential that the dye mixes completely with the blood, but this might not occur if dye is injected into, for example, the right atrium with sampling from the pulmonary artery.)

The amount of dye injected is known, while the transit time and average concentration can be determined by analysing the dilution curve. As illustrated in **Fig. 3.12**, recirculation of dye causes a second peak, which interferes with accurate determination of transit time. This is overcome by plotting the curve logarithmically, so that the exponential disappearance of dye becomes a straight line, which can be extrapolated to the baseline. The average concentration of dye is determined by integrating the area under the curve.

Unfortunately, dye accumulates in the circulation, causing a progressive elevation of the baseline and this limits the number of times the measurement can be performed. The technique is less accurate when cardiac output is low since the curve is flat, the recirculation peak is more evident and the shape of the curve is difficult to define.

Finally, the densitometer has to be calibrated first by mixing a sample of the patient's blood with a known amount of dye.

Thermodilution

Many of the problems associated with dye dilution can be overcome by using cold liquid as the indicator

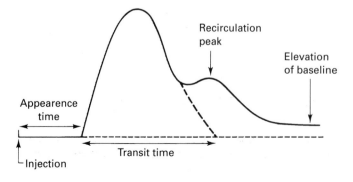

Fig. 3.12 Indicator dilution curve obtained using indocyanine green.

(Forrester *et al.*, 1972) and thermodilution cardiac output determination is now used extensively.

In practice, a modified Swan–Ganz catheter, with a lumen opening in the right atrium and a thermistor located a few cm from its tip, is inserted as described above. A known volume of liquid at a known temperature is injected as a bolus into the atrium. Subsequently, the injectate, which is completely mixed with blood during its passage through the right atrium and ventricle, passes into the pulmonary artery where the fall in temperature is detected by the thermistor (**Fig. 3.13**). The dilution curve is usually analysed by a computer, which provides a direct read-out of cardiac output.

Withdrawal of blood is not required and because the cold is rapidly dissipated in the tissues there is no recirculation peak and no elevation of the baseline. Measure-

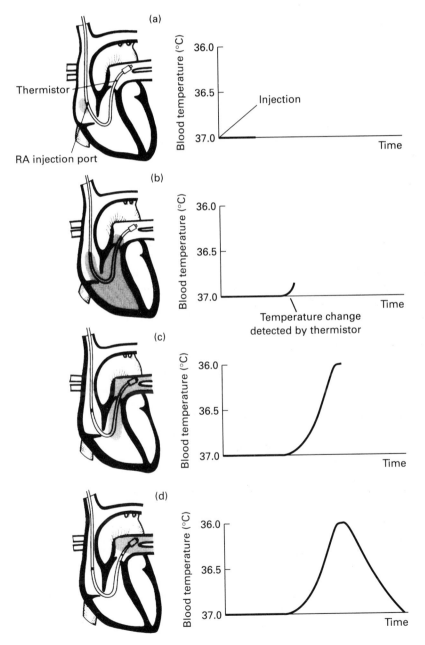

Fig. 3.13 Thermodilution method for cardiac output determination. Cold fluid injected into the right atrium (a), passes through the right ventricle and into the pulmonary artery where the temperature change is detected by the thermistor (b, c and d). Notice the absence of a recirculation peak and that there is no elevation of the baseline.

ments can therefore be repeated as often as required. Furthermore, the method is more accurate than dye dilution in low flow states, and the catheters are pre-calibrated.

Accuracy. The larger the volume of the injectate, and the lower its temperature, the greater is the *signal-to-noise ratio*. This increases accuracy and may be particularly important in ventilated patients in whom pulmonary artery temperature fluctuates during the respiratory cycle. Therefore, although it is possible to use as little as 5 ml of room temperature injectate, it is more usual to inject 10 ml of ice-cold 5% dextrose. The injectate is normally cooled in a container of iced water. Its temperature is measured by a thermistor placed just beyond the syringe. In all cases it is important to avoid warming the injectate by handling the barrel of the syringe. Inevitably, the injectate absorbs heat during its passage through the catheter and the necessary corrections are therefore incorporated into the formulae used to calculate cardiac output. For similar reasons, the first of each series of measurements should be rejected since the injectate will include warm fluid from within the catheter lumen.

Accuracy also depends on a *smooth injection*; it is therefore usual to record the shape of the dilution curve and to reject uneven curves. The mean of three consecutive cardiac output determinations that do not differ by more than 10% should be calculated. The repeatability of the method should be within ± 10% but, with care, greater accuracy can usually be achieved (Forrester *et al.*, 1972). Although repeatability can be improved by timing injections to coincide with the same point in the respiratory cycle, values obtained in this way are probably not a true reflection of overall cardiac output. To obtain a truly accurate value for mean cardiac output it may be necessary to perform a series of four measurements spread equally throughout the ventilatory cycle.

The technique is inaccurate in the presence of *intracardiac shunts* and *incompetence of the pulmonary or tricuspid valves*. Finally, recent observations suggest that inaccuracies may occur if injectate refluxes up the sidearm of the introducer sheath. Errors are greater when the injectate port is close to the tip of the introducer or is within the sheath, and are further increased when the sidearm of the sheath is open. It is therefore recommended that the injectate port should be located well downstream of the introducer sheath (i.e. the catheter should be inserted to a depth of > 45 cm) and that the introducer sidearm should be closed (Boyd *et al.*, 1994).

Complications. Bradycardia and *supraventricular tachycardias* have been reported in association with the injection of cold fluid. It is important to note the volumes of 5% dextrose injected, especially when cardiac output is measured repeatedly.

Continuous cardiac output determination

A 10 cm thermal filament is mounted on the pulmonary artery catheter close to the CVP lumen. Low heat energy is transmitted into the surrounding blood according to a pseudo-random binary sequence. The heat signal in the blood is processed over time and a 'thermodilution' curve is reconstructed from the temperature changes. A computer system produces a continuously updated (every 30–60 s), time-averaged value for cardiac output. Agreement with thermodilution cardiac output measurements appears to be sufficiently close for most clinical applications (Boldt *et al.*, 1994).

Lithium dilution (Linton *et al.*, 1993)

This recently described technique does not require pulmonary artery catheterization. A bolus of lithium chloride is administered via a central venous catheter and the change in arterial plasma lithium concentration is detected by a lithium-sensitive electrode. Cardiac output is derived from the lithium dilution curve. When compared to thermodilution this technique appears to be safe, simple and reasonably accurate.

Derived haemodynamic and oxygen transport variables

Measurement of cardiac output, intravascular pressures and heart rate permits calculation of a number of clinically important haemodynamic and oxygen transport variables (see **Appendices 1 and 2**, Chapter 2).

Determination of *pulmonary and systemic vascular resistances* may contribute to establishing a diagnosis (e.g. a low peripheral resistance is characteristic of septic shock), and provides a useful estimate of changes in right and left ventricular after-load. Calculation of the work performed by each ventricle (*right and left ventricular stroke work*) gives some indication of myocardial performance, especially if a *ventricular function curve* is constructed by relating changes in PAOP to alterations in stroke work. Construction of a ventricular function curve is also the best guide to the adequacy of a patient's circulating volume; fluid replacement can be considered to be optimal when further increases in PAOP do not improve left ventricular stroke work.

Haemodynamic assessment of a critically ill patient is

incomplete without analysis of arterial and mixed venous blood for blood gas tensions, acid–base status, the percentage saturation of haemoglobin with oxygen and oxygen contents (see Chapter 5). It is then possible to calculate oxygen delivery (DO_2) and oxygen consumption ($\dot{V}O_2$), which are important determinants of outcome from critical illness, as well as the arteriovenous oxygen content difference ($C_{a-v}O_2$), which together with the mixed venous oxygen saturation (S_vO_2) provides a guide to the relationship between tissue oxygen supply and utilization.

Indications for haemodynamic monitoring with a pulmonary artery catheter

Although it is often reasonable to assess a patient's response to simple measures before making the decision to catheterize the pulmonary artery it is clearly important not to delay until the situation has become irretrievable. In general, pulmonary artery catheters enable the clinician to optimize cardiac output and DO_2, while minimizing the risk of pulmonary oedema, and also allow the rational use of inotropes and vasoactive drugs. *Specific indications include* the following.

- Myocardial infarction—haemodynamically unstable, unresponsive to initial therapy. To differentiate hypovolaemia and cardiogenic shock.
- Shock—unresponsive to simple measures or when there is diagnostic uncertainty. To guide administration of fluid, inotropes and vasoactive agents and to optimize DO_2 and $\dot{V}O_2$.
- Pulmonary embolism—to establish the diagnosis, and assess its severity and to guide haemodynamic support.
- Pulmonary oedema—to differentiate cardiogenic from non-cardiogenic pulmonary oedema, to enable optimization of DO_2 and $\dot{V}O_2$ in adult respiratory distress syndrome (particularly when haemodynamically unstable and in those with ventricular dysfunction), and to guide haemodynamic support in cardiac failure.
- Haemodynamic instability when the diagnosis is unclear.
- High-risk surgical patients, particularly those with left ventricular dysfunction and/or ischaemic heart disease and those in whom massive volume losses are anticipated (e.g. routine use is recommended in liver transplantation). To optimize DO_2 and $\dot{V}O_2$.
- Major trauma—to guide volume replacement. To optimize DO_2 and $\dot{V}O_2$.
- Pre-eclampsia with hypertension, pulmonary oedema or oliguria.
- Chronic obstructive airways disease—patients with

cardiac failure, to exclude reversible causes of failure to wean from mechanical ventilation.
- Cardiac surgery in selected cases only; routine use is unnecessary.

Benefits of haemodynamic monitoring with a pulmonary artery catheter

There can be no doubt that the use of pulmonary artery catheters has made an enormous contribution to our understanding of the pathophysiology of critical illness, but their clinical value, in particular their influence on outcome, has been disputed (Robin 1985; Matthay & Chatterjee 1988; Sibbald & Sprung 1988). Although it is clear that clinical haemodynamic assessment is frequently inaccurate, that pulmonary artery catheterization improves diagnostic accuracy, and that clinically relevant information is obtained, which often prompts changes in treatment (Bailey *et al.*, 1990; Eisenberg *et al.*, 1984), it has been less easy to demonstrate convincingly that this has resulted in improved outcome. Not only are there formidable difficulties in performing well-designed studies with sufficient numbers of patients to demonstrate changes in mortality, but more accurate diagnosis can only have a major influence on survival when unequivocally effective treatment is available for the underlying disorder. Moreover, increasingly sophisticated haemodynamic manipulation may not necessarily influence the final outcome. Nevertheless, since the procedure is safe in experienced hands and is comparatively cheap, it is our view that used selectively, and provided data are accurately collected and correctly interpreted the benefits of pulmonary artery catheterization far outweigh the risks.

Assessment of tissue perfusion and oxygenation

CLINICAL EVALUATION

In the more straightforward cases it is possible to gain a fairly accurate idea of tissue perfusion, and by implication cardiac output and circulating volume, from an examination of the skin. When perfusion is poor the skin is cold, pale and blue with an increased capillary filling time. In the most seriously ill patients this may be associated with profuse sweating and the skin then feels ice-cold and 'clammy'. Conversely when the peripheries are pink and warm, with rapid capillary refill, circulating volume and tissue perfusion are probably adequate. Clinical examination can, however, be misleading (Bailey *et al.*, 1990), especially in patients with sepsis or septic shock in whom severe cardiovascular derangement and tissue hypoxia may be present despite apparently well-perfused extremities.

CORE–PERIPHERAL TEMPERATURE GRADIENT

A more objective assessment of peripheral perfusion can be obtained by recording peripheral temperature, usually from the extensor surface of the great toe. This technique is cheap, safe and is conventionally thought to be a good guide to tissue perfusion provided it is related to a reference value. Often the core temperature is measured simultaneously (e.g. from a nasopharyngeal probe or the thermistor of a pulmonary artery catheter), in which case an increased core–peripheral temperature gradient is considered to be indicative of poor perfusion. Others recommend that toe temperature should be related to room temperature. A fall in peripheral temperature is often the first sign of a deterioration in cardiovascular function and, because vasoconstriction is an early compensatory response, may occur before changes in other variables such as heart rate, blood pressure or central venous pressure. There is, however, recent evidence suggesting that in shock the core–peripheral temperature gradient is not a good guide to either the cardiac output or the systemic vascular resistance and that changes in this gradient do not correlate with alterations in either of these variables (Woods *et al.*, 1987).

MIXED VENOUS OXYGEN SATURATION $(S_{\bar{v}}O_2)$, ARTERIOVENOUS OXYGEN CONTENT DIFFERENCE $(C_{a-v}O_2)$ AND OXYGEN EXTRACTION RATIO (OER)

The $S_{\bar{v}}O_2$ can be determined intermittently using a bench oximeter or continuously using a modified fibre-optic pulmonary artery catheter (see Chapter 5). Because there is streaming of blood from the upper and lower halves of the body within the right atrium, true mixed venous blood can only be obtained from the pulmonary artery. At the level of P_{O_2} encountered in venous blood the oxyhaemoglobin dissociation curve is essentially linear and the normal range for $S_{\bar{v}}O_2$ is 70–85%.

In general $S_{\bar{v}}O_2$ is a reflection of tissue oxygenation, a fall implying that the supply of oxygen to the tissues is inadequate; values less than 50% are commonly associated with the onset of anaerobic metabolism. Reductions in $S_{\bar{v}}O_2$ frequently precede changes in other monitored variables and it has been suggested that continuous $S_{\bar{v}}O_2$ monitoring can provide a useful early indication of decompensation. Nevertheless, the clinical indications for continuous $S_{\bar{v}}O_2$ monitoring have not yet been clearly defined.

Changes in $S_{\bar{v}}O_2$ require careful interpretation; they must not be considered in isolation and should prompt measurement of other variables to ascertain the cause. The various possibilities can easily be appreciated by rearranging the Fick equation to give:

$$C_{\bar{v}}O_2 = C_aO_2 - \frac{\dot{V}O_2}{\dot{Q}_t}$$

A fall in $S_{\bar{v}}O_2$ may, therefore, be secondary to arterial hypoxaemia, a reduction in haemoglobin concentration, a fall in cardiac output, an increase in oxygen consumption or any combination of these.

Conversely $S_{\bar{v}}O_2$ will rise if oxygen delivery exceeds oxygen consumption.

Monitoring $S_{\bar{v}}O_2$ can also be misleading. In sepsis, for example, tissue hypoxia is largely due to impaired extraction or utilization of oxygen and $S_{\bar{v}}O_2$ is therefore frequently normal or high. In addition, at a critical level of D_{O_2} below which the tissues are unable to extract more oxygen, further reductions in D_{O_2} are associated not with the expected fall in $S_{\bar{v}}O_2$, but with a reduction in $\dot{V}_{O_2}$. It seems that in many critically ill patients this relationship applies at levels of D_{O_2} normally considered adequate—*'pathological supply dependency'* (see Chapter 4). Under these circumstances maintenance of a normal $S_{\bar{v}}O_2$ cannot be accepted as indicating that tissue oxygenation is satisfactory.

It must also be appreciated that $S_{\bar{v}}O_2$ is the weighted average of blood draining all the various vascular beds, and hypoxia in one region may be masked by luxury perfusion in another. Finally, a high $S_{\bar{v}}O_2$ may be the result of a left-to-right intracardiac shunt.

The normal $C_{a-v}O_2$ is approximately 4–5 vol%. A widening $C_{a-v}O_2$ indicates that the tissues are receiving insufficient oxygen to satisfy their requirements, whereas a narrow $C_{a-v}O_2$ is seen in high output states and those with impaired tissue oxygen utilization.

The OER is the proportion of delivered oxygen extracted by the tissues:

$$\frac{(C_aO_2 - C_{\bar{v}}O_2)}{C_aO_2}$$

the normal value being 0.22–0.30.

This index has the advantage of taking both the haemoglobin concentration and arterial oxygenation into consideration; it is therefore influenced only by changes in cardiac output and oxygen consumption. An increased OER indicates inadequate oxygen supply, while a narrow OER suggests a reduced metabolic rate or impaired oxygen utilization/extraction.

INTRA-MUCOSAL pH

The earliest compensatory response to hypovolaemia or a low cardiac output and the last to resolve following resuscitation is splanchnic vasoconstriction, whilst in sepsis, gut mucosal ischaemia may be precipitated by disturbed microcirculatory flow combined with increased oxygen requirements (see Chapter 4). Theoretically, therefore, the development of a mucosal acidosis should be a valuable early sign of 'compensated' shock, which might precede other signs of impaired tissue perfusion by many hours, and changes in mucosal pH might provide an excellent guide to the adequacy of resuscitation. Moreover, a persistently low intramucosal pH is likely to be a marker of the ischaemic mucosal injury which seems to predispose patients to the development of sepsis and multiple organ failure (see Chapter 4), a suggestion supported by studies showing that a low mucosal pH in the intraoperative period is associated with an increased risk of postoperative complications (Mythen & Webb, 1994), and that persistent mucosal acidosis is related to major morbidity after abdominal aortic surgery (Björck & Hedberg, 1994).

Intramucosal pH (pHi) can be estimated by placing a catheter with a saline-filled, silastic balloon at its tip in either the sigmoid colon as originally described or, more usually in clinical practice, in the stomach (*gastric tonometry*). In the latter instance an H_2-receptor antagonist is usually administered to minimize gastric acid secretion. The $P\text{CO}_2$ of the saline within the balloon equilibrates with intraluminal fluid, and then with mucosal $P\text{CO}_2$ over a period of about 30 minutes. The carbon dioxide tension in samples of saline withdrawn from the balloon can be determined intermittently. It is assumed that the bicarbonate concentration in arterial blood approximates that in the tissues and that mucosal pH can be derived using the Henderson–Hassebach equation.

This method more accurately reflects the pH in the superficial rather than the deeper mucosal layers; it also underestimates the severity of the acidosis in low-flow states because of the discrepancy between tissue and arterial bicarbonate which develops under these circumstances. In some situations (e.g. in patients undergoing abdominal aortic surgery), monitoring in the sigmoid colon may be superior to gastric tonometry (Björck & Hedberg, 1994).

The precise role of pHi monitoring in clinical practice has not yet been clearly defined; some authors, for example, have concluded that the information derived from gastric tonometry can be obtained more simply by determining the base deficit in arterial blood (Boyd *et al.*, 1993). On the other hand, in a larger study of patients with acute circulatory failure, gastric pHi was found to be a more reliable guide to the adequacy of tissue oxygenation than arterial pH, base deficit or lactate levels, and only gastric pHi at 24 hours independently predicted outcome (Maynard *et al.*, 1993). Similarly, in patients with sepsis, only gastric pHi contributed to the prediction of both multiple organ failure and death (Marik, 1993). There is also some evidence to support the suggestion that the use of gastric pHi measurements to guide therapy can improve outcome in critically ill patients, provided a significant mucosal acidosis has not developed before admission to intensive care (Gutierrez *et al.*, 1992).

LACTIC ACIDOSIS

Ultimately the consequence of impaired tissue perfusion is cellular hypoxia, anaerobic glycolysis and the production of lactic acid (see Chapters 4 and 5). The development of a metabolic acidosis and elevated blood lactate levels therefore usually indicates imbalance between oxygen supply and demand. This is, however, a relatively late and insensitive marker of reduced perfusion, and the absence of a metabolic acidosis does not exclude regional blood flow abnormalities.

REFERENCES

Bailey JM, Levy JH, Kopel MA, Tobia V & Grabenkort WR (1990) Relationship between clinical evaluation of peripheral perfusion and global hemodynamics in adults after cardiac surgery. *Critical Care Medicine* 18: 1353–1356.

Band JD & Maki DG (1979) Infections caused by arterial catheters used for hemodynamic monitoring. *American Journal of Medicine* 67: 735–741.

Björck M & Hedberg B (1994) Early detection of major complications after abdominal aortic surgery: predictive value of sigmoid colon and gastric intramucosal pH monitoring. *British Journal of Surgery* 81: 25–30.

Boldt J, Menges T, Wollbruck M, Hammermann H & Hempelmann G (1994) Is continuous cardiac output measurement using thermodilution reliable in the critically ill patient? *Critical Care Medicine* 22: 1913–1918.

Boyd O, Mackay CJ, Lamb G, Bland JM, Grounds RM & Bennett ED (1993) Comparison of clinical information gained from routine blood-gas analysis and from gastric tonometry for intramural pH. *Lancet* **341**: 142–146.

Boyd O, Mackay CJ, Newman P, Bennett ED & Grounds RM (1994) Effects of insertion depth and use of the sidearm of the introducer sheath of pulmonary artery catheters in cardiac output measurement. *Critical Care Medicine* **22**: 1132–1135.

Calvin JE, Driedger AA & Sibbald WJ (1981) Does the pulmonary capillary wedge pressure predict left ventricular preload in critically ill patients? *Critical Care Medicine* 9: 437–443.

Editorial (1986) Central vein catheterisation. *Lancet* **ii**: 669–670.

Eisenberg PR, Jaffe AS & Schuster DP (1984) Clinical evaluation compared to pulmonary artery catheterization in the hemodynamic assessment of critically ill patients. *Critical Care Medicine* **12**: 549-553.

Expert Panel (1991) The use of the pulmonary artery catheter (ESICM). *Intensive Care Medicine* **17**: I-VIII.

Forrester JS, Ganz W, Diamond G *et al.* (1972) Thermodilution cardiac output determination with a single flow-directed catheter. *American Heart Journal* **83**: 306-311.

Guttierrez G, Palizas F, Doglio G, *et al.* (1992) Gastric intramucosal pH as a therapeutic index of tissue oxygenation in critically ill patients. *Lancet* **339**: 195-199.

Kane PB, Askanazi J, Neville JF Jr, *et al.* (1978) Artefacts in the measurement of pulmonary artery wedge pressure. *Critical Care Medicine* **6**: 36-38.

Lappas D, Lell WA, Gabel JC, Civetta JM & Lowenstein E (1973) Indirect measurement of left-atrial pressure in surgical patients—pulmonary capillary wedge and pulmonary artery diastolic pressures compared with left-atrial pressure. *Anesthesiology* **38**: 394-397.

Linton RAF, Band DM & Haire KM (1993) A new method of measuring cardiac output in man using lithium dilution. *British Journal of Anaesthesia* **71**: 262-266.

Lozman J, Powers SR Jr, Older T *et al.* (1974) Correlation of pulmonary wedge and left atrial pressures. A study in the patient receiving positive end expiratory pressure ventilation. *Archives of Surgery* **109**: 270-277.

Mansfield PF, Hohn DC, Forrage BD, Gregurich MA & Ota DM (1994) Complications and failures of subclavian-vein catheterization. *New England Journal of Medicine* **331**: 1735-1738.

Marik PE (1993) Gastric intramucosal pH. A better predictor of multiorgan dysfunction syndrome and death than oxygen-derived variables in patients with sepsis. *Chest* **104**: 225-229.

Matthay MA & Chatterjee K (1988) Bedside catheterization of the pulmonary artery: risks compared with benefits. *Annals of Internal Medicine* **109**: 826-834.

Maynard N, Bihari D, Beale R, *et al.* (1993) Assessment of splanchnic oxygenation by gastric tonometry in patients with acute circulatory failure. *Journal of the American Medical Association* **270**: 1203-1210.

Mythen MG & Webb AR (1994) Intra-operative gut mucosal hypoperfusion is associated with increased post-operative complications and cost. *Intensive Care Medicine* **20**: 99-104.

Pace NL (1977) A critique of flow-directed pulmonary arterial catheterization. *Anaesthiology* **47**: 455-465.

Parker MM, Cunnion RE & Parrillo JE (1985) Echocardiography and nuclear cardiac imaging in the critical care unit. *Journal of the American Medical Association* **254**: 2935-2939.

Robin ED (1985) The cult of the Swan–Ganz catheter. Overuse and abuse of pulmonary flow catheters. *Annals of Internal Medicine* **103**: 445-449.

Russell JA, Joel M, Hudson RJ, Mangano DT & Schlobohm RM (1983) Prospective evaluation of radial and femoral artery catheterization sites in critically ill adults. *Critical Care Medicine* **11**: 936-939.

Sibbald WJ & Sprung CL (1988) The pulmonary artery catheter. The debate continues. *Chest* **94**: 899-901.

Singer M & Bennett ED (1991) Noninvasive optimization of left ventricular filling using esophageal Doppler. *Critical Care Medicine* **19**: 1132-1137.

Singer M, Allen MJ, Webb AR & Bennett ED (1991) Effects of alterations in left ventricular filling, contractility, and systemic vascular resistance on the ascending aortic blood velocity wave-form of normal subjects. *Critical Care Medicine* **19**: 1138-1145.

Sise MJ, Hollingsworth P, Brimm JE, *et al.* (1981) Complications of the flow-directed pulmonary artery catheter: a prospective analysis in 219 patients. *Critical Care Medicine* **9**: 315-318.

Swan HJC, Ganz W, Forrester J, *et al.* (1970) Catheterization of the heart in man with use of a flow-directed balloon-tipped catheter. *New England Journal of Medicine* **283**: 447-451.

Sykes MK (1963) Venous pressure as a clinical indication of adequacy of transfusion. *Annals of the Royal College of Surgeons* **33**: 185-197.

Sznajder JI, Zveibil FR, Bitterman H, Weiner P & Bursztein S (1986) Central vein catheterization. Failure and complication rates by three percutaneous approaches. *Archives of Internal Medicine* **146**: 259-261.

Thomas F, Burke JP, Parker J, *et al.* (1983) The risk of infection related to radial *vs* femoral sites for arterial catheterisation. *Critical Care Medicine* **11**: 807-812.

Timmins AC, Giles M, Nathan AW & Hinds CJ (1994) Clinical validation of a radionuclide detector to measure ejection fraction in critically ill patients. *British Journal of Anaesthesia* **72**: 523-528.

Willeford KL & Reitan JA (1994) Neutral head position for placement of internal jugular vein catheters. *Anaesthesia* **49**: 202-204.

Woods I, Wilkins RG, Edwards JD, Martin PD & Faragher EB (1987) Danger of using core/peripheral temperature gradient as a guide to therapy in shock. *Critical Care Medicine* **15**: 850-852.

Young JD & McQuillan P (1993) Comparison of thoracic electrical bioimpedance and thermodilution for the measurement of cardiac index in patients with severe sepsis. *British Journal of Anaesthesia* **70**: 58-62.

4 Shock

DEFINITION

The word 'shock' probably entered the English language in the sixteenth century, derived from the French word 'choc' meaning a sudden or violent blow between two armed forces or warriors. It was not used medically until 1743 in the French text of le Dran's 'A treatise of reflections drawn from experiences with gunshot wounds', and later, in 1831, Latto used the term to describe the effects of cholera on circulatory function.

In current medical practice, shock can be defined as *'acute circulatory failure with inadequate or inappropriately distributed tissue perfusion resulting in generalized cellular hypoxia'*. The various causes of shock can be classified as shown in **Table 4.1**.

CAUSES

Abnormalities of tissue perfusion may result from:

- pump failure;
- mechanical impediments to forward flow;
- loss of circulating volume;
- abnormalities of the peripheral circulation;
- a combination of these factors.

Cardiogenic shock

In cardiogenic shock, cardiac output falls because of an abnormality of the heart itself, most commonly as a result of an *acute myocardial infarction*. Cardiogenic shock may develop if more than 40% of the left ventricular myocardium is damaged, while infarction of more than 70% is usually rapidly fatal. Cardiogenic shock may also occur as a result of:

- acute aortic incompetence;
- acute ischaemic mitral regurgitation;
- left ventricular aneurysm.

It may be also seen after cardiac surgery and as a result of traumatic myocardial contusion. Myocardial depression may also complicate other forms of shock.

Table 4.1 Causes of shock.

Cardiogenic
Obstructive
Hypovolaemic (exogenous losses, endogenous losses)
Distributive (vascular dilatation, sequestration, arteriovenous shunting, maldistribution of flow)

Obstructive shock

In obstructive shock, the fall in cardiac output is caused by a mechanical obstruction to the circulation (e.g. a *pulmonary embolus*), or by restriction of cardiac filling, as occurs in *tamponade*.

Hypovolaemic shock

In hypovolaemic shock, the circulating volume is reduced, venous return to the heart falls and there is a reduction in stroke volume, cardiac output and blood pressure. Hypovolaemia may be due to *exogenous losses*, as occurs with haemorrhage and burns, or *endogenous losses*. In the latter, fluid is lost into the interstitial spaces through leaky capillaries or into body cavities such as the bowel (e.g. as in intestinal obstruction).

Distributive shock

Vascular dilatation, arteriovenous shunting, sequestration of blood in venous capacitance vessels and maldistribution of flow may lead to shock due to relative hypovolaemia, a reduction in peripheral resistance and impaired oxygen utilization, as occurs for example in those with *sepsis* and *anaphylaxis*. True hypovolaemia supervenes in these cases because of the fluid losses resulting from the increase in capillary permeability. In septic shock, there may also be a primary disturbance of cellular metabolism.

PATHOPHYSIOLOGY

Sympathoadrenal response to shock

Hypotension stimulates the baroreceptors and, to a lesser extent, the chemoreceptors, causing increased sympathetic nervous activity with 'spill over' of noradrenaline into the circulation. Later, this is augmented by the release of catecholamines (predominantly adrenaline) from the adrenal medulla. The resulting vasoconstriction, together with positive inotropic and chronotropic effects, helps to restore blood pressure and cardiac output (**Fig. 4.1**).

Opioid peptides containing the enkephalin sequence, which are widely distributed throughout the body, particularly within the sympathetic nervous system, have been identified within the same chromaffin cells as catecholamines and are also released into the circulation in shock (Evans *et al.*, 1984).

The reduction in perfusion of the renal cortex stimulates the juxtaglomerular apparatus to release renin. This converts angiotensinogen to angiotensin I, which is in turn converted to the potent vasoconstrictor, angiotensin II, in the lungs. In addition, angiotensin II stimulates secretion of aldosterone by the adrenal cortex causing sodium and water retention. This helps to restore the circulating volume (**Fig. 4.2**).

Neuroendocrine response to shock

Pituitary hormones are also released during shock so that circulating levels of adrenocorticotrophic hormone (ACTH), growth hormone (GH) and vasopressin (antidiuretic hormone, ADH) are elevated. β-endorphin is derived from the same precursor molecule as ACTH (pro-opiomelanocortin) and plasma levels of this peptide also increase in response to stressful stimuli such as shock. It has been suggested that this or other endogenous opioid peptides (e.g. the enkephalins), may be partly responsible for some of the cardiovascular changes seen in shock (Hinds, 1985).

Characteristically plasma cortisol increases markedly in shock, the normal circadian rhythm is lost and secretory peaks may occur at intervals. Although there is often considerable variation in cortisol levels, the extent and duration of the rise is generally related to the severity of the illness. The relationship between circulating cortisol and outcome is unclear, but there is some evidence that patients with sepsis who have a blunted response to ACTH have a worse prognosis (Rothwell *et al.*, 1991) and it is possible that such patients might benefit from steroid replacement. The cause of adrenocortical insufficiency in shock is not clear, but may be related to altered adrenal perfusion, ischaemic injury or mediator-induced adrenal damage.

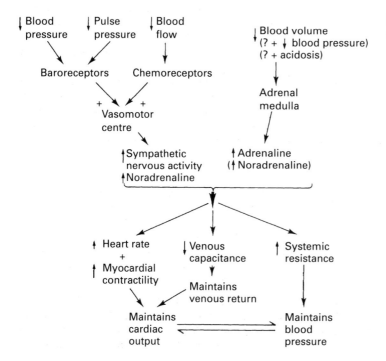

Fig. 4.1 The sympathoadrenal response to shock.

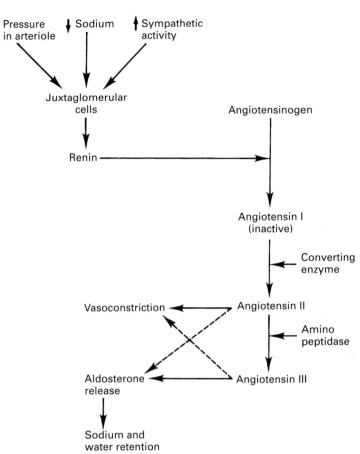

Fig. 4.2 The renin–angiotensin system in shock.

Release of inflammatory mediators

The presence of severe infection (often associated with bacteraemia or endotoxaemia) or large areas of devitalized tissue (e.g. following major trauma or extensive surgery), or prolonged episodes of hypoperfusion, can trigger a massive inflammatory response with systemic activation of leucocytes and release of a variety of potentially damaging 'mediators'.

Although clearly beneficial when targeted against local areas of infection or necrotic tissue, dissemination of this response is responsible for the haemodynamic changes and microvascular abnormalities and possibly intracellular defects, which together culminate in organ damage (**Fig. 4.3**).

MICROORGANISMS AND THEIR TOXIC PRODUCTS

In sepsis/septic shock the inflammatory cascade is triggered by the presence of microorganisms and/or their toxic products in the bloodstream. In other forms of shock ischaemic damage to the bowel mucosa may be associated with bacteraemia/endotoxaemia (see later). Whereas some bacteria produce a single toxin that is principally responsible for the disease (e.g. tetanus, cholera and botulism), others (e.g. staphylococci and streptococci) produce an array of *exotoxins* (e.g. as in toxic shock syndrome, see later). Some organisms, such as *Pseudomonas*, produce both exotoxins (high molecular weight, heat-labile, antigenic proteins) and *endotoxin*, a more heat-stable lipopolysaccharide (LPS) derived from the cell wall of Gram-negative bacteria (**Fig. 4.4**).

Endotoxin consists of:

- a lipid moiety (lipid A), which is structurally highly conserved and is thought to be responsible for most if not all of its biological activity;
- a core polysaccharide;
- oligosaccharide side chains, which differ considerably between strains and confer '0'-antigen specificity to the molecule.

The lipid A portion of LPS can be bound by a protein normally present in human serum *lipopolysaccharide-binding protein* (LBP), the concentration of which increases by around 100 times during the acute phase

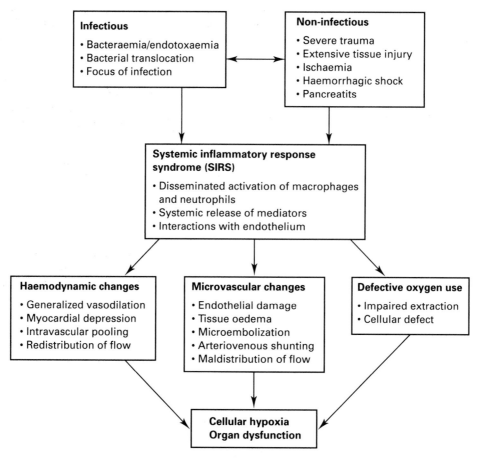

Fig. 4.3 Aetiology of multiple organ dysfunction syndrome (MODS).

response to infection. In the case of intact Gram-negative bacteria, binding of LBP to membrane LPS enhances opsonization by neutrophils and cells of the reticuloendothelial system (RES), whereas when LBP binds with free endotoxin it forms a complex, which is a much more potent inflammatory stimulant than endotoxin alone (see later).

Administration of endotoxin to both animals and humans (Suffredini *et al.*, 1989a) can reproduce many of the manifestations of septic shock and endotoxin is considered to be an important trigger of this condition. Certainly intermittent endotoxaemia is common in those with septic shock and is associated with the more severe manifestations of the syndrome including myocardial depression and multiple organ failure (Danner *et al.*, 1991). These authors also detected endotoxin in the blood of some patients with septic shock due to Gram-positive bacteria or *Candida* and speculated that this may have been related to undetected Gram-negative bacteraemia or release of endotoxin from elsewhere (e.g. the bowel lumen, see later).

Other bacterial cell wall components and toxins can also trigger septic shock, and probably because they all act through the final common pathway outlined below, the haemodynamic changes in Gram-negative and Gram-positive sepsis are indistinguishable (Ahmed *et al.*, 1991).

ACTIVATION OF THE COMPLEMENT CASCADE

Complement activation through the alternative pathway seems to be one of the earliest features of septic shock and may precede the haemodynamic alterations. Activation of the classical pathway probably occurs later, coinciding with the onset of shock. Complement activation may not be an important feature of hypovolaemic or cardiogenic shock (Leon *et al.*, 1982).

One of the many functions of the complement system is to attract and *activate leucocytes*, which then adhere to the endothelium, migrate into the extravascular compartment and release inflammatory mediators such as *proteases* (e.g. elastase) and *toxic oxygen radicals*. These can produce local tissue damage. For example, the free radical superoxide (O_2^-) can participate in a number of chemical reactions, yielding hydrogen per-

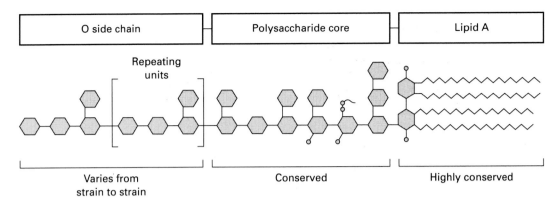

Fig. 4.4 Structure of endotoxin.

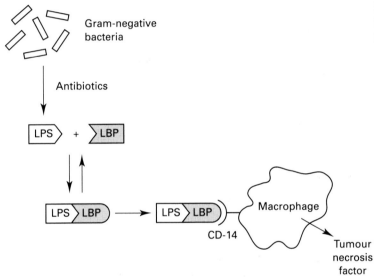

Fig. 4.5 Induction of cytokine synthesis by the lipopolysaccharide–lipopolysaccharide-binding protein (LPS–LBP) complex.

oxide (H_2O_2) and hydroxyl radicals (OH·), which can damage cell membranes, interfere with the function of a number of enzyme systems, activate prostaglandin metabolism, upregulate adhesion molecules (see later) and increase capillary permeability.

CYTOKINES

Cytokines are polypeptide messengers released by activated lymphocytes and macrophages and endothelium. They influence thermoregulation, endocrine function and metabolic responses, and also play an important role in immune function. For example interleukin-1 (IL-1) stimulates helper T cells to produce IL-2, which promotes the growth and proliferation of cytotoxic T cells, while tumour necrosis factor (TNF) enhances phagocytosis and neutrophil adherence, and also activates neutrophil degranulation.

Cytokines are important mediators of the systemic inflammatory response in shock; their synthesis is induced, for example, when the LPS–LBP complex interacts with the CD14 receptor on the cell surface of macrophages (**Fig. 4.5**).

Tumour necrosis factor (TNF) can be detected in the circulation shortly after the administration of endotoxin to human volunteers (Michie *et al.*, 1988a) and induces similar metabolic responses to endotoxin when given to humans (Michie *et al.*, 1988b). It is thought to play a pivotal role as an initiator of the host response to infection, many of its effects being mediated via the cyclo-oxygenase pathway (Michie *et al.*, 1988a).

The *IL-1 response* occurs shortly after TNF release (Hesse *et al.*, 1988). IL-1 shares many of the biological properties of TNF and the two cytokines act synergistically, in part through induction of cyclo-oxygenase, platelet activating factor and nitric oxide (NO) synthase (see later). Recent evidence suggests that both are required to elicit the full spectrum of acute haemodynamic and metabolic disturbances associated with bacterial infection (Ohlsson *et al.*, 1990).

Subsequently, *other cytokines including IL-6 and IL-8*, appear in the circulation. These cytokines are, however, less severely proinflammatory, being more involved in reparative processes such as neutrophil activation/chemotaxis (IL-8) and the enhanced production of acute phase reactants (IL-6). They may also fulfil an important role as downregulators of TNF and IL-1 production.

It is important to appreciate that the cytokine network is extremely complex, with many endogenous self-regulating mechanisms and interactions with other systems. Moreover, naturally occurring *soluble TNF receptors* are thought to be shed from cell surfaces in response to many of the same stimuli that induce TNF production; these may act as circulating inhibitory proteins to diminish the biological activity of TNF. An endogenous inhibitory protein that binds competitively to the IL-1 receptor has also been identified (Ohlsson *et al.*, 1990; Spinas *et al.*, 1990). It is conceivable that critical illness is associated with a reduction in the levels of these endogenous antagonists and that this reduces the patient's tolerance to further septic challenges.

ARACHIDONIC ACID METABOLITES (Feuerstein & Hallenbeck, 1987)

Arachidonic acid is an essential fatty acid, derived from the increased breakdown of membrane phospholipid. It is metabolized via the cyclo-oxygenase pathway to form prostaglandins and via the lipoxygenase pathway to produce leukotrienes (**Fig. 4.6**).

There are a large number of prostaglandins, each of which has distinct physiological effects: some cause vasoconstriction, others are vasodilators, some activate platelets, others inhibit platelet aggregation. Some prostaglandins also increase vascular permeability. Those members of the family considered to be of particular importance in shock are:

- prostacyclin (PGI$_2$), which is a vasodilator and inhibits platelet aggregation;
- thromboxane, which causes pulmonary vasoconstriction and activates platelets;
- PGF$_{2\alpha}$, which may be responsible for the early phase of pulmonary hypertension commonly seen in experimental septic shock.

Clearly, the net effect of the release of these substances in an individual patient depends on the relative concentrations of each particular prostaglandin.

The role of leukotrienes in shock is less certain, but they may be responsible for increased vascular permeability, coronary vasoconstriction and a reduction in cardiac output.

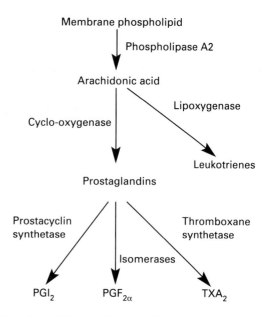

Fig. 4.6 Arachidonic acid metabolites.

PLATELET ACTIVATING FACTOR

Platelet activating factor (PAF) is a vasoactive lipid released from various cell populations such as leucocytes and macrophages. Its effects, which are caused both directly and indirectly through the secondary release of other mediators, include:

- hypotension;
- increased vascular permeability;
- platelet aggregation.

LYSOSOMAL ENZYMES

Lysosomal enzymes are released not only when cells die, but also in response to hypoxia, ischaemia, sepsis and acidosis. As well as being directly cytotoxic, they can cause myocardial depression and coronary vasoconstriction. Furthermore, lysosomal enzymes can convert *inactive kininogens*, which are usually combined with α2-globulin, to *vasoactive kinins* such as bradykinin. These substances can cause:

- vasodilatation;
- increased capillary permeability;
- myocardial depression;
- activation of clotting mechanisms.

INDUCED HISTAMINE

Induced histamine is distinct from the preformed 'mast cell' histamine that is released in many allergic phenomena, and the effects of induced histamine cannot be prevented by administering conventional antihistamines. Release of induced histamine may make a small contribution to the increase in vascular permeability in sepsis, but is unlikely to be relevant in shock of other aetiologies.

ENDOTHELIUM-DERIVED VASOACTIVE MEDIATORS (Editorial, 1991)

It is now recognized that the vascular endothelium is not only a physical barrier between blood and the vessel wall, but is also a highly complex organ involved in the regulation of blood vessel tone, vascular permeability, coagulation, angiogenesis, leucocyte and platelet reactivity, phagocytosis of bacteria and the metabolism of many vascular mediators.

Endothelial cells synthesize a number of endothelium-derived vasoactive mediators, which contribute to the regulation of blood vessel tone and the fluidity of the blood. These include:

- prostacyclin;
- endothelin-1;
- endothelium-derived relaxing factor (EDRF)—nitric oxide (NO).

EDRF is synthesized from the terminal guanidino-nitrogen atoms of the amino acid L-arginine under the influence of NO synthases (NOS). NO produces vasodilation and inhibition of platelet aggregation and adhesion by activating guanylate cyclase in the underlying vascular smooth muscle to form cyclic GMP. There is now evidence for the existence of several distinct NOS.

- 'Constitutive' NOS is present in endothelial cells, is responsible for the basal release of NO and may be involved in the physiological regulation of vascular tone, blood pressure and tissue perfusion.
- The 'inducible' enzyme, on the other hand, is induced in vascular endothelial and smooth muscle cells and monocytes within 4–18 hours of stimulation with certain cytokines, such as TNF, and endotoxin. The resulting prolonged increase in NO formation is now believed to be responsible for the sustained vasodilatation, hypotension and hyporeactivity to adrenergic agonists that characterizes septic shock. This mechanism may also be involved in severe haemorrhagic/traumatic shock.

Circulating levels of *endothelin-1*, a potent endogenous vasoconstrictor, are increased in cardiogenic shock and following severe trauma. Under these circumstances it may augment vascular resistance and maintain perfusion pressure (Koller *et al.*, 1991), although the exact physiological and pathological role of the endothelins is not yet well understood.

ADHESION MOLECULES

Adhesion of neutrophils to the vessel wall and subsequent extravascular migration of activated leucocytes is a key component of the sequence of events leading to endothelial injury, tissue damage and organ dysfunction. This process is mediated by inducible intercellular adhesion molecules (ICAMs) found on the surface of leucocytes and endothelial cells. Expression of these molecules can be induced by LPS and by inflammatory cytokines such as IL-1 and TNF. Three separate families of molecules are involved in promoting leucocyte-endothelial interaction.

- Selectins (P, E and L selectin): these are initial 'capture' molecules and initiate the process of leucocyte rolling on vascular endothelium.
- Immunoglobulin superfamily—ICAM-1, vascular cell adhesion molecule-1 (VCAM-1): these are involved in the formation of a more secure bond, which leads to leucocyte migration into the tissues.
- Integrins.

Soluble forms of adhesion molecules have been identified in peripheral blood and may serve as an indirect measure of the state of endothelial activation. In a recent study circulating levels of E-selectin, ICAM-1 and VCAM-1 were found to be higher in patients with sepsis and organ dysfunction than in control patients. High levels of E-selectin in particular were associated with a very poor prognosis (Cowley *et al.*, 1994).

Haemodynamic changes

CARDIOGENIC SHOCK

The clinical features of cardiogenic shock are seen when the cardiac index falls to around 1.8 l/min/m^2 or less. Heart rate and systemic vascular resistance increase in an attempt to maintain blood pressure. This may lead to a vicious circle in which increasing myocardial oxygen consumption causes an extension of ischaemic areas with a further reduction in cardiac output. Ventricular filling pressures are usually high, although relative hypovolaemia is sometimes precipitated by therapy with vasodilators or diuretics combined with volume losses into the lungs, and may co-exist with persisting chest radiographic evidence of pulmonary oedema (Timmis *et al.*, 1981). The patient may then benefit from cautious volume expansion. Cardiogenic shock may also be associated with a low pulmonary artery occlusion pressure (PAOP) in those with right ventricular infarction. When cardiogenic shock is caused by a ventricular septal defect, valvular incompetence or a ventricular aneurysm, a proportion of ventricular ejection fails to reach the systemic circulation.

OBSTRUCTIVE SHOCK

Cardiac tamponade

Increasing intrapericardial pressure progressively reduces ventricular volumes and increases diastolic pressures. This is associated with corresponding increases in right and left atrial pressures, although sometimes, for example following cardiac surgery, one or other filling pressure may rise earlier, and to a greater extent, than the other. Cardiac transmural pressures fall and in extreme tamponade may become negative, in which case the ventricles probably fill by diastolic suction. Ultimately the ventricles may fill only during atrial systole, particularly at rapid heart rates. Reduced ventricular filling leads to a reduction in ventricular systolic pressure, stroke volume and cardiac output. There is a compensatory tachycardia and vasoconstriction, while ejection fraction is initially maintained or even increased. Eventually compensation fails and blood pressure falls. In extreme tamponade the rise in diastolic pressures may precipitate myocardial ischaemia, although in less severe cases the reduction in coronary flow may be offset by decreased myocardial work.

HYPOVOLAEMIC SHOCK

Cardiac output falls as a result of the reduction in ventricular pre-load and there is a compensatory rise in systemic vascular resistance, venoconstriction and tachycardia. Blood flow is diverted away from less important areas in order to maintain perfusion of vital organs. The pulse pressure is narrowed and tachycardia almost invariably precedes the development of hypotension. Blood pressure is usually maintained until the circulating blood volume is reduced by more than 20–25%. Ventricular filling pressures—central venous pressure (CVP) and PAOP—are usually low although their response to a fluid challenge provides a more accurate assessment of the extent of volume losses. Later in the evolution of severe hypovolaemic shock there may be a paradoxical bradycardia. In some cases myocardial contractility is impaired by ischaemia, infarction, pre-existing cardiac disease or, later, by the effects of complicating sepsis (see later).

DISTRIBUTIVE SHOCK

Septic shock (Parrillo et al., 1990)

The dominant haemodynamic feature of septic shock is *peripheral vascular failure*; persistent vasodilation, refractory to vasoconstrictors is characteristic of non-survivors (Groeneveld et al., 1986). Provided hypovolaemia has been corrected, cardiac output is usually high, a low cardiac index being uncommon even in the very late stages of septic shock (Parrillo et al., 1990). Nevertheless it is now recognized that *myocardial depression* is a common feature and is usually manifested as a decreased ejection fraction, with a reduced left ventricular stroke work, which responds poorly to volume loading (Parker et al., 1984; Ellrodt et al., 1985; Ognibene et al., 1988; Suffredini et al., 1989a). Despite the reduced ejection fraction, stroke volume is generally maintained by ventricular dilatation, probably related to increased myocardial compliance (Parker et al., 1984; Ognibene et al., 1988; Suffredini et al., 1989a), and tachycardia is responsible for the high cardiac output.

As well as this global myocardial dysfunction *reversible segmental left ventricular abnormalities* have also been noted in patients with septic shock, most often in those with underlying heart disease (Ellrodt et al., 1985). Although in this study there were no differences in left ventricular ejection fraction, left ventricular stroke work or the frequency of segmental dysfunction between survivors and non-survivors (Ellrodt et al., 1985), others have noted that reversible ventricular dilatation with a reduced ejection fraction is seen more commonly in those who survive (Parrillo et al., 1990). The latter observation may be explained by a greater degree of myocardial oedema, or right ventricular distension, which could impede left ventricular dilatation in non-survivors. Moreover, extreme vasodilatation in non-survivors would tend to minimize the reduction in ejection fraction and the degree of ventricular dilatation. It has been suggested that because myocardial dysfunction can be ameliorated by inotropic support it is not an important determinant of outcome in septic shock, but this issue has yet to be resolved. Whereas some authors have noted that cardiac output and oxygen delivery are higher in survivors (Tuchschmidt et al., 1989), others have been unable to demonstrate such a relationship (Dhainaut et al., 1987).

Similar abnormalities also affect the right ventricle in septic shock (Parker et al., 1990), and in some cases right ventricular failure associated with pulmonary hypertension and coronary hypoperfusion may prevent an increase in cardiac output in response to volume loading (Schneider et al., 1988).

It seems unlikely that these alterations in ventricular performance are attributable to global myocardial ischaemia since coronary blood flow is normal or increased and the myocardial oxygen content difference is narrowed in patients with septic shock (Cunnion *et al.*, 1986). These findings do not, however, exclude focal myocardial ischaemia due to regional reductions in flow (Dhainaut *et al.*, 1987) or microcirculatory abnormalities. Ischaemia may also occur in those with pre-existing coronary artery disease.

Ventricular performance may be impaired in septic shock by a circulating *myocardial depressant substance*, the presence of which correlates quantitatively with the decrease in left ventricular ejection fraction (Parrillo *et al.*, 1985). Other factors that may contribute to myocardial depression in shock include acidosis, hypoxaemia and myocardial oedema.

Microcirculatory changes

In *septic shock* there is:

- vasodilatation;
- maldistribution of flow;
- arteriovenous shunting;
- increased capillary permeability with interstitial oedema.

Although these microvascular abnormalities may largely account for the reduced oxygen extraction often seen in patients with sepsis, there may also be a *primary defect in cellular oxygen utilization*.

In the initial stages of other forms of shock, and sometimes when hypovolaemia supervenes in sepsis and anaphylaxis, increased sympathetic activity causes constriction of precapillary arterioles and, to a lesser extent, the postcapillary venules. This helps to maintain systemic blood pressure. Furthermore, the hydrostatic pressure within the capillaries falls and fluid is mobilized from the extravascular space into the intravascular compartment. This *'transcapillary refill'*, combined with the salt and water retention described above, to some extent restores the circulating volume and promotes flow by reducing viscosity. If shock persists, the accumulation of metabolites, such as lactic acid and carbon dioxide, combined with the release of vasoactive substances, causes relaxation of the precapillary sphincters, while the postcapillary venules, which are more sensitive to hypoxic damage, become relatively unresponsive to these substances and remain constricted. Blood is therefore sequestered within the dilated capillary bed and fluid is forced into the interstitial spaces, causing *interstitial oedema, haemoconcentration* and an *increase in viscosity*. Blood also becomes more viscous at low flow rates since the streaming effect, which normally channels red blood cells (RBCs) down the centre of vessels, is reduced. In addition, RBCs become less elliptical and there is reversible aggregation of RBCs and platelets.

This reduction in flow through the microcirculation, combined with the increase in viscosity, renders shocked patients highly susceptible to procoagulant stimuli. The release of ADP from platelets in response to the presence of particulate matter, noradrenaline, proaggregant mediators (e.g. platelet activating factor) and thrombin, together with the reduced flow and increased viscosity, leads to *platelet aggregation* and *clot formation* within the capillary bed.

In addition, cell damage caused, for example, by the effects of endotoxin and antigen–antibody complexes on the capillary endothelium, leads to the release of tissue thromboplastins. The production of PGI_2, which inhibits platelet aggregation, by the capillary endothelium may be impaired, and factor XII may be activated by endotoxin both directly and through alteration of the endothelial cells. Activated factor XII cleaves factor XI to XIa, which triggers the intrinsic coagulation pathway. Tissue plasminogen activator is released early in response to endotoxin and activated plasmin limits the extent of thrombosis. Later increased fibrinolysis may be offset by the release of a plasminogen activator inhibitor (Suffredini *et al.*, 1989b).

Cells supplied by capillaries blocked by this process of *disseminated intravascular coagulation (DIC)* (Hewitt & Davies, 1983) inevitably become hypoxic and eventually die. Tissue ischaemia is further exacerbated as capillaries are compressed by interstitial oedema. This process therefore causes serious damage to vital organs in shock.

Finally, because clotting factors and platelets are consumed they are unavailable for haemostasis elsewhere and a coagulation defect results—hence the alternative name for DIC of *'consumption coagulopathy'*. This leads to abnormal bleeding (e.g. from surgical wounds or venepuncture sites), haematuria, bleeding from the nose or gums and ecchymoses. The platelet count is reduced, the prothrombin time prolonged and fibrin/fibrinogen degradation products (FDPs) are elevated; in some a *microangiopathic haemolytic anaemia* develops. This process occurs earlier and is most severe in septic shock.

Capillary endothelial injury is mediated by a number of factors, particularly in septic shock, including DIC, microemboli, release of vasoactive compounds, and complement activation, as well as by the adhesion and extravascular migration of leucocytes (see above and Chapter 6, adult respiratory distress syndrome). Capillary permeability is thereby increased so that fluid is lost into the interstitial space causing further hypovolaemia, interstitial oedema and organ dysfunction.

REPERFUSION INJURY

If resuscitation is successful and flow through the microcirculation is restored, tissue damage may be exacerbated by activation of phospholipase A_2 and the generation of large quantities of oxygen-free radicals. During the period of ischaemia, xanthine dehydrogenase is converted to xanthine oxidase and ATP is catabolized to hypoxanthine. When oxygen again becomes available hypoxanthine is rapidly converted to uric acid under the influence of xanthine oxidase, in the process generating large amounts of free radicals (**Fig. 4.7**). The gut mucosa is especially vulnerable to this 'reperfusion injury' (Schoenberg & Beger, 1993).

Supply dependency

A number of studies have suggested that in apparently stable critically ill patients, especially those with adult respiratory distress syndrome (ARDS), multiple organ failure and sepsis, oxygen consumption ($\dot{V}O_2$) often rises if oxygen delivery (DO_2) is actively increased (e.g. with fluid loading, prostacyclin, catecholamines or blood transfusion) and falls in response to reductions in oxygen transport (e.g. induced by the application of

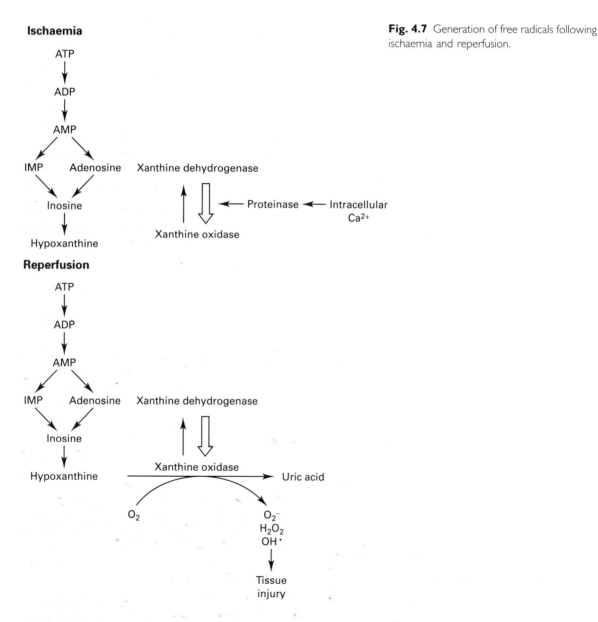

Fig. 4.7 Generation of free radicals following ischaemia and reperfusion.

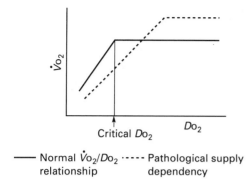

Fig. 4.8 Relationship between oxygen delivery (Do_2) and oxygen consumption ($\dot{V}o_2$).

positive end-expiratory pressure—PEEP) (Danek *et al.*, 1980; Haupt *et al.*, 1985; Gilbert *et al.*, 1986; Kruse *et al.*, 1990). This linear relationship between $\dot{V}o_2$ and Do_2, termed 'supply dependency,' contrasts with normal physiology where in resting subjects $\dot{V}o_2$ remains constant once a critical Do_2 is exceeded and exercise-induced increases in $\dot{V}o_2$ are met by an appropriate increase in Do_2 (**Fig. 4.8**).

Pathological supply dependency is probably largely a consequence of maldistribution of flow in the microcirculation, predominantly related to inappropriate vasodilation, but is probably exacerbated by microemboli, interstitial oedema, localized vasoconstriction and arteriovenous shunting. These microcirculatory disturbances may be combined with defective cellular oxygen utilization. As a result oxygen extraction is impaired, mixed venous oxygen saturation ($S_{\bar{v}}o_2$) rises, arteriovenous oxygen content difference ($C_{a-\bar{v}}o_2$) is narrowed, and the slope of the $\dot{V}o_2/Do_2$ relationship is flattened and moved to the right. In addition $\dot{V}o_2$ is often increased as a result of the hypermetabolic response to illness or injury.

It might be anticipated that these abnormalities would be associated with an oxygen debt and it is perhaps not surprising, therefore, that in some studies supply dependency has been accompanied by lactic acidosis (Haupt *et al.*, 1985; Gilbert *et al.*, 1986; Kruse *et al.*, 1990). Others, however, have not been able to confirm a relationship between supply dependency and lactic acidosis (Ronco *et al.*, 1991; Phang *et al.*, 1994). It has also proved difficult to demonstrate that the critical Do_2 can be exceeded and the 'plateau' attained in apparently supply dependent patients. Not surprisingly, therefore this phenomenon has given rise to considerable controversy and for a number of reasons studies investigating $Do_2/\dot{V}o_2$ relationships should be interpreted cautiously.

- Do_2 is calculated as the product of $\dot{Q}_t$ and C_ao_2 and in many studies $\dot{V}o_2$ has been derived using the reverse Fick equation, that is $\dot{V}o_2 = \dot{Q}_t \times (C_ao_2 - C_{\bar{v}}o_2)$. The presence of the shared variables $\dot{Q}_t$ and C_ao_2 may give

rise to 'mathematical coupling' in which, for example, an erroneously high determination of $\dot{Q}_t$ will translate into increases in both Do_2 and $\dot{V}o_2$. Although the magnitude and relevance of this effect has been disputed in one study of patients with ARDS, $\dot{V}o_2$ determined by analysis of expired gas did not change when Do_2 was increased by blood transfusion whereas calculated $\dot{V}o_2$ did (Ronco *et al.*, 1991). More recently the same group of investigators have produced further evidence to suggest that mathematical coupling of random error in the measurement of shared variables could explain finding dependence of Fick $\dot{V}o_2$ on Do_2 in clinically resuscitated patients with ARDS (Phang *et al.*, 1994).

- Importantly $\dot{V}o_2$ may vary spontaneously (Villar *et al.*, 1990), as well as in response to minor disturbances and therapeutic interventions such as chest physiotherapy (Weissman & Kemper, 1991) and the associated appropriate increase in Do_2 may then be wrongly interpreted as indicating supply dependency.
- In septic shock the $\dot{V}o_2$ response to an increase in oxygen transport may vary from time to time in the same patient (Palazzo & Suter, 1991).
- The critical Do_2 for anaerobic metabolism in critically ill patients may be considerably lower than previously reported and may not be altered by sepsis (Ronco *et al.*, 1993).
- The relationship between pathological supply dependency and prognosis remains unclear (Bihari *et al.*, 1987; Palazzo & Suter, 1991).

Organ dysfunction

The most vital organs of the body, such as the brain and heart, are relatively protected from the ill effects of alterations in blood pressure by their ability, within certain limits, to maintain blood flow at a constant level despite changes in perfusion pressure (**Fig. 4.9**). This *autoregulation* is an intrinsic property of some vascular smooth muscle and is independent of its innervation. It is lost when the vessels become rigid (e.g. due to atheroma), and the limits for autoregulation are reset at higher levels in those with pre-existing hypertension (see **Fig. 4.9**).

Because sympathetic tone is often high in shocked patients, the autoregulation curve is shifted to the right (i.e. tissue flow will fall at higher pressures than in normal subjects). Later in the evolution of shock, vasoparesis may occur (see above), and under these circumstances autoregulation may fail (i.e. flow becomes passive and pressure-dependent). Furthermore, dilatation of healthy vessels in the presence of atheroma elsewhere may 'steal' blood from areas supplied by diseased

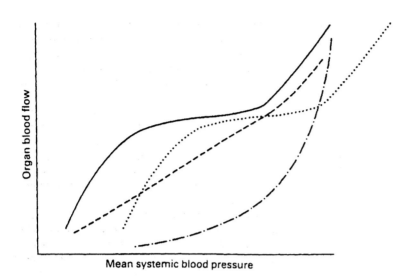

Fig. 4.9 Autoregulation of organ blood flow. Flow to vital organs is normally maintained constant over a wide range of perfusion pressures (——). When vessels are rigid (e.g. due to atheroma), flow is linearly related to pressure (– – –). Passive flow (– · –) occurs in distensible vessels (e.g. normal arterioles in skin) and those in ischaemic areas with toxic arteriolar paralysis. In hypertensive subjects (...) the limits for autoregulation are reset at a higher level.

vessels. This can cause, for example, symptoms of cerebral ischaemia, particularly in the elderly.

HEART

In cardiogenic shock, disease of the myocardium is, of course, the primary abnormality. Despite the ability of the coronary circulation to autoregulate, and the reduction in myocardial oxygen consumption which usually occurs when blood pressure falls, myocardial dysfunction may develop during prolonged severe shock of any aetiology (see above).

Myocardial ischaemia, affecting particularly the vulnerable endocardial layer, may be an important cause of this reduction in cardiac performance although its contribution to myocardial depression in septic shock is uncertain (see above). When systemic blood pressure falls below a certain critical level, myocardial blood flow is inevitably reduced, especially when the ability of the coronary circulation to autoregulate is impaired by atheroma. Myocardial ischaemia could be exacerbated by coronary 'steal', a reduction in the distensibility of collateral vessels and obstruction of capillary flow by myocardial oedema. Furthermore, the local effects of cellular hypoxia can cause abnormalities of excitation and contraction with the development of arrhythmias and impaired myocardial function. Circulating myocardial depressant substances may also contribute to cardiac dysfunction in shock (see above).

LUNGS

In the early stages of shock, the reduction in pulmonary blood flow and perfusion pressure leads to *V/Q inequalities* with an increased dead space, while in hyperdynamic patients the *V/Q* ratio will be low. The patient usually develops a tachypnoea in response to the metabolic acidosis and chemoreceptor stimulation, so that P_aCO_2 is often reduced while P_aO_2 may be either normal or low. Later *respiratory muscle fatigue* may supervene, in part because of reduced perfusion; rarely a reduction in cerebral blood flow may *depress the respiratory centre*.

Patients in whom shock is severe and prolonged may develop respiratory failure 12–48 hours after the initial episode. Previously, this was referred to as the *'shock lung syndrome'*, and it is one cause of ARDS (see Chapter 6). The development of ARDS in shock is almost invariably associated with sepsis and is a rare sequel of pure hypovolaemia. Similarly, sepsis is frequently associated with respiratory abnormalities.

Finally, respiratory failure associated with shock may be caused or exacerbated by other factors such as:

- aspiration of gastric contents;
- fluid overload;
- lung contusion;
- thermal inhalation injury;
- pulmonary infection;
- oxygen toxicity.

(These subjects are discussed elsewhere.)

KIDNEYS

Oliguria is almost invariable in the shocked patient and may be prerenal, renal or postrenal. Prerenal oliguria will respond to volume expansion and this should be achieved as rapidly as possible to prevent progression to established acute renal failure. In the early stages autoregulation maintains the glomerular filtration rate (GFR) and oliguria is related to increased antidiuretic hormone (ADH) and aldosterone levels. Subsequently oliguria may be exacerbated by a fall in GFR. Postrenal causes, such as *urethral damage in trauma patients*, must also be excluded (see Chapter 12).

A few patients with septic shock may develop an inappropriate polyuria despite hypovolaemia. In patients with septic shock receiving inotropic support, renal vascular resistance remained unchanged while renal blood flow varied from markedly reduced to slightly increased (Brenner *et al.*, 1990). As the shock resolved renal blood flow tended to increase. These authors concluded that sepsis-induced renal dysfunction may occur despite normal values for total renal blood flow.

LIVER

The liver is to some extent protected from ischaemic damage, not only by its ability to autoregulate, but also by its dual blood supply. Nevertheless, the reduction in hepatic arterial and portal flow frequently leads to a *benign and reversible conjugated hyperbilirubin-aemia* and also *impairs the reticuloendothelial function* of the liver. The latter exacerbates bacteraemia/endotoxaemia. Hepatic hypoxia may also lead to increased lactate production, a raised blood ammonia and elevated aminotransferases. In the most severe cases overt hepatic failure (see Chapter 13) may develop and this is often irreversible.

SPLANCHNIC CIRCULATION (Haglund *et al.*, 1987)

In *hypovolaemic* and *cardiogenic shock*, marked compensatory vasoconstriction in the splanchnic bed redistributes flow to more immediately vital organs and may increase the circulating blood volume by as much as 30%. In *septic shock*, particularly when volume replacement has been adequate, splanchnic flow is markedly increased and parallels changes in cardiac output. These changes in splanchnic vascular resistance cause substantial alterations in total peripheral resistance and may account for almost all of the increase seen in hypovolaemic and cardiogenic shock.

When the reduction in intestinal perfusion pressure and/or blood flow is only modest, autoregulation and a compensatory increase in oxygen extraction normally prevent mucosal injury, and following brief episodes of more serious reduction in flow damage may be limited to an increase in capillary permeability, caused largely by free radicals generated during reperfusion (see above). More prolonged episodes of hypoperfusion are, however, associated with significant ischaemic injury, which is initially confined to the superficial layer of the mucosa. Characteristically mucosal damage starts as a small lesion at the tip of the villous; the villous may then become denuded. Finally the entire villous layer becomes necrotic. Gastrointestinal injury in low output shock and following partial ischaemia never involves the deeper layers and is substantially exacerbated by reperfusion (see above).

Ischaemic mucosal injury in *sepsis* when splanchnic flow is increased may be explained by maldistribution of microcirculatory flow and by a marked increase in splanchnic oxygen demand (Ruokonen *et al.*, 1993). As a result of the latter, oxygen extraction may rise and portal venous Po_2 falls, and this may contribute to hepatic hypoxia.

Complete vascular occlusion produces a rapid progression of injury from increased mucosal permeability seen after only about 30 minutes to complete loss of villi at one hour, transmucosal necrosis after four hours and transmural infarction within 8–16 hours. Reperfusion injury does not appear to play an important role.

In severe shock of any aetiology, including endotoxin challenge, loss of mucosal integrity within the gastrointestinal tract may allow increased bacterial translocation (Deitch *et al.*, 1987) and passage of endotoxin into the portal venous system. Activation of liver macrophages and systemic bacteraemia/endotoxaemia combine to amplify the systemic inflammatory response, thereby contributing to the development and persistence of sepsis and multiple organ failure (see later).

Mucosal vasoconstriction (e.g. in response to hypovolaemia) increases the susceptibility of the gastric mucosa to acid-mediated damage and this may result in subclinical or, less often, frank bleeding. In sepsis, a reduction in gastric mucosal flow is not consistently found, but ischaemia may result from an increased oxygen demand and impaired oxygen extraction. Splanchnic ischaemia may also damage the pancreas ('shock pancreas') (Lamy *et al.*, 1987) with the systemic release of pancreatic enzymes and 'myocardial depressant factor'.

CENTRAL NERVOUS SYSTEM (Hasselgren & Fischer, 1986)

Although the central nervous system is well protected from the ill effects of hypotension by autoregulation and the cerebral vasodilation induced when patients are hypoxic or hypercarbic (see Chapter 14), reversible cerebral dysfunction is a common feature of shock.

Patients with severe sepsis are particularly liable to develop acute disturbances of cerebral function. This may present as restlessness, irritability, agitation, disorientation, confusion, lethargy, somnolence, stupor or even coma and may be due to:

● inadequate cerebral perfusion;

- metabolic disturbances—electrolyte imbalance, acid-base disorders, hypo- or hyperglycaemia, hypo- or hyperthermia, hypoxaemia, endocrine disturbances;
- the direct cerebral effects of endotoxin;
- the effects of drug administration;
- meningo-encephalitis (occasionally).

A number of striking similarities are seen between the hypercatabolic response to sepsis and the metabolic changes associated with the encephalopathy of liver failure (see Chapter 13); there is some evidence that *'septic encephalopathy'* can be attributed to similar alterations in plasma and brain amino acid profiles. In sepsis, increased muscle protein breakdown combined with impaired hepatic metabolism leads to elevated plasma levels of sulphur-containing and aromatic amino acids (AAA), the increase in sulphur-containing amino acids being somewhat greater than in hepatic encephalopathy. Plasma levels of branched chain amino acids (BCAA) are normal or, in some cases, slightly reduced, perhaps because of increased oxidation in muscle and fat. Combined with altered amino acid transport across the blood–brain barrier, these changes lead to increased concentrations of AAA within the brain. Consequently, the activity of serotinergic pathways is increased, cerebral concentrations of catecholaminergic neurotransmitters falls and levels of 'false neurotransmitters' such as octopamine and phenylethanolamine increase.

These alterations in the profile of cerebral neurotransmitters could account for many of the features of septic encephalopathy, but other mechanisms, such as changes in the number and activity of receptors, may also be involved.

There is some evidence that administration of BCAA to patients with sepsis can be beneficial. They are an excellent energy source, reduce muscle protein breakdown, restore immune competence and, when combined with glucose, may normalize the plasma amino acid profile, as well as competing with AAAs for transport across the blood–brain barrier. Brain amino acid and neurotransmitter profiles may be returned to normal and this could improve or reverse the encephalopathy.

There seems to be an association between the severity of the encephalopathy and prognosis in sepsis. In those who survive, however, a full recovery of cerebral function can be anticipated unless hypotension is particularly severe and prolonged, there is pre-existing cerebrovascular disease or the patient has a cerebrovascular accident.

Metabolic changes

Gluconeogenesis and triglyceride formation are stimulated by increased glucagon and catecholamine levels, while hepatic mobilization of glucose from glycogen is increased. Catecholamines inhibit insulin release and reduce peripheral glucose uptake. Combined with elevated circulating levels of other insulin antagonists such as cortisol and growth hormone these changes ensure that the majority of shocked patients are hyperglycaemic. Occasionally hypoglycaemia is precipitated by depletion of hepatic glycogen stores and inhibition of gluconeogenesis. This is more common in those with underlying liver disease. Free fatty acid synthesis is also increased leading to hypertriglyceridaemia.

Muscle proteolysis is initiated to provide energy, especially from BCAAs, and hepatic protein synthesis is preferentially augmented to produce the 'acute phase reactants'. The latter are thought to be important components of the host defence system: C-reactive protein, for example, is involved in opsonization and complement activation, α-1-antitrypsin is an important protease inhibitor and caeruloplasmin is a free radical scavenger.

Once the supply of oxygen to the cells becomes insufficient for continuation of the tricarboxylic acid (TCA) cycle, production of energy in the form of ATP becomes dependent on anaerobic metabolism. Under these circumstances, glucose is metabolized in the normal way to pyruvate, but is then converted to lactate instead of entering the Kreb's cycle. The H^+ ions thereby released cause a metabolic acidosis (type A lactic acidosis, see Chapter 5). This pathway is relatively inefficient in terms of energy production. Eventually, because of reduced availability of ATP, the sodium pump fails, cells swell due to accumulation of salt and water, and potassium losses increase. In the final stages, release of lysosomal enzymes may contribute to cell death while the rise in cytosolic calcium levels is probably a terminal event related to failure of the calcium pump.

CLINICAL PRESENTATION OF SHOCK

Hypovolaemic shock

The aetiology of hypovolaemic shock is usually clinically obvious (e.g. trauma, surgery, burns or intestinal obstruction), although gastrointestinal haemorrhage may be concealed, at least initially.

Signs of inadequate tissue perfusion in shock include:

- cold, pale, slate-grey skin;
- increased capillary filling time;
- oliguria or anuria;
- confusion and restlessness (in severe cases).

Increased sympathetic activity produces vasoconstriction, which although helping to maintain blood pressure, further reduces tissue blood flow and causes:

- tachycardia;

- a narrowed pulse pressure;
- sweating.

Sometimes pre-existing heart disease or the administration of β-blockers limits the tachycardia. As shock becomes more severe, the skin changes spread further proximally and *extreme hypovolaemia may be associated with bradycardia*. Hypotension is an unreliable sign, particularly in hypovolaemic shock, since blood pressure may be maintained despite the loss of up to 25% of the circulating volume. On the other hand, such a patient will exhibit all the signs of compensatory sympathetic activity just described. It is therefore not adequate simply to restore blood pressure in shock and treatment must be continued until the tachycardia has settled, peripheral perfusion is improved and urine flow is adequate.

In the initial stages of shock, the patient is often tachypnoeic, either due to associated chest or lung injury or in an attempt to compensate for a metabolic acidosis. The development of a tachypnoea some time after the onset of shock is often the first sign of the development of ARDS or the fat embolism syndrome.

Cardiogenic shock

Cardiogenic shock has been defined as a systolic blood pressure less than 90 mm Hg (or a fall of more than 30 mm Hg from the pre-morbid value) with evidence of reduced perfusion such as oliguria (urine output < 20 ml/h), impaired mental function and peripheral vasoconstriction. Hypotension due to vasovagal reactions, serious arrhythmias, drug reactions or hypovolaemia must first be excluded.

The clinical features of cardiogenic shock are the same as those described for hypovolaemic shock with the addition of the signs of myocardial failure. These may include an elevated jugular venous pressure (JVP), basal crepitations, pulsus alternans and a 'triple' rhythm. In some cases there may be frank pulmonary oedema with severe dyspnoea and central cyanosis. Clinical examination may also reveal the aetiology of cardiogenic shock (e.g. a systolic murmur appearing after a myocardial infarction suggests mitral regurgitation).

Obstructive shock

CARDIAC TAMPONADE

The clinical features of cardiac tamponade resemble those of congestive cardiac failure, except that the lungs are nearly always clear (possibly because the reduction in right ventricular ejection prevents pulmonary engorgement). Most patients are relatively or absolutely hypotensive and the neck veins are distended. When tamponade is due to massive haemorrhage (e.g. due to penetrating cardiac injury or aortic rupture) shock is the dominant feature.

Heart sounds are usually muffled, but are often better heard over the base of the heart. Sometimes there is relative accentuation of the pulmonary component of the second heart sound and in those with inflammatory or neoplastic lesions there may be a pericardial rub. The apex beat may be impalpable. *Kussmaul's sign* (inspiratory expansion of the neck veins) should be absent unless there is epicardial constriction as well as fluid in the pericardium. The possibility of constrictive pericarditis should also be suspected if a third heart sound is heard before or after drainage. In those with clinically significant tamponade without extreme hypotension, *pulsus paradoxus* (an inspiratory decline in systolic blood pressure which exceeds 10 mm Hg) is normally palpable at any available artery. Pulsus paradoxus may be absent or minimal when there is significant constriction and in those with left ventricular hypertrophy, severe left heart failure, atrial septal defect or severe aortic regurgitation. Right heart tamponade, which may be due to loculated blood after cardiac surgery, is generally not associated with pulsus paradoxus.

Sepsis and septic shock

SEPSIS

This can be defined as the systemic inflammatory response to the presence of infection; it is being diagnosed with increasing frequency and is now one of the commonest causes of death in critically ill patients. Although this may be partly explained by a greater awareness of the condition, there has undoubtedly been a dramatic increase in the true incidence of sepsis caused by a progressive rise in the number of susceptible patients due to:

- an enlarging older population;
- increased use of cytotoxics, corticosteroids and radiotherapy;
- prolonged survival of patients with diseases that compromise immunity, such as malignancy, diabetes mellitus and critical illness, and transplant recipients;
- the more widespread use of invasive techniques such as intravascular cannulation, parenteral nutrition, urinary tract instrumentation and radical surgery.

The exact *incidence of sepsis* is difficult to determine, but it has been estimated that there may be in the region of 400,000 cases of sepsis in the USA each year, with 200,000 episodes of septic shock and 100,000 deaths from the disease (Parrillo *et al.*, 1990). In the UK there could be around 60,000 episodes of sepsis each year.

The success of attempts to reduce the high mortality associated with sepsis hinges on early recognition of life-threatening infection, preferably before shock develops. Prompt institution of specific treatment and supportive measures (see later) may then prevent the development of dangerous sequelae such as septic shock and vital organ failure, and improve outcome.

Signs of sepsis include:

- pyrexia or hypothermia;
- rigors;
- sweating;
- nausea;
- vomiting;
- tachypnoea;
- tachycardia;
- hyperdynamic circulation (warm, pink peripheries, rapid capillary refill and a bounding pulse).

Other manifestations of sepsis include:

- leucocytosis, leucopenia, a leukaemoid reaction, eosinopenia;
- hyperglycaemia, and in more severe cases hypoglycaemia.

It has been recommended that the term *severe sepsis* (previously called 'sepsis syndrome', Bone, 1991) be used when these signs are combined with hypotension or evidence of hypoperfusion and organ dysfunction such as hypoxaemia, oliguria, lactic acidosis or altered mental function (confusion, irritability, lethargy and coma) (Bone *et al.*, 1992; Members of the American College of Chest Physicians/Society of Critical Care Medicine Consensus Conference Committee, 1992).

Mild *liver dysfunction* with jaundice and a coagulopathy with thrombocytopenia/DIC often complicate more serious cases. The clinical signs of DIC include excessive bleeding from wounds and vascular cannulation sites, sometimes combined with a purpuric rash. Particularly severe DIC classically occurs in meningococcal septicaemia and may be associated with bilateral adrenal haemorrhage, hypoadrenalism and profound hypotension.

The diagnosis of sepsis is often difficult and a high index of suspicion is required if cases are not to be missed or diagnosed too late. The classical signs may not be present, particularly in the elderly, and mild confusion, tachycardia, tachypnoea, glucose intolerance and a rising plasma creatinine, for example, may be the only clues, sometimes associated with unexplained hypotension.

SEPTIC SHOCK

Septic shock can be defined as hypotension complicating severe sepsis despite adequate fluid resuscitation.

Patients with septic shock are usually clinically hyperdynamic ('warm shock'), but occasionally there is cutaneous vasoconstriction with cold, pale, blue extremities. Conventionally this clinical picture of 'cold shock' is interpreted as indicating a 'low output' state related to hypovolaemia or myocardial depression with compensatory vasoconstriction, but invasive monitoring may reveal a low total systemic vascular resistance and a high cardiac output. Nevertheless in some patients volume replacement, combined with inotropic support when indicated, is associated with an increased cardiac output and improved peripheral perfusion. It has been suggested that the terms 'warm' and 'cold' shock are unhelpful and should be discarded (Bone, 1991).

Much of the confusion in the literature, particularly in relation to the outcome of septic shock, has been attributed to a failure to distinguish between readily reversible episodes of hypotension and the much more serious *refractory shock*. The latter has been defined as shock unresponsive to conventional therapy (intravenous fluids with inotropic and/or vasoactive agents) within 1 hour (Bone, 1991).

SYSTEMIC INFLAMMATORY RESPONSE SYNDROME

The clinical signs of sepsis may or may not be associated with bacteraemia (defined as the presence of viable bacteria in the circulating blood), and in one prospective study only 45% of those with sepsis syndrome were found to be bacteraemic (Bone *et al.*, 1989). Some cases may be related to infection with fungi, pathogenic viruses or rickettsia, but similar or even identical physiological responses can be produced by non-infectious processes such as pancreatitis, severe trauma, extensive tissue injury, ischaemia and haemorrhagic shock. It has been recommended, therefore, that the term *systemic inflammatory response syndrome (SIRS)* be used to describe the disseminated inflammation that can complicate this diverse range of disorders and that the term 'sepsis' should be reserved for those patients with 'SIRS' who have a documented infection (**Fig. 4.10**).

To avoid confusion, ensure reliable communication and allow meaningful evaluation of the efficacy of new treatments, standard terminology for SIRS, sepsis, severe sepsis, septic shock and refractory shock has been proposed (**Table 4.2**). It has also been suggested that septicaemia is an imprecise term and to avoid confusion should no longer be used (Bone, 1991; Bone *et al.*, 1992; Members of the American College of Chest Physicians/Society of Critical Care Medicine Consensus Conference Committee, 1992).

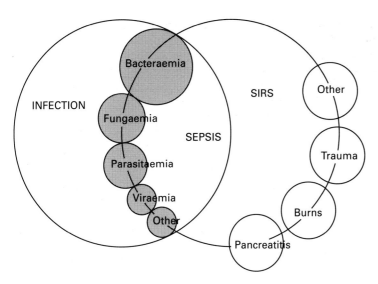

Fig. 4.10 Systemic inflammatory response syndrome (SIRS), sepsis and infection. From the American College of Chest Physicians/Society of Critical Care Medicine Consensus Conference, 1992.

Table 4.2 Recommended standard terminology.

Systemic inflammatory response syndrome (SIRS)

The systemic inflammatory response to a variety of severe clinical insults. The response is manifested by two or more of the following:

- Temperature > 38°C or < 36°C
- Heart rate > 90 beats/min
- Respiratory rate > 20 breaths/min or P_aCO_2 < 4.3 kPa
- White cell count > 12000 cells/mm^3, < 4000 cells/mm^3 or > 10% immature forms

Sepsis

SIRS resulting from documented infection.

Severe sepsis

Sepsis associated with organ dysfunction, hypoperfusion or hypotension. Hypoperfusion and perfusion abnormalities may include, but are not limited to, lactic acidosis, oliguria or an acute alteration in mental state.

Septic shock

Severe sepsis with hypotension (systolic BP < 90 mm Hg or a reduction of > 40 mm Hg from baseline) in the absence of other causes for hypotension) despite adequate fluid resuscitation. (Patients receiving inotropic or vasopressor agents may not be hypotensive when perfusion abnormalities are documented.)

Refractory shock

Shock unresponsive to conventional therapy (intravenous fluids and inotropic/vasoactive agents) within one hour.

TOXIC SHOCK SYNDROME (Williams, 1990)

Toxic shock syndrome is caused by infection with a toxin-producing *Staphylococcus aureus*, although severe streptococcal infection may present similarly (Stevens *et al.*, 1989). An epidemic of toxic shock syndrome in the late 1970s and early 1980s was probably related to the marketing of hyperabsorbable tampons. Although most cases occur in women aged 15–34 years, usually during menstruation. The syndrome also occurs in men. Other causes include:

- surgical wound infection;
- conjunctivitis;
- cellulitis;
- abscesses;
- fasciitis;
- infected burns;
- septic abortion;
- osteomyelitis;
- empyema.

The *clinical features* are the same whatever the source of toxin. The diagnosis is based on the presence of:

- fever (at least 38.9°C);
- rash;
- hypotension;
- evidence of involvement of at least three systems.

The rash is a macular erythema, which blanches on pressure and may be generalized, patchy or localized. About 1–2 weeks after the onset there may be desquamation. Involvement of other systems is indicated by:

- diarrhoea, vomiting;
- myalgia, elevated creatine phosphokinase (CPK), rhabdomyolysis;
- impaired renal function;
- leucocytosis, thrombocytopenia, DIC;
- confusion, drowsiness;
- erythema of conjunctivae, oropharynx or tongue.

Abdominal pain may be associated with abnormal liver function or evidence of pancreatitis. Vaginal hyperaemia, desquamation and ulceration may be seen. Some patients develop ARDS.

MONITORING AND LABORATORY INVESTIGATIONS IN SHOCK (Table 4.3)

Monitoring is discussed in Chapters 3 and 5, but some further aspects of monitoring the shocked patient will be mentioned here.

Cardiovascular monitoring and investigations

If mistakes are to be avoided, frequent clinical examination is essential, even in the most fully monitored patients. It is usually possible to make some assessment of volume losses in hypovolaemic shock, although such approximations can be grossly inaccurate; in major trauma, for example, losses are often considerably underestimated.

Examination of skin colour, temperature, capillary refill time and the presence or absence of sweating, together with the rate and character of the pulse provides a rapid guide to the severity of shock and the response to treatment. In straightforward cases such as a fit young man with moderate haemorrhage following a road traffic accident (RTA), invasive monitoring may be unnecessary. Clinical assessment combined with frequent blood pressure measurement using a sphygmo-

---

Table 4.3   Monitoring and laboratory investigations in shock.

Cardiovascular	
Clinical assessment	Peripheral perfusion
	Rate and character of pulse
Non-invasive monitoring	ECG
	Blood pressure
	Core–peripheral temperature gradient
	Echocardiography/radionuclide imaging
Invasive monitoring	Intra-arterial blood pressure
	Central venous pressure
	Urine output
	Pulmonary artery flotation catheter (in selected patients including those with major haemorrhage, severe trauma, septic shock, massive pulmonary embolus, myocardial problems, ARDS)
Respiratory	
Clinical assessment	Respiratory rate
Investigations	Chest radiograph
	Blood gas analysis
Investigations	
Biochemistry	Acid–base
	Blood lactate
	Urea and electrolytes
	Blood sugar
	Liver function tests
Haematology	Haemoglobin concentration/packed cell volume
	Coagulation studies
	White blood cell count
Microbiology (in sepsis/septic shock)	Blood cultures
	Urine, sputum, cerebrospinal fluid (in selected cases) and pus for microscopy, culture and sensitivities

manometer may be sufficient. An ECG is non-invasive and allows detection of arrhythmias and myocardial ischaemia.

The more seriously ill and those who fail to respond to initial treatment will require invasive monitoring including *CVP measurement* and *intra-arterial pressure* recording. As discussed in Chapter 3, measurement of the *core-peripheral temperature gradient* (or the big toe temperature related to ambient temperature) together with the *hourly urine output*, provide a useful guide to the adequacy of cardiac output and tissue perfusion in hypovolaemic shock. It has been suggested that *gastric tonometry* is a particularly sensitive indicator of the adequacy of tissue perfusion (see Chapter 3). *Pulmonary artery catheterization* may be indicated in selected cases, including patients with:

- major haemorrhage (e.g. > 8 unit transfusion);
- severe trauma;
- septic shock;
- myocardial problems;
- ARDS;
- massive pulmonary embolism.

Echocardiography or, when available, *radionuclide imaging*, may be used to assess ventricular performance and exclude complications such as mitral valve prolapse (see Chapter 3).

Respiratory monitoring and investigation

The *respiratory rate* must be recorded at frequent intervals and should gradually decrease as the metabolic acidosis resolves. The subsequent development of tachypnoea is an indication that all is not well, and may herald the onset of fat embolism or ARDS.

A *chest radiograph* must always be taken and may initially reveal:

- unsuspected rib fractures;
- pneumothorax;
- haemothorax;
- widening of the mediastinum (suggestive of aortic dissection).

The onset of ARDS will be associated at first with ill-defined diffuse shadowing or a 'ground glass' appearance on the chest radiograph, which may later progress to a mottled appearance with areas of consolidation in an 'alveolar' pattern. Air bronchograms may also be seen (see Chapter 6).

Blood gas analysis may reveal hypoxia with a normal or low $P_a CO_2$. A rising $P_a CO_2$, severe hypoxia, increasing tachypnoea and exhaustion suggest that respiratory support will be required.

Biochemical investigations

Serial determination of *blood lactate levels* provides a guide to the severity of shock, the response to therapy and the prognosis (Bakker *et al.*, 1991). A proportion of septic patients will have a metabolic alkalosis. In some, this may be related to identifiable causes such as massive blood transfusion or hypokalaemia, but in others the aetiology is unclear.

Urea and electrolytes should always be measured since they provide a baseline, which may be useful in the event of subsequent deterioration. They may also reveal unsuspected problems such as pre-existing renal dysfunction. Shocked patients may develop either hypo- or hyperglycaemia (see above) and *blood sugar* levels should always be estimated.

Liver function tests are of importance later since hepatic dysfunction may follow the period of impaired perfusion, and breakdown of transfused blood and haematomas increases bilirubin levels. Total protein and albumin levels should be measured frequently because the albumin concentration is an important determinant of plasma colloid osmotic pressure (COP). The latter can be measured directly using an 'oncometer' and may influence the development of pulmonary oedema (see Chapter 2).

Haematological investigations

The *haemoglobin (Hb) concentration* and *packed cell volume (PCV)* (microhaematocrit) should always be measured although they do not provide a reliable guide to the extent of blood and fluid losses because of the variable degree of haemoconcentration that may occur. They are, however, useful when deciding which solution to use for volume replacement (see later).

Thrombocytopenia and *coagulopathies* may occur, either as a result of transfusing large amounts of stored blood or the development of DIC. A falling platelet count is often the first indication of the latter and the diagnosis may be confirmed by measuring circulating levels of FDPs.

In septic shock, the *white blood cell count* is often raised, with a left shift and toxic granulation, although sometimes the patient is leucopenic. A rising white cell count some time after an episode of shock may indicate the development of sepsis (e.g. an intra-abdominal abscess in a patient with multiple injuries).

Microbiological investigations

In patients with sepsis or septic shock, every effort must be made to identify the source of infection and the causative organism. Samples of urine, sputum, cerebrospinal fluid (when indicated) and pus from drainage sites should be sent to the laboratory for microscopy and culture. *Blood cultures* should also be performed, although they may be negative even when the clinical diagnosis is beyond doubt.

In some cases, the presence of endotoxin in the circulation can be detected using the *'Limulus lysate' test*, even when blood cultures are negative. This test uses an extract of amoebocytes present in the haemolymph of the horseshoe crab (*Limulus polyphemus*), which forms a solid gel within 24 hours of being exposed to endotoxin. This technique has been modified by the introduction of synthetic substrates, which bypass the gelation steps and release a chromophore. The use of these chromogenic substrates increases the sensitivity and specificity of the method and may allow quantification of endotoxaemia (Scully, 1984). This test is usually used only for research.

If an organism is isolated and appropriate antibiotics are administered, the prognosis of septic shock is improved (Kreger *et al.*, 1980). It should be remembered that shock may be the result of infection with rickettsiae, viruses or fungi, as well as bacteria.

MANAGEMENT

General considerations

In all forms of shock, the aim of treatment is to restore oxygen delivery to the tissues (**Fig. 4.11**, see Chapter 2), while at the same time correcting the underlying cause (e.g. by surgical intervention to arrest haemorrhage or eradicate infection). Delay in making the diagnosis and initiating treatment as well as suboptimal resuscitation contribute to the development of vital organ failure and must be avoided. Early recognition of sepsis (see above) allows treatment to be initiated before shock and vital organ damage supervene.

It is important to remember that shocked patients may require analgesia since this is easily overlooked in the heat of the moment. Because of the sluggish muscle blood flow, opiates should be administered in small divided doses intravenously (e.g. morphine 2.5 mg i.v.).

SEPTIC SHOCK/SEPSIS

A thorough clinical examination should first be performed to identify the source of infection, followed by conventional chest and abdominal radiography. In difficult cases, more sophisticated imaging techniques may prove useful. For example, portable real-time *ultrasonography* is non-invasive and can be used at the bedside to localize fluid collections in the chest and abdomen.

It can also demonstrate gallstones, obstruction to the biliary tree and pyonephrosis. Once the collection has been identified, the ultrasound image can be used to guide diagnostic and therapeutic needle aspiration. This can be particularly useful in the case of a loculated empyema. Unfortunately, the ultrasound image is distorted by neighbouring gas-filled structures such as the stomach and large bowel. So, although ultrasound can visualize a right subphrenic abscess satisfactorily, it is less valuable when fluid is suspected in the left subphrenic or paracolic regions. Under these circumstances, a *CT scan* may be more useful, although this will involve moving the patient from the intensive care unit and can therefore be hazardous for unstable patients. CT scanning can also be used to guide percutaneous needle aspiration of fluid collections. *Gallium-67 citrate and indium-labelled white cells* have been used to detect inflammatory foci. They do not, however, differentiate a sterile inflammatory response from septic collections, nor is localization sufficiently accurate to allow needle aspiration.

In patients with intra-abdominal sepsis or abscess formation in any site, an aggressive approach to *surgical exploration* and *drainage of pus* must be adopted. If there is any doubt about the origin of sepsis, all intravascular catheters should be removed and their tips sent for culture. In *toxic shock syndrome*, the tampon, if present, must be removed. This alone may lead to resolution of infection. In *necrotizing fasciitis* (see Chapter 11), radical surgical excision of infected tissue is essential. There is evidence that an *'open abdomen'* approach to the management of severe intra-abdominal sepsis, perhaps with daily laparotomies using a 'zipper' in the abdominal wall, can improve outcome (Garcia-Sabrido *et al.*, 1988).

Appropriate antibiotic therapy is vital in sepsis and should be guided by the source of infection, whether it was acquired in the hospital or in the community, and known local patterns of sensitivity (see Chapter 11).

Respiratory support

The first priority in all acutely ill patients is to *secure the airway*. This often simply requires insertion of an oropharyngeal airway, but in some cases endotracheal intubation may be necessary. The latter also protects the lungs from inhalation of blood, vomit and other debris and is often essential in those with severe facial injuries. Very rarely, emergency cricothyrotomy (Chapter 7) may be required.

All shocked patients should receive supplementary oxygen, and those with severe chest and/or head injuries may require immediate intubation and *mechanical ventilation*. Because of the adverse haemodynamic effects of positive pressure ventilation (Chapter 7), it is

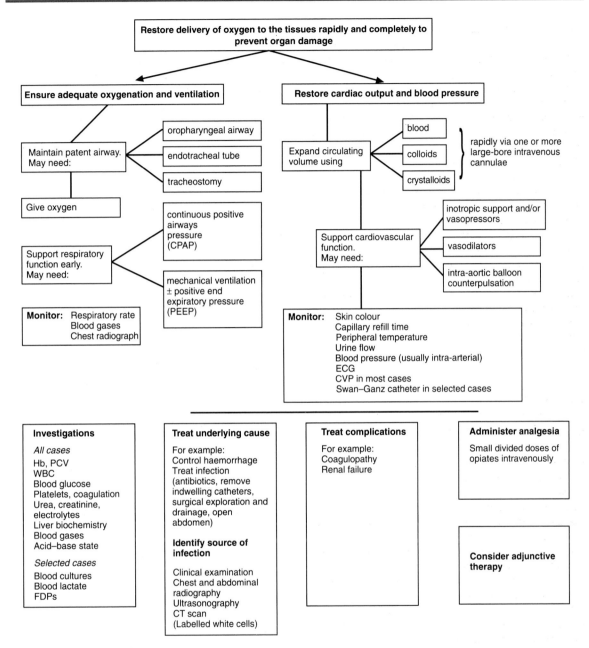

Fig. 4.11 Management of shock.

important (when time allows) to optimize the patient's cardiovascular performance (e.g. by restoring circulating volume) before instituting artificial ventilation. Later, intermittent positive pressure ventilation (IPPV), often combined with PEEP, may be necessary in those patients who develop ARDS.

There is some evidence that the introduction of a standardized treatment regimen that includes the early institution of IPPV and aggressive surgery can improve outcome from septic shock (Ledingham & McArdle, 1978). Because mechanical ventilation abolishes the work of breathing and reduces oxygen consumption it

may also be beneficial in cardiogenic shock (see Chapter 7).

Cardiovascular support

Whatever the aetiology of the haemodynamic disturbance, tissue blood flow must be restored by achieving and maintaining an adequate cardiac output as well as by ensuring that systemic blood pressure is sufficient to maintain perfusion of vital organs. Traditionally a mean arterial pressure (MAP) ≥ 60 mm Hg has been considered to be adequate, but there is some evidence to suggest that 80 mm Hg may be a more appropriate target, and many now believe that the aim should always be to achieve the patient's premorbid blood pressure.

As well as controlling heart rate, the three determinants of stroke volume (pre-load, contractility and after-load) must be manipulated appropriately.

PRE-LOAD AND VOLUME REPLACEMENT

Optimization of pre-load is the most efficient way of increasing cardiac output. Volume replacement is obviously of primary importance in hypovolaemic shock, but is also required in anaphylaxis (see below) and septic shock because of vasodilatation, sequestration of blood and loss of circulating volume due to the increase in capillary permeability. In obstructive shock, high filling pressures may be required to maintain an adequate stroke volume, while even in cardiogenic shock, careful volume expansion may occasionally lead to a useful increase in cardiac output. On the other hand, patients with severe cardiac failure in whom ventricular filling pressures may be markedly elevated can benefit from measures to reduce pre-load (and after-load), such as the administration of diuretics and vasodilators (see later).

A crude clinical assessment of the extent of the volume deficit is usually possible, although, as mentioned previously, these estimates can be very inaccurate. Blood losses are often underestimated, particularly when there are scalp and facial wounds because bandaging merely disguises the extent of the haemorrhage in these very vascular areas. Measurement of Hb, PCV, and urea and electrolytes is usually unhelpful in the early stages of resuscitation.

The clinical response to transfusion (slowing heart rate, improved tissue perfusion and rising blood pressure) may be a sufficient guide to the volume required, but monitoring of CVP and/or PAOP will often be necessary. It is important to appreciate that isolated readings of CVP or PAOP are generally unhelpful and do not provide a meaningful measure of the circulating volume (see also Chapter 2). Ideally volume replacement should be titrated to achieve the PAOP (or CVP) that produces optimum ventricular stroke work. In hypovolaemic and septic shock, a PAOP of around 12 mm Hg is usually associated with peak left ventricular stroke work (Packman & Rackow, 1983). When interpreting these variables, it is important to appreciate that ventricular compliance is often reduced in shock. In view of the increased capillary permeability, particularly in those with sepsis, it is sometimes sensible to limit volume requirements by using inotropic support and vasopressors to achieve the desired cardiac output and MAP.

The circulating volume must be replaced as quickly as possible (i.e. within minutes not hours) since rapid restoration of cardiac output and perfusion pressure reduces the chances of serious organ damage, particularly the development of acute renal failure. Therefore, in many patients with severe haemorrhagic shock, two or more large-bore intravenous cannulae will be required so that fluid can be transfused rapidly under pressure. Careful monitoring will ensure that despite this aggressive approach, volume overload does not occur.

Failure to respond to fluid replacement should prompt a careful search for complications such as tension pneumothorax, cardiac tamponade or significant continued bleeding.

The clinical use of a 'G-suit' (*military antishock trousers—MAST*) to limit blood loss and reduce venous pooling in victims of massive trauma was first described in Vietnam. Although the application of MAST helps to maintain blood pressure, it can interfere with ventilation, and deflation may be associated with profound hypotension. The use of MAST remains controversial, but they may help to tamponade intra-abdominal haemorrhage in some cases, especially in those with pelvic fractures or severe retroperitoneal haemorrhage.

In patients with massive rapid blood loss, salvaging and retransfusion of shed blood (*Autotransfusion*) can be extremely useful. The safest technique is probably to use a red cell saver, which washes the cells prior to reinfusion and avoids the risks of coagulopathy and air embolism. Filtration systems are cheaper and have been improved, while post-cardiac surgery chest drainage blood is defibrinated and can be easily retransfused.

Choice of fluid for volume replacement

Blood. In haemorrhagic shock it would seem logical to replenish the circulating volume with whole blood as soon as it becomes available. In other forms of shock, transfusion of plasma-reduced blood or concentrated red cells may be required to maintain the Hb concentration at acceptable levels. In extreme emergencies, uncrossmatched O-negative blood can be used, but an emergency crossmatch can be performed in only 30 minutes and is almost as safe as the standard procedure. Donor blood is usually separated into its various components and it is therefore necessary to transfuse concentrated red cells or plasma-reduced blood to maintain adequate levels of Hb, and use plasma or a plasma substitute for volume replacement. It has been suggested that limited normovolaemic haemodilution (PCV 25–30%) might improve tissue oxygen delivery since the reduction in oxygen-carrying capacity may be offset by an increase in cardiac output and improved distribution of flow through the microcirculation. Moreover, there is evidence that transfusing old red blood cells to patients with sepsis fails to improve oxygen uptake and may precipitate splanchnic ischaemia, perhaps because poorly deformable transfused cells cause microcirculatory occlusion (Marik & Sibbald, 1993).

Blood transfusion may be complicated by:

- incompatibility reactions;
- immunosuppression;
- pyrexia due to contained pyrogens;
- transmission of diseases such as viral hepatitis and human immunodeficiency virus (HIV).

It has been estimated that in the USA the risk of acquiring HIV for a patient receiving an average blood transfusion is approximately 1 in 28,000 (Cumming *et al.*, 1989). Most recipients of HIV-infected blood become seropositive and AIDS develops in about half of these patients within seven years (Ward *et al.*, 1989).

Other special problems may arise when large volumes of stored blood are transfused rapidly. These include the following:

- *Hypothermia.* Bank blood is stored at 4°C and if large volumes are transfused, the patient will become hypothermic. Furthermore, peripheral venoconstriction may slow the rate of the infusion, and cold blood transfused rapidly through a centrally placed cannula can induce arrhythmias. Some therefore recommend that blood should be warmed during transfusion.
- *Microembolism.* Stored blood contains microaggregates, consisting mainly of dead platelets and leucocytes. The majority are not removed by the filters present in normal giving sets, which have a pore size of approximately 120 μm. Some consider microemboli to be a contributory factor to the development of ARDS and suggest that pulmonary dysfunction in trauma patients may be prevented or ameliorated by removing these microaggregates with 40 μm filters (Reul *et al.*, 1973). Others have suggested, however, that hypoxaemia in trauma patients is more dependent on the nature and severity of the injury than massive blood transfusion (Collins *et al.*, 1978), and the value of routine filtration remains unproven. The disadvantages of such filters include the cost and slowing the rate of transfusion, but some still recommend their use, particularly when large volumes of blood are administered. It has been suggested that fine-screen filtration reduces the incidence of febrile reactions to transfused blood by removing most of the leucocytes (Schned & Silver, 1981). Fresh blood should not be filtered since this will remove functioning platelets and possibly viable clotting factors.
- *Coagulopathy.* Stored blood has essentially no effective platelets and is deficient in clotting factors. Consequently, with large transfusions, a coagulation defect may develop. This should be treated by replacing clotting factors with fresh frozen plasma (FFP) and the administration of platelet concentrates. Very

occasionally, cryoprecipitate can be used to correct a proven deficiency of factor VIII.

- *Metabolic acidosis/alkalosis.* Stored blood is now preserved in citrate/phosphate/dextrose (CPD), which is less acidic than the acid/citrate/dextrose (ACD) solution used previously. Metabolic acidosis attributable solely to blood transfusion is unusual and in any case rarely requires correction (see below). Patients will often develop a metabolic alkalosis 24–48 hours after a large blood transfusion, probably largely due to citrate metabolism, and this will be exacerbated if the preceding acidosis has been corrected with intravenous sodium bicarbonate.
- *Hypocalcaemia.* Stored blood is anticoagulated using citrate, which binds the calcium ions required for clotting. When this blood is transfused rapidly, excess citrate may reduce total body ionized calcium levels, causing myocardial depression. This is uncommon in practice, but if necessary can be corrected by administering 10 ml of 10% calcium chloride intravenously. Routine administration of calcium is not recommended.
- *Increased oxygen affinity.* As mentioned in Chapter 2, the position of the oxyhaemoglobin dissociation curve is influenced by the concentration of 2,3-diphosphoglycerate (DPG) in the red cell. In stored blood, the red cell 2,3-DPG content is reduced so that the curve is shifted to the left. The oxygen affinity of Hb is therefore increased and oxygen delivery is impaired. This effect is less marked with CPD blood. Red cell levels of 2,3-DPG are substantially restored within 12 hours of transfusion.
- *Hyperkalaemia.* Potassium levels in stored blood rise progressively. When the blood is warmed prior to transfusion, however, the cells begin to metabolize, the sodium pump becomes active and potassium levels fall. Hyperkalaemia is rarely a problem with massive transfusions.

Recently, nutrient additive solutions have been developed that allow red cell storage in the absence of plasma. In this way plasma extraction from donor blood is maximized, the shelf-life of the red cell suspensions is prolonged and transfusion is facilitated by the reduction in viscosity. The most commonly used additive is SAG (saline, adenine, glucose) to which mannitol (M) is now added to reduce spontaneous lysis (*SAGM blood*). One possible disadvantage of these suspensions is that macroaggregates may form progressively and ways of minimizing this problem are currently being investigated.

In view of these complications of blood transfusion, particularly the risk of transmitting disease, as well as the expense, many centres are attempting to reduce their use of stored blood. It is well recognized that previously fit patients who have an episode of haemorrhagic shock can survive with extremely low Hb concentrations provided their circulating volume, and thus their ability to maintain an adequate cardiac output, is maintained. It is, however, a matter of opinion whether a modest degree of anaemia (Hb 10 g/dl, PCV 30%) is advantageous because of improved flow through the microcirculation or is disadvantageous because tissue oxygen delivery can only be maintained by an increased cardiac output or hypervolaemia.

Because of these considerations as well as the trend towards 'component' therapy mentioned before, the use of crystalloid solutions, plasma, plasma substitutes and oxygen-carrying solutions is assuming greater importance in the management of shock.

Crystalloid solutions. Although crystalloid solutions (e.g. normal (0.9%) saline, Ringers–lactate) are cheap (**Table 4.4**), convenient to use and free of side-effects, the use of large volumes of these fluids should in general be avoided. They are rapidly distributed across the intravascular and interstitial spaces, and volumes of crystalloid 2–4 times that of colloid are required to achieve an equivalent haemodynamic response (Virgilio *et al.*, 1979; Rackow *et al.*, 1983). Moreover, volume expansion is transitory, COP is reduced (Virgilio *et al.*, 1979; Rackow *et al.*, 1983), fluid accumulates in the interstitial spaces, and pulmonary oedema may be precipitated (Rackow *et al.*, 1983). It has also been suggested that the development of peripheral oedema may impair tissue oxygenation, delay wound healing and decrease gastrointestinal motility and absorptive capacity.

In one study of patients undergoing intra-abdominal vascular surgery, pulmonary function on the first postoperative day was significantly worse in the group receiving crystalloid than in those given colloid (Skillman *et al.*, 1975). Nevertheless, others have demonstrated that such patients tolerate large volumes of crystalloid well (Virgilio *et al.*, 1979) and it appears that

any excess fluid is rapidly mobilized once the stress response abates. Moreover, in hypovolaemic shock both the interstitial and intracellular compartments are eventually depleted as fluid moves into the intravascular space and crystalloid solutions can be used to correct these deficits. Although volume replacement with predominantly crystalloid solutions is therefore advocated by some authorities for the uncomplicated previously healthy patient with traumatic or perioperative hypovolaemia, a more reasonable approach is to use crystalloids initially, but to use colloids as well if there is a continued need for volume replacement in excess of about one litre.

It is worth noting that 5% dextrose equilibrates with both the interstitial and intracellular spaces and is useless for expanding the intravascular compartment. Conversely *hyperosmotic sodium chloride* draws large volumes of intracellular water into the extracellular space and some have suggested that this fluid may be valuable in the early stages of resuscitation. Hyperosmotic saline may reduce myocardial oedema and the risk of subendocardial ischaemia. There is, however, little evidence that it is more effective than conventional fluid replacement and major limiting factors include hypernatraemia, reduced intracellular volume and hyperosmolality.

Colloidal solutions. These produce a greater and more sustained increase in plasma volume with associated improvements in cardiovascular function, oxygen transport and oxygen consumption. They also increase colloid osmotic pressure (Rackow *et al.*, 1983) and if the circulating volume is promptly restored with colloids, depletion of the interstitial and intravascular spaces can be avoided. When capillary permeability is increased, however, these substances may escape from the intravascular compartment and increase interstitial oncotic pressure, thereby enhancing oedema formation (Holcroft & Trunkey, 1974; Weaver *et al.*, 1978) and slowing its resolution. Colloidal solutions may also inhibit a saline diuresis (Weaver *et al.*, 1978). A meta-analysis of clinical trials did little to resolve the controversy. Although there was a tendency in favour of crystalloid resuscitation in trauma patients, whereas the use of colloids seemed to be associated with improved outcome in non-septic and elective surgical patients, none of the differences in mortality were statistically significant (Velanovich, 1989). In the authors' view, all forms of fluid replacement can be hazardous, particularly when capillary permeability is increased, but in most critically ill patients colloids should be used in preference to administering large volumes of crystalloid. Colloids include the following.

- *Natural colloids.* Human albumin solution (HAS) is prepared by fractionating donor plasma and is heat-treated to inactivate contaminating viruses. It has a

Table 4.4 Comparison of cost of fluids used for volume replacement.

Fluid	Cost (£)/500 ml (approximate)
Normal saline	0.78
Ringers-lactate	1.25
Haemaccel	3.43
Gelofusine	3.56
Dextran 70	4.90
Elohes	9.75
Hespan	16.72
Albumin 4.5%	29.50
Albumin 20%	142.50

similar colloid osmotic pressure to plasma and is now widely available, although expensive. In normal subjects, HAS will expand the circulating volume by an amount roughly equivalent to the volume infused. It has a half-life in the circulation of 10–15 days, although in those with increased capillary permeability this is considerably reduced. As HAS has the same sodium content as plasma, this may be a disadvantage in those at risk of developing hypernatraemia. Although anaphylactoid reactions are rare, they do occur in less than 1% of cases. HAS should not be used for routine volume replacement, particularly if losses are continuing, since other cheaper solutions (see **Table 4.4**) are equally effective in the short term. In a recent randomized comparison the use of albumin rather than 3.5% polygeline (see below) for volume replacement had no influence on mortality, length of stay in intensive care or the incidence of pulmonary oedema and renal failure (Stockwell *et al.*, 1992a & b). Clinically significant hypoalbuminaemia may be associated with hypovolaemia, oedema, pleural effusions and ascites. Under these circumstances administration of albumin in combination with diuretics may be indicated. In those who are hypernatraemic and/or at risk of fluid overload concentrated 20% albumin may be used. HAS is also an appropriate replacement fluid for patients undergoing plasma exchange.

- *Dextrans*. These are polymolecular polysaccharides contained in either 5% dextrose or normal saline. Low-molecular weight dextran (mol. wt 40,000) has a powerful osmotic effect so that fluid moves from the extravascular to the intravascular compartment, thereby expanding the circulating volume by approximately twice the volume infused. Although viscosity is reduced, this may be counterbalanced by a decrease in the flexibility of the red cells. Dextran 40 is rapidly excreted by the kidneys and its effect is therefore relatively short-lived. It can form a complex with fibrinogen, thereby inducing a coagulopathy. It also coats the red cell membrane so that blood must be taken for crossmatching before giving it. Dextran 70 (mol. wt 70,000) is also hyperoncotic, although less so than dextran 40, and also interferes with crossmatching. It has a longer half-life, however, and is probably the most suitable dextran for routine use. There is a small risk of delayed allergic reactions to all the dextrans. Anaphylactic reactions, which are extremely violent and life-threatening, are increasing in frequency.

- *Polygelatin solutions (Haemaccel, Gelofusine)*. These have an average mol. wt of 35,000 and are iso-osmotic with plasma. The only important difference between the two solutions is that Haemaccel has about ten times more calcium (6.3 mmol/l) and potassium (5.1 mmol/l) than Gelofusine. They do not interfere with crossmatching. It appears that large volumes of polygelatins can be given with impunity since coagulation defects do not occur and they do not impair renal function. They are also cheap. Because they readily cross the glomerular basement membrane their half-life in the circulation is only 4–5 hours and they can promote a diuresis. There is also some evidence that high molecular weight gelatin complexes may leak out of the capillaries, exacerbating pulmonary oedema. Moreover, administration of large volumes of gelatins represents a considerable saline load. These solutions are particularly useful during the acute phase of resuscitation, especially when volume losses are continuing, but in many patients colloids with a longer half-life will be required later to achieve haemodynamic stability. The incidence of allergic reactions (0.5–10%) is probably greater than with the dextrans.

- *Hydroxyethyl starches (HES)*. These are rather more expensive than the gelatins, but cheaper than HAS (see **Table 4.4**). Elimination of HES occurs via the kidneys following hydrolysis by amylase. HES are also stored transiently in the reticuloendothelial system, but apparently without causing functional impairment. The commonly used HES have a mean mol. wt of approximately 450,000 and a half-life of about 12 hours. Volume expansion is equivalent to, or slightly greater than, the volume infused. The reported incidence of allergic reactions is approximately 0.1%. There is some concern that infusion of large volumes may precipitate a coagulopathy, partly by decreasing factor VIII activity and prolonging the partial thromboplastin time (Stump *et al.*, 1985).

Oxygen-carrying blood substitutes (Urbaniak, 1991). The ideal solution for volume replacement in shock would have an oncotic pressure similar to plasma with a long half-life, no risk of transmissible disease, zero incidence of allergic reactions, no requirement for crossmatching and a long shelf-life at room temperature. It would also carry oxygen. Some progress was made towards attaining the latter objective with the development of *fluorocarbon emulsions* (Fluosol-DA20); these contain HES, electrolytes and an emulsifying agent. Unfortunately they have a linear oxygen dissociation curve and only contribute significantly to oxygen delivery when alveolar oxygen tension is relatively high. Furthermore, they have a short intravascular half-life and are associated with a number of adverse reactions, including pulmonary toxicity, possibly related to complement activation and cytokine release initiated by the detergent used to maintain emulsion stability. These solutions are not therefore considered suitable for clinical use and are not commercially available.

Hb solutions also have potential as oxygen-delivering resuscitation fluids. The use of pure 'stroma-free' Hb was limited by nephrotoxicity, hypotensive reactions, a short intravascular half-life and high oxygen affinity. More recent developments have included polymerizing pyridoxalated stroma-free Hb with glutaraldehyde, encapsulating Hb inside synthetic lipid membranes, and the production of recombinant Hbs. None of these approaches has yet produced a clinically acceptable blood substitute.

INOTROPIC AND VASOACTIVE AGENTS

As discussed above, myocardial contractility may be impaired either as the primary abnormality (cardiogenic shock) or as a secondary phenomenon in severe hypovolaemic, anaphylactic or septic shock.

Before instituting specific measures to stimulate the myocardium, however, it is important to identify and if possible correct any of the various associated abnormalities that can impair cardiac performance. These include:

● hypoxia;
● hypocalcaemia;
● the effects of some drugs (e.g. β-blockers, antiarrhythmics and sedatives).

Correction of metabolic acidosis

Conventionally extreme acidosis is also said to depress myocardial contractility and may limit the response to vasopressor agents, although in dogs infused with lactic acid to achieve a pH ≤ 7.2 cardiac output was unaffected (Arieff *et al.*, 1983) and attempted correction of acidosis with intravenous sodium bicarbonate may be detrimental. Additional carbon dioxide is generated and, because carbon dioxide, but not the bicarbonate ion, readily diffuses across the cell membrane, intracellular pH is further reduced. Moreover, when compared to sodium chloride administration infusion of bicarbonate in hypoxic dogs was associated with a reduction in MAP and cardiac output, and a greater increase in lactate levels (Graf *et al.*, 1985). Other potential disadvantages of bicarbonate therapy include sodium overload, hyperosmolality, and a left shift of the oxyhaemoglobin dissociation curve. Also ionized calcium levels may be reduced and, in combination with the fall in intracellular pH may be responsible for impaired myocardial performance.

In a prospective, randomized, controlled, cross-over clinical study both sodium bicarbonate and sodium chloride produced slight increases in PAOP and cardiac output, while MAP was unchanged. Sodium bicarbonate

significantly increased pH and plasma bicarbonate, but unlike sodium chloride, decreased ionized calcium and increased both $P_a\text{CO}_2$ and end-tidal carbon dioxide. The response to infused catecholamines was unaffected (Cooper *et al.*, 1990). In general, therefore, treatment of lactic acidosis should concentrate on correcting the cause, while acidosis may be most safely controlled by hyperventilation. Administration of bicarbonate may still be useful in renal tubular acidosis and in acidosis due to gastrointestinal losses of bicarbonate.

Some alternative agents for correcting lactic acidosis have been described including *dichloroacetate* and *carbicarb*. Dichloroacetate stimulates pyruvate dehydrogenase, the enzyme responsible for catalysing the oxidation of pyruvate to acetyl CoA. In a controlled trial, dichloroacetate treatment of patients with severe lactic acidosis produced unimpressive changes in arterial blood lactate and pH and failed to alter haemodynamics or survival (Stacpoole *et al.*, 1992). Carbicarb is an equimolar solution of sodium bicarbonate and disodium carbonate. This buffer can raise pH without increasing carbon dioxide levels and may improve haemodynamics (Bersin & Arieff, 1988). Its role in the treatment of lactic acidosis has yet to be clarified.

'Goal directed' therapy

If the signs of shock persist despite adequate volume replacement, and perfusion of vital organs is jeopardized, pressor agents may be administered to improve cardiac output and blood pressure. Although conventionally the objective has been to achieve normal haemodynamics it is clear that survival of patients with septic or traumatic shock (as well as following major surgery and those with ARDS) is associated with elevated values for cardiac output, $D\text{O}_2$ and $\dot{V}\text{O}_2$ (Shoemaker *et al.*, 1973; Tuchschmidt *et al.*, 1989; Russell *et al.*, 1990).

It would seem that in order to recover from major acute illness or injury patients must sustain a hypermetabolic state by increasing cardiac output and $D\text{O}_2$ to satisfy the increased cellular oxygen requirements and compensate for impaired oxygen extraction (see supply dependency above). Some have therefore advocated that in high-risk surgical patients treatment should be directed at increasing cardiac output, $D\text{O}_2$ and $\dot{V}\text{O}_2$ until they equal or exceed the median values found in survivors (i.e. cardiac index $> 4.5 \, \text{l/min/m}^2$, $D\text{O}_2 > 600 \, \text{ml/min/m}^2$ and $\dot{V}\text{O}_2 > 170 \, \text{ml/min/m}^2$) in order to replenish tissue oxygen and prevent organ dysfunction (Shoemaker *et al.*, 1973). In one study early institution of treatment aimed at achieving these survivor values was shown to improve survival after major surgery (Shoemaker *et al.*, 1988), and in another the use of dopexamine (see later) to increase perioperative oxygen delivery reduced mortality in high-risk patients (Boyd *et al.*, 1993). Other authors have suggested that elevation of systemic D_{O_2} and $\dot{V}_{O_2}$ to levels that some have called 'supranormal' might also improve outcome in patients with septic shock (Edwards *et al.*, 1989; Tuchschmidt *et al.*, 1992) as well as in heterogeneous groups of critically ill patients (Yu *et al.*, 1993) and trauma victims (Fleming *et al.*, 1992).

In some patients, however, it may prove impossible to achieve target values for $\dot{V}_{O_2}$, partly because reduced cardiac reserves limit the increase in D_{O_2}, but mainly because of flow maldistribution and an inability of the tissues to extract or use oxygen. As a result increases in D_{O_2} are accompanied by a rising $S_{\bar{v}}_{O_2}$ and a fall in oxygen extraction; lactate levels remain elevated. In such patients the prognosis is very poor (Hayes *et al.*, 1993), and the use of high doses of inotropic vasoactive agents may be associated with an increased incidence of complications such as myocardial ischaemia, tachyarrhythmias and maldistribution of tissue flow. Moreover, a recent prospective, randomized, controlled trial in a heterogeneous group of critically ill patients demonstrated that, provided volume replacement is adequate, perfusion pressure is well maintained (MAP > 80 mm Hg) and cardiac output is kept within the normal range, outcome is not improved by instituting treatment with dobutamine at the time of admission to the intensive care unit in an attempt to achieve survivor values of D_{O_2} and $\dot{V}_{O_2}$ (Hayes *et al.*, 1994). In these patients it was often impossible to increase $\dot{V}_{O_2}$ and it seemed that aggressive attempts to boost oxygen consumption may in some cases have been detrimental. Although unselective targeting of 'supranormal' D_{O_2} and $\dot{V}_{O_2}$ following admission to intensive care cannot therefore be recommended, some still believe that less aggressive treatment more precisely tailored to an individual patient's requirements may be more effective. It is also possible that there are advantages to targeting D_{O_2} rather than $\dot{V}_{O_2}$, that alternative inotropic agents may be more efficacious, and that certain subgroups of patients, such as trauma patients, may benefit from such treatment.

Others believe that the ability to achieve the recommended target values simply indicates an adequate physiological reserve and therefore a good prognosis. This suggestion is supported by a recent study demonstrating the prognostic value of the responses of D_{O_2} and $\dot{V}_{O_2}$ to a short infusion of dobutamine in patients with sepsis syndrome and normal lactate levels (Vallet *et al.*, 1993).

Nevertheless most would agree that early institution of aggressive haemodynamic support, in particular adequate volume replacement (see above) combined with the rational use of inotropic and/or vasoactive agents, can improve outcome from critical illness and is likely to be particularly efficacious when instituted peroperatively in high-risk surgical patients. The authors believe that in the majority of high-risk patients such treatment should be guided by haemodynamic monitoring using a pulmonary artery catheter.

Choice of inotropic/vasoactive agent

The rational selection of an appropriate pressor agent depends on a thorough understanding of the cardiovascular effects of the available drugs, combined with an accurate assessment of the haemodynamic disturbance. The effects of a particular agent in an individual patient are unpredictable and the response must therefore be closely monitored so that the regimen can be altered appropriately if necessary. In most cases this requires pulmonary artery catheterization, measurement of cardiac output and calculation of derived variables (see Chapter 3). In some patients, inotropes are administered to redistribute blood flow (e.g. dopamine to increase renal blood flow, dopexamine to improve splanchnic perfusion), and in others inotropic support can be usefully combined with the administration of a vasodilator (see below). All inotropic agents should be given via a large central vein.

The most popular of the currently available inotropes are discussed below.

Adrenaline

Adrenaline stimulates both α- and β-receptors, but at low doses β effects seem to predominate. This produces a tachycardia with an increase in cardiac index and a fall in peripheral resistance, while at higher doses, α-mediated vasoconstriction develops. If the latter produces useful increases in cardiac output and perfusion pressure, urine output may nevertheless increase and renal failure may be avoided. As the dose is further increased, however, cardiac output may actually fall and be associated with signs of marked vasoconstriction, tachycardia and the development of a metabolic acidosis. Under these circumstances, the reduction in renal blood flow usually causes oliguria and may precipitate acute renal failure.

Despite these disadvantages, adrenaline remains an extremely useful inotrope. It is very potent and may prove successful when other agents have failed, particularly following cardiac surgery. This may be because it stimulates myocardial α-receptors. It can also be useful in patients with severe hypotension associated with a low systemic resistance, and it is increasingly accepted as a cheap effective means of reversing hypotension and increasing oxygen delivery in septic shock resistant to dopamine (Bollaert *et al.*, 1990). To avoid oliguria, renal failure and metabolic acidosis, the minimum effective dose should be used, and its administration should be discontinued as soon as possible. It is possible that the addition of 'low-dose' dopamine to the regimen may help to preserve renal function (see below).

Noradrenaline

Noradrenaline is predominantly an α-agonist. It may be of value in severe hypotension associated with a low systemic resistance (e.g. in intractable septic shock, Meadows *et al.*, 1988). Administration of noradrenaline to such patients is associated with an increase in systemic vascular resistance, while cardiac output is unchanged or increased. When blood pressure is restored to above a critical threshold, urine flow and creatinine clearance increase (Martin *et al.*, 1990). The combination of dopamine with noradrenaline may further enhance renal blood flow. There is a risk of producing excessive vasoconstriction with impaired organ perfusion, peripheral ischaemia and increased after-load. Administration of high doses of noradrenaline has been implicated as a contributory factor in the development of symmetrical peripheral gangrene (Hayes *et al.*, 1992). Noradrenaline administration should therefore normally be accompanied by full haemodyamic monitoring including determination of cardiac output and calculation of the systemic vascular resistance.

Isoprenaline

This β-stimulant has both inotropic and chronotropic effects, and also reduces peripheral resistance by dilating skin and muscle blood vessels (Holloway *et al.*, 1975). This latter effect means that much of the increased flow is diverted away from vital organs such as the kidneys and may account for the oliguria that can be associated with its use. Most of the increase in cardiac output produced by isoprenaline is due to the tachycardia (Holloway *et al.*, 1975) and this, together with the development of arrhythmias, seriously limits its value. There are now few indications for isoprenaline in the critically ill adult.

Salbutamol

Salbutamol is predominantly a β₂-stimulant and therefore dilates vessels in skeletal muscle and splanchnic beds. It can cause a marked tachycardia, may precipitate arrhythmias, and has only minimal effects on stroke volume. In general, its cardiac effects are less violent than those of isoprenaline and it may therefore occasionally prove useful in post-cardiac surgery patients, especially those with bradycardia.

Dopamine

Compared with isoprenaline, dopamine, which is a precursor of noradrenaline, causes less tachycardia, is less arrhythmogenic and has a relatively greater effect on stroke volume (Holloway *et al.*, 1975). Dopamine acts on β₁ and, to a lesser extent β₂ receptors, α-receptors and dopaminergic DA1 and DA2 receptors. When used in low doses, peripheral resistance falls, largely due to DA1 receptor-mediated dilatation of splanchnic and renal vasculature. Renal and hepatic blood flow increase (Schmid *et al.*, 1979), urine output is improved (Davis *et al.*, 1982), and it is possible that failure of these vital organs is thereby prevented (see Chapter 12). The importance of the renal vasodilator effect of dopamine has, however, been questioned and it has been suggested that the increased urine output is largely attributable to the rise in cardiac output, combined with a decrease in aldosterone concentrations and inhibition of tubular sodium reabsorption mediated via DA1-stimulation. Dopamine also increases noradrenaline release and at higher doses vasoconstriction occurs, increasing after-load and raising ventricular filling pressures. This can be dangerous in patients with cardiac failure in whom LAP is already high. There is also some evidence to suggest that the use of dopamine to achieve a target MAP > 75 mm Hg may precipitate gut mucosal ischaemia, whereas noradrenaline can improve splanchnic oxygenation (Marik & Mohedin, 1994), and in an animal model of haemorrhagic shock even low-dose dopamine hastened the onset of splanchnic ischaemia (Segal *et al.*, 1992). In some patients the dose of dopamine is limited by β-receptor effects such as tachycardia and arrhythmias.

Dopexamine

Dopexamine is an analogue of dopamine and activates β₂ receptors as well as DA1 and DA2 receptors. It is more potent at DA1 than DA2 receptors and also inhibits neuronal re-uptake of noradrenaline. Dopexamine is a very weak positive inotrope, but is a powerful splanchnic vasodilator, reducing afterload and improving blood flow to vital organs, including the kidney. It is an effective natriuretic and diuretic agent. At higher doses a fall in diastolic pressure and MAP may reduce regional blood flow. In septic shock, dopexamine can increase cardiac index and heart rate, but causes further reductions in systemic vascular resistance (Colardyn *et al.*, 1989). It has been suggested that this agent is likely to be most useful in the management of low-output left ventricular failure, although it may also prove to be a valuable adjunct to the perioperative management of high-risk patients (Boyd *et al.*, 1993).

Dobutamine

Dobutamine is closely related to dopamine and similarly causes less tachycardia and arrhythmias than isoprenaline. When compared with dopamine, however, the relative effects of the two agents on heart rate and rhythm are a matter of dispute. Dobutamine has no specific effect on the renal vasculature, although urine output often increases as cardiac output and blood pressure improve. The advantage of dobutamine lies in its ability to reduce systemic resistance, as well as improve cardiac performance, thereby decreasing both after-load and ventricular filling pressures. Dobutamine is therefore useful in patients with cardiogenic shock and cardiac failure. In septic shock the addition of dobutamine to a standard protocol increased cardiac output, Do_2 and $\dot{V}o_2$, while in some cases systemic vascular resistance fell (Vincent *et al.*, 1990). Dobutamine may be particularly useful in septic patients with fluid overload or myocardial failure (Jardin *et al.*, 1981).

Enoximone

Enoximone is active both orally and intravenously, and is a phosphodiesterase III inhibitor with inotropic and vasodilator properties. Myocardial oxygen demand is not greatly increased, but there is a danger that excessive vasodilatation may precipitate or worsen systemic hypotension. The effects of enoximone may be additive with those of catecholamines and the addition of this agent to standard adrenergic support can markedly increase cardiac output and stroke volume in cardiogenic shock (Vincent *et al.*, 1988). Because enoximone acts beyond the β-receptor it may be useful in patients wit- receptor 'down-regulation' and in those receiving β blockers.

A disadvantage of all these agents

When used in patients with respiratory failure all these agents increase venous admixture; this may be due simply to passive opening of pulmonary vessels by the increased flow and pressure or to a specific reversal of the hypoxic vasoconstrictor response.

Receptor 'down-regulation'

Many of the most seriously ill patients become increasingly resistant to the effects of pressor agents, an observation attributed to 'down-regulation' of adrenergic receptors. This may be due to a reduction in receptor numbers, or a decreased affinity of the receptor for its ligand induced by overstimulation or by a direct effect of inflammatory mediators on the cell membrane. The resultant vascular hyporeactivity to both endogenous and exogenous catecholamines is a particular feature of septic shock.

Summary

Some still consider dopamine to be the inotrope of choice in most critically ill patients, largely because of its effects on splanchnic blood flow. Dobutamine is equally popular and is particularly indicated in cases where the vasoconstriction caused by dopamine could be dangerous (i.e. in those with cardiac disease and septic patients with fluid overload or myocardial failure). The combination of dobutamine and noradrenaline is currently popular for the management of patients who are shocked with a low systemic vascular resistance. Dobutamine is given to achieve an optimal cardiac output, while noradrenaline is used to restore an adequate blood pressure by limiting the degree of vasodilatation. This combination of agents has been shown to be an effective means of achieving survivor values for Do_2 and $\dot{V}o_2$, and maintaining perfusion pressure in patients with septic shock (Edwards *et al.*, 1989).

Adrenaline, because of its potency, remains a useful agent in those patients unresponsive to other measures, especially after cardiac surgery, and is a cheap effective agent for the management of septic shock (Bollaert *et al.*, 1990).

Finally, *digoxin* has been shown to exert a positive inotropic effect in patients with severe sepsis and cardiac failure (Nasraway *et al.*, 1989), although its use solely for its inotropic properties remains controversial.

VASODILATOR THERAPY, AFTER-LOAD AND PRE-LOAD REDUCTION

In selected patients, after-load reduction may be used to increase stroke volume and decrease myocardial oxygen requirements by reducing systolic wall tension. Vasodilatation also decreases heart size and diastolic ventricular wall tension so that coronary blood flow is improved. The relative magnitude of the falls in pre-load and after-load depends on the pre-existing haemodynamic disturbance, concurrent volume replacement and the agent selected (see later).

Vasodilator therapy is most beneficial in patients with cardiac failure in whom the ventricular function curve is flat, and falls in pre-load have only a limited effect on stroke volume. This form of treatment, combined in selected cases with inotropic support, can therefore sometimes be useful in cardiogenic shock and in patients with pulmonary oedema associated with low cardiac output, mitral regurgitation or an acute ventricular septal defect. Furthermore, because of their ability to improve the myocardial oxygen supply : demand ratio, vasodilators can be used to control angina and limit ischaemic damage following myocardial infarction. They may also be valuable in shocked patients who remain vasoconstricted and oliguric despite restoration of an adequate blood pressure, and in controlling hypertension (e.g. in post-cardiac surgery patients).

Vasodilator therapy is potentially dangerous and vasodilatation should be achieved cautiously, guided by continuous haemodynamic monitoring, usually including pulmonary artery catheterization or direct measurement of LAP. The circulating volume must be adequate before treatment is started and, except in those with cardiac failure, falls in pre-load should be prevented to avoid serious reductions in cardiac output and blood pressure. If diastolic pressure is allowed to fall, coronary blood flow may be jeopardized and myocardial ischaemia may be precipitated, particularly if a reflex tachycardia develops in response to the hypotension. Provided myocardial performance is not impaired, it is therefore sometimes appropriate to control the tachycardia with a β-blocker. It is also important to appreciate that currently available vasodilators reverse hypoxic pulmonary vasoconstriction and increase intrapulmonary shunt (D'Oliveira et al., 1981).

The selection of an appropriate agent in an individual patient depends on a careful assessment of the haemodynamic disturbance and on whether the effect required is predominantly a reduction in pre-load, after-load or both.

Adrenergic blockers

Adrenergic blockers predominantly dilate arterioles and therefore mainly influence after-load. Phenoxybenzamine is unsuitable for use in the critically ill because of its slow onset of action (1–2 hours to maximum effect) and prolonged duration of effect (2–3 days). Phentolamine is very potent with a rapid onset and short duration of action (15–20 minutes). It can be used to control blood pressure acutely in hypertensive crises, but may produce a marked tachycardia and is too expensive to administer as a continuous infusion.

Direct-acting vasodilators

Direct-acting vasodilators are the agents most commonly used to achieve vasodilatation in the critically ill.

Hydralazine. This predominantly affects arterial resistance vessels. It therefore reduces after-load and blood pressure while cardiac output and heart rate increase. Renal and limb blood flow are also increased. Hydrala-

zine can be administered orally to patients with chronic cardiac failure, but in intensive care practice it is usually given as an intravenous bolus (5–10 mg) to control acute increases in blood pressure, particularly after cardiac surgery.

Sodium nitroprusside (SNP). This dilates both arterioles and venous capacitance vessels, and the pulmonary vasculature. It therefore reduces the after-load and pre-load of both ventricles and can improve cardiac output and the myocardial oxygen supply : demand ratio. Some authorities have suggested, however, that SNP can exacerbate myocardial ischaemia by producing a 'steal' phenomenon in the coronary circulation (Chiariello et al., 1976). The increased cardiac output is preferentially distributed to musculoskeletal regions. If arterial pressure falls, hepatic and renal blood flow are unchanged, whereas if pressure is maintained, splanchnic flow increases slightly.

The effects of SNP are rapid in onset and spontaneously reversible within a few minutes of discontinuing the infusion. Moreover, tachyphylaxis is not a problem.

An overdose of SNP can cause cyanide poisoning with histotoxic hypoxia caused by inhibition of cytochrome oxidase, the terminal enzyme of the respiratory chain. This is manifested as a metabolic acidosis and a fall in the arteriovenous ($C_{a-v}O_2$) oxygen content difference. These effects should not inhibit the clinical use of SNP since they are only seen when a gross overdose has been administered and are easily avoided with care. In the short term (a few hours) infusions should be limited to a total dose of 1.5 mg/kg. There is only limited information concerning the safe dosage for long-term administration (several hours to days, or even weeks), although it has been suggested that maximum infusion rates of approximately 4 μg/kg/min (certainly less than 8 μg/kg/min) and a total dose of 70 mg SNP/kg over periods of up to two weeks are the maximum allowable without risking toxic effects (Vesey & Cole, 1985). Although thiocyanate (SCN) accumulation is not a concern during hypotensive anaesthesia, high plasma levels may be achieved during long-term administration, with possible toxic consequences. Monitoring of SCN levels is therefore recommended during infusions lasting more than three days, particularly in the presence of renal insufficiency (Vesey & Cole, 1985). Treatment of cyanide toxicity is discussed in Chapter 18. SNP is broken down during prolonged exposure to light; this problem can be avoided by making up the solution in relatively small quantities or by protecting it with silver foil.

Nitroglycerine (glyceryl trinitrate, GTN) and isosorbide dinitrate (ISDN). These agents are predominantly venodilators. They can therefore cause marked reductions in pre-load, which may be associated with falls in cardiac output and compensatory vasoconstriction. Even when there is an overall reduction in systemic vascular resistance, renal blood flow may fall. When cardiac output is increased, most of the additional flow is distributed to musculoskeletal regions. They are of most value in patients with cardiac failure in whom pre-load reduction may reduce ventricular wall tension and improve coronary perfusion without adversely affecting cardiac performance. Furthermore, these agents may reverse myocardial ischaemia by increasing and redistributing coronary blood flow. They can therefore be used to control angina and limit infarct size. GTN and ISDN are therefore often used in preference to SNP in patients with cardiac failure and/or myocardial ischaemia (Kaplan & Jones, 1979). Finally, both GTN and ISDN reduce pulmonary vascular resistance, an effect that can occasionally be exploited in patients with a low cardiac output secondary to pulmonary hypertension.

Nifedipine. This calcium channel blocker can be administered orally or sublingually to control hypertension. It is a particularly potent peripheral smooth muscle relaxant that causes a reduction in systemic vascular resistance and an increase in cardiac output. Most of the increased flow is distributed to musculoskeletal beds, with lesser increases in hepatic, splanchnic and renal flow.

Angiotension converting enzyme (ACE) inhibitors. ACE inhibitors such as captopril and enalapril reduce systemic vascular resistance and generally increase renal blood flow by reducing angiotension-induced arteriolar tone. This effect is, however, more pronounced in the efferent vessels, and glomerular filtration rate may therefore remain unchanged or fall despite the increased flow. Nevertheless, sodium excretion usually increases, largely due to a reduction in aldosterone release. ACE inhibitors can be useful when weaning patients with cardiac failure from intravenous vasodilators.

MECHANICAL CIRCULATORY ASSISTANCE

Intra-aortic balloon counterpulsation (Swanton, 1984)

Various techniques for mechanically supporting the failing myocardium have been described; of these, intra-aortic balloon counterpulsation (IABCP) has proved most practical and is now widely used.

A catheter with an inflatable sausage-shaped balloon is inserted via a femoral artery using a percutaneous Seldinger technique and passed into the aorta until its tip lies just distal to the left subclavian artery (**Fig. 4.12**). Early in diastole, the balloon is rapidly inflated so that the pressure in the aortic root rises and coronary

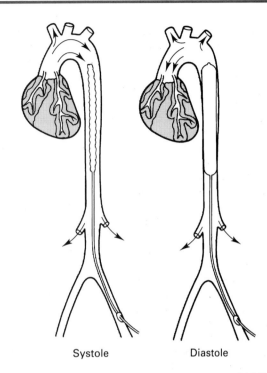

Systole   Diastole

Fig. 4.12 Intra-aortic balloon counterpulsation (IABCP). Rapid deflation of the balloon occurs at the onset of systole and causes a reduction in after-load. Early in diastole the balloon is rapidly inflated to increase the pressure in the aortic root and enhance coronary blood flow.

blood flow is increased. Rapid deflation of the balloon is timed to occur at the onset of systole (usually triggered by the R wave on the ECG) and this leads to a reduction in after-load. Pre-load, pulmonary artery pressure and pulmonary vascular resistance may also be reduced. The reduction in left ventricular work reduces myocardial oxygen requirements and this, combined with the increased coronary blood flow, may result in a reversal of ischaemic changes and limitation of infarct size. IABCP may not, however, increase coronary blood flow distal to significant stenoses. Improved myocardial performance, together with the reduction in after-load, can lead to an increased cardiac output. Inflation and deflation of the balloon must be precisely timed to achieve effective counterpulsation (**Fig. 4.13**).

The only absolute *contraindications* to IABCP are *aortic aneurysms* (or other severe disease of the descending aorta) and *marked aortic regurgitation*. Relative contraindications include arrhythmias and extreme tachycardias, both of which limit the ability of the device to trigger balloon deflation accurately.

Complications of IABCP include:

- failure to pass the balloon;
- aortic dissection;
- limb ischaemia;
- thrombosis;

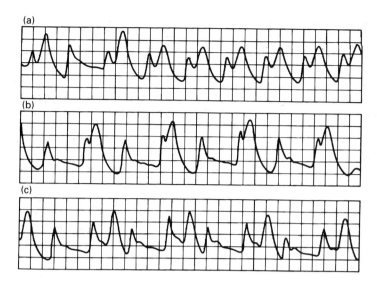

(a)

(b)

(c)

Fig. 4.13 (a) The effect of intra-aortic balloon counterpulsation (IABCP) on the arterial pressure trace. Note the increased diastolic pressure, the slight fall in systolic pressure (due to after-load reduction) and reduced end-diastolic pressure (due to rapid balloon deflation). (b) It is important that the balloon inflates immediately the aortic valve closes (i.e. on the dicrotic notch). In this case the balloon is inflating too early. This impedes left ventricular ejection. (c) In this case balloon inflation is delayed.

- embolism;
- infection.

IABCP has proved most useful for weaning patients from cardiopulmonary bypass and for those who develop myocardial ischaemia in the perioperative period. It may also be used to support patients in cardiogenic shock who have surgically correctable lesions, such as ischaemic ventricular septal defects or mitral regurgitation, while they are being prepared for surgery. In patients with severe ischaemia (e.g. those with unstable angina) IABCP may relieve pain and possibly prevent infarction while preparations are made for coronary artery vein grafting or percutaneous transluminal coronary angioplasty (PTCA). The use of IABCP for the treatment of cardiogenic shock complicating myocardial infarction without a surgically correctable lesion has been less successful, although some feel that this may be due partly to delay in instituting IABCP and extension of the infarct caused by the previous use of inotropes. There is only limited experience with the use of IABCP in myocardial failure complicating septic shock, but it seems that the technique may be life-saving in those with reversible global myocardial dysfunction complicating anaphylaxis (Raper & Fisher, 1988).

Other ventricular assist devices

Centrifugal pumps can be used to bypass and 'off-load' the right or, more often, the left ventricle while maintaining adequate systemic blood flow. Such devices are usually used as a means of discontinuing cardiopulmonary bypass in the hope that ventricular function will improve significantly over the ensuing 48–72 hours. They may also be used as a 'bridge' to cardiac transplantation. Alternative devices include *mechanical hearts*,

used to support potential cardiac transplant recipients and *arteriovenous pumps*.

Haematological problems

The most commonly encountered haematological problem in shock is a coagulation defect, usually due to massive blood transfusion and/or consumption coagulopathy (DIC), the latter being particularly common in sepsis. This can usually be corrected with transfusions of FFP, occasionally combined with platelets, or fresh blood. DIC should be prevented or reversed by aggressive treatment of the underlying condition. Heparinization has been recommended, but this is potentially extremely dangerous, particularly in trauma and postoperative patients, and is rarely indicated. Later, coagulation may be impaired secondary to the development of renal and/or hepatic failure.

Renal function

Established acute renal failure still has a high mortality and its prevention is therefore a priority when treating shock.

Prevention of acute intrinsic renal failure is best achieved by restoring cardiac output, blood pressure and renal blood flow as rapidly as possible, combined with early and aggressive management of oliguria (see Chapter 12).

MULTIPLE ORGAN FAILURE

Although it is now usually possible to support patients through the early stages of shock, trauma or other life-threatening illnesses, a disappointingly high proportion subsequently develop progressive failure of several vital organs (DeCamp & Demling, 1988; Barton & Cerra, 1989). Once three or more organs have failed the mortality is extremely high (more than 80% in most series), and sequential multiple organ failure (MOF) is now the commonest mode of death in intensive care patients, accounting for as many as 75% of all deaths in surgical intensive care units (Barton & Cerra, 1989). Moreover, these patients spend long periods in intensive care and consume a large proportion of available resources.

Definition

Currently there is no consensus on the definition of MOF syndrome and criteria for failure of individual organs differ. Because the extent of organ dysfunction can vary both between patients and within the same patient over time the term *multiple organ dysfunction syndrome* (MODS) has recently been suggested to indicate the wide range of severity and dynamic nature of this disorder (Bone *et al.*, 1992; Members of the American College of Chest Physicians/Society of Critical Care Medicine Consensus Conference, 1992). Organ dysfunction is defined as *'the presence of altered organ function in an acutely ill patient such that homeostasis cannot be maintained without intervention'*. Transient impairment of organ function rapidly responsive to short-term measures should probably be excluded from this definition.

Aetiology

There are two distinct, but not mutually exclusive, pathways by which MODS may develop (**Fig. 4.14**).

- In *primary MODS* there is a direct insult to an individual organ (e.g. pulmonary aspiration, lung contusion or renal damage due to rhabdomyolysis), which fails early as a result of an inflammatory response, confined, at least in the early stages, to the affected organ.
- The aetiology of *secondary MODS* is complex, but in general terms organ damage is thought to be precipitated by systemic dissemination of the inflammatory

response associated with the haemodynamic disturbance, microcirculatory abnormalities and defective oxygen utilization described earlier in this chapter (see **Fig. 4.3**). Secondary MODS can therefore be viewed as a complication of SIRS (see above) and can be considered as representing the more severe end of the spectrum of illness in patients with SIRS/sepsis. Secondary MODS usually evolves after a latent period from the initiating event, which is most commonly infectious (usually bacterial, but sometimes viral, fungal or parasitic), but may be non-infectious (e.g. the presence of extensive wounds or necrotic tissue). Secondary MODS may therefore follow sepsis, trauma, shock, major surgery and many other serious illnesses (e.g. pancreatitis, perforation of the gastro-intestinal tract, pneumonia), or may arise in response to SIRS precipitated by primary MODS.

Clinical features

Characteristic features of patients with MODS include:

- an increased metabolic rate;
- a hyperdynamic circulation;
- hyperventilation;
- an impaired immune response;
- evidence of persistent or recurrent sepsis with fever (almost invariable);
- septic shock (common).

Sequential failure of interdependent organs occurs progressively over weeks, although the pattern of organ dysfunction is variable.

In most cases the lung is the first organ to be affected, usually with the development of ARDS, and this is associated with cardiovascular instability and deteriorating renal function. Secondary pulmonary infection complicating ARDS frequently acts as a further stimulus to the inflammatory response. Gastrointestinal failure is common, with an inability to tolerate enteral feeding and abdominal distension due to paralytic ileus. Disruption of the muscosal barrier (see above) is associated with portal bacteraemia/endotoxaemia and activation of liver macrophages, which release inflammatory mediators into the venous circulation. This may initiate or perpetuate pulmonary damage; lung macrophages are

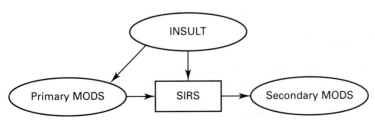

Fig. 4.14 Pathways for the development of multiple organ dysfunction syndrome (MODS).

activated with systemic release of mediators and a vicious cycle of events ensues. This has led to the gut being described as *'the motor of MOF'*. Hepatic metabolism is markedly increased in the early stages, but later liver dysfunction, partly attributable to Kupffer cell activation, is associated with jaundice, elevated liver enzymes and a decreased albumin level. Gastrointestinal haemorrhage, ischaemic colitis, acalculous cholecystitis and pancreatitis may also occur (see Chapter 15), as may coagulopathies. Features of central nervous system dysfunction (see above) include impaired conscious level and disorientation, progressing to coma. The metabolic derangement is associated with elevated blood sugar levels, catabolism and wasting. Although characteristically these patients initially have a hyperdynamic circulation, eventually cardiovascular collapse supervenes, culminating in hypometabolism and failure of tissue oxygenation.

Treatment

Treatment of established MODS is supportive. The principles of cardiovascular support are discussed earlier in this chapter, and respiratory, renal, hepatic and nutritional support in the appropriate chapters elsewhere. Prevention of organ failure in those at risk is therefore crucial. Aggressive early resuscitation is essential, and activation of macrophages must be prevented or minimized by early excision of devitalized tissue and drainage of infection. Preservation of the integrity of the gut mucosal barrier by maximizing splanchnic perfusion and early enteral feeding is also important. Early recognition of organ dysfunction and prompt intervention may be associated with reversal of organ impairment and an improved outcome.

ADJUNCTIVE THERAPY IN SHOCK AND SEPSIS

The persistently high mortality associated with sepsis and septic shock has stimulated a search for additional forms of treatment that, when used in conjunction with conventional therapy would assist shock reversal, prevent or minimize organ damage and improve outcome. Because many of the manifestations of sepsis, including the haemodynamic changes and vital organ damage, are mediated by an uncontrolled dissemination of the inflammatory cascade, it has been postulated that mortality might be reduced by inhibiting the mediators of this response (see above). Despite encouraging results in animal models, however, this approach has, for a number of reasons, proved generally disappointing. One explanation has been that unselective suppression of inflammatory pathways may prevent the beneficial as

well as the adverse effects of mediators and could, for example, impair the patient's ability to eradicate infection, while increasing susceptibility to secondary sepsis. On the other hand it has been suggested that, because many agents are targeted against only one component of the inflammatory response, the use of multiple therapy is likely to be more effective than administration of a single 'magic bullet'. Other problems have included the currently incomplete understanding of the pathophysiology of sepsis and the uncritical extrapolation of results obtained in animal models to clinical practice.

Corticosteroids

Corticosteroids are powerful anti-inflammatory agents and have a number of potentially beneficial actions in shock, including:

- inhibition of complement-induced granulocyte activation;
- reduction in the liberation of free arachidonic acid from membrane phospholipid;
- stabilization of lysosomal membranes;
- inhibition of cytokine synthesis.

Prior administration of corticosteroids can also prevent the induction of the enzyme responsible for the synthesis of NO (see below).

The use of high-dose corticosteroids (usually methylprednisolone 30 mg/kg) in shock has therefore been extensively investigated. The results of animal studies suggested that pharmacological doses of corticosteroids could reduce mortality, particularly in septic shock, provided they were administered sufficiently early (Hinshaw *et al.*, 1980), and initial clinical studies, albeit much criticized, were also encouraging (Schumer, 1976). For many years, therefore, high-dose corticosteroids were widely used in the management of shock and it is only comparatively recently that large well-designed clinical trials have demonstrated that large doses of methylprednisolone do not improve outcome in severe sepsis or septic shock, even when administered within a few hours of the diagnosis (Bone *et al.*, 1987; The Veterans Administration Systemic Sepsis Cooperative Study Group, 1987). Indeed there is evidence that in some cases mortality may be increased (Bone *et al.*, 1987), probably because of a higher incidence of deaths attributable to infective complications in those given corticosteroids. Although still a subject for debate, most now believe that pharmacological doses of corticosteroids should not be administered to patients with shock or sepsis.

Non-steroidal anti-inflammatory agents

(Feuerstein & Hallenbeck, 1987)

Inhibition of cyclooxygenase with non-steroidal anti-inflammatory agents (NSAIDS) such as meclofenamate, aspirin, indomethacin or ibuprofen, limits formation of eicosanoids from arachidonic acid and may be associated with beneficial effects in animal shock models. In patients with sepsis syndrome, ibuprofen has been shown to reduce arachidonic acid metabolism significantly, with an associated fall in body temperature, heart rate and peak airway pressure, as well as a trend towards more rapid shock reversal (Bernard et al., 1991). These agents are, however, relatively unselective and will inhibit formation of eicosanoids with potentially advantageous actions (e.g. prostacyclin) as well as those with deleterious effects such as thromboxane and leukotrienes.

More specific agents that inhibit lipoxygenase or antagonize leukotrienes are also available. Their role in the management of patients with shock remains to be established.

Prostacyclin

Some of the vasodilator eicosanoids (such as PGE_1 and prostacyclin) may have beneficial effects in patients with sepsis/MODS, in particular by enhancing oxygen uptake in response to increases in Do_2 (Bihari et al., 1987). They will also inhibit platelet aggregation. Nevertheless their role in clinical practice is uncertain (see also Chapter 7).

Opiate antagonists (Hinds, 1985)

Although a number of investigators have demonstrated a pressor response to naloxone in shock, as well as a reduction in inotrope requirements, in one controlled study (De Maria et al., 1985) both treatment and placebo groups showed a similar increase in blood pressure and naloxone has not yet been shown to improve outcome. In addition, as with steroids, there are a number of possible adverse effects of opiate antagonism in shock including:

- tachyarrhythmias;
- pulmonary oedema;
- seizures;
- most importantly, reversal of analgesia and sedation.

Administration of partial agonists may produce similar haemodynamic improvement without reversing analgesia (Donaldson et al., 1988). The clinical use of opiate antagonists or partial agonists cannot currently be recommended.

Monoclonal antibodies and immunotherapy (Hinds, 1992)

There is reason to hope that monoclonal antibodies, which can be precisely targeted against individual mediators or their receptors and have minimal potential for adverse effects, may allow more effective manipulation of the systemic response to infection. For example, antibodies have been raised against TNF as well as its receptor. Administering antibodies to TNF has produced encouraging results in some animal models of septic shock (Tracey et al., 1987), although in others administration of TNF antagonists has had no effect or been deleterious. Preliminary results from phase III clinical studies of murine monoclonal anti-TNFα antibody suggest some benefit in patients with septic shock, although the use of a dimeric TNF receptor fusion protein in high doses may be associated with a worse outcome. The role of anti-TNF treatments in the management of sepsis/septic shock will remain unclear until these and other studies have been completed and published. In general, because cytokines play an important role in host resistance, inhibition could, as with steroids, impair the patient's immune capabilities. Conversely inhibiting only one of the many cytokines involved in the response to infection might not be sufficient to influence outcome.

An alternative approach, which might overcome these problems, would be to target the toxic products of the infecting organism rather than the mediators of the inflammatory response. It is now possible to direct treatment specifically against circulating endotoxin, although compared to manipulation of the inflammatory cascade this approach has the obvious disadvantage of being limited to cases of Gram-negative bacteraemia or endotoxaemia.

Studies in the early 1980s indicated that immunotherapy with human polyclonal antiserum or plasma directed against endotoxin core determinants could reduce mortality in Gram-negative bacteraemia (Ziegler et al., 1982) and protect high-risk patients from septic shock (Baumgartner et al., 1985). The use of polyclonal antiserum is, however, unsatisfactory because the antibody content is variable, there is a potential for transmitting infection and an individual can donate serum only once. These difficulties have been circumvented by the production of monoclonal antibodies such as HA-1A, a human monoclonal IgM antibody that binds to Lipid A. In a prospective randomized controlled trial (Ziegler et al., 1991) HA-1A significantly reduced 28-day mortality in patients with Gram-negative bacteraemia. The validity of these findings has, however, been seriously questioned and, particularly in view of the financial implications (it has been estimated that the annual cost of administration of HA-1A to all patients with Gram-negative sepsis could exceed $1 billion in the USA), introducing treatment with monoclonal antibodies directed against endotoxin has been delayed until further studies have been completed and some of the uncertainties resolved.

In the future it should be possible to produce monoclonal antibodies against other toxic products of infecting organisms, as well as other components of the inflammatory cascade and their receptors. Antibodies have been raised, for example, against each protein in the contact system, and it may be possible to target adhesion molecules with specific monoclonal antibodies. Treatment with a combination of monoclonal antibodies, perhaps tailored to the particular clinical situation, should then be feasible. In some circumstances prophylactic administration may be indicated, while in others treatment may have to be given repeatedly. Early administration is likely to be more effective, and appropriately timed treatment might be used to prevent the deterioration sometimes associated with the first dose of antibiotics.

Platelet activating factor antagonists

Administration of platelet activating factor (PAF) antagonists can produce beneficial effects in animal models of shock, including reversal of hypotension (Toth & Mirulaschek, 1986). In a recent prospective randomized controlled trial administration of a PAF-receptor antagonist failed to reduce mortality significantly in patients with severe sepsis, although outcome was significantly improved in the subgroup with Gram-negative sepsis. The authors concluded that this agent seems to be a safe and promising treatment for patients with severe Gram-negative sepsis (Dhainault et al., 1994).

Protease inhibitors (Colman, 1989)

Because the interaction between factor XII, plasma kininogens and prekallikrein can trigger hypotension, DIC and neutrophil activation, recombinant or synthetic protease inhibitors could be beneficial in shock.

Nitric oxide synthase inhibitors

Experimental studies have demonstrated that the vascular hyporeactivity to adrenergic agonists and the peripheral vascular failure associated with endotoxaemia can be reversed by inhibiting NO synthesis with L-arginine analogues, and prevented by inhibiting the induction of a cytokine-inducible NO synthase with dexamethasone. The concept that increased NO formation contributes to circulatory failure in human shock is supported by only very limited clinical experience. Petros

et al. (1991) have reported that intravenous administration of the arginine analogue L-NMMA (L-N-methylarginine) to two patients with refractory shock was associated with a rapid dose-dependent increase in blood pressure and systemic vascular resistance, while Lorente et al. (1993) found that administration of N-nitro-L-arginine to patients with sepsis syndrome produced vasoconstriction and a fall in cardiac output. There are also concerns about the effects of inhibiting NO production on renal perfusion, coagulation and immune function. Further studies of these agents are clearly required.

Plasma exchange/haemofiltration
(Groeneveld, 1990)

It has been suggested that plasma exchange may benefit patients with sepsis and MODS, perhaps because various toxins and mediators are removed from the circulation. Others have claimed that continuous high-volume arteriovenous haemofiltration, sometimes supplemented by plasma exchange or dialysis, can improve outcome in these patients. The beneficial effects on cardiorespiratory function and survival in these studies seem to be independent of alterations in fluid balance and have been attributed to mediator clearance. So far, however, clinical evidence is largely anecdotal and no prospective controlled trials have been performed.

Pentoxifylline

Pentoxifylline is a xanthine derivative that increases intracellular cyclic AMP levels and inhibits TNF production by mononuclear cells. In human volunteers it blocks the endotoxin-induced increase in circulating levels of TNF, but not IL-6 (Zabel et al., 1989). Pentoxifylline might, therefore, have beneficial effects in clinical endotoxin shock, although there is concern that abrupt discontinuation of this agent may precipitate hyperresponsiveness to LPS.

Cytokine antagonists, soluble receptors and receptor antagonists

Recent evidence suggests that natural control of the proinflammatory effects of cytokines is exerted by endogenous cytokine antagonists and by soluble forms of cytokine receptors, which are shed into the circulation and excreted in the urine. Administration of soluble receptors might bind cytokines, prevent activation of effector cells and facilitate clearance of cytokines from the circulation.

Another approach that may prove valuable is the

administration of recombinant cytokine receptor antagonists. For example, a specific human IL-1 receptor antagonist (rh IL-1ra) has been shown to reduce mortality in experimental endotoxin shock (Ohlsson *et al.*, 1990), although the results of a recent randomized double-blind controlled trial failed to show a statistically significant increase in survival for all patients receiving the study medication. There was, however, some suggestion that rh IL-1ra produced a dose-related increase in survival in those with sepsis and organ dysfunction and/or a predicted risk of death of 24% or more (Fisher *et al.*, 1994).

Finally there is some evidence to suggest that an inhibitor of TNF processing that would inhibit release of this cytokine without interfering with its cell-associated activity, might be a particularly effective treatment for sepsis (Mohler *et al.*, 1994).

Bactericidal permeability increasing protein

Bactericidal permeability increasing protein (BPI) is a human protein derived from neutrophil granules that binds to lipid A and may prevent macrophage activation. A recombinant amino terminal fragment of BPI has been shown to prevent haemodynamic responses to endotoxin in rats (Ammons & Kung, 1993).

N-acetylcysteine

N-acetylcysteine has antioxidant properties and being a sulphydryl donor may contribute to the regeneration of NO and glutathione. In liver failure *N*-acetylcysteine can increase cardiac output, D_{O_2}, $\dot{V}_{O_2}$ and oxygen extraction (see Chapter 13), and in patients with septic shock seemed to improve tissue oxygenation in about half of those treated (Spies *et al.*, 1994). It remains to be seen whether this agent can improve outcome.

ANAPHYLACTIC SHOCK

Pathogenesis

Anaphylactic shock is an acute reaction to a foreign substance to which the patient has already been sensitized (immediate, or Type I, hypersensitivity) and commonly follows the administration of a drug, blood product, plasma substitute or contrast media. It may also occur in response to an insect sting or the ingestion of a particular food or food additive. Clinically indistinguishable 'anaphylactoid' reactions in which the mechanism is non-immunological or undetermined may

also occur. Similar symptoms may also be produced by direct drug effects, physical factors or exercise, and in some cases a causative agent cannot be identified.

Sensitization follows exposure to an allergenic substance, which either alone or in combination with a hapten, stimulates synthesis of IgE; this binds to the surface of mast cells or basophils. On re-exposure the antigen interacts with the IgE on the cell surface, leading to mast cell degranulation and release of histamine, slow-reacting substance of anaphylaxis (SRS-A), eosinophilic chemotactic factor of anaphylaxis (ECF-A) and PAF. Intravenous hypnotic agents and contrast media may activate complement C3. As well as the haemodynamic changes, these mediators may precipitate smooth muscle contraction and increased glandular secretion.

Clinical features

There is a latent period between exposure and the development of symptoms, which is usually less than 30 minutes if the agent has been given parenterally. Reactions may be transient or protracted and vary in severity from mild to fatal.

The commonest feature is *profound vasodilatation* with *hypotension* and *tachycardia*. The combination of vasodilatation and hypovolaemia due to *increased capillary permeability* leads to a reduction in ventricular filling pressures and a fall in cardiac output. Myocardial function may also be impaired (Raper & Fisher, 1988). These haemodynamic changes may occur in isolation, but are often accompanied by *cutaneous manifestations* such as:

- an erythematous blush;
- generalized urticaria;
- angioedema;
- conjunctival injection;
- pallor and cyanosis.

Loss of protein-rich fluid into the tissues through the 'leaky' capillaries appears as *oedema*, often most obvious in the face but, more dangerously, may also cause laryngeal obstruction. There may also be:

- bronchospasm;
- rhinitis;
- nausea;
- vomiting;
- abdominal cramps;
- diarrhoea.

Other features may include:

- pulmonary oedema;
- coughing;
- arthralgia;
- paraesthesiae, convulsions, coma;
- clotting abnormalities.

The patient may complain of a metallic taste, a choking sensation and apprehension.

Management (Table 4.5)

The drug of first choice for severe anaphylactic reactions is *adrenaline* (0.5–1.0 mg intramuscularly or if muscle blood flow is thought to be compromised by shock, a slow intravenous injection of 0.5 mg given over 5 minutes. This may be followed by a continuous intravenous infusion). This agent increases intracellular levels of cyclic AMP in leucocytes and mast cells and inhibits further release of histamine and SRS-A. Adrenaline will also increase myocardial contractility and peripheral vascular tone, and relax bronchial smooth muscle. Occasionally cardiopulmonary resuscitation (see Chapter 8) will be required. If bronchospasm is unresponsive to adrenaline alone *aminophylline* should be administered as a slow intravenous bolus and *noradrenaline* can be given for profound refractory vasodilatation. Steroids are of no proven benefit and should be reserved for patients with refractory bronchospasm. Antihistamines are only indicated in protracted cases and those with angioedema.

Follow up of these patients is essential. The responsible agent must be determined or confirmed by *in vitro* or *in vivo* testing. Hypersensitization should be considered for food, pollen and bee sting allergies. The patient should wear a 'medic-alert' bracelet and be given a note stating the nature of the reaction and the causative agent. Patients and their next of kin can be given appropriate drugs and instructed in their use.

Table 4.5 Management of anaphylaxis.

Adrenaline 0.5–1.0 mg intramuscularly (or as a slow intravenous injection of 0.5 mg given over 5 minutes. This may be followed by a continuous intravenous infusion).
Oxygen and airway (may require tracheal intubation/cricothyrotomy)
Establish venous access
Expand circulating volume
May require mechanical ventilation

Intravenous aminophylline for bronchospasm unresponsive to adrenaline

Noradrenaline for profound refractory vasodilatation

Steroids only for refactory bronchospasm

Antihistamine only in protracted cases and those with angioedema

Consider IABCP for severe myocardial failure

PULMONARY EMBOLISM

Pulmonary emboli usually originate from thromboses in the deep veins of the lower limbs, pelvis or inferior vena cava. Much less often thrombi in the upper limbs, right atrium or ventricle may be the source. Frequently these venous thrombi are asymptomatic. Risk factors include:

- heart failure;
- cancer;
- hip fractures;
- prolonged bed rest;
- age over 65 years;
- obesity;
- oestrogen therapy.

Symptoms

Symptoms include a sudden onset of dyspnoea, chest pain (substernal or pleuritic), apprehension and a non-productive cough. Massive pulmonary embolism may precipitate syncope. Later pulmonary infarction may be associated with pleuritic pain and haemoptysis.

Haemodynamic changes

Massive pulmonary embolism precipitates systemic hypotension and shock. Cardiac output falls, systemic vascular resistance is increased, and there is usually a tachycardia; bradycardia is an ominous sign. Mean pulmonary artery pressure is increased by about 5 mm Hg when more than 50% of the pulmonary vasculature is acutely obstructed. CVP is elevated and the right ventricle dilates, but PAOP is often low.

Physical signs

Physical signs include tachypnoea, cyanosis and tachycardia. The rise in pulmonary artery pressure may be associated with splitting of the second heart sound and a loud pulmonary component, right ventricular heave and a gallop rhythm. The JVP may be elevated with a prominent 'a' wave. There may be clinical evidence of deep vein thrombosis and a slight fever.

The commonest ECG finding is non-specific ST depression and T wave inversion in the anterior leads. P pulmonale, right bundle branch block and atrial arrhythmias may also be seen. The classic pattern of S_1, Q_3, T_3 is unusual.

The chest radiograph may be normal or may show focal pulmonary oligaemia, localized infiltrates, consolidation, a raised diaphragm, pleural effusion or large pulmonary arteries.

When pulmonary embolism is suspected specific investigations may include a *V/Q* scan (see Chapter 5) and pulmonary angiography. In selected patients, lower limb venography or I^{131}-labelled fibrinogen uptake may be indicated.

Treatment (Table 4.6)

RESUSCITATION

Oxygen should be administered in high concentrations; patients with severe respiratory distress may require mechanical ventilation. Haemodynamic support centres on maintaining right ventricular perfusion. Expansion of the circulating volume should therefore be combined with inotropic support using an agent that will maintain systemic blood pressure and thereby preserve right ventricular perfusion in the face of elevated right ventricular pressures.

DEFINITIVE TREATMENT

Definitive treatment is directed towards preventing further thrombus formation and proximal embolization. Thrombolysis and physical removal of emboli may also be indicated.

Heparin

New thrombus formation can be inhibited by administering heparin (an intravenous bolus of 5000–10,000 units followed by a continuous intravenous infusion at 1000–2000 units/hour). The dose should be adjusted to maintain the activated partial thromboplastin time at 1.5–2.5 times the control value. Heparin administration has the additional advantage of limiting the rise in pulmonary artery pressure by inhibiting the release of serotinin and histamine from platelets. Prolonged treatment may be complicated by thrombocytopenia.

Warfarin

Usually heparin is continued for 7–10 days and is followed by *warfarin* administration, overlapping by at least 5 days to counteract the hypercoagulability that may occur during the early stages of warfarin treatment. The loading dose of warfarin is normally around 10 mg/day for 2 days followed by a maintenance dose of about 3–9 mg/day. The dose must, however, be closely monitored and adjusted to maintain the prothrombin time at about 2–3 times the control value. Oral warfarin therapy should be continued for 1.5–2 months in those with deep venous thrombosis, for 3–6 months following pulmonary embolism, and for longer in particularly high-risk cases. If acute reversal of warfarin therapy is essential it is best achieved by administering FFP. Longer

Table 4.6	Management of pulmonary embolism.
Resuscitation	Oxygen and airway May require mechanical ventilation Expand circulating volume Inotrope/vasopressor to maintain right ventricular perfusion
Definitive treatment	**Heparin** (intravenous bolus 5000–10,000 units, followed by 1000–2000 units/h for 7–10 days), followed by warfarin (overlapping by at least 5 days) (loading dose of around 10 mg/day for 2 days, followed by maintenance dose of 3–9 mg/day) **Thrombolytic therapy** (e.g. streptokinase 250,000 units intravenously over 30 mins, followed by infusion of 100,000 units/h for 24 h) should be considered when there is haemodynamic instability, the perfusion defect involves one or more lobes of the lung, or there is extensive proximal deep vein thrombosis. Commence heparin infusion when streptokinase is discontinued (usually after 24 hours, but 3–7 days of streptokinase may be more effective) **Vena caval filter** if there are recurrent pulmonary emboli despite anticoagulation, large free-floating thrombi in the iliofemoral veins, the patient cannot tolerate anticoagulation, or following pulmonary embolectomy **Pulmonary embolectomy** may be indicated when profoundly shocked due to massive embolus when streptokinase is contraindicated or fails

lasting reversal of anticoagulation can be produced by giving vitamin K.

Thrombolytic therapy

Thrombolysis (e.g. with *streptokinase*) should be considered for pulmonary embolism associated with haemodynamic instability and when the perfusion defect involves one or more lobes of the lung, as well as in some patients with extensive proximal deep vein thrombosis. A loading dose of 250,000 units should be administered intravenously over 30 minutes, followed by an infusion of 100,000 units/hour for 24 hours. There is, however, some evidence that a longer period of treatment (3-7 days) may be more effective. Treatment should be monitored using the thrombin time, which should be maintained at 2-4 times the control value. A heparin infusion should be started when the streptokinase is discontinued.

Streptokinase is pyrogenic and antigenic. Immunological reactions can be controlled with antihistamines and hydrocortisone; adrenaline and resuscitation equipment should be immediately available. There is also a significant risk of haemorrhage with streptokinase. If serious bleeding occurs it should be discontinued, FFP should be administered and the fibrinolytic activity of streptokinase antagonized by ε-aminocaproic acid or aprotinin. New clot-specific thrombolytic agents such as recombinant tissue plasminogen activator cause less systemic fibrinogenolysis and may have some advantage.

Vena caval filters

In patients who have either recurrent pulmonary emboli despite anticoagulation or large free-floating thrombi in the iliofemoral veins, a filter can be positioned in the inferior vena cava to prevent pulmonary embolism. Filters may also be used in patients who cannot tolerate anticoagulation and immediately following pulmonary embolectomy.

Pulmonary embolectomy

The value of pulmonary embolectomy is uncertain. It may be indicated in a patient who is profoundly shocked due to massive pulmonary embolism when streptokinase is contraindicated or fails.

Percutaneous catheter fragmentation

In patients with acute massive pulmonary embolism it may be possible to restore cardiac output rapidly by using a conventional cardiac catheter to break up the embolus and disperse the fragments distally (Brady *et al.*, 1991).

REFERENCES

Ahmed AJ, Knise JA, Haupt MT, Chandrasekar PH & Carlson RW (1991) Hemodynamic responses to Gram-positive versus Gram-negative sepsis in critically ill patients with and without circulatory shock. *Critical Care Medicine* **19**: 1520-1525.

Ammons WS & Kung AHC (1993) Recombinant amino terminal fragment of bactericidal/ permeability-increasing protein prevents haemodynamic responses to endotoxin. *Circulatory Shock* **41**: 176-184.

Arieff AI, Gertz EW, Park R et al. (1983) Lactic acidosis and the cardiovascular system in the dog. *Clinical Science* **64**: 573-580.

Bakker J, Coffenils M, Leon M, Gris P & Vincent J-L (1991) Blood lactate levels are superior to oxygen-derived variables in predicting outcome in human septic shock. *Chest* **99**: 956-962.

Barton R & Cerra FB (1989) The hypermetabolism. Multiple organ failure syndrome. *Chest* **96**: 1153-1160.

Baumgartner J-D, Glauser MP, McCutchan JA et al. (1985) Prevention of Gram-negative shock and death in surgical patients by antibody to endotoxin core glycolipid. *Lancet* **ii**: 59-63.

Bernard GR, Reines HD, Halushka PV et al. (1991) Prostacyclin and thromboxane A$_2$ formation is increased in human sepsis syndrome. Effects of cyclooxygenase inhibition. *American Review of Respiratory Disease* **144**: 1095-1101.

Bersin RM & Arieff AI (1988) Improved hemodynamic function during hypoxia with Carbicarb, a new agent for the management of acidosis. *Circulation* **77**: 227-233.

Bihari D, Smithies M, Gimson A & Tinker J (1987) The effects of vasodilatation with prostacyclin on oxygen delivery and uptake in critically ill patients. *New England Journal of Medicine* **317**: 397-403.

Bollaert PE, Bauer P, Audibert G, Lambert H & Larcan A (1990) Effects of epinephrine on hemodynamics and oxygen metabolism in dopamine-resistant septic shock. *Chest* **98**: 949-953.

Bone RC (1991) Sepsis, sepsis syndrome, multi-organ failure: a plea for comparable definitions. *Annals of Internal Medicine* **114**: 332-333.

Bone RC, Fisher CJ Jr, Clemmer TP, Slotman GJ, Metz CA, Balk RA & The Methylprednisolone Severe Sepsis Study Group (1987) A controlled clinical trial of high-dose methylprednisolone in the treatment of severe sepsis and septic shock. *New England Journal of Medicine* **317**: 653-658.

Bone RC, Fisher CJ Jr, Clemmer TP, Slotman CJ, Metz CA, & The Methylprednisolone Severe Sepsis Study Group (1989) Sepsis syndrome: a valid clinical entity. *Critical Care Medicine* **17**: 389-393.

Bone RC, Sprung CL & Sibbald WJ (1992) Definitions for sepsis and organ failure. *Critical Care Medicine* **20**: 724-726.

Boyd O, Grounds RM & Bennett ED (1993) A randomized clinical trial of the effect of deliberate perioperative increase of oxygen delivery on mortality in high-risk surgical patients. *Journal of the American Medical Association* **270**: 2699-2707.

Brady AJB, Crake T & Oakley CM (1991) Percutaneous catheter fragmentation and distal dispersion of proximal pulmonary embolus. *Lancet* **338**: 1186-1189.

Brenner M, Schaer GL, Mallory DL, Suffredini AF & Parrillo JE (1990) Detection of renal blood flow abnormalities in septic and critically ill patients using a newly designed indwelling thermodilution renal vein catheter. *Chest* **98**: 170-179.

Chiariello M, Gold HK, Leinbach RC, Davis MA & Maroko PR (1976) Comparison between the effects of nitroprusside and nitroglycerin on ischemic injury during acute myocardial infarction. *Circulation* **54**: 766-773.

Colardyn FC, Vandenbogaerde JF, Vogelaers DP & Verbeke JH (1989) Use of dopexamine hydrochloride in patients with septic shock. *Critical Care Medicine* **17**: 999-1003.

Collins JA, James PM, Bredenberg CE et al. (1978) The relationship between transfusion and hypoxemia in combat casualties. *Annals of Surgery* **188**: 513-520.

Colman RW (1989) The role of plasma proteases in septic shock. *New England Journal of Medicine* **320**: 1207-1209.

Cooper DJ, Walley KR, Wiggs BR & Russell JA (1990) Bicarbonate does not improve hemodynamics in critically ill patients who have lactic acidosis. A prospective, controlled clinical study. *Annals of Internal Medicine* **112**: 492-498.

Cowley HC, Heney D, Gearing AJH, Hemingway I & Webster NR (1994) Increased circulating adhesion molecule concentrations in patients with the systemic inflammatory response syndrome: a prospective cohort study. *Critical Care Medicine* **22**: 651-657.

Cumming PD, Wallace EV, Schorr JB & Dodd RY (1989) Exposure of patients to human immunodeficiency virus through the transfusion of blood components that test antibody-negative. *New England Journal of Medicine* **321**: 941-946.

Cunnion RE, Schaer GL, Parker MM, Natanson C & Parrillo JE (1986) The coronary circulation in human septic shock. *Circulation* **73**: 637-644.

Danek SJ, Lynch JP, Weg JG & Dantzer DR (1980) The dependence of oxygen uptake on oxygen delivery in the adult respiratory distress syndrome. *American Review of Respiratory Disease* **122**: 387-395.

Danner RL, Elin RJ, Hosseini JM, Wesley RA, Reilly JM & Parrillo JE (1991) Endotoxemia in human septic shock. *Chest* **99**: 169-175.

Davis RF, Lappas DG, Kirklin JK, Buckley MJ & Lowenstein E (1982) Acute oliguria after cardiopulmonary bypass: renal functional improvement with low-dose dopamine infusion. *Critical Care Medicine* **10**: 852-856.

DeCamp MM & Demling RH (1988) Posttraumatic multisystem organ failure. *Journal of the American Medical Association* **260**: 530-534.

Deitch EA, Berg R & Specian R (1987) Endotoxin promotes the translocation of bacteria from the gut. *Archives of Surgery* **122**: 185-190.

De Maria A, Craven DE, Hefferman JJ, McIntosh TK, Grindlinger GA & McCabe WR (1985) Naloxone versus placebo in treatment of septic shock. *Lancet* **i**: 1363-1365.

Dhainaut JF, Huyghebaert MF, Mansalkier JF et al. (1987) Coronary haemodynamics and myocardial metabolism of lactate, free fatty acids, glucose and ketones in patients with septic shock. *Circulation* **75**: 533-541.

Dhainaut J-FA, Tenaillon A, Tulzo Y et al. (1994) Platelet-activating factor receptor antagonist BN 52021 in the treatment of severe sepsis: a randomized, double-blind, placebo-controlled, multicenter clinical trial. BN 52021 Sepsis Study Group. *Critical Care Medicine* **22**: 1720-1728.

D'Oliveira M, Sykes MK, Chakrabarti MK, Orchard C & Keslin J (1981) Depression of hypoxic pulmonary vasoconstriction by sodium nitroprusside and nitroglycerine. *British Journal of Anaesthesia* **53**: 11-18.

Donaldson MDJ, Vesey CJ, Wilks M & Hinds CJ (1988) Beneficial effects of buprenorphine (a partial opiate agonist) in porcine *Escherichia coli* septicaemia: a comparison with naloxone. *Circulatory Shock* **25**: 209-221.

Editorial (1991) Nitric oxide in the clinical arena. *Lancet* **338**: 1560-1562.

Edwards JD, Brown GCS, Nightingale P, Slater RM & Farragher EB (1989) Use of survivors' cardiorespiratory values as therapeutic goals in septic shock. *Critical Care Medicine* **17**: 1098-1103.

Ellrodt AG, Riedinger MS, Kimchi A, Berman DS, Maddahi, J, Swan HJC & Murata GH (1985) Left ventricular performance in septic shock: reversible segmental and global abnormalities. *American Heart Journal* **110**: 402-409.

Evans SF, Medbak S, Hinds CJ, Tomlin SJ, Varley JG & Rees LH (1984) Plasma levels and biochemical characterisation of circulating met-enkephalin in canine endotoxin shock. *Life Sciences* **34**: 1481-1486.

Feuerstein G & Hallenbeck JM (1987) Prostaglandins, leukotrienes and platelet activating factor in shock. *Annual Review of Pharmacological Toxicology* **27**: 301-313.

Fisher CJ Jr, Dhainault J-FA, Opal SM et al. (1994) Recombinant human interleukin 1 receptor antagonist in the treatment of patients with sepsis syndrome. *Journal of the American Medical Association* **271**: 1836-1843.

Fleming A, Bishop M, Shoemaker W et al. (1992) Prospective trial of supranormal values as goals of resuscitation in severe trauma. *Archives of Surgery* **127**: 1175-1181.

Garcia-Sabrido JL, Tallado JM, Christou NV, Polo JR & Valdecantos E (1988) Treatment of severe intra-abdominal sepsis and/or necrotic foci by an 'open abdomen' approach. Zipper and zipper-mesh techniques. *Archives of Surgery* **123**: 152-156.

Gilbert EM, Haupt MT, Mandanas RY, Huanniga AJ & Carlson RW (1986) The effect of fluid loading, blood transfusion, and catecholamine infusion on oxygen delivery and consumption in patients with sepsis. *American Review of Respiratory Disease* **134**: 873-878.

Graf H, Leach W & Arieff AI (1985) Evidence for the detrimental effect of bicarbonate therapy in hypoxic lactic acidosis. *Science* **227**: 754-756.

Groeneveld ABJ (1990) Septic shock and multiple organ failure: treatment with haemofiltration? *Intensive Care Medicine* **16**: 489-490.

Groeneveld ABJ, Bronsveld W & Thijs LG (1986) Hemodynamic determinants of mortality in human septic shock. *Surgery* **99**: 140-153.

Haglund U, Bulkley GB & Granger DN (1987) On the pathophysiology of intestinal ischemic injury. Clinical review. *Acta Chirurgica Scandinavica* **153**: 321-324.

Hasselgren P-O & Fischer JE (1986) Septic encephalopathy. Etiology and management. *Intensive Care Medicine* **12**: 13-16.

Haupt MT, Gilbert EM & Carlson RW (1985) Fluid loading increases oxygen consumption in septic patients with lactic acidosis. *American Review of Respiratory Disease* **131**: 912-916.

Hayes MA, Yau EHS, Hinds CJ & Watson JD (1992) Symmetrical peripheral gangrene: association with noradrenaline administration. *Intensive Care Medicine* **18**: 433-436.

Hayes MA, Yau EHS, Timmins AC, Hinds CJ & Watson D (1993) Response of critically ill patients to treatment aimed at achieving supranormal oxygen delivery and consumption. Relationship to outcome. *Chest* **103**: 886-895.

Hayes MA, Timmins AC, Yau EHS, Palazzo M, Hinds CJ & Watson D (1994) Elevation of systemic oxygen delivery in the treatment of critically ill patients. *New England Journal of Medicine* **330**: 1717-1722.

Hesse DG, Tracey KJ, Fong Y, Manogue KR, Palladino MA Jr, Cerami A, Shires GT & Lowry SF (1988) Cytokine appearance in human endotoxemia and primate bacteremia. *Surgery Gynecology and Obstetrics* **166**: 147-153.

Hewitt PE & Davies SC (1983) The current state of DIC. *Intensive Care Medicine* **9**: 249-252.

Hinds CJ (1985) Opiate antagonists in shock. *British Journal of Hospital Medicine* **34**: 233-234.

Hinds CJ (1992) Monoclonal antibodies in sepsis and septic shock. *British Medical Journal* **304**: 132-133.

Hinshaw LB, Archer LT, Beller-Todd BK *et al.* (1980) Survival of primates in LD100 septic shock following steroid/antibiotic therapy. *Journal of Surgical Research* **28**: 151-170.

Holcroft JW & Trunkey DD (1974) Extravascular lung water following hemorrhagic shock in the baboon: comparison between resuscitation with Ringer's lactate and Plasmanate. *Annals of Surgery* **180**: 408-417.

Holloway EL, Stinson EB, Derby GC & Harrison DC (1975) Action of drugs in patients early after cardiac surgery 1. Comparison of isoproterenol and dopamine. *American Journal of Cardiology* **35**: 656-659.

Jardin F, Sportiche M, Bazin M, Bourokba A & Margairaz A (1981) Dobutamine: a hemodynamic evaluation in human septic shock. *Critical Care Medicine* **9**: 329-332.

Kaplan JA & Jones EL (1979) Vasodilator therapy during coronary artery surgery. Comparison of nitroglycerin and nitroprusside. *Journal of Thoracic and Cardiovascular Surgery* **77**: 301-309.

Koller J, Mai P, Wieser C, Pomaroli A, Puscheridorf B & Herold M (1991) Endothelin and big endothelin concentrations in injured patients. *New England Journal of Medicine* **325**: 1518.

Kreger BE, Craven DE & McCabe WR (1980) Gram-negative bacteremia iv. Re-evaluation of clinical features and treatment in 612 patients. *American Journal of Medicine* **68**: 344-355.

Kruse JA, Haupt MT, Puri VK & Carlson RW (1990) Lactate levels as predictors of the relationship between oxygen delivery and consumption in ARDS. *Chest* **98**: 959-962.

Lamy M, Faymonville ME & Deby-Dupont G (1987) Shock pancreas: a new entity? In: Vincent JL (ed) *Update in Intensive Care and Emergency Medicine*, pp. 148-154. Springer-Verlag, Berlin.

Ledingham IMcA & McArdle CS (1978) Prospective study of the treatment of septic shock. *Lancet* **i**: 1194-1197.

Leon C, Rodrigo MJ, Tomasa A *et al.* (1982) Complement activation in septic shock due to gram-negative and gram-positive bacteria. *Critical Care Medicine* **10**: 308-310.

Lorente JA, Landin L, De Pablo R, Renes E & Liste D (1993) L-arginine pathway in the sepsis syndrome. *Critical Care Medicine* **21**: 1287-1295.

Marik PE & Mohedin M (1994) The contrasting effects of dopamine and norepinephrine on systemic and splanchinic oxygenation utilization in hyperdynamic sepsis. *Journal of the American Medical Association* **272**: 1354-1357.

Marik PE & Sibbald WJ (1993) Effect of stored blood transfusion on oxygen delivery in patients with sepsis. *Journal of the American Medical Association* **269**: 3024-3029.

Martin C, Eon B, Saux P, Aknin P & Gollin F (1990) Renal effects of norepinephrine used to treat septic shock patients. *Critical Care Medicine* **18**: 282-285.

Meadows D, Edwards JD, Wilkins RG & Nightingale P (1988) Reversal of intractable septic shock with norepirephrine therapy. *Critical Care Medicine* **16**: 663-666.

Members of the American College of Chest Physicians/Society of Critical Care Medicine Consensus Conference Committee (1992) Definitions for sepsis and organ failure and guidelines for the use of innovative therapies in sepsis. *Critical Care Medicine* **20**: 864-874.

Michie HR, Manogue KR, Spriggs DR *et al.* (1988a) Detection of circulating tumor necrosis factor after endotoxin administration. *New England Journal of Medicine* **318**: 1481-1486.

Michie HR, Spriggs DR, Manogue KR, *et al.* (1988b) Tumor necrosis factor and endotoxin induce similar metabolic responses in human beings. *Surgery* **104**: 280-286.

Mohler KM, Sleath PR, Fitzner JM *et al.* (1994) Protection against a lethal dose of endotoxin by an inhibitor of tumour necrosis factor processing. *Nature* **370**: 218-220.

Nasraway SA, Rackow EC, Astez ME, Karras G & Weil MH (1989) Inotropic response to digoxin and dopamine in patients with severe sepsis, cardiac failure and systemic hyperperfusion. *Chest* **95**: 612-615.

Ognibene FP, Parker MM, Natanson C, Shelhamer JH & Parrillo JE (1988) Depressed left ventricular performance. Response to volume infusion in patients with sepsis and septic shock. *Chest* **93**: 903-910.

Ohlsson K, Björk P, Bergenfeldt M, Hageman R & Thompson RC (1990) Interleukin-1 receptor antagonist reduces mortality from endotoxin shock. *Nature* **348**: 550-552.

Packman M & Rackow EC (1983) Optimum left heart filling pressure during fluid resuscitation of patients with hypovolemic and septic shock. *Critical Care Medicine* **11**: 165-169.

Palazzo MG & Suter PM (1991) Delivery dependent oxygen consumption in patients with septic shock: daily variations, relationship with outcome and the sick-euthyroid syndrome. *Intensive Care Medicine* **17**: 325-332.

Parker MM, Shelhamer JH, Bacharach SL *et al.* (1984) Profound but reversible myocardial depression in patients with septic shock. *Annals of Internal Medicine* **100**: 483-490.

Parker MM, McCarthy KE, Ognibene FP & Parrillo JE (1990) Right ventricular dysfunction and dilatation, similar to left ventricular changes, characterize the cardiac depression of septic shock in humans. *Chest* **97**: 126-131.

Parrillo JE, Burch C, Shelhamer JH, Parker MM, Natanson C &

Schuette W (1985) A circulating myocardial depressant substance in humans with septic shock. *Journal of Clinical Investigations* **76**: 1539-1553.

Parrillo JE, Parker MM, Natanson C *et al.* (1990) Septic shock in humans. Advances in the understanding of pathogenesis, cardiovascular dysfunction and therapy. *Annals of Internal Medicine* **113**: 227-242.

Petros A, Bennett D & Vallance P (1991) Effect of nitric oxide synthase inhibitors on hypotension in patients with septic shock. *Lancet* **338**: 1557-1558.

Phang PT, Cunningham KF, Ronco JJ, Wiggs BR & Russell JA (1994) Mathematical coupling explains dependence of oxygen consumption on oxygen delivery in ARDS. *American Journal of Respiratory Critical Care Medicine* **150**: 318-323.

Rackow EC, Falk JL, Fein A *et al.* (1983) Fluid resuscitation in circulatory shock: a comparison of the cardiorespiratory effects of albumin, hetastarch, and saline solutions in patients with hypovolemic and septic shock. *Critical Care Medicine* **11**: 839-850.

Raper RF & Fisher MM (1988) Profound reversible myocardial depression following human anaphylaxis. *Lancet* **i**: 386-388.

Reul GJ Jr, Greenberg SD, Lefrak EA *et al.* (1973) Prevention of post-traumatic pulmonary insufficiency. Fine screen filtration of blood. *Archives of Surgery* **106**: 386-394.

Ronco JJ, Phang PT, Walley KR, Wiggs B, Fenwick JC & Russell JA (1991) Oxygen consumption is independent of changes in oxygen delivery in severe adult respiratory distress syndrome. *American Review of Respiratory Disease* **143**: 1267-1273.

Ronco JJ, Fenwick JC, Tweedale MG, Wiggs BR, Phang PT, Cooper DJ, Cunningham KG, Russell JA & Walley KR (1993) Identification of the critical oxygen delivery for anaerobic metabolism in critically ill septic and nonseptic humans. *Journal of the American Medical Association* **270**: 1724-1730.

Rothwell PM, Udwadia ZF & Lawler PG (1991) Cortisol response to corticotrophin and survival in septic shock. *Lancet* **337**: 582-583.

Ruokonen R, Takala J, Kari A, Saxén H, Mertsola J & Hansen EJ (1993) Regional blood flow and oxygen transport in septic shock. *Critical Care Medicine* **21**: 1296-1303.

Russell JA, Roneo JJ, Lockhat D, Belzberg A, Kiess M & Dodek PM (1990) Oxygen delivery and consumption and ventricular preload are greater in survivors than in nonsurvivors of the adult respiratory distress syndrome. *American Review of Respiratory Disease* **141**: 659-665.

Schmid E, Angehrn W, Althaus F, Gattiker R & Rothlin M (1979) The effect of dopamine on hepatic–splanchnic blood flow after open heart surgery. *Intensive Care Medicine* **5**: 183-188.

Schneider AJ, Teule GJJ, Groeneveld ABJ, Nauta JJP, Heidendal GAK & Thijs LG (1988) Biventricular performance during volume loading in patients with early septic shock, with emphasis on the right ventricle: a combined hemodynamic and radionuclide study. *American Heart Journal* **116**: 103-112.

Schned AR & Silver H (1981) The use of microaggregate filtration in the prevention of febrile transfusion reactions. *Transfusion* **21**: 675-681.

Schoenberg MH & Beger HG (1993) Reperfusion injury after intestinal ischemia. *Critical Care Medicine* **21**: 1376-1386.

Schumer W (1976) Steroids in the treatment of clinical septic shock. *Annals of Surgery* **184**: 333-341.

Scully MF (1984) Measurement of endotoxaemia by the *Limulus* test. *Intensive Care Medicine* **10**: 1-2.

Segal JM, Phang PT & Walley KR (1992) Low-dose dopamine hastens onset of gut ischemia in a porcine model of hemorrhagic shock. *Journal of Applied Physiology* **73**: 1159-1164.

Shoemaker WC, Montgomery ES, Kaplan E & Elwyn DH (1973) Physiologic patterns in surviving and nonsurviving shock patients. *Archives of Surgery* **106**: 630-636.

Shoemaker WC, Appel PL, Kram HB, Waxman K & Lees TS (1988) Prospective trial of supranormal values of survivors as therapeutic goals in high risk surgical patients. *Chest* **94**: 1176-1186.

Skillman JJ, Restall DS & Salzman EW (1975) Randomized trial of albumin *vs* electrolyte solutions during abdominal aortic operations. *Surgery* **78**: 291-303.

Spies CD, Reinhart K, Witt I, *et al.* (1994) Influence of N-acetyl-cysteine on indirect indicators of tissue oxygenation in septic shock patients: results from a prospective, randomized, double-blind study. *Critical Care Medicine* **22**: 1738-1746.

Spinas GA, Bloesch D, Kaufmann MT, Keller U & Dayer JM (1990) Induction of plasma inhibitors of interleukin 1 and TNF activity by endotoxin administration to normal humans. *American Journal of Physiology* **234**: R 993-997.

Stacpoole PW, Wright EC, Baumgartner TG *et al.* (1992) A controlled clinical trial of dichloroacetate for treatment of lactic acidosis in adults. *New England Journal of Medicine* **327**: 1564-1569.

Stevens DL, Tanner MH, Winship J *et al.* (1989) Severe group A streptococcal infections associated with a toxic shock-like syndrome and scarlet fever toxin A. *New England Journal of Medicine* **321**: 1-7.

Stockwell MA, Soni N & Riley B (1992a) Colloid solutions in the critically ill. *Anaesthesia* **47**: 3-6.

Stockwell MA, Scott A, Day A, Riley B & Soni N (1992b) Colloid solutions in the critically ill. *Anaesthesia* **47**: 7-9.

Stump DC, Strauss RG, Henriksen RA, Petersen RE & Saunder R (1985) Effects of hydroxyethyl starch on blood coagulation, particularly factor VIII. *Transfusion* **25**: 349-354.

Suffredini AF, Fromm RE, Parker MM *et al.* (1989a) The cardiovascular response of normal humans to the administration of endotoxin. *New England Journal of Medicine* **321**: 280-287.

Suffredini AF, Harpel PC & Parrillo JE (1989b) Promotion and subsequent inhibition of plasminogen activation after administration of intravenous endotoxin to normal subjects. *New England Journal of Medicine* **320**: 1165-1172.

Swanton RH (1984) Who requires balloon pumping? *Intensive Care Medicine* **10**: 271-273.

Timmis AD, Fowler MB, Burwood RJ, Gishen P, Vincent R & Chamberlain DA (1981) Pulmonary oedema without critical increase in left atrial pressure in acute myocardial infarction. *British Medical Journal* **283**: 636-638.

Toth PD & Mikulaschek AW (1986) Effects of a platelet-activating factor antagonist, CV-3988, on different shock models in the rat. *Cirulatory Shock* **20**: 193-203.

Tracey KJ, Fong Y, Hesse DG *et al.* (1987) Anti-cachectin/TNF monoclonal antibodies prevent septic shock during lethal bacteraemia. *Nature* **330**: 662-664.

Tuchschmidt J, Fried J, Swinney R & Sharma OP (1989) Early

haemodynamic correlates of survival in patients with septic shock. *Critical Care Medicine* **17**: 719-723.

Tuchschmidt J, Fried J, Aztiz M & Rackow E (1992) Elevation of cardiac output and oxygen delivery improves outcome in septic shock. *Chest* **102**: 216-220.

Urbaniak SJ (1991) Artificial blood. *British Medical Journal* **303**: 1348-1350.

Velanovich V (1989) Crystalloid versus colloid fluid resuscitation. A meta-analysis of mortality. *Surgery* **105**: 65-71.

Vallet B, Chopin C, Curtis SE *et al.* (1993) Prognostic value of the dobutamine test in patients with sepsis syndrome and normal lactate values: a prospective, multicenter study. *Critical Care Medicine* **21**: 1868-1875.

Vesey CJ & Cole PV (1985) Blood cyanide and thiocyanate concentrations produced by long-term therapy with sodium nitroprusside. *British Journal of Anaesthesia* **57**: 148-155.

The Veterans Administration Systemic Sepsis Cooperative Study Group (1987) Effect of high-dose glucocorticoid therapy on mortality in patients with clinical signs of systemic sepsis. *New England Journal of Medicine* **317**: 659-665.

Villar J, Slutsky AS, Hew E & Aberman A (1990) Oxygen transport and oxygen consumption in critically ill patients. *Chest* **98**: 687-692.

Vincent J-L, Carlier E, Berrè J, Armistead CW Jr, Kahn RJ, Coussaert E & Cantraine F (1988) Administration of enoximone in cardiogenic shock. *American Journal of Cardiology* **62**: 419-423.

Vincent J-L, Roman A & Kahn RJ (1990) Dobutamine administration in septic shock: addition to a standard protocol. *Critical Care Medicine* **18**: 689-693.

Virgilio RW, Rice CL, Smith DE *et al.* (1979) Crystalloid vs colloid resuscitation: is one better? A randomized clinical study. *Surgery* **85**: 129-139.

Ward JW, Bush TJ, Perkins HA *et al.* (1989) The natural history of transfusion-associated infection with human immunodeficiency virus. *New England Journal of Medicine* **321**: 947-952.

Weaver DW, Ledgerwood AM, Lucas CE *et al.* (1978) Pulmonary effects of albumin resuscitation for severe hypovolemic shock. *Archives of Surgery* **113**: 387-392.

Weissman C & Kemper M (1991) The oxygen uptake–oxygen delivery relationship during ICU interventions. *Chest* **99**: 430-435.

Williams GR (1990) The toxic shock sydrome. *British Medical Journal* **300**: 960.

Yu M, Levy MM, Smith P, Takiguchi SA, Miyasaki A & Myers SA (1993) Effect of maximizing oxygen delivery on morbidity and mortality rates in critically ill patients: a prospective, randomized controlled study. *Critical Care Medicine* **21**: 830-838.

Zabel P, Wolteb DT, Schönharting MM & Schade UF (1989) Oxpentifylline in endotoxaemia. *Lancet* **i**: 1474-1477.

Ziegler EJ, McCutchan JA, Fierer J *et al.* (1982) Treatment of Gram-negative bacteremia and shock with human antiserum to a mutant *Escherichia coli*. *New England Journal of Medicine* **307**: 1225-1230.

Ziegler EJ, Fisher CJ Jr, Sprung CL, Straube RC, Sadoff JC, Foulke GE *et al.* (1991) Treatment of Gram-negative bacteremia and septic shock with HA-1A human monoclonal antibody against endotoxin. *New England Journal of Medicine* **324**: 429-436.

5 Assessment and Monitoring of Respiratory Function

Vital management decisions, such as the institution of mechanical ventilation and the initiation of weaning from respiratory support, depend on the ability to assess respiratory function accurately. Respiratory monitoring is also required to evaluate the patient's response to treatment and optimize ventilatory support. Clinical assessment is of the utmost importance. Signs of severe respiratory distress include:

- the use of accessory muscles of respiration;
- suprasternal and intercostal recession;
- paradoxical or asynchronous movement of the rib cage and abdomen;
- respiratory alternans;
- tachypnoea;
- tachycardia;
- sweating;
- pulsus paradoxus;
- inability to speak.

Together with a subjective assessment of the degree of exhaustion, these signs are often the best guides to the need for respiratory support.

The most sensitive indicator of increasing respiratory difficulty is a rising respiratory rate, although errors of up to four breaths/minute may easily occur when respiratory frequency is determined by observing chest wall movement over 15 seconds and multiplying the number of excursions by four (Tobin, 1992).

Carbon dioxide retention may be suspected in a patient with a bounding pulse, warm, vasodilated peripheries, a tremor of the outstretched hand and an impaired conscious level, but the presence or absence of cyanosis is an unreliable guide to the adequacy of oxygenation. The final decision as to when to wean a patient from artificial ventilation is often largely based on clinical judgement, although many objective criteria have been described (see later and Chapter 7).

The history and clinical examination can be supplemented by measurements of tidal volume (V_T) and vital capacity (VC) and these, together with the pulse rate, blood pressure and respiratory rate, should be recorded at regular intervals so that the patient's progress can be observed and any deterioration detected immediately. Blood gas analysis is essential and a chest radiograph should always be obtained. In some cases maximum mouth pressures may be helpful, and in those with airways obstruction, maximum expiratory flow rates should be recorded. An assessment of lung mechanics can also be valuable in selected cases. More sophisticated investigations, such as the determination of alveolar–capillary permeability, are occasionally indicated, but are usually confined to research applications.

These techniques for assessing respiratory function are performed intermittently. Continuous monitoring (e.g. with pulse oximetry and capnography) is required to detect the rapid changes that may occur either in response to alterations in treatment or spontaneously.

MEASUREMENT OF LUNG VOLUMES

THE VITAL CAPACITY

The vital capacity (VC) provides an indication of the patient's ability to inspire deeply, maintain lung expansion and cough. It is particularly useful when assessing patients with respiratory inadequacy due to neuromuscular problems. The VC depends on:

- the power of the respiratory muscles;
- the elastic properties of the chest wall and lung parenchyma;
- the size and patency of the airways at low lung volumes;
- the volume of the lungs, which varies with sex and body size.

There are many causes of a reduced VC (**Table 5.1**), all of which can, if severe, eventually lead to a fall in V_T. V_T is therefore a less sensitive indicator of deterioration than VC, while minute ventilation (the product of V_T and respiratory rate) rises initially and falls precipitously only at a late stage when the patient is exhausted.

The normal VC is 65-75 ml/kg and V_T is 7 ml/kg (about 500 ml). In general a $V_T < 5$ ml/kg or a VC < 15 ml/kg are indicative of serious respiratory difficulty.

Table 5.1 Causes of a reduced vital capacity.
Diseases of chest wall, pleura, lung parenchyma, nerves, muscles
Pleural effusion, haemothorax, pneumothorax
Loss of lung tissue (e.g. lung resection)
Replacement of lung tissue (e.g. tumour)
Premature airway closure (e.g. chronic airflow limitation)
Abdominal distension

FUNCTIONAL RESIDUAL CAPACITY

Functional residual capacity (FRC) can be measured using helium dilution, nitrogen washout or a body plethysmograph. These techniques are difficult or impossible in ventilated intensive care patients and are generally used only for research. FRC falls when:

- the abdomen is distended;
- there are painful thoracic or abdominal wounds;
- in the supine position;
- lung volume is reduced by pulmonary pathology.

Wright's respirometer

The V_T, minute volume and VC can be measured most easily at the bedside using a Wright's respirometer (**Fig. 5.1**). Access to the airway is required, but this is easily achieved in intubated patients by attaching the device to the catheter mount. In the spontaneously breathing, unintubated patient a mouthpiece can be used or a mask can be closely applied to the patient's face. There is therefore inevitably some degree of interference with

the patient's airway and this has the disadvantage of interrupting the oxygen supply, as well as potentially altering the respiratory pattern.

The Wright's respirometer is a delicate instrument and is easily damaged if dropped. Because of the inertia of the vane and the resistance of the device, it under-reads at low flows. On the other hand, at high flows, the momentum of the vane causes the instrument to over-read.

Accuracy is also affected by condensation of water vapour and, to a lesser extent, by alterations in the composition of respired gas. Nevertheless, in clinical practice errors are rarely greater than 10%. The dead space and resistance of the device are low and it is therefore well tolerated by spontaneously breathing patients. Electronic versions are also available.

Pneumotachograph

Whereas the Wright's respirometer is a unidirectional device that only measures expired volumes, the pneumotachograph records flows in both inspiration and expiration (**Fig. 5.2**). Flow rates are calculated from the measured pressure difference across the fixed resistance; inspired and expired volumes are obtained by integrating these flows.

The best known pneumotachograph is the *Fleisch head*, in which the resistance is formed by a piece of

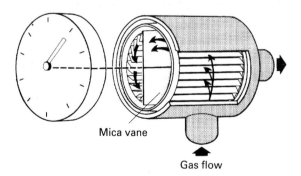

Fig. 5.1 Wright's respirometer. Gas flowing into the device is channelled through a series of tangential slits and rotates the lightweight mica vane. The latter is connected to the pointer on the dial by gears.

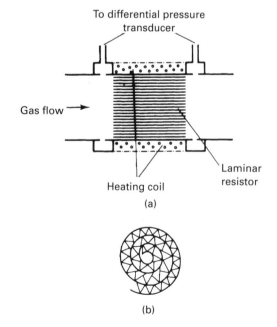

Fig. 5.2 Fleisch pneumotachograph head (see text). (a) Longitudinal section. (b) Cross-section to show corrugated foil wound into spiral. From Sykes & Vickers (1973), with permission.

corrugated foil wound into a spiral. This creates a large number of parallel-sided tubes, which ensure laminar flow. Condensation of water vapour on the foil, which can alter its resistance and create turbulent flow, is prevented by surrounding the device with a heating coil. Mucus traps are also required to prevent obstruction. Although alterations in the composition and temperature of the gas mixture interfere with the measurement, when used carefully an accuracy of $\pm 5\%$ is possible.

Considerable care and attention to detail are required when using pneumotachographs and they have not proved suitable for routine clinical use. Alternatives have therefore been described. These have included the use of a *heated wire mesh* to provide the resistance, in which case flow is turbulent and sophisticated electronics are required to produce a linear output; and lightweight devices with a *variable orifice*, which are unaffected by water vapour, allow tracheal secretions to pass easily and are relatively insensitive to temperature changes.

Heated wire or thermistor

Another approach to the measurement of inspired and expired volumes is to place a heated wire or a thermistor in the gas stream. The magnitude of temperature changes is then dependent on gas flow rates.

Vortex spirometer

The vortex spirometer generates vortices in the gas stream. These are detected and counted by an ultrasonic beam, the number of vortices being dependent on gas flow rate. These vortex spirometers are said to be accurate over a wide range of flows and are largely unaffected by gas composition, humidity or temperature.

ASSESSING AIRWAYS OBSTRUCTION

Clinical evaluation of the severity of airflow obstruction is notoriously inaccurate. The patient's progress, and in particular response to treatment, can be assessed objectively by serial measurement of *expiratory flow rates*. These depend not only on the resistance of the intrathoracic airways, but also on lung elastic recoil; they are therefore greatest at high lung volumes (when airways resistance is least and elastic recoil maximal) and decrease progressively throughout expiration. Because increasing expiratory force leads to collapse of the distal airways, flow rates are largely independent of muscular effort. Expiratory flow rates are, however, reduced by extreme weakness. Improvement in expiratory flow

rates following administration of bronchodilators distinguishes reversible from irreversible airways obstruction.

Timed measurements of a forced vital capacity

Timed measurements of forced vital capacity (FVC) can be performed at the bedside using a *vitalograph* and provide an accurate, reproducible measure of airway calibre. The portion of the FVC exhaled in the first second is termed the *forced expiratory volume in one second (FEV_1)*, and this is best expressed as a percentage of the FVC.

Normally the FEV_1 is 50–60 ml/kg and represents 70–80% of the FVC. In those with airways obstruction the FEV_1 is reduced to a greater extent than the FVC and the FEV_1/FVC ratio falls below 70%. In restrictive disorders, on the other hand, both FEV_1 and FVC are reduced and the ratio is unchanged or increased.

The Wright's peak flow meter

Wright's peak flow meter (**Fig. 5.3**) is a cheap and convenient means of assessing airways obstruction at the bedside. *Peak expiratory flow rate (PEFR)* is, however, relatively effort dependent and is less reproducible than the FEV_1. Although it is useful for assessing the severity of airways obstruction and the response to treatment it is not sufficiently specific to be diagnostic of airflow limitation. The normal PEFR is 450–700 l/min in adult males and 300–500 l/min in adult females. In severe airways obstruction values as low as 60 l/min may be recorded.

MAXIMUM MOUTH PRESSURES

Maximum inspiratory and expiratory pressures can be measured at the mouth or via an endotracheal/ tracheostomy tube using an aneroid manometer or a pressure transducer. They are useful indices of the power of the inspiratory and expiratory muscles respectively, although they do depend on patient cooperation.

- Maximum expiratory pressure is not often measured in intensive care patients.
- *Maximum inspiratory pressure* (MIP) is usually measured during a maximum inspiratory effort against an occluded airway at RV or FRC.

The normal value for MIP varies with age and sex, exceeding $- 90$ cm H_2O in young females and $- 130$ cm H_2O in young males. Values less than $- 25$ cm H_2O suggest that spontaneous ventilation is likely to be inadequate (see also Chapter 7).

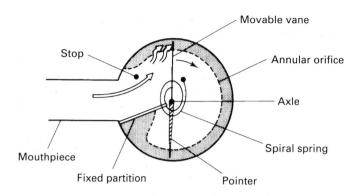

Fig. 5.3 Wright's peak flow meter. From Sykes & Vickers (1973), with permission. The patient makes a forced expiration. The expired gas is deflected onto the rotating vane, which is moved against the resistance offered by the spiral spring. As the vane rotates the annular orifice opens progressively allowing gas to escape to the outside. The maximum deflection of the vane depends on the peak flow rate. The vane is maintained in this position by a ratchet.

ASSESSMENT OF LUNG MECHANICS

In mechanically ventilated patients effective static compliance (see Chapter 2) (C_{es}) can be calculated from:

$$C_{es} = \frac{V_{et}}{P_{plat} - PEEP_A - PEEP_i}$$

where V_{et} is exhaled tidal volume, P_{plat} is plateau airway pressure, $PEEP_A$ = applied positive end-expiratory pressure (PEEP) and $PEEP_i$ is intrinsic PEEP.

Dynamic compliance (C_{dyn}) (see Chapter 2) is given by:

$$C_{dyn} = \frac{V_{et}}{PIP - PEEP_A - PEEP_i}$$

where PIP is peak inspiratory pressure.

Airway resistance can be calculated from

$$R_{aw} = \frac{PIP - P_{plat}}{Peak\ flow}$$

MEASURING WORK OF BREATHING

To measure the work of breathing requires simultaneous measurement of the transpulmonary pressure change (i.e. airway pressure – intrapleural pressure) and V_T. Because an oesophageal balloon has to be inserted, the work of breathing is usually assessed clinically.

NON-INVASIVE MONITORING OF VENTILATION

There have been a number of attempts to develop a satisfactory method for continuously monitoring respiratory function that does not intrude on the airway. One example, which appears to have potential for use in the spontaneously breathing patient, is the *inductance plethysmograph* (Tobin, 1992). The inductive elements are formed by two coils of insulated wire sewn onto bands placed around the rib cage and abdomen.

Changes in thoracic and abdominal volumes alter the inductance of the coil. Provided the device is correctly calibrated it can provide accurate measurements of respiratory timing and thoracic abdominal coordination, as well as a reasonably accurate assessment of changes in V_T (Tobin, 1992).

When using such non-invasive devices, the most valuable information is obtained by analysing changes in the pattern of respiration (e.g. the increasing respiratory rate, the later reduction in V_T, and the loss of the normal breath-to-breath variation in V_T during the onset of acute respiratory failure). The reverse trend may be seen during weaning from artificial ventilation.

MONITORING INSPIRED AND EXPIRED GAS COMPOSITION

Oxygen

Usually the inspired oxygen concentration which is commonly expressed as a fraction of one, (F_IO_2), is measured using either a polarographic or a fuel cell method. Determination of the expired oxygen fraction is less frequently required.

Fuel cells produce a voltage that is proportional to the partial pressure of oxygen (PO_2) to which they are exposed. They are unaffected by water vapour, but have a slow response time and are relatively inaccurate. Furthermore, they are depleted by continued exposure to oxygen and this limits their life span.

Polarographic electrodes also normally have a slow response time, although this can be increased electronically to allow breath-by-breath analysis.

Paramagnetic analysers are extremely accurate, but require careful calibration. They are affected by water vapour and, again, the response time is slow. They are only suitable for the intermittent analysis of discrete samples of dried gas and consequently their use is generally confined to research.

Mass spectrometers (Gothard et al., 1980) are also very accurate and have the added advantages of a rapid response time and the ability to analyse gas concentrations in the presence of water vapour. They are therefore well suited to the continuous analysis of both inspired and expired gas concentrations in ventilated patients, but are expensive, bulky and require considerable expertise during operation and maintenance. These difficulties have limited their introduction into clinical intensive care practice.

Carbon dioxide

Traditionally, the fractional concentration of carbon dioxide in mixed expired gas ($F_E CO_2$) is determined by analysing a Douglas bag collection with an infrared carbon dioxide analyser. $F_E CO_2$ has to be measured in order to determine V_D/V_T and the amount of carbon dioxide excreted per unit time ($\dot{V}CO_2$) as described in Chapter 2.

CAPNOGRAPHY

Continuous breath-by-breath analysis of expired carbon dioxide, using either an infra-red analyser or a mass spectrometer, may also provide clinically useful information. The infra-red absorption technique is inexpensive and simple to use. Expired gas is either sampled from a sidestream port and analysed by a remote sensor or the sensor is positioned in the mainstream of expired gas. The disadvantage of sidestream sampling is that the tubing may become occluded by mucus and water vapour. Mainstream sensors also have a faster response time.

Variations in the carbon dioxide waveform can indicate:

- changes in the production or transport of carbon dioxide;
- alterations in lung function;
- apparatus malfunction.

Changes in the wave form are not, however, diagnostic and other clinical observations are usually required to determine the underlying cause.

The end-tidal carbon dioxide tension ($P_{E'}CO_2$) is perhaps of more clinical value. It can be considered to reflect the partial pressure of alveolar carbon dioxide ($P_A CO_2$) and therefore the partial pressure of arterial carbon dioxide ($P_a CO_2$). $P_{E'}CO_2$ can therefore be used as an immediate guide to the patient's ventilation requirements bearing in mind the normal gradient between alveolar and arterial carbon dioxide tensions. The discrepancy between $P_{E'}CO_2$ and $P_a CO_2$ does, however, increase as lung function deteriorates and changes in $P_{E'}CO_2$ may also be caused by alterations in the distribution of ventilation.

MEASUREMENT OF RESPIRATORY GAS EXCHANGE

Direct measurements of oxygen consumption $\dot{V}O_2$ and $\dot{V}CO_2$ by analysing respiratory gases can be used to estimate energy expenditure and to calculate alveolar/dead space ventilation and cardiac output by the Fick principle (see Chapter 3). Determination of respiratory $\dot{V}O_2$ is also important when evaluating the relationship between oxygen supply and demand (see Chapter 4).

Traditionally $\dot{V}O_2$ has been determined by collecting expired gas in a Douglas bag over a timed period. The volume of gas in the bag is measured most accurately using a wet gas meter. $F_I O_2$ and $F_E O_2$ are determined using one of the methods already described (e.g. a paramagnetic analyser). If the subject is breathing air, $F_I O_2$ is, of course, known to be 20.98% and need not be measured. Often, the inspired volume is not measured directly, but is derived using a standard formula. $\dot{V}O_2$ is then calculated from:

$$\dot{V}O_2 = (\dot{V}_I \times F_I O_2) - (\dot{V}_E \times F_E O_2).$$

This technique is, however, relatively complicated and time-consuming and the principle on which the method is based applies only under steady-state conditions, when respiratory $\dot{V}O_2$ is identical to tissue $\dot{V}O_2$. This is extremely difficult to achieve clinically, particularly in artificially ventilated subjects. Also determination of $\dot{V}O_2$ becomes progressively less accurate as $F_I O_2$ increases.

Various alternative means of measuring $\dot{V}O_2$, which overcome some of these difficulties are available and may be more appropriate for clinical use. For example, a pneumotachnograph can be used to measure inspired and expired volumes continuously as described previously. This can be combined with continuous determination of $F_I O_2$ and $F_E O_2$ to obtain $\dot{V}O_2$. $\dot{V}CO_2$ can also be determined if $F_E CO_2$ is measured ($F_I CO_2$ can be assumed to be zero). This allows calculation of the respiratory quotient (RQ).

Probably the most suitable device for use in critically ill patients is the *Deltatrac* (Datex/Instrumentarium, Helsinki, Finland). This system measures the difference between $F_I O_2$ and $F_E O_2$ using a fast-response, paramagnetic differential oxygen sensor; $F_E CO_2$ is measured with an infra-red carbon dioxide analyser. Expired air is collected through an inbuilt mixing chamber and flow is measured by gas dilution. Spontaneously breathing patients can be studied using a canopy system (Takala *et al.*, 1989).

BLOOD GAS ANALYSIS AND ACID–BASE DISTURBANCES

In the early days of intensive care, blood gas analysis was performed using the equilibration technique. This method, developed over 20 years ago by Professor Astrup, was a relatively time-consuming procedure and required some degree of technical expertise. Combined with the reluctance of clinicians to puncture arteries, this meant that blood gas analysis was only rarely performed.

The original Astrup trolleys consisted of a pH electrode and a microtonometer, but some of the later versions also included a direct reading 'Clark' electrode for the determination of blood oxygen tension. Subsequently, the equilibration technique was superseded by the commercial development of the direct reading PCO_2 electrode and all three were then miniaturized sufficiently to be incorporated in a single cuvette, allowing measurements to be performed on one blood sample. Following the introduction of the microprocessor, automation of most of the processes involved became feasible and modern automated blood gas analysers were soon available commercially. At the same time, there was an increasing acceptance of the ease and relative safety of arterial puncture and cannulation. Consequently, arterial blood gas analysis is now one of the most commonly performed objective tests of respiratory function.

Accuracy of blood gas analysis

Automation of measurement, calculation and display can give a false impression of reliability and accuracy. This may lead to an uncritical acceptance of the results obtained. The clinician must therefore be aware of the potential sources of error when performing blood gas analysis and of the ways in which these can be minimized.

SAMPLING

In the past, it was recommended that glass syringes should be used to obtain the arterial sample. These were said to have two advantages:

- the plunger moves freely, allowing arterial blood to flow into the syringe under its own pressure;
- glass is an efficient barrier to diffusion of gases out of the sample.

In fact, most clinicians find an ordinary plastic syringe, with a continuous negative pressure applied to the plunger, quite satisfactory, and in practice diffusion of gases into the wall of the syringe is not a problem.

On the other hand, *continuing metabolism of white blood cells*, and to a lesser extent reticulocytes, can cause significant reductions in PO_2 and pH, combined with increases in PCO_2, particularly when the initial tension is high. If the sample cannot be analysed immedi-

ately, metabolism can be slowed by immersing the syringe in iced water, having first sealed the end with a plastic cap (Biswas *et al.*, 1982).

To prevent clot formation within the analyser, the sample must be adequately anticoagulated. On the other hand, *excessive dilution of the blood with heparin*, which is acidic, will significantly reduce its PCO_2, although dilution probably has little effect on pH or PO_2 (Bradley, 1972). Therefore, heparin should be used in a concentration of 1000 u/ml, and the volume limited to that contained within the dead space of the syringe (i.e. approximately 0.1 ml). Although this will adequately anticoagulate a 2 ml sample, it is not sufficient for the unnecessarily large volumes of blood sometimes presented for analysis.

Even with the most careful technique, air almost inevitably enters the sample. The gas tensions within these *air bubbles* will equilibrate with those in the blood, thereby lowering the PCO_2 and usually raising the PO_2 of the sample. Provided they are ejected immediately, however, their effect is insignificant. Nevertheless, errors will arise if bubbles taking up more than 0.5–1% of the sample volume are not removed, particularly if the sample is stored at room temperature (Biswas *et al.*, 1982).

MEASUREMENT ERRORS

pH electrodes

Although the traditional pH notation is still used extensively, many now refer to the hydrogen ion concentration ($[H^+]$) in nmol/l. The measurement of pH is particularly prone to error, the commonest cause of erroneous readings being contamination of the electrode with blood proteins.

PCO_2 electrodes

PCO_2 measurements are generally very accurate. When errors do arise they are usually associated with the development of holes in the electrode membrane or, less often, loss of the silver chloride coating on the reference electrode. The membrane can be replaced relatively easily, but in the latter instance a new electrode is required. Since holes in the membrane occur fairly frequently, there is usually no time for protein contamination to become a problem.

PO_2 electrodes

The current output of the oxygen electrode is less for blood than for a gas with an identical PO_2. This discrepancy is called the 'blood gas factor' and is peculiar to oxygen electrodes. It is thought to be due to consumption of oxygen by the electrode from blood immediately adjacent to the tip of the cathode. This generates a gradient of oxygen tension across the sample and causes the electrode to under-read. The blood gas factor has a proportionately greater effect on the absolute value of Po_2 at higher oxygen tensions. Furthermore, loss of oxygen into the plastic walls of the cuvette and tubing increases as Po_2 rises; therefore, considerable care is necessary to obtain accurate measurements of oxygen tension when Po_2 is high. As with the other electrodes, protein contamination may also cause problems.

QUALITY CONTROL AND MAINTENANCE

It is essential that on-site equipment that is used extensively out of hours by both medical and nursing staff is subject to strict quality control procedures and regular maintenance. Although automated blood gas analysers are self-calibrating, they should be checked regularly with quality control material, preferably daily. Ampoules containing buffered liquid of known pH and blood gas tensions are available for this purpose. The discrepancy between the measured and the known standard values can then be recorded. Any deviation of these figures outside the predetermined limits indicates a significant fault in the relevant electrode. This can then be remedied (e.g. by replacing the membrane). In practice, however, it is more usual to avoid problems by changing the membranes regularly. Although buffered liquids can detect the majority of errors associated with the O_2 and CO_2 electrodes, they may fail to demonstrate protein contamination of the pH electrode. The latter can be detected with tonometered calf serum, although it is usually easier and simpler to clean the electrode at regular intervals.

Interpretation of blood gases and acid–base status

The normal values and ranges obtained when blood gas analysis is performed are shown in **Table 5.2**. As well as direct measurements of H^+ activity (expressed as pH

or $[H^+]$), Po_2 and Pco_2, other values relevant to the assessment of the patient's oxygenation and acid–base status are calculated by the microprocessor contained within the analyser.

TOTAL, OR ACTUAL, BICARBONATE CONCENTRATION

Total or actual bicarbonate concentration is influenced by alterations in the amount of carbon dioxide, and by metabolic changes in the amounts of acid and alkali in the blood. It is calculated from the Henderson–Hasselbach equation (see later).

STANDARD BICARBONATE

The standard bicarbonate concentration can be derived to assess the contribution of metabolic factors and disregard changes due to alterations in Pco_2. This is the amount of bicarbonate that would be present in a particular blood sample if the Pco_2 was 5.3 kPa (40 mm Hg), the temperature was 37°C and the blood was fully oxygenated at sea level.

BASE DEFICIT

Base deficit is simply a convenient number for calculating the amount of sodium bicarbonate required to correct a metabolic acidosis. It is calculated as the amount of base that needs to be added to or subtracted from each litre of extracellular fluid to return the pH to a value of 7.4 at Pco_2 of 5.3 kPa (40 mm Hg) at 37°C. Most often, the clinician is given the base excess, which is negative if there is a base deficit (i.e. a metabolic acidosis) and positive if there is a metabolic alkalosis.

SATURATION OF HAEMOGLOBIN WITH OXYGEN

Modern automated blood gas analysers can also calculate the saturation of haemoglobin with oxygen using one of the mathematical formulae describing the oxy-

Table 5.2 Normal values for measurements obtained when blood gas analysis is performed.

H^+	35–45 nmol/l (7.35–7.45 pH units)
Po_2 Pco_2	10–13.3 kPa (75–100 mm Hg) 4.8–6.1 kPa (36–46 mm Hg)
Actual HCO_3^- Standard HCO_3^- Base deficit	22–26 mmol/l 22–26 mmol/l ± 2.5
Percentage saturation	95–100

haemoglobin dissociation curve. When performing this calculation they usually assume that the curve is normally positioned, although in some the P_{50} can be specified by the operator. Percentage saturation is closely related to the oxygen content of the blood, which, as discussed in Chapter 2, can be of more clinical relevance than the Po_2. Some analysers will actually calculate oxygen content, either assuming a value for the haemoglobin concentration or by using a value entered by the operator. The calculation also assumes that all the haemoglobin is available to bind oxygen, (i.e. there is no met- or carboxyhaemoglobin present).

The interpretation of these results can be considered in two separate parts: disturbances of carbon dioxide homeostasis and acid–base balance, and alterations in oxygenation. In all cases, the following details must be known:

- The history.
- The age of the patient.
- The F_iO_2.
- Any other relevant treatment (e.g. the administration of sodium bicarbonate and the ventilator settings for those on mechanical ventilation).

Disturbances of acid–base balance

All enzyme reactions have optimum values for pH at which the reaction proceeds most rapidly. Alterations in pH can, therefore, theoretically lead to a state of 'metabolic chaos' in which some reactions proceed faster than they should, while others slow down. The pH also affects the degree of ionization of various molecules (e.g. an alkalosis causes ionized calcium to bind to protein and may precipitate tetany). The distribution of ions across cell membranes is also influenced by the quantity of H^+ ions in the body and this applies particularly to potassium (see Chapter 10). Severe metabolic acidosis can cause cerebral and myocardial depression (see Chapter 4), while the respiratory centre is stimulated initially, but is subsequently depressed as the acidosis becomes more severe. A marked metabolic alkalosis may combine with an associated hypokalaemia to depress cardiac function. As discussed in Chapter 2, changes in both pH and Pco_2 cause shifts of the oxyhaemoglobin dissociation curve.

The body therefore resists changes in pH using a variety of buffer systems, as well as by regulating the renal excretion of non-volatile acids and bases and adjusting alveolar ventilation to control the arterial carbon dioxide tension.

BUFFER SYSTEMS

A buffer is a mixture of a weak acid (which, in contrast to a strong acid, is only partially dissociated in water)

and its conjugate base. In the body, the main buffer systems are carbonic acid/bicarbonate, phosphates and proteins.

- For the phosphate system: $H_2PO_4^- \rightleftharpoons H^+ + HPO_4^{2-}$.
- For the carbonic acid/bicarbonate system : $H_2CO_3 \rightleftharpoons H^+ + HCO_3^-$.

At equilibrium the law of mass action applies and states that the product of the concentrations of H^+ and HCO_3^- divided by the concentration of H_2CO_3 will remain constant. That is

$$K = \frac{[H^+]\,[HCO_3^-]}{[H_2CO_3]}$$

Henderson rearranged this equation to allow calculation of the $[H^+]$:

$$[H^+] = \frac{K[H_2CO_3]}{[HCO_3^-]}$$

Later Hasselbach modified this equation using the pH nomenclature:

$$pH = pK + \frac{\log\,[HCO_3^-]}{[H_2CO_3]}$$

Buffer systems are most effective when they are maximally dissociated, that is when the pH is close to their dissociation constant (pK). Protein is an effective intracellular buffer because its pK is similar to the intracellular pH (7.0), while the pK of haemoglobin is 7.4. The pK of the phosphate system is 6.8, but that of the bicarbonate system is only 6.1. Nevertheless, the latter is of most interest to clinicians because it is present in large amounts, its components can be measured and it is influenced by renal and respiratory compensatory mechanisms.

$$\begin{array}{ccccc} H^+ + & \underset{\substack{\text{Ionic} \\ \text{dissociation}}}{\rightleftharpoons} & H_2CO_3 & \underset{\substack{\text{Carbonic} \\ \text{anhydrase}}}{\rightleftharpoons} & CO_2 + H_2O \quad \textit{Kidneys} \\ HCO_3^- & & & & \text{(in solution)} \\ & & & & \downarrow \\ & & & & CO_2 \text{ (gas} \quad \textit{Lungs} \\ & & & & \text{phase)} \end{array}$$

Alterations in alveolar ventilation can compensate rapidly for metabolic abnormalities, while renal mechanisms operate over a longer time course and can also compensate for respiratory disturbances. Renal regulation of H^+ balance is achieved by reabsorption or excretion of filtered HCO_3^-, excretion of ammonia or excretion of titratable acidity. Electrical neutrality is usually maintained by reabsorption of Na^+.

Since $[H_2CO_3]$ is proportional to the P_aCO_2 the Henderson-Hasselbach equation can be rewritten as:

$$[H^+] \propto \frac{Pco_2}{[HCO_3^-]}$$

Pco_2 can therefore be plotted against $[H^+]$ (or pH) and the various acid-base disturbances described in relation to this (**Fig. 5.4**). Both acidosis and alkalosis can occur, and either may be metabolic (i.e. primarily affecting the bicarbonate component of the system) or respiratory (i.e. primarily affecting P_{CO_2}). Compensatory changes may also be apparent. In clinical practice, arterial [H$^+$] values outside the range 126 nmol/l–18 nmol/l (pH 6.9–7.7) are very rarely encountered.

RESPIRATORY ACIDOSIS

Respiratory acidosis is caused by retention of carbon dioxide; the P_{CO_2} and [H$^+$] rise (see **Fig. 5.4**. Sometimes there is a small increase in HCO$_3^-$. A chronically raised P_{CO_2} is compensated by renal retention of bicarbonate and [H$^+$] returns towards normal. A constant arterial bicarbonate concentration is then usually established within 2–5 days. This represents a primary respiratory acidosis with a compensatory metabolic alkalosis. It is worth recognizing that because treatment such as the administration of diuretics can exacerbate hypochloraemia and produce further retention of bicarbonate, [H$^+$] may be on the low side of normal, even when carbon dioxide retention is the primary abnormality.

Common causes of respiratory acidosis include ventilatory failure and chronic obstructive airways disease (COAD, type II respiratory failure—see Chapter 6).

RESPIRATORY ALKALOSIS

In respiratory alkalosis the reverse occurs with a fall in P_{CO_2} and [H$^+$] (see **Fig. 5.4**), often with a small reduction in bicarbonate concentration. If hypocarbia persists some degree of renal compensation may occur, producing a metabolic acidosis, although in practice this is unusual. A respiratory alkalosis is often produced intentionally or unintentionally when patients are artificially ventilated; it may also be seen in hypoxaemic (type I) respiratory failure (see Chapter 6) and in those living at altitude.

METABOLIC ACIDOSIS

Metabolic acidosis may be due to excessive acid production, most commonly lactic acid, during an episode of shock or following cardiac arrest. Another common cause is diabetic ketoacidosis. A metabolic acidosis may also develop in chronic renal failure, or following either the administration of acid substances, or the loss of large amounts of alkali (e.g. from the lower gastrointestinal tract or in renal tubular acidosis). Respiratory compensation for a metabolic acidosis is usually slightly delayed because the blood–brain barrier initially prevents the respiratory centre from sensing the increased blood [H$^+$]. Following this short delay, however, the patient

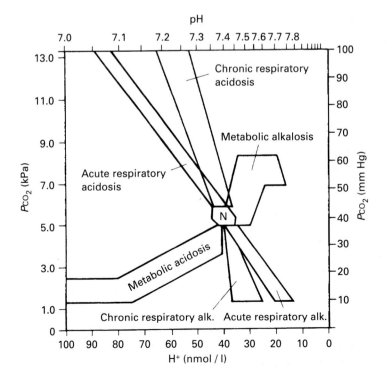

Fig. 5.4 Diagram representing disturbances of acid–base balance (95% confidence limits). The area of normal values is labelled N. From Goldberg *et al.* (1973), with permission. © 1973, American Medical Association.

hyperventilates and 'blows off' carbon dioxide to produce a compensatory respiratory alkalosis. As can be seen from **Fig. 5.4**, there is a limit to this respiratory compensation since values for P_aCO_2 less than about 1.5 kPa (11 mm Hg) are in practice never achieved. It should also be noted that respiratory compensation cannot occur if the patient's ventilation is controlled.

Anion gap

When the aetiology of a metabolic acidosis is not clinically obvious, calculation of the 'anion gap' may help to differentiate between the various causes. This is calculated as the difference between the sum of the bicarbonate and chloride concentrations and the sum of the sodium and potassium concentrations. Normally, the sum of the unmeasured anions (sulphates, phosphates, plasma proteins and anions of organic acids) ranges from 5 to 12 mmol/l. When the acidosis is due to a loss of base, the 'anion gap' will be normal. Conversely, a metabolic acidosis with an increased 'anion gap' results from a gain of acid (e.g. in ketoacidosis, renal failure, poisoning with methanol, salicylates, or ethylene glycol (antifreeze), and in lactic acidosis).

Lactic acidosis

Lactic acidosis may be due to increased production and/or decreased removal of lactic acid. The principal sources of lactic acid are skeletal muscle, brain and erythrocytes; lactate ions are converted to glucose or oxidized by the liver and kidney. Two types of lactic acidosis have been identified, designated type A and type B.

Type A lactic acidosis. This is more common and is due to inadequate tissue perfusion, cellular hypoxia and anaerobic glycolysis. The ability of the liver to remove the excess lactic acid is often impaired by underperfusion as well as by severe acidosis, and in extreme cases the liver may actually produce, rather than consume, lactate. The clinical picture is usually dominated by the underlying cause and treatment is directed at reversing tissue hypoxia (see Chapter 4).

Type B lactic acidosis. This occurs in the absence of tissue hypoxia. In the past, the most common cause was the administration of phenformin to patients with impaired renal or hepatic function. Other causes include diabetic ketoacidosis (see Chapter 16), severe liver disease (see Chapter 13), intravenous infusion of sorbitol or fructose, ethanol ingestion, methanol poisoning (see Chapter 18), acute infections and rare hereditary disorders (e.g. glucose-6-phosphate dehydrogenase

deficiency). Renal failure is commonly present, but is probably not a cause in itself. The patient usually presents with marked hyperventilation, which may progress to drowsiness, vomiting and eventually coma. Blood pressure is normal, there is no cyanosis and the patient is well perfused.

Treatment of severe type B lactic acidosis involves removal of the precipitating cause and the intravenous administration of sodium bicarbonate; it may prove to be extremely difficult to reverse the acidosis and very large amounts of bicarbonate may be required (e.g. 1000 mmol). Therefore, some recommend that the first 2–3 litres are given as an isotonic (1.4%) solution, followed by 8.4% sodium bicarbonate. The large volumes of fluid required may precipitate volume overload and pulmonary oedema (Vaziri *et al.*, 1979. Peritoneal dialysis with bicarbonate-buffered solution or haemodiafiltration has been advocated for resistant cases (Vaziri *et al.*, 1979).

METABOLIC ALKALOSIS

Metabolic alkalosis can be caused by loss of acid (e.g. from the stomach with nasogastric suction or in high intestinal obstruction) or by excessive administration of absorbable alkali. Overzealous treatment with intravenous sodium bicarbonate is frequently implicated. In such cases of metabolic alkalosis the urinary chloride concentration is usually low. Some less-common causes of metabolic alkalosis in which urinary chloride is high include hyperaldosteronism, Cushing's syndrome, ingestion of liquorice and severe potassium deficiency. Depletion of the extracellular fluid volume and a reduction in total body potassium are both important precipitating factors in the development of metabolic alkalosis. Contraction of the extracellular compartment causes increased sodium reabsorption in exchange for hydrogen ions. The latter are lost in the urine and bicarbonate reabsorption is increased. Similarly, potassium depletion stimulates the kidneys to retain potassium in exchange for hydrogen ions. Diuretics are frequently implicated in both extracellular fluid volume depletion and hypokalaemia.

Treatment consists of correcting the underlying cause; specific treatment is rarely required. If severe alkalosis persists despite restoring the extracellular fluid volume and correction of potassium depletion, the carbonic anhydrase inhibitor acetazolamide or, very occasionally, intravenous hydrochloric acid may be indicated.

Respiratory compensation for a metabolic alkalosis is often slight and it is rare to encounter a $P_aCO_2 > 6.5$ kPa (50 mm Hg), even with severe alkalosis.

INTERPRETING THE ACID–BASE STATE OF A PATIENT

Proceed as follows:

- Look at the [H⁺] to see whether the patient is acidotic or alkalotic.
- Look at the standard bicarbonate and the base excess. If the standard bicarbonate is low and the base excess is negative (i.e. there is a base deficit) there is a metabolic acid
  the base (
  alosis.
- Look at th
  piratory c
  respirator
  ory alkalo
- Although
  by the dir
  the case.
  then only
  context ir

It should
severe circu
be consider
venous bloo
particularly
anical ventil
istration of
The importa
tice is not y
a widened a
ful indicator
venous bloo
base status.

Alteratio

Having inter
be evaluated
to remember that in most situations it is the oxygen content of the arterial blood (C_aO_2) that matters and that this is determined by the percentage saturation of haemoglobin with oxygen. The latter is related to the P_O_2 by the oxyhaemoglobin dissociation curve. The clinical significance of this is discussed in Chapter 2, but it is most important to look at the P_O_2 in conjunction with the percentage saturation; in general, if the latter is greater than 95%, oxygenation can be considered to be adequate. Remember that P_aO_2 is influenced by factors other than pulmonary function, including alterations in the mixed venous oxygen tension (P_vO_2) caused by changing metabolic rate and/or cardiac output, and shifts in the position of the dissociation curve (see Chapter 2).

DETERMINATION OF OXYGEN CONTENT

As discussed above, the derived values for oxygen content produced by automated blood gas analysers are not sufficiently accurate even for clinical use. Direct measurement of oxygen content, or its calculation from accurately determined values for haemoglobin and oxygen saturation, is therefore often required, usually in
r to derive other important variables such as V_O_2
percentage venous admixture.

clinical practice, oxygen content is usually calcu-
from accurately determined values for haemo-
in and oxygen saturation. These can be measured
g a *photometric technique*. The automated bench
eters designed for this purpose are relatively robust
easy to operate and can therefore be used on-site
taff who have been instructed in their use. They
sure the optical absorbance of haemolysed blood at
at four separate wavelengths, thereby providing
es for carboxy- and methaemoglobin as well as
haemoglobin. These values, together with derived
gen content, are then displayed digitally.

VIVO BLOOD GAS MEASUREMENT

re are obvious potential clinical advantages in mon-
ng blood gas tensions continuously rather than
rmittently. The instantaneous detection of changes
lood gas tensions allows rapid evaluation and adjust-
t of therapy, as well as immediate recognition of
riorating cardiorespiratory function. The effects of
entially dangerous manoeuvres (e.g. hypoxaemia
urring during endotracheal suction) or accidents
h as circuit disconnection are also immediately
arent.
travascular blood gas tensions can be monitored
tinuously using miniaturized electrodes or mass
ctrometry, while oxygen saturation can be determ-
d using fibre-optic oximeters. Blood gas tensions and
oxygen saturation can also be estimated continuously
using transcutaneous electrodes or oximetry.

Electrode systems

Techniques for continuous *in vivo* determination of oxygen tension are usually based on miniaturized Clark electrodes. Usually these devices incorporate a lumen to allow discrete samples of arterial blood to be obtained intermittently.

Although the linear response of these electrodes is good when compared with bench analysis, they have a tendency to drift and are influenced by changes in body temperature. They therefore have to be calibrated at regular intervals against conventionally analysed arterial samples. Because fresh blood is continuously flowing past the electrode membrane, the blood gas factor is normally small and can be ignored, although in low-flow states this may become a significant source of error.

Such electrodes have been widely used to monitor P_aO_2 continuously in neonates, in whom it is essential to control P_aO_2 within narrow limits at all times to avoid cerebral hypoxia on the one hand and retrolental fibroplasia on the other. They have also been used for continuous monitoring of venous oxygen tension, and in critically ill adults a sustained fall in $P_{\bar{v}}O_2$ to below 5.3 kPa (40 mm Hg) was found to be a reliable indicator of respiratory or cardiovascular deterioration, which was not always clinically obvious (Armstrong et al., 1978). Nevertheless, although a reduction in $P_{\bar{v}}O_2$ implies that tissue oxygenation is impaired, a normal or high value does not necessarily indicate that oxygenation is adequate. Despite the potential advantages of intravascular PO_2 electrodes, their use has not yet become established in adult intensive care practice.

The development of intravascular electrodes for determining PCO_2 has been beset by technical problems, mainly the difficulty of miniaturizing glass electrodes and their fragility. These have prevented their introduction into the intensive care unit for long-term monitoring, although they have been used for limited periods in anaesthetized subjects.

Mass spectrometry

As well as being used for the measurement of inspired and expired gas concentrations as outlined above, mass spectrometers have been used to continuously monitor intravascular blood gas tensions. Indwelling, fine-bore, semi-flexible stainless steel catheters, which are impermeable to the analysed gases, are normally used for sampling. The tip of the catheter is perforated and covered with a gas-permeable membrane, across which blood gases equilibrate. The proximal end is connected to a vacuum system, which aspirates these gases into the mass spectrometer.

The main advantage of this technique is that several gases can be analysed simultaneously. Clearly, this system will remove gases from the layer of blood adjacent to the membrane, thereby creating a significant 'blood gas factor'. It also requires previous calibration against in vitro blood gas analysis. To date, the cost and complexity of this technique, together with the need for frequent expert maintenance of the apparatus, has limited its introduction into clinical practice.

Fibre-optic spectrophotometry

The technique of in vivo oximetry uses an intravascular fibre-optic catheter and is based on the same principles as those used in the bench oximeters described above. A beam of light consisting of a number of precisely known wavelengths is generated, usually by a light-emitting diode, and transmitted down one of two bundles of optical fibres. Light reflected from the red cells is returned to a photodiode detector along the other bundle of fibres. In this way, the percentage saturation of haemoglobin with oxygen can be measured continuously and accurately in vivo. Although fibre-optic spectrophotometers are generally very stable, the signal may be distorted by deposition of fibrin or if the tip of the catheter impinges on the vessel wall.

These devices can be positioned relatively easily in the pulmonary artery and have been used successfully for continuous determination of mixed venous oxygen saturation ($S_{\bar{v}}O_2$). Fibre-optic oximeters have now been incorporated into Swan–Ganz catheters and this has facilitated their introduction into routine clinical practice.

Transcutaneous blood gas measurement
(Shoemaker & Vidyasalgar, 1981; Eberhard et al., 1981)

TRANSCUTANEOUS PO_2 ($P_{tc}O_2$)

As with continuous intravascular PO_2 determination, most of the initial experience with measurement of $P_{tc}O_2$ was gained in neonates. The principle of the method is based on increasing the diffusion of oxygen from the blood in the subdermal capillary loops to the skin surface, where its partial pressure can be measured with a conventional Clark electrode housed behind a membrane. The oxygen tension gradient from capillary to skin surface is clearly dependent on P_aO_2 but is also influenced by many other factors including:

- skin thickness;
- tissue blood flow;
- tissue oxygen consumption;
- the position of the oxyhaemoglobin dissociation curve.

Transcutaneous electrodes therefore incorporate a heating element, which is maintained at 44–45°C and warms the underlying skin to approximately 43°C. This increases skin permeability and blood flow, and also facilitates unloading of oxygen from haemoglobin by shifting the dissociation curve to the right. These effects are, however, to some extent offset by a local increase in VO_2. Nevertheless, provided tissue blood flow is adequate, it is usually possible to obtain a reasonable linear correlation between $P_{tc}O_2$ and P_aO_2.

Accurate results are very dependent on adequate skin blood flow so that in patients with low cardiac output $P_{tc}O_2$ is a poor indicator of P_aO_2. Although in neonates $P_{tc}O_2$ usually closely reflects P_aO_2, many feel that in adults, even when peripheral perfusion is good, $P_{tc}O_2$ should only be used as an indicator of trends in P_aO_2.

Although the response time is rapid in infants (10–15 seconds) this increases to 45–60 seconds in adults and the reading will take 5–15 minutes to reach a plateau following application of the electrode. Finally the area of skin underlying the electrode can be damaged by excessive heating.

POLAROGRAPHIC OXYGEN SENSORS

A polarographic oxygen sensor that can be applied to the conjunctiva has been described (Fatt & Deutsch, 1983). These devices eliminate the need to heat the skin and have a faster response time than transcutaneous electrodes. Although it was initially thought that conjunctival sensors would be less dependent on perfusion, they have since been found to be sensitive to local and systemic alterations in flow. Some consider them to be of use during resuscitation and transport.

TRANSCUTANEOUS P_{CO_2} ($P_{tc}CO_2$)

Most transcutaneous carbon dioxide electrodes consist of a conventional glass pH electrode combined with a heating element. Carbon dioxide is, of course, more soluble than oxygen and is produced, rather than consumed, by the tissues. Furthermore, heating the skin increases local carbon dioxide production and capillary P_{CO_2}. Therefore, $P_{tc}O_2$ is consistently higher than P_aCO_2 and the difference between the two varies considerably from patient to patient depending on skin characteristics. However, changes in $P_{tc}CO_2$ do follow the trend of alterations in P_aCO_2, although in shock $P_{tc}CO_2$ can be very high and the discrepancy between P_aCO_2 and $P_{tc}CO_2$ is increased.

Pulse oximetry (Taylor & Whitwam, 1986)

Light weight oximeters that measure the changing amount of light transmitted through pulsating arterial blood and provide a continuous non-invasive assessment of arterial oxygen saturation (S_aO_2) can be applied to an ear lobe or finger. These devices are reliable, do not require calibration, are easy to use and have superseded transcutaneous blood gas electrodes for continuous monitoring of oxygenation in adult intensive care prac-

tice. They automatically compensate for variations in skin thickness, slight differences in skin pigmentation and small changes in peripheral perfusion. The signal is, however, very susceptible to noise and movement artefact may cause difficulties.

The accuracy of oximeters varies, but in general the 95% confidence limits are roughly ± 4% when S_aO_2 is greater than 80%; below this value they tend to over-read. Poor peripheral perfusion, oedema, venous congestion and abnormal haemoglobins lead to inaccuracies. Elevated carboxyhaemoglobin levels, for example, result in falsely high readings; this may be important in recently admitted heavy smokers and in carbon monoxide poisoning. Jaundice may result in falsely low values for S_aO_2.

It is important to appreciate that pulse oximetry is not a sensitive guide to changes in oxygenation because, assuming an error of ± 4%, a reading of 95% could represent either a true value of 91% (i.e. P_aO_2 approximately 8 kPa) or 99% (i.e. P_aO_2 approximately 20 kPa); S_aO_2 becomes a useful indicator of P_aO_2 only when it has fallen below 90% (a P_aO_2 of about 8 kPa), and pulse oximetry cannot be used to monitor P_aO_2 when the upper level of P_aO_2 is critical (e.g. in neonates). Clearly an S_aO_2 within normal limits in a patient receiving supplemental oxygen in no way excludes the possibility of hypoventilation (Hutton & Clutton-Brock, 1993).

DUAL OXIMETRY (Räsänen et al., 1987)

Continuous monitoring of S_aO_2 and S_vO_2 has been advocated as a means of obtaining real-time assessment of changes in peripheral oxygen extraction and pulmonary gas exchange. Thus, for example, the development of hypoxaemia with convergence of S_aO_2 and S_vO_2 indicates worsening gas exchange with a fall in extraction, whereas divergence of S_aO_2 and S_vO_2 implies increased peripheral oxygen use.

OTHER INDICES OF PULMONARY FUNCTION

In the most severely ill patients, more sophisticated indices of pulmonary gas exchange may occasionally prove useful (e.g. in following a patient's progress and response to therapy or deciding when to wean a patient from artificial ventilation).

Alveolar–arterial oxygen difference ($P_{A-a}O_2$)

$P_{A-a}O_2$ can be determined by measuring P_aO_2 and calculating P_AO_2 from the alveolar air equation (see Chapter

2). This requires accurate determination of the F_1O_2, barometric pressure and P_aCO_2. The RQ can be assumed to be 0.8. The $P_{A-a}O_2$ has certain limitations as an index of pulmonary function for the following reasons.

- It is influenced by the P_AO_2 so that even in normal subjects $P_{A-a}O_2$ increases as F_1O_2 rises.
- It is influenced by the $P_{\bar{v}}O_2$ (i.e. it will alter if cardiac output, metabolic rate, oxygen extraction or the position of the dissociation curve change).

Some feel that it is useful to determine the $P_{A-a}O_2$ with the patient breathing 100% oxygen. This can then be compared with predicted values under these circumstances and with values obtained in the same patient breathing air. However, breathing pure oxygen, even for short periods, can in itself impair lung function and this practice should in general be avoided.

Percentage venous admixture and dead space

Because of the limitations of $P_{A-a}O_2$ just described, it is more satisfactory to calculate percentage venous admixture. Physiological dead space is often calculated at the same time to provide the 'three compartment' analysis of respiratory function described in Chapter 2.

This three-compartment analysis does not, however, provide any information about the relative contribution of true shunt and V/Q disturbance to the total venous admixture, nor does it describe the nature of the V/Q inequality. Methods have been developed using the intravenous injection of inert tracer gases of different solubilities, which can, when analysed by computer produce a description of alveolar V/Q distributions. These techniques are generally not used in clinical practice.

Iso-shunt lines

When hypoxaemia is due to pulmonary venous admixture and the patient is in a reasonably steady state, a series of lines can be plotted relating P_aO_2 to F_1O_2, each line representing the relationship for a particular value of venous admixture. It was at one time suggested that these 'iso-shunt' lines might be used to limit the frequency of blood gas analysis needed to control oxygen therapy (Benatar *et al.*, 1973).

The $P_aO_2 : F_1O_2$ ratio

The $P_aO_2 : F_1O_2$ ratio can be used as a simple index of the severity of lung dysfunction. It does not take into account fluctuations in P_aCO_2.

Alveolar–capillary permeability

Techniques for determining alveolar–capillary permeability have been developed largely as research tools and are rarely used clinically.

Epithelial permeability can be assessed by recording the clearance of an inhaled aerosol of technetium[99m]-DTPA (diethylene triamine pentacetic acid) from the lungs using a gamma camera or an externally placed scintillation counter. Tc[99m]-DTPA is an inert γ-emitter with a short half-life of about six hours; it is assumed that the endothelium is freely permeable to this small molecule and that changes in clearance therefore reflect alterations in epithelial integrity. Tc[99m]-DTPA clearance is increased in smokers, as well as in adult respiratory distress syndrome (ARDS), and the technique can be used to distinguish cardiogenic from non-cardiogenic pulmonary oedema (see Chapter 6).

Endothelial permeability can be assessed by measuring the accumulation in the lung of an intravascular radiotracer such as Tc[99m] or iodine[131]-labelled albumin or transferrin. In ARDS this method appears to be less sensitive, but more specific than the measurement of DTPA clearance. Specificity and sensitivity can be increased by using a double isotope technique (e.g. by simultaneously labelling red blood cells to provide an intravascular marker).

A less sensitive and more invasive technique is to measure the accumulation of I[131]-labelled albumin in bronchoalveolar secretions.

Extravascular lung water (Staub, 1986)

Techniques for the determination of extravascular lung water include the *thermodilution double indicator method* (Noble *et al.*, 1980) and *double radiotracer indicator dilution*. The latter involves injection into the right atrium of two radiotracers (one of which remains intravascular, while the other diffuses freely through the extravascular spaces) followed by sampling of arterial blood to obtain time activity curves. These techniques provide a poor estimate of the severity of ARDS.

Ventilation–perfusion scans

Lung perfusion can be assessed by determining the distribution of intravenous Tc[99m]-labelled microspheres. Although segmental perfusion defects in the appropriate clinical setting are suggestive of pulmonary embolism, hypoxic pulmonary vasoconstriction in lung regions where ventilation is reduced or absent (e.g. in areas of collapse and/or consolidation) may complicate interpretation. The diagnosis of pulmonary embolism is supported by excluding obvious lung pathology in the region of interest on plain chest radiography or by demonstrating normal ventilation in areas of reduced perfusion using, for example, aerosolized xenon[133] (V/Q scan). Ventilation scanning can, however, be difficult, if not impossible, in critically ill patients, especially when an endotracheal tube is in place.

REFERENCES

Adroguè HJ, Rashad MN, Gorin AB, Yacoub J & Madias NE (1989) Assessing acid-base status in circulatory failure. Differences between arterial and central venous blood. *New England Journal of Medicine* **320**: 1312-1316.

Armstrong RF, Walker JS, St Andrew D *et al.* (1978) Continuous monitoring of mixed venous oxygen tension P_vO_2 in cardiorespiratory disorders. *Lancet* **i**: 632-634.

Benatar SR, Hewlett AM & Nunn JF (1973) The use of iso-shunt lines for control of oxygen therapy. *British Journal of Anaesthesia* **45**: 711-718.

Biswas CK, Ramos JM, Agroyannis B & Kerr DNS (1982) Blood gas analysis: effect of air bubbles in syringe and delay in estimation. *British Medical Journal* **284**: 923-927.

Bradley JG (1972) Errors in the measurement of blood PCO_2 due to dilution of the sample with heparin solution. *British Journal of Anaesthesia* **44**: 231-232.

Eberhard P, Mindt W & Schafer R (1981) Cutaneous blood gas monitoring in the adult. *Critical Care Medicine* **9**: 702-705.

Fatt I & Deutsch TA (1983) The relation of conjunctival PO_2 to capillary bed PO_2. *Critical Care Medicine* **11**: 445-448.

Goldberg M, Green SB, Moss ML *et al.* (1973) Computer-based instruction and diagnosis of acid-base disorders. A systematic approach. *Journal of the American Medical Association* **223**: 269-275.

Gothard JWW, Busst CM, Branthwaite MA, Davies NJH & Denison DM (1980) Applications of respiratory mass spectrometry to intensive care. *Anaesthesia* **35**: 890-895.

Hutton P & Clutton-Brock T (1993) The benefits and pitfalls of pulse oximetry. *British Medical Journal* **307**: 457-458.

Noble WH, Kay JC, Maret KH & Caskanette G (1980) Reappraisal of extravascular lung thermal volume as a measure of pulmonary edema. *Journal of Applied Physiology* **48**: 120-129.

Räsänen J, Downs JB, Malec DJ, DeHaven B & Seidman P (1987) Estimation of oxygen utilization by dual oximetry. *Annals of Surgery* **206**: 621-623.

Shoemaker WC & Vidyasagar D (1981) Physiological and clinical significance of $P_{tc}O_2$ and $P_{tc}O_2$ measurements. *Critical Care Medicine* **9**: 689-690.

Staub NC (1986) Clinical use of lung water measurements. Report of a workshop. *Chest* **90**: 588-594.

Sykes MK & Vickers MD (1973) *Principles of Measurement for Anaesthetists*. Oxford, Blackwell Scientific, pp. 126-131.

Takala J, Keinänen O, Väisänen P & Kari A (1989) Measurement of gas exchange in intensive care: laboratory and clinical validation of a new device. *Critical Care Medicine* **17**: 1041-1047.

Taylor MB & Whitwam JG (1986) The current status of pulse oximetry. *Anaesthesia* **41**: 943-949.

Tobin MJ (1992) Breathing pattern analysis. *Intensive Care Medicine* **18**: 193-201.

Vaziri ND, Ness R, Wellikson L, Barton C & Greep N (1979) Bicarbonate buffered peritoneal dialysis. An effective adjunct in the treatment of lactic acidosis. *American Journal of Medicine* **67**: 392-396.

6 Respiratory Failure

DEFINITION

Respiratory failure occurs when pulmonary gas exchange is sufficiently impaired to cause hypoxaemia with or without hypercarbia.

TYPES, MECHANISMS AND CLINICAL FEATURES

The respiratory system consists of a gas exchanging organ (the lungs) and a ventilatory pump (respiratory muscles/thorax), either or both of which can fail and precipitate respiratory failure.

Acute hypoxaemic (Type I) respiratory failure

Acute hypoxaemic (Type I) respiratory failure (ARF) is caused by diseases that interfere with gas exchange by damaging lung tissue. Hypoxaemia is due to right-to-left shunts, ventilation/perfusion (V/Q) mismatch or, most often, a combination of these two. As discussed in Chapter 2, barriers to diffusion are almost never an important cause of hypoxaemia. An increase in right-to-left shunt occurs when alveoli are completely collapsed, become totally consolidated or are filled with oedema fluid. V/Q inequalities result from pulmonary parenchymal disease that causes regional variations in compliance, an increased scatter of time constants (see Chapter 2) and/or abnormalities of perfusion. Also, functional residual capacity (FRC) is reduced so that tidal exchange takes place below closing volume (i.e. airway closure occurs throughout the respiratory cycle), and this is associated with an increase in the number of relatively underventilated lung units.

Initially, there is usually an increase in total ventilation, which compensates for the increased dead space (V_D) and maintains P_aCO_2 at normal levels. Indeed, relative hyperventilation, possibly in response to severe hypoxaemia and/or stimulation of irritant and mechanoreceptors within the lungs, may cause a reduction in P_aCO_2. The degree of hypoxaemia is limited by constriction of vessels supplying those alveoli with a low PO_2—'*hypoxic pulmonary vasoconstriction*'—although the intensity of this response is very variable and appears to be genetically determined (see Chapter 2).

As well as the impairment of gas exchanging properties, the lungs deteriorate mechanically with a reduction in compliance (associated with the fall in FRC, see Chapter 2) and/or an increase in resistance, so that the work and metabolic cost of breathing is increased. Under these circumstances, patients find it easier to breathe rapidly with a low tidal volume (V_T). Finally, these patients are often pyrexial, with a raised metabolic rate, and this further increases both oxygen consumption ($\dot{V}O_2$) and the volume of carbon dioxide that has to be excreted. Therefore the characteristic clinical features of ARF include:

- hypoxia;
- hypocarbia;
- tachypnoea;
- small V_T.

In contrast to the normal pattern of ventilation, there is little moment to moment variation in either respiratory rate or V_T.

Ventilatory (Type II) respiratory failure

Ventilatory failure occurs when alveolar ventilation is insufficient to excrete the volume of carbon dioxide being produced by tissue metabolism. Carbon dioxide is therefore retained, producing an increase in both arterial and alveolar PCO_2. Due to the operation of the alveolar gas equation (see Chapter 2, equation 2.16), this inevitably leads to a fall in alveolar oxygen tension (P_AO_2) and hypoxaemia, even in patients with normal lungs. Inadequate alveolar ventilation may be due to:

- reduced ventilatory effort;
- inability to overcome an increased resistance to ventilation;
- failure to compensate for an increase in V_D and/or carbon dioxide production;
- a combination of these factors.

The respiratory muscles have a large reserve, however, and considerable impairment of function may be present without ventilatory failure. Characteristic clinical features of pure ventilatory failure, therefore, include:

- hypercarbia;
- hypoxia;
- a reduced rate and/or depth of breathing.

These patients may suffer from an extremely distressing sensation of breathlessness, even when ventilation is apparently adequate (e.g. judged by blood gas values).

Mixed respiratory failure

Often, the two types of respiratory failure are combined to produce a mixed picture. As discussed above, acute diseases of the pulmonary parenchyma initially cause purely hypoxaemic respiratory failure. In some cases, however, exhaustion eventually supervenes; the patient is then unable to overcome the mechanical impairment of lung function and cannot compensate for the increased V_D and carbon dioxide production. At this stage, the arterial carbon dioxide tension (P_aCO_2) begins to rise and mixed respiratory failure develops.

Ventilatory failure is often complicated by the subsequent development of pulmonary abnormalities. This is because these patients are unable to cough adequately, sigh or take deep breaths, and are therefore at risk of alveolar collapse, retention of secretions and secondary infection. In addition, in those with an associated bulbar palsy, aspiration can occur and further damage the lungs.

Respiratory muscle dysfunction

Respiratory muscle fatigue (see Chapter 2) has been demonstrated in healthy subjects submitted to high inspiratory resistive loads and may also play a role in the development of respiratory failure, although overt respiratory muscle fatigue is probably unusual and the underlying mechanisms are not yet fully understood. Increased fatiguability of the sternomastoid muscle has, however, been demonstrated in patients with severe respiratory disease on admission to hospital (Efthimiou et al., 1987), and this appeared to resolve as the patient recovered. It was suggested that respiratory muscle fatigue had contributed to hypercapnia in these patients, although the exact significance of these findings remains unclear. It has also been postulated that 'chronic' respiratory muscle fatigue, a poorly understood phenomenon, may contribute to the development of hypercapnia in chronic respiratory failure.

Predisposing factors to the development of respiratory muscle fatigue include:

- an increased load (e.g. imposed by airways obstruction, a reduction in lung compliance or chest wall abnormalities);
- muscle weakness related to neuromuscular disorders

(see later in this chapter and chapter 7), disuse atrophy, malnutrition, generalized wasting, or old age.

Muscle dysfunction may be exacerbated by:

- sepsis;
- metabolic disturbances;
- hypoxaemia;
- hypercarbia;
- hyperinflation (see later).

In addition, profound *reductions in respiratory muscle blood flow*, such as may occur in cardiogenic shock, can lead to impaired respiratory muscle contraction in the face of increased excitation, especially when combined with the increased demands imposed by compensatory hyperventilation and pulmonary oedema (Aubier et al., 1981).

Mechanisms that may mediate fatigue include:

- inhibition of neural drive;
- impaired neuromuscular transmission;
- excessive force and duration of contraction;
- impaired excitation/contraction coupling;
- depletion of muscle energy stores;
- failure of the contractile machinery.

Two types of muscle fatigue can be identified:

- *high frequency fatigue*, which is thought to be due to impaired neuromuscular transmission and/or propagation of the action potential;
- *low frequency fatigue*, which may reflect impaired excitation contraction coupling.

Although high-frequency nerve stimulation generates maximum muscle tension, the force of contraction rapidly falls when it persists. If this high-frequency fatigue were allowed to develop in the respiratory muscles there would be a rapid and catastrophic loss of ventilatory capacity. Lower frequency stimulation produces less initial force, but tension is well maintained and soon exceeds that generated by high-frequency stimulation. Low-frequency fatigue of respiratory muscles, which experimentally is long-lasting and associated with muscle fibre damage, may be an important component of ventilatory failure, but it requires massive overload to develop and has proved difficult to demonstrate clinically. It may be that both low-frequency fatigue, with consequent muscle damage, and high-frequency fatigue, with the rapid onset of extreme respiratory failure, do not readily occur because the central nervous system will not (or cannot) drive the peripheral contractile apparatus sufficiently hard (Moxham, 1990).

The role of *central fatigue* in respiratory failure is uncertain, but it may be that respiratory drive is modified to avoid central, high-frequency and low-frequency fatigue and thereby optimize ventilation, albeit at the cost of hypercapnia. Ventilatory failure may therefore be the result of a reduction in central drive, which is intended to protect the respiratory muscles from over-load and fatigue. For example, during weaning from mechanical ventilation, if the load is excessive and unsustainable, patients breathe rapidly with a low V_T. This reduces the work of breathing, but at the expense of carbon dioxide retention.

Clinical features of respiratory muscle fatigue

It has been suggested that tachypnoea, asynchronous or paradoxical respiration, respiratory alternans and finally a rising P_aCO_2 with a reduction in respiratory rate and minute volume are indicative of respiratory muscle fatigue. In *asynchronous respiration* there is a discrepancy in the rate of movement of the thoracic and abdominal compartments, while in *paradoxical respiration* they move in opposite directions. *Respiratory alternans* is caused by recruitment and derecruitment of the accessory/intercostal muscles and the diaphragm, leading to an increase in the breath-to-breath variation in the relative contribution of the rib cage and abdomen to V_T.

At present, however, there is no convincing evidence that any particular constellation of physical signs can serve as sensitive or specific markers of respiratory muscle fatigue. The detection of an abnormal pattern of thoraco-abdominal motion does, however, suggest a significantly increased respiratory load. Objective measures of respiratory muscle strength and fatigue are discussed in Chapter 5.

CAUSES OF RESPIRATORY FAILURE

Respiratory failure is commonly precipitated by:

- surgical operations (particularly upper abdominal or thoracic);
- acute respiratory tract infections;
- the administration of depressant drugs.

The causes of respiratory failure can best be considered according to anatomical location (**Fig. 6.1**).

Respiratory centre

Causes of depression of the respiratory centre commonly seen in the intensive care unit include:

- raised intracranial pressure or direct trauma (e.g. head injury);
- infections (e.g. meningo-encephalitis);
- vascular lesions;
- drug overdose (e.g. narcotics, barbiturates).

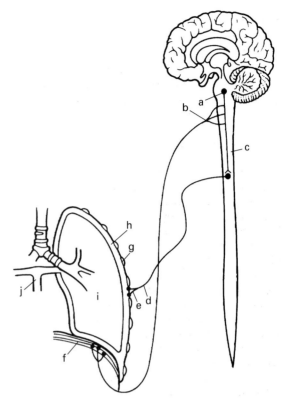

Fig. 6.1 Respiratory failure according to anatomical location: (a) respiratory centre; (b) phrenic nerve; (c) spinal cord; (d) motor nerves; (e) neuromuscular junction; (f) muscle; (g) chest wall; (h) pleura; (i) lungs and airways; (j) pulmonary circulation.

Patients in traumatic coma with intracranial hypertension may also have associated pulmonary oedema, lung contusion or aspiration pneumonia. Frequently, the laryngeal reflexes are also depressed and in some cases there may be a true bulbar palsy. Both predispose the patient to aspiration pneumonitis. Severe hypoxia and extreme hypercarbia can also reduce the responsiveness of the respiratory centre.

SLEEP-RELATED RESPIRATORY DISTURBANCES

Central sleep apnoea

In central sleep apnoea, there is periodic cessation of spontaneous impulse formation during sleep, which leads to repeated episodes of apnoea with absent respiratory efforts.

Complaints of dyspnoea and other respiratory findings are rarely prominent. Patients may present with:

- lethargy;
- headache;

- daytime sleepiness;
- unexplained polycythaemia;
- pulmonary hypertension;
- cor pulmonale.

Patients with *primary alveolar hypoventilation*, in whom there is a blunted ventilatory response to hypoxia and hypercarbia in the absence of abnormal lung function, may present with similar signs and symptoms.

Obstructive sleep apnoea

Patients with obstructive sleep apnoea suffer from intermittent functional upper airway obstruction during sleep, which is thought to be due to episodic loss of pharyngeal tone. This is associated with loud snoring, frequent apnoeic episodes, especially during rapid eye movement (REM) sleep, with severe hypoxaemia and repeated nocturnal awakening or arousal. Although traditionally associated with obesity, many patients are not significantly overweight. The condition is also associated with chronic obstructive pulmonary disease (COPD) and a reduced size of the pharyngeal opening, even when the patient is awake.

Occasionally obstructive sleep apnoea is associated with:

- daytime hypersomnolence:
- poor concentration;
- morning headache;
- impotence;
- systemic/pulmonary hypertension;
- unexplained cor pulmonale;
- polycythaemia.

The diagnosis is made when a sleep study demonstrates frequent severe apnoeic episodes associated with marked oxygen desaturation and vigorous respiratory efforts.

Correctable factors include:

- encroachment in the pharynx (obesity, acromegaly, enlarged tonsils);
- nasal obstruction (nasal deformities, rhinitis, polyps, adenoids);
- respiratory depressant drugs (alcohol, sedatives, strong analgesics).

Spinal cord

Very rarely, lesions of the high cervical cord or brain stem may interrupt the pathways involved in automatic breathing, while leaving the conscious pathways intact. Because these unfortunate patients therefore have to remember to breathe, long periods of apnoea occur, even when the subject is awake, and serious carbon dioxide retention occurs when they fall asleep. The hypercarbia increases cerebral blood flow, causing headaches, nightmares and disturbed sleep patterns. This condition has been called *'Ondine's curse'*, after a water nymph who, according to German mythology, cursed her husband by abolishing all his automatic functions. When he finally became exhausted and fell asleep, he died.

Traumatic damage to the spinal cord at or above the origin of the phrenic nerve (C3, C4, C5) causes severe ventilatory failure since only the accessory muscles are spared. Partial lesions are common, while cord damage below this level causes less respiratory impairment since diaphragmatic breathing remains intact (see also Chapter 9).

Poliomyelitis has its major impact on the anterior horn cells in the spinal cord and/or the motor nuclei of the cranial nerves and, in some cases, the respiratory centre itself is involved. The patient may therefore have a bulbar paralysis, in which case airway protection is vital, or spinal polio, which may cause weakness of the respiratory muscles and ventilatory failure. Sometimes both bulbar and spinal motor nuclei are affected.

If the spasms of *tetanus* are prolonged and severe, they may interfere with ventilation, but in any case treatment of the most severe cases consists of heavy sedation, paralysis and artificial ventilation (see Chapter 14). There is also some evidence that tetanus causes respiratory depression by a direct effect on the brain stem.

Motor neurone disease is a progressive disorder affecting the cerebral cortex, brain stem and spinal cord and is manifested as muscular atrophy with spasticity and hyperreflexia. It is a disease of middle age, which usually progresses inexorably and relatively rapidly (2–5 years) until death supervenes from respiratory failure, often associated with aspiration pneumonia. There is no known treatment and mechanical ventilation is often inappropriate.

Motor nerves

In *Guillain-Barré syndrome*, lower motor neurone weakness develops a few days, or even weeks, after a 'flu-like' illness. Usually the lower limbs are affected first, but later weakness may spread to the muscles of the face and trunk. A significant proportion of patients with this syndrome then develop ventilatory failure and require artificial ventilation (see Chapter 14).

Neuromuscular junction

Although *myasthenia gravis* may affect any voluntary muscle, ventilatory failure is unusual except during acute exacerbations ('myasthenic crisis'), overdosage with anticholinesterases ('cholinergic crisis') or post-operatively (following thymectomy) (see Chapter 14).

Botulism is an extremely rare form of food poisoning in which botulinum toxin prevents the release of acetylcholine from motor nerve endings, causing flaccid paralysis and ventilatory failure.

Organophosphorus compounds have been developed as chemical weapons and are used as insecticides. They are long-acting anticholinesterases and produce respiratory depression, bronchospasm, salivation, bradycardia, hypertension and convulsions (see Chapter 18).

Failure to reverse the effects of *neuromuscular blocking agents* used during anaesthesia is an occasional cause of admission to intensive care units for artificial ventilation.

Chest wall

If a segment of chest wall becomes unstable (e.g. due to *multiple rib fractures*), particularly when associated with lung contusion, it may be impossible to sustain adequate ventilation (see Chapter 9). Similarly, if the thorax is deformed (e.g. due to kyphoscoliosis), lung expansion will be impaired. These patients may eventually develop ventilatory failure and are prone to recurrent chest infections. On the other hand, ventilatory failure is unusual when chest movement is restricted, but the thorax is uniform (e.g. as in ankylosing spondylitis).

Rarely, patients with *myopathies* or *myositis* may develop respiratory failure. Artificial ventilation may be required and can allow time for the diagnosis to be established (e.g. by muscle biopsy).

Pleura

Pneumothorax, haemothorax, pleural effusion and *empyema* may all cause or exacerbate respiratory failure.

Lungs and airways

As discussed above, diseases affecting primarily the lungs and airways initially cause hypoxaemic respiratory failure, but may later progress to the mixed type. Causes of ARF include pneumonia, asthma, left ventricular failure and adult respiratory distress syndrome (ARDS) (see below). Examples of chronic type I respiratory failure include emphysema and fibrosing lung disease. The commonest cause of mixed respiratory failure is COPD. Upper airway obstruction is usually well tolerated initially, but can rapidly progress to frank respiratory failure.

Pulmonary circulation

As well as mechanically obstructing the circulation (see Chapter 4), acute pulmonary embolism can cause *V/Q* inequalities, possibly via reflex mechanisms, with hypoxaemia and tachypnoea. Recurrent pulmonary emboli eventually produce chronic pulmonary hypertension and respiratory failure.

PRINCIPLES OF MANAGEMENT

Clearly, the specific treatment of respiratory failure will vary according to the underlying cause, but the same general principles apply in all cases.

- Hypoxaemia should be corrected;
- The load on the respiratory muscles should be reduced by improving lung mechanics and controlling fever.
- Ventilatory pump capacity should be optimized.

The importance of chest wall stiffness and decreased abdominal compliance in increasing the respiratory load are sometimes not fully appreciated. Since it seems unlikely that overt high- or low-frequency fatigue are allowed to develop in respiratory failure, specific therapy to counteract fatigue is probably of little value (Moxham, 1990).

Respiratory failure must not be considered in isolation. Not only do hypoxia and hypercarbia adversely affect cardiovascular performance, but a low cardiac output is associated with a reduction in P_vO_2, exacerbating the adverse effects of a given degree of shunt on arterial oxygenation. Low cardiac output is also associated with a decrease in respiratory muscle blood flow, anaerobic metabolism in respiratory muscles (which exacerbates lactic acidosis) and respiratory muscle fatigue (Aubier *et al.*, 1982). Many drugs that act on the cardiovascular system, such as dopamine and sodium nitroprusside, have been shown to increase pulmonary venous admixture, probably by reversing hypoxic pulmonary vasoconstriction. Myocardial failure often causes pulmonary congestion with increased shunting, and hypotension may lead to an increased V_D, particularly during intermittent positive pressure ventilation (IPPV). Finally, the increased work and metabolic cost of breathing increases the load on the myocardium and respiratory system.

Oxygen therapy

INDICATIONS

Oxygen therapy is always indicated in patients with *acute hypoxaemic or mixed respiratory failure*. For reasons discussed previously it is most effective when the main abnormality is V/Q mismatch, but is less efficacious in the presence of a fixed right-to-left shunt (see Chapter 2).

In patients with *pure ventilatory failure*, the primary abnormality is retention of carbon dioxide; specific treatment is therefore directed towards lowering P_aCO_2 and P_ACO_2. The administration of oxygen is, however, a useful first step when managing these patients since it effectively reverses the hypoxia, which is the inevitable consequence of the elevated P_ACO_2.

Patients with *carbon monoxide poisoning* will also benefit from oxygen administration. By increasing P_aO_2, the dissociation of carboxyhaemoglobin is accelerated and the increase in dissolved oxygen improves tissue oxygenation.

METHODS OF OXYGEN ADMINISTRATION

In mechanically ventilated patients, the inspired oxygen concentration (F_IO_2) is easily measured (see Chapter 5) and can be maintained at the desired level by mixing air and oxygen in appropriate proportions. This also applies to spontaneously breathing patients with endotracheal tubes or a tracheostomy connected either to a T-piece or a continuous positive airway pressure (CPAP) circuit (see Chapter 7).

In the non-intubated spontaneously breathing patient, measuring F_IO_2 is not usually a practical proposition. Fortunately, in the majority of patients, the precise concentration of oxygen delivered is not crucial and a 'variable performance' device, such as a *simple face mask* or *nasal cannulae* (**Fig. 6.2**) will suffice. With these devices, the patient entrains a variable amount of air to supplement the flow of oxygen during inspiration, and it is not possible to predict with any degree of accuracy the concentration of oxygen being delivered to the patient's lungs. Furthermore, the F_IO_2 varies during the respiratory cycle and is dependent on the oxygen flow rate,

as well as the patient's V_T and respiratory rate (Goldstein *et al.*, 1982). Since the peak inspiratory flow rate may be as much as 30 l/min, considerable volumes of air may be entrained at this point in the respiratory cycle. On the other hand, if the patient hypoventilates, the F_IO_2 will rise. With these devices, the F_IO_2 probably varies from about 0.35–0.55% with oxygen flows of 6–10 l/min.

Nasal cannulae are often preferred to face masks because they are less claustrophobic and do not interfere with sleep, feeding or speaking. They may, however, cause ulceration of the nasal or pharyngeal mucosa, and in some cases are associated with abdominal distension caused by swallowing oxygen. Although oxygen flow rates of 0.5–15 l/min can be used through nasal cannulae, high flow rates (more than 2–4 l/min) are very uncomfortable; it may then be preferable to administer additional oxygen via a face mask. This has the added advantage that if the mask is removed (e.g. to perform mouth care), the patient continues to receive some supplemental oxygen.

If more accurate administration of oxygen is required, a *'fixed performance'* device should be used. There are three ways of delivering a known constant F_IO_2.

Firstly, a gas mixture of the required oxygen concentration can be delivered to the patient via a tight-fitting face mask and a circuit containing a reservoir bag and a one-way valve. The reservoir bag partially collapses during inspiration and supplements the fresh gas flow; during expiration, the bag is refilled. Because there is no entrainment of air, the F_IO_2 is known and remains constant throughout the respiratory cycle. As with the use of tight-fitting face masks for the application of CPAP, these are generally poorly tolerated and can produce pressure necrosis of the facial skin.

The second method involves the application of the Venturi principle (see **Fig. 6.2c**), producing *'high air flow with oxygen enrichment'* (HAFOE) (Campbell, 1960a, b). If oxygen is delivered through an injector at a given flow rate, a fixed amount of air will be entrained

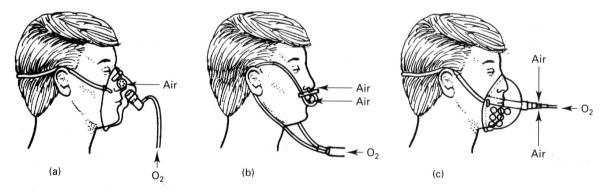

Fig. 6.2 Methods of administering supplemental oxygen to an unintubated patient: (a) simple face mask; (b) nasal cannulae, both (a) and (b) are variable performance devices; (c) Venturi mask is a fixed performance device.

and the F_IO_2 can be accurately predicted. Relatively low flows of oxygen entrain large volumes of air and this, combined with the large volume of the mask, ensures that the patient's requirements for fresh gas are satisfied even at peak inspiration. Masks are available that will deliver 24%, 28%, 34% and 60% oxygen. For example, a 24% Ventimask uses an oxygen flow rate of only 2 l/min, but produces a total fresh gas flow of 50 l/min downstream of the injector. The design of the mask is crucial, particularly with regard to its volume, and some commercially available devices are unsatisfactory (Campbell, 1982).

Finally, *oxygen tents* can be used as fixed-performance devices and have proved to be particularly useful in children. They require a high fresh gas flow with a preset F_IO_2. Re-breathing is prevented by allowing gas to escape around the lower unsealed edges of the tent.

PHYSIOLOGICAL EFFECTS OF OXYGEN THERAPY

In normal subjects, breathing oxygen causes a reduction in minute ventilation of approximately 10%, probably due to a decrease in chemoreceptor drive. The consequent rise in P_aCO_2 is exacerbated by a reduction in the buffering capacity of oxygenated haemoglobin. V_D may be increased by redistribution of pulmonary blood flow, and absorption collapse (see below) can increase venous admixture. In some cases, reversal of hypoxic pulmonary vasoconstriction may be associated with a fall in pulmonary vascular resistance, while cardiac output may decrease in association with a rise in peripheral resistance. Occasionally, administration of oxygen to those with ARF leads to a transient deterioration in conscious level. This is thought to be due to an acute reduction in cerebral blood flow when the reversal of hypoxia leaves the cerebral vasoconstrictor effect of hypocarbia unopposed.

OXYGEN TOXICITY

Although oxygen is present in the air we breathe, and is essential to life, the possibility that prolonged administration of high concentrations of this gas may have toxic effects has been recognized for many years. As long ago as 1775, Joseph Priestley introduced the concept of oxygen toxicity, and a century later hyperbaric oxygen was shown to cause convulsions in birds. In 1899, Lorrain-Smith demonstrated that mice and other small animals developed pulmonary complications when exposed to high Po_2. It was not until the 1920s, however, that the therapeutic use of oxygen became common practice and the possibility of oxygen toxicity began to concern clinicians. Even now, the relevance of oxygen-induced lung damage in clinical practice remains controversial.

Experimental work (Kapanci *et al.*, 1969) has shown that mammalian lungs continuously exposed to high concentrations of oxygen develop pulmonary capillary endothelial cell swelling with the formation of interstitial oedema and hyaline membranes. Type I alveolar lining cells are also injured during this early phase of oxygen-induced lung damage. Later, this 'exudative phase' progresses to a 'proliferative phase' with hyperplasia of type II alveolar lining cells (granular pneumocytes), septal thickening, capillary hyperplasia and infiltration with fibroblasts. There may also be damage to the bronchial epithelium and interference with ciliary activity. If the animal recovers, the lungs show focal scarring and septal fibrosis, with dilatation and proliferation of pulmonary capillaries.

The evidence that high concentrations of oxygen cause lung damage in humans is less conclusive. Nevertheless, volunteers exposed to high concentrations of oxygen for more than 24 hours develop tracheobronchitis (manifested as substernal pain), with a reduction in vital capacity (VC), lung compliance and pulmonary diffusing capacity (Comroe *et al.*, 1945; Caldwell *et al.*, 1966). Mucociliary clearance and macrophage function are impaired within a few hours of breathing 100% oxygen. It is more difficult to prove that oxygen damages the lungs of patients who receive high concentrations to correct hypoxaemia since clearly such patients already have underlying lung disease, the histological appearances of which are often non-specific. In addition, there are no pathognomonic chest radiographic or pathological appearances of oxygen-induced lung damage. Finally, there are obvious difficulties in devising a study with a suitable control group. Despite these problems, two prospective controlled studies have been performed. In one (Singer *et al.*, 1970), post-cardiac surgery patients were ventilated with either 100% oxygen or less than 50% oxygen for approximately 24 hours. There were no differences in intrapulmonary shunt, effective compliance, V_D/V_T ratio or clinical course between the two groups. The other study (Barber *et al.*, 1970), performed in patients with irreversible brain damage, showed that after 30–40 hours, P_aO_2 was lower, while intrapulmonary shunt and the V_D/V_T ratio were greater in those ventilated with 100% oxygen than in the control group. Radiographic appearances and measurement of total lung weight supported these findings, although there were no noteworthy histological differences between the two groups. These investigations suggest that 100% oxygen can cause some deterioration in lung function, but only if administered for more than 24 hours.

The mechanisms by which oxygen damages the lungs are unclear, although it seems probable that the formation of free radicals of oxygen is an important cause of direct cellular damage (Deneke & Fanburg, 1982). Interestingly, this is also one of the postulated causes of the lung lesion in ARDS, and in both instances production of oxygen radicals by activated polymorphonuclear leucocytes may be important. A number of drugs, including paraquat and bleomycin, increase the rate of production of oxygen-free radicals and may exacerbate oxygen-induced lung injury. Other factors such as a deficiency of vitamins E and C, old age, hypermetabolic states, hyperthyroidism and adrenocortical excess may predispose to oxygen toxicity, while enzymes such as superoxide dismutase are generally protective.

High inspired concentrations of oxygen will also displace nitrogen from the lungs, and this may be associated with *'absorption collapse'* of underventilated lung units. The contribution of reduced surfactant production to atelectasis in this situation is uncertain. Finally, inadequate humidification of oxygen will exacerbate pulmonary problems by drying both the bronchial mucosa, which impairs the mucociliary transport mechanism, and the bronchial secretions.

Other adverse effects of high concentrations of oxygen include retrolental fibroplasia and exacerbation of barotrauma-induced bronchopulmonary dysplasia in neonates, while hyperbaric oxygen can precipitate convulsions.

Although it is clear that retrolental fibroplasia is caused by excessively high P_aO_2, it seems that lung damage is related more to P_AO_2 than to the P_aO_2. It is also worth noting that it is the normal areas of lung that are exposed to the highest PO_2 and that it is therefore these areas that may be most damaged by the use of high F_IO_2. Finally it has been suggested that P_aO_2 may modify oxygen tolerance and that patients with pulmonary disease may be more resistant to oxygen-induced lung injury.

In conclusion, it seems reasonable to assume that administration of oxygen can damage the lungs and that the extent of the injury depends on the duration of exposure and the concentration of oxygen. It is therefore important to use the lowest F_IO_2 compatible with adequate arterial oxygenation. Conventionally, the aim is to achieve at least 90%, and preferably 95%, saturation of haemoglobin with oxygen. It must be remembered, however, that at levels of saturation approaching 90% the patient is close to the steep portion of the oxyhaemoglobin dissociation curve where small falls in P_aO_2 cause significant reductions in oxygen content. Although there is only limited information on safe levels for oxygen therapy, long-term administration of an F_IO_2 ≤ 0.5 or of 100% oxygen for less than 24 hours, is traditionally considered to be acceptable. *Dangerous hypoxia should never be tolerated through a fear of oxygen toxicity.*

MONITORING THE EFFECTS OF OXYGEN THERAPY

Some clinical improvement may be obvious following the administration of oxygen (e.g. reversal of cyanosis, slowing of the respiratory rate and a reduction in respiratory distress). Arterial blood gas analysis is, however, essential for proper assessment of the effects of treatment, and ideally a baseline sample should be obtained first with the patient breathing air. In most cases, the aim is to achieve a P_aO_2 within normal limits and more than 95% saturation of haemoglobin with oxygen. It is pointless to administer oxygen in concentrations that produce a higher than normal P_aO_2 since, because of the shape of the dissociation curve, oxygen content is not significantly increased. If potentially toxic concentrations of oxygen are required to achieve a normal P_aO_2, lower values may be accepted provided that oxygen content, and by implication oxygen delivery (DO_2), remains acceptable. In particular, more than 90% saturation of haemoglobin with oxygen can sometimes be considered adequate, and this may be achieved at P_aO_2 values as low as 8 kPa (60 mm Hg). Compensatory mechanisms such as polycythaemia, a shift of the dissociation curve, an increase in cardiac output and a redistribution of blood flow may preserve cellular oxygen delivery despite severe arterial hypoxaemia.

Clinical assessment of cellular oxygenation is difficult, although a reduction in $P_{\bar{v}}O_2$ or mixed venous oxygen saturation ($S_{\bar{v}}O_2$) is thought to be a reasonable indication that tissue oxygenation is impaired (see Chapters 2, 3 and 5). Other indices such as the development of lactic acidosis are too insensitive to be of value in assessing oxygen therapy. It is also worth re-emphasizing that when PO_2 is low, the patient is operating on the steep part of the oxyhaemoglobin dissociation curve and small increases in PO_2 will produce clinically useful improvements in oxygen content. This fact is utilized when administering oxygen to patients who are dependent on a hypoxic drive to respiration in whom too great an increase in P_aO_2 may cause dangerous carbon dioxide retention.

Control of secretions

Many patients with respiratory failure produce large quantities of bronchial secretions, which are often infected. In order to prevent sputum retention, with its attendant dangers of pulmonary collapse and perpetuation of infection, these secretions must be cleared.

HYDRATION

Patients with severe respiratory failure are often unable to drink and lose large quantities of fluid due to pyrexia, hyperventilation and the excessive work of breathing. Dehydration is therefore frequent, and as a result secretions may become more tenacious. This can be avoided by humidifying inspired gases and, more importantly, by achieving adequate systemic hydration with intravenous crystalloid solutions. On the other hand, lung water is frequently increased in patients with respiratory failure, particularly in ARDS, and in these patients fluid restriction is essential.

MUCOLYTIC AGENTS

A number of mucolytic agents have been developed that can reduce sputum viscosity *in vitro*. For example, various cysteine analogues have been described that reduce the number of cross-linking disulphide bridges in polymeric mucus glycoproteins to produce less viscid thiomonomers. There is, however, no good clinical evidence that these agents are of benefit.

CHEST PHYSIOTHERAPY (Selsby & Jones, 1990)

Conventional chest physiotherapy uses *postural drainage, percussion* and *vibration* (PDPV) in an attempt to mobilize secretions and expand collapsed lung segments. In those with copious sputum production these techniques, usually in combination with *directed coughing*, may be associated with an enhanced clearance of secretions and improved lung function. Patients with acute exacerbations of COPD, but without excessive secretions, do not, however, benefit from PDPV and chest physiotherapy may even be associated with worsening airways obstruction, although this can usually be prevented by prior administration of a bronchodilator. The *'forced expiratory technique'* (FET), which involves expiring forcefully from mid to low lung volumes while maintaining an open glottis (*'puffing exercises'*) has been shown to be superior to both directed coughing and PDPV in enhancing sputum clearance; it may be most effective when combined with postural drainage. It would appear that PDPV is of no value, and may even be detrimental, in patients with acute primary pneumonia.

Critically ill patients are particularly at risk during physiotherapy, not only because they often have severe lung disease, but also because of associated problems such as cardiovascular instability and raised intracranial pressure. In particular, numerous studies have demonstrated that PDPV and tracheal suctioning can precipitate dangerous hypoxaemia, which may last for an hour or more after treatment. The most likely mechanism for this hypoxaemia is atelectasis, which may be exacerbated by repetitive coughing and increased oxygen requirements in lightly sedated, unparalysed patients, as well as ventilator disconnection. Moreover, positive end-expiratory pressure (PEEP) is lost during disconnection and this is associated with an immediate increase in shunt, which can take as long as 60 minutes

to recover. Closed suctioning systems, which obviate the need to disconnect the ventilator, and self-inflating bags incorporating a PEEP valve are now available and may be useful in selected cases.

Current evidence suggests that chest physiotherapy is indicated for critically ill patients with excessive secretions or acute atelectasis, but is likely to be of little value in those with pulmonary oedema (either cardiogenic or associated with ARDS) or pulmonary consolidation without copious secretions. In patients with acute lobar collapse, PDPV and *fibre-optic bronchoscopy* are usually equally effective, but success is more likely in the absence of an air bronchogram (i.e. when bronchial obstruction has led to distal collapse) than in those with an air bronchogram (indicative of peripheral collapse/consolidation). The value of prophylactic chest physiotherapy in mechanically ventilated patients is uncertain.

ENDOTRACHEAL INTUBATION AND TRACHEOSTOMY

When chest physiotherapy fails to clear copious secretions and the patient, who is often exhausted, confused and uncooperative, continues to deteriorate, direct access to the airway is required for effective tracheobronchial suction. In the most urgent cases, endotracheal intubation is usually the safest technique but, when time allows, a 'minitracheostomy', which involves inserting a small diameter tube into the trachea via the cricothyroid membrane, should be performed (see Chapter 7). This technique facilitates the clearance of secretions in those who are unable to cough effectively, and in some cases the need for intubation and mechanical ventilation can be averted. Glottic function is maintained. Minitracheostomy is contraindicated in those who are unable to protect their own airway. A formal tracheostomy may be required at a later stage (see Chapter 7).

RESPIRATORY STIMULANTS

A variety of analeptic agents have been used to increase alveolar ventilation in patients with carbon dioxide retention, as well as to arouse those who are drowsy, stimulating them to cough and cooperate with physiotherapy. The safety margin with these agents is, however, small. For example *nikethamide*, which has a short duration of action, may precipitate hypertension, tachycardia, sweating, vomiting, tremors, rigidity and convulsions, especially when administered repeatedly. *Doxapram* is a more potent and selective agent with a wider safety margin. Its respiratory stimulant effect is mediated by both peripheral and central chemoreceptors, and when given slowly it may be possible to achieve peripherally mediated stimulation while largely avoiding unwanted central effects.

Although analeptics may produce short-term improvements in ventilatory function, it appears that the central respiratory drive is usually adjusted appropriately to deal most effectively with the load (see earlier in this chapter) and there is a danger that respiratory stimulants will accelerate the onset of muscle fatigue. Since there is little evidence to suggest that doxapram reduces the need for intubation and mechanical ventilation in respiratory failure, its use is not generally recommended. There is, however, some evidence that a short-term infusion of doxapram, or even a single slow bolus intravenous dose given in the recovery area, may reduce the incidence of postoperative pulmonary complications in high-risk cases (Jansen et al., 1990). When ventilatory failure is due to drug-induced central depression, therapeutic stimulation of respiratory drive, often with a specific antagonist such as naloxone, is clearly indicated.

In patients with chronic ventilatory failure, *medroxyprogesterone* stimulates respiration centrally and can significantly correct carbon dioxide retention during both wakefulness and sleep. *Acetazolamide* achieves a similar effect mediated by an increase in hydrogen ion concentration [H^+] acting at both peripheral and medullary chemoreceptors, although in some patients this response is not sustained (Skatrud & Dempsey, 1983). These two agents may be useful in selected patients with chronic carbon dioxide retention and nocturnal hypoventilation. Antidepressants such as *protriptyline* are capable of suppressing REM sleep and augmenting upper airway respiratory muscle activity. They may therefore be useful as a means of reducing the number of REM-related apnoeic episodes.

Control of infection

When respiratory failure has been precipitated by pulmonary infection, except when this is due to a virus, appropriate antibiotic therapy should be commenced. Ideally, the causative organism should be isolated, and its sensitivity to various antibiotics determined, before treatment is started; in practice, this is often not possible. Many patients have been receiving one or more antibiotics before admission to the intensive care unit, and in the remainder it is not usually practicable to await the results of bacteriological investigations before starting treatment. The identification of the rarer causes of pneumonia such as *Mycoplasma, Legionella* and *Pneumocystis carinii*, can be difficult and time-consuming. It is, however, important to obtain a sputum sample and blood culture before initiating or changing antibiotic therapy. A Gram stain of sputum may give a valuable clue to the aetiology of the pneumonia; later, the results of culture and sensitivities may lead to appropriate modification of the antibiotic regimen. Isolation of an organism from both sputum and blood strongly suggests that this is the pathogen. In the absence of bacteriological information, a reasonable antibiotic regimen should be selected on the basis of the most likely infecting organisms (see Chapter 11).

Treatment of airways obstruction

In asthma, reversal of airways obstruction is clearly fundamental, but many patients with COPD may also have an element of reversible airflow limitation.

β-STIMULANTS

In the past, isoprenaline was used extensively as a bronchodilator. This agent is, however, a non-selective β-stimulant and its use was often complicated by the development of tachycardia and/or arrhythmias. More selective β_2 agonists such as *salbutamol* and *terbutaline* are now therefore preferred, although even these can produce β_1 effects in high doses.

β-stimulants can be given orally, but are more effective when administered as a nebulized aerosol. The nebulizing dose of salbutamol is 2.5–5 mg every four hours. In resistant cases, more frequent administration may prove effective. A continuous intravenous infusion can be used when inhaled bronchodilators alone fail to reverse severe airway obstruction (Williams & Seaton, 1977), alternatively the subcutaneous route has been advocated. Salbutamol can be given as a loading dose of up to 500 μg over one hour, followed by an infusion at 5–20 μg/min. Side-effects include:

- tachycardia;
- tremor;
- hypokalaemia;
- hyperglycaemia;
- lactic acidosis.

Adrenaline can be given subcutaneously (0.1–0.5 mg, repeated if necessary two or three times at 30-minute intervals) or intravenously, and may be effective when other agents have failed. Compared to β_2 agonists it has the additional advantage of further increasing airway diameter as a result of vasoconstriction and mucosal shrinkage.

IPRATROPIUM BROMIDE

Ipratropium bromide is an anticholinergic bronchodilator with no systemic atropine-like effects that does not inhibit mucociliary clearance. It may be useful when nebulized in combination with β_2 stimulants.

THEOPHYLLINES

Phosphodiesterase inhibitors increase intracellular levels of cyclic AMP, but there is some doubt as to whether this mediates their bronchodilator effect. These agents may also increase cardiac output and improve respiratory muscle function, although muscle fatigue may be potentiated by increased energy consumption. Theophyllines have a relatively slow onset of action.

In the UK, *aminophylline*, which contains 80% theophylline, is the most commonly used member of this group of drugs and can be given intravenously, orally or as a suppository. This agent has a low therapeutic ratio and the dose has to be carefully controlled to avoid side-effects such as:

- tachycardia;
- arrhythmias;
- sweating;
- tremor;
- nausea;
- vomiting;
- insomnia;
- seizures.

Aminophylline can also *exacerbate V/Q mismatch*, possibly by reversing hypoxic pulmonary vasoconstriction. Some therefore recommend measurement of plasma levels, which is technically difficult, or the use of nomograms to control the dose. The therapeutic range lies between 5 and 20 µg/ml; life threatening arrhythmias and convulsions may occur at levels greater than 40 µg/ml. The intravenous loading dose of aminophylline is 5-6 mg/kg over 20-30 minutes and this can be followed by an infusion at 0.5 mg/kg/h in patients not previously treated with theophylline. This dose should be reduced in patients with infection, cirrhosis, congestive heart failure or COPD, and in those receiving cimetidine, ciprofloxacin, erythromycin or benzodiazepines. The dose may need to be increased in younger patients, smokers without COPD, and regular alcohol consumers without liver impairment. Because it may prove difficult to find the optimal dose for an individual patient, aminophylline should only be used in those who are unresponsive to other agents.

STEROIDS

Mucosal inflammation is an important component of airways obstruction in asthma, as well as in many patients with acute exacerbations of COPD. Parenteral steroids (e.g. hydrocortisone 200 mg intravenously six-hourly followed by a continuous intravenous infusion at 0.5 mg/kg/h) are therefore often used in combination with β-stimulants to suppress mucosal inflammation and help relieve airways obstruction. As well as their ability to suppress delayed hypersensitivity reactions and the inflammatory response, corticosteroids can increase cyclic AMP levels and restore the responsiveness of the bronchial tree to catecholamines (Shenfield et al., 1975). The onset of these effects is, however, slow (3-6 h; maximal effect in 6-12 h), and such large doses of corticosteroids might be deleterious in the presence of infection. In less severe cases, inhaled/nebulized steroids or, in those who are able to take medication by mouth, oral administration of steroids may be preferred.

β-stimulants, steroids and aminophylline can all increase urinary potassium losses.

VOLATILE ANAESTHETIC AGENTS

Both halothane and ether have bronchodilator properties and may be useful in the occasional patient when conventional treatment has failed (Robertson et al., 1985). Ether is, however, explosive in the presence of oxygen and can damage some ventilators.

KETAMINE

Ketamine is an intravenous anaesthetic agent that increases circulating catecholamines and may be a useful sedative in severe asthma.

Control of lung water

In many patients with respiratory failure, alveolar-capillary permeability is increased, lowering the threshold for the development of pulmonary oedema. This is most obvious in those with ARDS (see later); it is a less-prominent feature of pneumonia and obstructive airways disease, but is an important contributory factor in many cases of postoperative respiratory failure. As discussed in Chapter 2, lung water is likely to be further increased if plasma oncotic pressure falls and/or pulmonary vascular pressures rise. The tendency to develop 'wet lungs' may also be exacerbated by the use of positive pressure ventilation, with or without the application of PEEP (see Chapter 7).

To minimize the increase in lung water, fluids should be restricted, and it is often necessary to administer diuretics. Serum albumin should, if possible, be maintained within normal limits. This is often difficult to achieve, even with frequent administration of concentrated albumin solutions and an aggressive approach to nutritional support, partly because these patients are often extremely catabolic, but also because of a persistent leakage of plasma proteins into the interstitial spaces (see also Chapters 4 and 7 for a discussion of the relative merits of colloids or crystalloids for volume replacement in patients at risk of developing ARDS or in whom the condition is established). Finally, left atrial pressure (LAP), usually inferred from measurement of pulmonary artery occlusion pressure (PAOP), should be manipulated to produce the optimal cardiac output and Do_2, while avoiding increased hydrostatic pressures, which might contribute to the development of pulmonary oedema. In general, this means that PAOP should be maintained at 10–15 mm Hg, although in ARDS, lower values (e.g. ≤ 8 mm Hg) may be a more appropriate target. Some authorities attempt to take account of oncotic effects and suggest that when the colloid osmotic pressure/PAOP gradient falls to below 7 mm Hg there is an increased risk of pulmonary oedema (Puri *et al.*, 1980). There is evidence that in patients with increased extravascular lung water, fluid restriction and diuresis, guided by measurements of PAOP and cardiac output, is associated with a reduction in pulmonary oedema, days on a ventilator and days in intensive care (Mitchell *et al.*, 1992).

Optimizing ventilatory pump capacity

Respiratory muscle weakness has many causes including:

- malnutrition;
- catabolism;
- immobility;
- metabolic disturbances;
- old age;
- steroid myopathy;
- various acquired neuromuscular disorders (Coakley *et al.*, 1993) (see Chapter 7).

Hypophosphataemia, hypokalaemia, hypomagnesaemia, hypoxaemia and hypercapnia must all be corrected. Relief of airways obstruction will be associated with a reduction in lung volume and may restore the respiratory muscles to a more mechanically advant-

ageous position (see later in this chapter). Adequate nutrition is clearly important, but the role of enhanced nutrition, the administration of growth factors (see Chapter 10) and muscle training is uncertain. Sepsis, especially when accompanied by shock, markedly impairs respiratory muscle contractility and enhances fatigue (Hussain *et al.*, 1985).

Mechanical ventilatory support

If the patient continues to deteriorate or fails to respond to the measures outlined above, mechanical ventilatory support should be considered (see Chapter 7).

The value of *resting the respiratory muscles* with assisted ventilation is uncertain. In those with chronic ventilatory failure, long-term nocturnal ventilation improves daytime P_AO_2 and P_ACO_2 and may improve respiratory muscle strength. The mechanism for this improvement is unclear, but may be related to improved sleep quality, control of cor pulmonale, better V/Q matching, resetting of central respiratory controllers and increases in lung and/or chest wall compliance. There is only limited evidence that rest relieves fatigue and improves muscle function in either chronic or acute respiratory failure (Efthimiou *et al.*, 1987; Moxham, 1990).

INDICATIONS

Indications for instituting mechanical ventilatory support in respiratory failure vary according to the underlying disease process (see later). In *hypoxaemic and mixed respiratory failure*, the decision is made largely on clinical grounds, aided by blood gas analysis and sometimes simple bedside tests of respiratory function (e.g. V_T and maximum inspiratory force, **Table 6.1**). If the clinical signs of severe respiratory distress (e.g. tachypnoea > 40/min, asynchronous or paradoxical breathing, respiratory alternans, inability to speak, sweating) persist despite maximal treatment and the patient appears exhausted, particularly if this is associated with confusion, restlessness and agitation, venti-

---

Table 6.1 Objective guidelines for instituting ventilatory support.

Respiratory rate	> 40/min
Tidal volume (V_T)	< 5 ml/kg
Vital capacity (VC)	< 15 ml/kg
Maximum inspiratory force	< 25 cm H_2O
Arterial oxygen tension (P_aO_2)	< 8 kPa (60 mm Hg)
Alveolar-arterial oxygen difference ($P_{A-a}O_2$)	> 47 kPa (350 mm Hg)
Arterial carbon dioxide tension (P_aCO_2)	> 8 kPa (60 mm Hg)
V_D/V_T	> 0.6

latory support is usually required. Worsening blood gases may confirm that the situation is deteriorating, a rising $P_a\text{CO}_2$ (> 8 kPa) and/or extreme hypoxaemia with $P_a\text{O}_2$ < 8 kPa and alveolar–arterial oxygen difference $(P_{A-a}\text{O}_2)$ > 47 kPa (350 mm Hg) despite oxygen therapy being particularly significant in relation to the need for artificial ventilation. By this stage, bedside tests of respiratory function are rarely helpful.

In contrast, the decision to institute artificial ventilation in patients with *ventilatory failure* is influenced more by the results of blood gas analysis and bedside tests of respiratory function, in particular the VC, than by clinical assessment. Normally, artificial ventilation should be instituted in a patient with ventilatory failure when the VC has fallen to less than 10–15 ml/kg, since this may reduce the incidence of complications such as atelectasis and infection, as well as prevent respiratory arrest. V_T and respiratory rate, on the other hand, are relatively insensitive indicators of the need for artificial ventilation in ventilatory failure because they change only late in the course of the disease. A high $P_a\text{CO}_2$, particularly if it is rising, is generally an indication for urgent artificial ventilation in these patients.

Treatment as outlined above, particularly the control of lung water, must continue once IPPV has been instituted. Additional measures that may be useful include reduction of oxygen requirements (e.g. by heavy sedation, paralysis and cooling), together with maintenance of an adequate cardiac output and haemoglobin level, the ultimate goal being to improve tissue oxygenation and prevent organ damage (see Chapter 4).

POSITIVE END-EXPIRATORY PRESSURE

If, despite these measures, it proves impossible to achieve adequate oxygenation of arterial blood without raising $F_I\text{O}_2$ to potentially dangerous levels (see above), the application of a PEEP should be considered (see Chapter 7).

CONTINUOUS POSITIVE AIRWAY PRESSURE

Patients with ARF who are not exhausted and/or hypoventilating may be allowed to continue to breathe spontaneously while a positive pressure is applied to the airway via an endotracheal tube (see chapter 7). In those patients who can protect their own airway, and in whom retention of secretions is not a problem, CPAP may be applied using a tight-fitting face mask. In selected cases, this technique is a valuable means of avoiding mechanical ventilation.

Other special techniques for respiratory support (e.g. high-frequency ventilation, pressure-control inverse ratio ventilation, extracorporeal membrane oxygenation/ carbon dioxide removal) may be useful in selected cases. These are considered in Chapter 7.

SOME COMMON CAUSES OF RESPIRATORY FAILURE IN THE INTENSIVE CARE UNIT

Postoperative respiratory failure

PATHOPHYSIOLOGY

Surgery and anaesthesia can precipitate atelectasis in dependent lung regions with reductions in FRC, forced expiratory volume in one second (FEV_1), forced vital capacity (FVC) and compliance associated with premature small airway closure, impaired ability to cough, and muscle splinting. The pattern of breathing also alters with a reduction in V_T and an increased respiratory rate. Diaphragmatic tone and movement are reduced, breathing becomes predominantly thoracic, and the overall activity of the abdominal muscles is increased, particularly during expiration. The reduction in FRC may therefore be largely explained by a cranial shift of the diaphragm combined with loss of lung volume due to mucus plugs and alveolar collapse. There is a close relationship between the fall in FRC, the increase in pulmonary shunt and the hypoxaemia, which is invariably present postoperatively and may persist for many days (Jones *et al.*, 1990). Frequent superimposed episodes of more severe hypoxaemia occur during sleep in those given opiates and are related to periods of apnoea with airways obstruction, in part due to hypotonia of the muscles of the upper airway. Later hypoxia is common during the prolonged periods of REM sleep that are necessary to compensate for the lack of REM sleep in the early postoperative period.

These abnormalities of lung function are particularly severe following upper abdominal surgery, when FRC may fall to as little as 20% of the preoperative value, and VC and FEV_1 are reduced by approximately 60% in the immediate postoperative period. Similar, but slightly less severe, changes occur after thoracic surgery. Lung function returns to normal over a period of 1–3 weeks.

Surgery and anaesthesia are also associated with depression of macrophage function and ciliary activity, while the lower respiratory tract may become colonized with bacteria. It is not surprising that in susceptible patients these changes are often associated with retention of secretions, basal lung collapse and superimposed infection (either an exacerbation of pre-existing bronchitis or secondary pneumonia), or that in some cases they precipitate respiratory failure (**Fig. 6.3**).

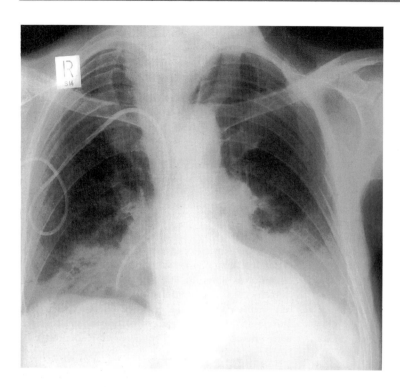

Fig. 6.3 Postoperative respiratory failure showing bilateral basal collapse/ consolidation.

PREDISPOSING FACTORS

Postoperative pulmonary complications are much more common in patients with pre-existing respiratory disease, particularly those in whom preoperative assessment of lung function demonstrates significant reductions in maximum breathing capacity and expiratory flow rates, or carbon dioxide retention (Tisi, 1979). Obesity, smoking and prolonged anaesthesia also predispose to postoperative pulmonary complications. Conversely, they are rare in previously fit patients with normal lung function. It is therefore logical to concentrate preventive measures on those patients known to be most at risk.

PREVENTION AND TREATMENT

In high-risk cases, surgery should be delayed in order to optimize respiratory function and minimize the risk of subsequent serious pulmonary complications. Therefore, patients with bronchiectasis or severe COPD, particularly if associated with cor pulmonale and polycythaemia, will often benefit from a period of intensive physiotherapy, with antibiotic treatment for active infection, before surgery. In some cases, bronchodilator therapy and/or corticosteroids may be beneficial. Similarly, patients with other forms of chronic respiratory disease will require preoperative treatment of any superimposed respiratory tract infections. Patients must be

persuaded to stop smoking, preferably several weeks before surgery.

In the postoperative period, simple but effective preventive measures include chest physiotherapy with deep breathing, coughing and exercises designed to improve respiratory muscle function. The administration of doxapram in the recovery room can reduce the incidence of postoperative complications in high-risk cases (Jansen *et al.*, 1990). If possible, the patient should be sat up at approximately 45 degrees because in this position diaphragmatic movement is not impeded by the abdominal contents and expansion of basal lung segments is improved. In some centres, the *'incentive spirometer'* is used to encourage deep breathing as an alternative to intermittent positive pressure breathing, while the application of mask CPAP may be a useful means of achieving re-expansion of collapsed lung segments, particularly in those in whom the major abnormality is a reduction in FRC (e.g. the obese patient who has recently undergone upper abdominal surgery). The provision of adequate analgesia is of paramount importance since pain will seriously inhibit the patient's ability to cough and expand the lungs (see Chapter 10).

Despite these measures, some patients will need endotracheal intubation, possibly combined with bronchoscopy, or a mini-tracheostomy to control bronchial secretions, while others will deteriorate further and require ventilatory support. Selected cases may therefore benefit from elective postoperative artificial ventilation.

Severe asthma

There is some evidence that both the absolute number of hospital admissions for severe asthma and the proportion who require mechanical ventilation have increased progressively since the 1960s (Williams, 1989), and the death rate from asthma appears to be increasing (McFadden, 1991). It seems likely that many of these deaths are preventable since a proportion of patients die before they reach hospital and a number of sudden and apparently unpredictable deaths occur after admission to hospital. Substandard hospital care is more common in fatal cases of asthma including inadequate monitoring, suboptimal use of inhaled β-agonists, administration of sedation, inadequate clinical assessment and failure to institute mechanical ventilation (Eason & Markowe, 1987).

AETIOLOGY

Factors precipitating severe asthma include exposure to high concentrations of allergen and respiratory infection (either bacterial or viral). Alterations in treatment regimens (e.g. a sudden reduction in the dose of corticosteroids) (James et al., 1977), an overdose of sedatives, desensitization procedures, provocation tests and anaesthesia may all provoke intense bronchospasm. The stimuli most often associated with fatal or near fatal airways obstruction include profound emotional upsets, serious atmospheric pollution, use of β-blockers and ingestion of non-steroidal anti-inflammatory drugs (NSAIDS) in sensitive subjects (McFadden, 1991). There is evidence that reduced chemosensitivity to hypoxia and blunted perception of dyspnoea may predispose patients to fatal asthma attacks (Kikuchi et al., 1994).

Aspirin-induced asthma is a common problem that affects 8–20% of adult asthmatics. The aetiology is not clear, but probably involves inhibition of cyclo-oxygenase, with preferential metabolism of arachidonic acid to produce bronchoconstrictor and pro-inflammatory leukotrienes rather than prostaglandins. An alternative explanation is that a chronic viral infection generates cytotoxic lymphocytes, which are normally suppressed by prostaglandins, but which will attack virus-infected respiratory tract cells when cyclo-oxygenase is inhibited (Power, 1993).

PATHOPHYSIOLOGY

The increased airway resistance in asthma is due to oedema of the bronchial mucosa and obstruction by thick, tenacious mucous plugs, as well as an increase in bronchomotor tone. Recent reports have emphasized the role of mucosal inflammation in producing airways obstruction (Djukanovic et al., 1990). Lung elastic recoil is reduced in association with persistent activity of the inspiratory muscles throughout expiration. Alveolar pressure remains positive at the end of expiration, a phenomenon known as *intrinsic or 'auto' PEEP*, and this may cause a 'dynamic' compression of the distal airways. Forced expiratory flow rates and VC are reduced, air trapping causes an increase in FRC and total lung capacity and the work of breathing is increased. Hyperinflation impairs respiratory muscle function (see later). Pulmonary vascular resistance increases, producing right ventricular strain and sometimes a fall in cardiac output. This will be exacerbated if, as is often the case, the patient is hypovolaemic.

CLINICAL FEATURES

An asthmatic attack can be considered severe if it is particularly prolonged (i.e. lasting several days) or if it is resistant to therapy. Such episodes are sometimes referred to as *'status asthmaticus'*, which has been defined as *'an acute asthmatic attack in which the degree of bronchial obstruction is either severe from the beginning or progressively increases in severity and is not relieved by conventional therapy.'*

Signs that the attack is particularly severe include:

- extreme dyspnoea causing an inability to speak, eat, drink or even sleep;
- use of accessory muscles;
- tachycardia;
- upright posture;
- mental confusion and exhaustion.

Pulsus paradoxus may be difficult to detect and is an unreliable sign, while in the most severe cases wheezing may be absent due to the marked reduction in air flow. Ventilatory failure with hypercarbia is associated with restlessness, anxiety and a bounding pulse. A silent chest, cyanosis and bradycardia indicate a very severe attack. It is important to appreciate that the degree of bronchospasm often worsens appreciably in the early hours ('early morning dips'), possibly because of the reduction in blood cortisol levels at this time (James et al., 1977) or the diurnal variation in catecholamine levels.

There is a spectrum of clinical presentations, but broadly two patterns can be defined.

- In one, very severe airways obstruction develops extremely rapidly, sometimes leading to death within minutes or at most a few hours. This *sudden asphyxic asthma* may develop in a previously symptomless patient, is commonest in young men and is often associated with marked bronchial reactivity. Patients frequently present comatose with a silent chest, a very high P_aCO_2 and a metabolic acidosis. Respiratory arrest is relatively common. These patients do, however, respond promptly to treatment.

- At the other end of the spectrum are those whose *respiratory failure develops slowly and progressively* with muscle fatigue and exhaustion. The presentation may, however, appear precipitate because symptoms are minimized by denial, underperception of breathlessness and behaviour modification until airway obstruction is very severe. These patients tend not to seek medical help and the severity of their disease is often underestimated; they are therefore frequently undertreated and poorly controlled. Response to treatment may be slow.

The clinical presentation of *aspirin-induced asthma* is characteristic. Initially there is a sudden onset of malaise, nasal obstruction and discharge, and sneezing, and frequently a productive cough. These symptoms then evolve over a few weeks into a persistent rhinitis with nasal polyps. Over the following months the patient develops sensitivity to NSAIDS manifested as acute bronchospasm, cutaneous flushing of the head and neck, rhinorrhoea, conjunctival irritation and, in a few cases, circulatory collapse and respiratory arrest. The asthma in such cases is generally severe, protracted and difficult to control. The combination of asthma, nasal polyps and aspirin intolerance has been termed the 'aspirin triad' (Power, 1993).

INVESTIGATIONS

A chest radiograph should always be obtained in patients hospitalized with acute severe asthma to exclude the rare possibility of a pneumothorax. Characteristically, the chest radiograph will show the features of pulmonary hyperinflation with hyperlucent lung fields, horizontal ribs, flat diaphragms and a vertical heart. Usually the patient is too breathless to perform lung function tests, but measurement of FVC, FEV_1, and peak expiratory flow rate (PEFR) may be used to assess the response to treatment. It is also important to appreciate that by performing such objective measurements in apparently less severe cases, the danger of underestimating the severity of the attack can be avoided. A PEFR < 40% of predicted or < 200 l/min suggests a severe attack.

An ECG may reveal tachycardia, arrhythmias, ST segment changes, P pulmonale in leads II and III and right axis deviation.

Initially, the patient is hypoxic due to *V/Q* mismatch, while relative hyperventilation induces hypocarbia. A normal or high P_aCO_2 is an ominous sign that the patient is tiring. A metabolic acidosis is relatively common and may be due to circulatory failure, a reduction in hepatic metabolism of lactate and an increase in circulating catecholamines (endogenous or exogenous).

MANAGEMENT

Patients with acute asthma are managed according to the principles outlined above with oxygen, rehydration, physiotherapy and bronchodilators. Current evidence suggests that in general β-agonists are more effective when nebulized than when given intravenously (Crompton, 1990), although in severe asthma it is possible that the intravenous route is more efficacious. In those with severe resistant asthma who fail to respond to nebulized β-agonists, intravenous administration of bronchodilators is therefore still recommended. Antibiotics should only be given when there is strong evidence of bacterial infection. Correction of the metabolic acidosis with sodium bicarbonate will be associated with a transient increase in carbon dioxide production and should, if possible, be avoided. There is some evidence that in those with severe airways obstruction, high F_IO_2 may precipitate or worsen hypercarbia and it is therefore prudent to initiate oxygen therapy in a controlled fashion, adjusted according to the results of blood gas analysis (McFadden, 1991). *Administration of sedatives, cough suppressants or β-blockers can cause rapid, and sometimes fatal, deterioration.*

Mechanical ventilation

Although ventilating patients with severe asthma is extremely hazardous, it is equally dangerous to procrastinate when the patient is exhausted. Some characteristic features of those requiring IPPV include:

- youth;
- a long history of asthma;
- previous hospital admissions in status;
- attacks lasting more than 24 hours before admission.

It can be difficult to assess which patients require ventilation, but some generally accepted criteria are:

- extreme exhaustion;
- increasing mental disturbance;
- coma;
- severe hypoxaemia;
- life-threatening respiratory acidosis:
- a P_aCO_2 that is higher than 8 kPa and rising despite aggressive therapy.

Patients who have a respiratory arrest will require immediate intubation and ventilation (see Chapter 8).

Selecting the pattern of ventilation. There are a number of important considerations when selecting an appropriate pattern of ventilation for an asthmatic patient. Because of the severe airway obstruction, a long expiratory phase is required to avoid overinflation of the lungs. On the other hand, the time constants of most lung units are markedly increased (see Chapter 2) and inspiration may have to be prolonged to allow adequate distribution of inspired gases. Therefore, a slow respiratory rate (e.g. 6–10 breaths/min), with long inspiratory and expiratory phases, is usually required. V_T may have to be limited (e.g. 8–10 ml/kg) to avoid high inflation pressures and the risk of barotrauma. For a given minute volume, hyperinflation is minimized by using a lower V_T and a higher respiratory rate. The inspiratory flow rate can be increased (e.g. > 80 l/min) to allow a longer expiratory phase, but this may adversely affect the distribution of ventilation (Tuxen & Lane, 1987). In severe cases, the minute volume is inevitably inadequate and it may be impossible to return P_aCO_2 to within normal limits. Although hypercarbia is a strong stimulus for the patient to breathe and 'fight' the ventilator, it has to be tolerated and the patient should be heavily sedated and, if necessary, paralysed (avoiding agents that might release histamine).

The use of PEEP in severe asthma is controversial since an 'intrinsic PEEP' associated with airway compression and lung hyperinflation, is already present. Nevertheless externally applied PEEP downstream from the compressed distal airways may overcome the obstruction to flow without increasing alveolar pressure (Marini, 1989). Although a few have recommended high levels of PEEP, most would suggest that only low levels (< 7.5 cm H_2O) should be used to avoid overdistension of near normal or partially obstructed lung units. In general, however, PEEP appears to be detrimental in severe asthma since it further increases lung volume, elevates intrathoracic and airway pressures and depresses the circulation (Tuxen, 1989). Nevertheless cautious application of low-level PEEP may be useful during spontaneous breathing.

Apart from increasing the risk of pneumothorax, overinflation of the lungs compresses the heart and attenuates the pulmonary vasculature, further increasing pulmonary vascular resistance. Eventually, the right ventricle fails and cardiac output falls. This may be a terminal event. The risk of this complication can be minimized by ensuring that expiration is completed before the next inspiration begins, either by auscultation or by disconnecting the patient from the ventilator and listening at the endotracheal tube. A rising central venous pressure (CVP) may be a useful indication of hyperinflation. In severe cases it may be necessary to disconnect the patient from the ventilator intermittently to allow lung deflation.

Similar considerations apply when ventilating patients with chronic airflow limitation (see below). Moreover, rapidly lowering the P_aCO_2 towards normal in these patients, some of whom have a compensatory metabolic alkalosis, may cause a marked increase in pH with a reduction in ionized calcium levels, cerebral vasoconstriction and a danger of fitting. There may also be a dramatic fall in cardiac output.

Bronchial lavage

Obstruction by tenacious mucus plugs is an important component of the increased airway resistance in severe asthma. Some authorities therefore recommend bronchial lavage in patients who require IPPV. This is almost invariably associated with severe hypoxia and hypercarbia and as a consequence is extremely hazardous. An alternative is to instil small quantities of saline into the endotracheal tube at regular intervals, although the efficacy of this technique is questionable.

Discontinuing respiratory support

Weaning and extubation of patients with reversible airway obstruction may precipitate a further episode of severe bronchospasm. A useful technique is to allow the patient to breathe 50% nitrous oxide in oxygen (Entonox) for ten minutes to provide temporary sedation before extubation. Alternatively, the patient can be sedated with, for example, a continuous infusion of propofol or chlormethiazole during this period.

Acute respiratory failure associated with chronic obstructive pulmonary disease

PATHOPHYSIOLOGY

Airflow limitation in patients with COPD is due to a combination of mucosal inflammation, bronchial gland hypertrophy, excessive secretions and bronchoconstriction, the latter being caused by stimulation of airway sensory receptors by inhaled irritants and the release of inflammatory mediators. In those with emphysema, loss of lung elasticity is associated with an increase in airways resistance due to reduced radial traction on the airway combined with an increase in dynamic compression during expiration; there is also a reduction in maximum expiratory flow associated with the fall in elastic recoil pressure. The combination of airflow limitation and reduced elastic recoil leads to pulmonary hyperinflation and a fall in lung compliance (see Chapter 2). The energy cost of breathing is increased, sometimes to as much as 15% of total body $\dot{V}O_2$, and ventilatory reserve is reduced; resting ventilation may then constitute as much as 40% of maximum ventilatory capacity.

Although hyperinflation tends to minimize airway obstruction, it adversely effects *inspiratory muscle function*. The decrease in muscle fibre length reduces the force of contraction while flattening of the diaphragm, associated with a decrease in its radius of curvature, reduces the efficiency of diaphragmatic pressure generation. Moreover, because of the orientation of the muscle fibres, diaphragmatic contraction may produce rib cage deflation rather than expansion. Similarly the horizontal position of the ribs makes it more difficult for the respiratory muscles to expand the thorax. In patients with stable COPD, however, it seems that compensatory mechanisms may counterbalance these deleterious effects of hyperinflation on diaphragm function (Rochester, 1991; Similouski *et al.*, 1991).

Pulmonary gas exchange is deranged in COPD due to a combination of V/Q mismatch (caused by airways obstruction, pulmonary parenchymal disease and disturbances of the pulmonary vasculature) and hypoventilation. In those with carbon dioxide retention, respiratory drive is usually increased; it is unclear whether a fall in V_T contributes to hypercarbia in stable COPD at rest. Those with acute respiratory failure who develop hypercarbia do, however, breathe at smaller tidal volumes and higher respiratory rates than those who remain eucapnic, probably in an attempt to avoid fatigue and minimize respiratory distress. It seems that as well as the deterioration in lung mechanics other factors are likely to contribute to carbon dioxide retention (e.g. hypercarbia can itself have a depressant effect on chemoreceptors). In addition, hypoventilation has the advantage that as P_ACO_2 rises a greater volume of carbon dioxide can be excreted at a given level of alveolar ventilation.

In some patients with COPD, alveolar destruction and distortion destroys the capillary bed and, combined with hypoxic pulmonary vasoconstriction, leads to *pulmonary hypertension* with secondary vascular changes. Cor pulmonale may develop and worsening hypoxia during an episode of respiratory failure may precipitate severe right heart failure.

CLINICAL PRESENTATION

Acute respiratory failure complicating COPD is usually precipitated by respiratory tract infection associated with worsening bronchospasm and retention of secretions. Deterioration may also be related to the administration of sedatives or narcotic analgesics, surgery, development of a pneumothorax, rib fractures due to trauma or excessive coughing, pulmonary embolism or congestive heart failure. In some cases, respiratory failure may simply represent the final stages of irreversible lung disease.

Clinically *hyperinflation* presents as:

- intercostal and supraclavicular recession;
- decreased distance between the cricoid cartilage and the sternal notch;
- reduced cardiac dullness;
- an increased antero–posterior diameter of the chest.

Cor pulmonale is recognized by detecting peripheral oedema, jugular venous distension and hepatomegaly.

Traditionally two distinct clinical types have been described;

- *pink puffers*, who present with hyperventilation, severe dyspnoea and relatively normal blood gases, and suffer predominantly from emphysema;
- *blue bloaters*, whose major abnormality is chronic bronchitis, and who are cyanosed with cor pulmonale, profuse secretions and little or no dyspnoea.

In practice the majority of patients lie somewhere between these two extremes and post-mortem studies have not supported this simplistic distinction.

As well as features suggestive of a precipitating infection (fever, purulent sputum, leucocytosis, clinical evidence of pulmonary consolidation, lung infiltrates on chest radiography) patients with acute exacerbations of COPD may present with:

- worsening wheeze;
- dyspnoea;
- tachypnoea;
- use of accessory muscles;
- intercostal and supraclavicular recession;
- pulsus paradoxus;
- 'pursed lip' breathing.

Other features include:

- cyanosis;
- rhonchi;
- prolonged expiration and expiratory wheeze.

Occasionally patients present with increasing hypercarbia and acidosis without dyspnoea (e.g. when their conscious level has been depressed by drugs or in the advanced stages of respiratory failure). Such cases are easily missed. *Cor pulmonale* may be evident as a loud pulmonary component to the second heart sound, a right ventricular heave, elevated jugular venous pulse and peripheral oedema. *Signs of acute hypercapnia* may also be present including anxiety, dyspnoea, confusion, transient psychosis, coma and, in some cases, tremors, myoclonic jerks, asterixis and seizures. In addition, cerebral vasodilatation leads to headaches, papilloedema, and occasionally focal neurological signs, while peripheral vasodilatation is associated with warm, flushed skin and a bounding pulse. As P_ACO_2 rises P_aO_2 inevitably falls (see Chapter 2) and some believe that many of these features of carbon dioxide narcosis are mediated more by hypoxia and acidosis than by the elevated PCO_2.

Complications associated with acute respiratory failure in patients with COPD include pulmonary embolism (which may occur in up to 25% of cases), pneumothorax, gastrointestinal haemorrhage and renal insufficiency. A wide variety of arrhythmias including premature atrial beats, atrial fibrillation, premature ventricular contractions and ventricular tachycardia are common.

INVESTIGATIONS

A *full blood count* may reveal polycythaemia, which is not only secondary to chronic hypoxia but is also a response to persistently elevated carboxyhaemoglobin levels caused by continued heavy cigarette smoking.

A *chest radiograph* should always be obtained to diagnose or exclude pneumothorax, lobar or segmental collapse, pneumonia or obvious left ventricular failure. The chest radiograph may suggest pulmonary hypertension with prominent proximal and attenuated distal vascular markings, and an enlarged right heart. Radiological features of emphysema include hyperinflation, flattened diaphragms, a vertical heart, vascular attenuation and bullae (**Fig. 6.4**).

The *ECG* may show features of right atrial and ventricular hypertrophy including P pulmonale, right axis deviation, dominant R waves in V_{1-2}, right bundle branch block and ST depression, as well as T wave flattening and inversion in V_{1-3}.

Pulmonary function tests characteristically show a fall in FEV_1, FVC, and the FEV_1/FVC ratio, a reduced diffusing capacity and an increased residual volume (RV), functional residual capacity (FRC) and total lung capacity (TLC).

Sputum should be sent for microscopy and culture.

TREATMENT

Routine treatment of acute exacerbations of COPD consists of:

- controlled oxygen therapy;
- elimination of infection with antibiotics (usually amoxycillin or cefuroxime, combined with erythromycin, see Chapter 11);
- physiotherapy;
- bronchodilators/corticosteroids for reversible airways obstruction.

Even in emphysematous patients whose airways obstruction is conventionally considered to be irrevers-

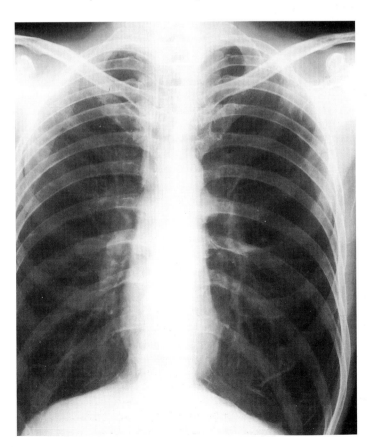

Fig. 6.4 Chest radiograph of a patient with emphysematous chronic obstructive pulmonary disease. Notice the hyperinflated lungs with low flat diaphragms and narrow cardiac silhouette.

ible, considerable improvement may be achieved with bronchodilators. *Diuretics* may be required in those with pulmonary hypertension and cor pulmonale or left ventricular failure.

The role of *inspiratory muscle training* in those with chronic respiratory failure is controversial, but it may improve muscle strength and thereby diminish the perception of respiratory effort. The objective of training should be to treat muscle weakness not fatigue, and preserve a normal pattern of breathing (Rochester, 1991).

Controlled oxygen therapy

Relief of life-threatening hypoxia is clearly the first priority and this can usually be achieved by administering supplemental oxygen and optimizing cardiac output. It is important to appreciate, however, that administration of oxygen is nearly always associated with a rise in P_aCO_2 due not only to a fall in minute ventilation, but probably also to reversal of hypoxic pulmonary vasoconstriction, which leads to worsening V/Q mismatch, and the Haldane effect (i.e. carbon dioxide dissociates from haemoglobin). In most cases this rise in P_aCO_2 is of no consequence, but in those with severe COPD, long-standing hypercarbia and a 'hypoxic' drive to respiration, oxygen therapy may significantly decrease alveolar ventilation and precipitate severe carbon dioxide retention. Because these patients are hypoxic they are operating on the steep portion of their oxyhaemoglobin dissociation curve and small increases in P_aO_2 not sufficient to cause significant carbon dioxide retention, will lead to useful increases in arterial oxygen content (C_aO_2). This forms the basis for 'controlled oxygen therapy' (Campbell, 1960a) using fixed performance masks ('Ventimask') delivering 24%, 28% or 34% oxygen. Careful monitoring is essential with frequent blood gas analysis to achieve the optimal effect. Although small increases in P_aCO_2 can be tolerated, the pH should not be allowed to fall below 7.25. If significant carbon dioxide retention does occur, it is important not to deprive the patient of supplemental oxygen since, because of the respiratory depression and the increase in P_ACO_2, P_aO_2 is likely to fall to a level lower than that on admission.

Mechanical ventilation

If the patient continues to deteriorate despite these measures, institution of mechanical ventilation should be considered. This decision is primarily clinical (see above) and intervention is often prompted by deteriorating mental status, ineffective cough or apnoea.

Selection of patients for mechanical ventilation. In general it is prudent to be cautious about embarking on mechanical ventilation in those with severe chronic respiratory failure because they are particularly susceptible to complications and in a proportion of cases weaning will prove to be impossible. Selection of suitable patients is based largely on an assessment of the severity and nature of the underlying chronic pulmonary disease. The patient's previous exercise tolerance and ability to lead an independent existence are perhaps the most important considerations. Those who were severely incapacitated (e.g. able to walk only a few yards on the flat) before the acute episode will be extremely difficult to wean from the ventilator. Conversely, if the patient was previously leading a full and active life an aggressive approach to treatment should be adopted. It is also important to enquire about previous admissions to hospital with respiratory failure and whether the patient has required mechanical ventilation in the past. If possible, the duration of any previous intensive care admissions and details of the weaning process should be ascertained. Polycythaemia and cor pulmonale suggest that the patient has been hypoxic for some time, while an elevated bicarbonate concentration indicates that hypercarbia has been present for at least a few days. In general, success is most likely in patients with a clearly reversible component to their lung pathology (e.g. superadded infection and/or reversible airways obstruction), whereas those with end-stage lung disease associated with unresponsive airflow limitation are unlikely to benefit from mechanical ventilation. Clearly if there is any doubt, as is frequently the case, the patient should be intubated and ventilated. Non-invasive mechanical ventilation may be useful as a means of avoiding endotracheal intubation (see Chapter 7) and there is some evidence that nasal IPPV reduces mortality when compared to 'conventional' therapy (Bott *et al.*, 1993).

General measures

Mechanically ventilated patients with COPD require prophylaxis against thromboembolism (usually subcutaneous heparin) and adequate nutritional support (usually via the enteral route). Hypophosphataemia, which can impair respiratory muscle function (Aubier *et al.*, 1985), is extremely common and may be related to an intracellular shift of phosphate secondary to correction of respiratory acidosis (Laaban *et al.*, 1989). Phosphate administration is indicated in those with severe hypophosphataemia, those with symptoms related to low phosphate levels, when there is pre-existing hypophosphataemia and in alcoholics. The benefits of phosphate administration in those with lesser degrees of hypophosphataemia are less clear. Hypokalaemia, hypomagnesaemia and hypocalcaemia may also adversely effect the performance of respiratory muscles and should be corrected.

PROGNOSIS

Approximately 80% of those patients with COPD who require mechanical ventilation should survive to leave hospital, but the two-year survival rate may be only 30%.

Upper airway obstruction

CAUSES

Upper airway obstruction is a life-threatening emergency and may be due to:

- an obstruction within the lumen of the airway;
- swelling originating from the wall of the airway;
- extrinsic compression.

  Causes include:

- trauma;
- foreign bodies;
- airway burns;
- tumours (e.g. lymphoma);
- haematomas (e.g. following carotid endarterectomy or thyroid surgery);
- infections such as epiglottitis, croup, tonsillar hypertrophy or abscess, retropharyngeal abscess, diphtheria.

Instrumentation of the respiratory tract may also be complicated by obstruction, for example endotracheal tubes can become blocked with secretions (see Chapter 7), and following extubation, laryngeal oedema or tracheal stenosis may compromise the airway.

CLINICAL FEATURES

Upper airway obstruction presents as:

- dyspnoea;
- stridor;
- wheeze;
- hoarseness;
- dysphonia:
- an unusual cough.

Initially symptoms may occur only on exertion, but as the obstruction worsens respiratory difficulty becomes evident even at rest. At first patients are usually able to compensate by increasing respiratory effort and the use of accessory muscles; V_T, respiratory rate and blood gases therefore often remain within normal limits. Once

exhaustion develops or the severity of the obstruction becomes insuperable, deterioration occurs very quickly. The patient becomes extremely alarmed and agitated, inspirations are gasping, activity of the accessory muscles becomes increasingly prominent and there is suprasternal and intercostal recession; these features may be combined with a persistent cough, corneal ecchymoses and subcutaneous emphysema. In the pre-terminal stages consciousness may be lost, the patient becomes hypoxic, hypercarbic and acidotic, cardiac arrhythmias develop and stridor usually diminishes.

In general the degree of stridor bears little relationship to the severity of the obstruction. Inspiratory stridor suggests supraglottic obstruction, while expiratory stridor is indicative of a lesion below the glottis; sometimes stridor is heard during both inspiration and expiration. In some cases the severity of symptoms is related to posture and *lying the patient supine may precipitate complete obstruction*.

Airways obstruction may be fixed or variable. *Fixed obstructions* (e.g. due to tumour or a stricture) are unaffected by dynamic changes in the cross-sectional area of the airways and airflow is reduced equally in inspiration and expiration. *Variable obstructions*, on the other hand, are influenced by the alterations in airway calibre that occur during the respiratory cycle. During inspiration the extrathoracic airway tends to collapse because the intraluminal pressure becomes negative compared to the atmosphere, whereas the intrathoracic airway has a tendency to expand because the pleural pressure becomes more negative than the intraluminal pressure. Although during normal quiet breathing these alterations are relatively small (less than 15%), during the increased respiratory effort induced by obstruction airway calibre may change by more than 50%. Therefore in a patient with a variable extrathoracic obstruction (e.g. due to vocal cord palsy or a goitre) the reduction in flow will be greater during inspiration while the reverse is true for a variable intrathoracic obstruction.

INVESTIGATIONS

Antero–posterior and lateral *radiographs* of the chest and neck, *tomography* and a *CT scan* may reveal the site, severity and nature of the obstruction. In some cases *endoscopy* will be required. *Blood gas analysis* should be performed. It is important not to endanger the patient's life by delaying relief of the obstruction or by leaving them unaccompanied while investigations are performed.

TREATMENT

Because flow through the obstruction is turbulent, resistance is dependent on the density of the inspired gas and may be reduced by administering a mixture of *helium* (which is less dense than air) in oxygen. Adequate *humidification* is essential. Often, this simply allows time to prepare for endotracheal intubation and/or tracheostomy or cricothyrotomy.

Ideally *endotracheal intubation* should only be performed by an experienced operator accompanied by a skilled assistant in an anaesthetic room or operating theatre. All the equipment that might be required to secure the airway must be immediately available including a full range of endotracheal tubes in varying sizes, adequate suction, bougies and stylets, as well as resuscitation equipment. A surgeon should be standing by in case urgent tracheostomy is necessary. Monitoring should include ECG and pulse oximetry.

Some consider *awake intubation* using topical anaesthesia, cricoid pressure and a fibre-optic intubating laryngoscope to be the safest option, but this is often not possible in a restless and uncooperative patient. The alternative is *inhalational induction of anaesthesia* using halothane in 100% oxygen or in a helium/oxygen mixture, followed by laryngoscopy and attempted intubation with the patient breathing spontaneously. This has the advantage that bubbles of saliva may form during expiration and indicate the position of the glottic opening. A transtracheal bougie, fibre-optic stylet or percutaneous retrograde cricothyroid guide wire may all prove useful.

If all else fails, *tracheostomy* should be performed, although this is extremely hazardous under these circumstances and *cricothyrotomy* may be the preferred technique. *Transtracheal jet ventilation* should only be used when expiration is unlikely to be significantly impeded. In some instances (e.g. severe head and neck trauma), an elective tracheostomy may be performed once the airway has been secured.

Specific treatment

Specific treatment of the obstruction may involve antibiotics, surgery, radiotherapy or chemotherapy. Extubation can be considered when the patient is awake and cooperative, with competent laryngeal reflexes and there is an air leak around the tube with the cuff deflated. Facilities for emergency reintubation must be immediately available. When mucosal swelling is contributing to airway narrowing, the obstruction may be relieved by administering nebulized adrenaline (1 ml of 1 : 1000 adrenaline diluted in 5 ml 0.9% saline); this may 'buy time' until more definitive treatment can be organized, and in some cases may circumvent the need for tracheal intubation (MacDonnell *et al.*, 1995). Over a longer time course the swelling may be reduced by dexamethasone 4 mg intravenously every six hours.

Pulmonary oedema

Pulmonary oedema is a recognized complication of severe upper airway obstruction (Oswalt *et al.*, 1977) and has been described most often in children with acute epiglottitis. It may be caused by the huge negative intrathoracic pressures generated to overcome the resistance to ventilation, leading to a marked reduction in the interstitial perimicrovascular pressure. A period of IPPV with PEEP is nearly always required in such cases, but resolution of the oedema is fairly rapid and weaning can usually commence within 24–48 hours. A similar mechanism may explain the pulmonary oedema that can develop when a lung that has been collapsed for some time (e.g. by a pneumothorax or pleural effusion) is re-expanded. It is thought that surfactant is inactivated during the period of lung collapse and that large negative pressures are therefore generated during reinflation.

Epiglottitis

CLINICAL FEATURES

Epiglottitis is caused almost exclusively by *Haemophilus influenzae* type B and usually affects children 1–6 years of age, although adult cases do occur. It has an acute onset with fever, toxaemia and noisy breathing. The child adopts a characteristic posture, sitting foward with an open mouth from which saliva dribbles, and usually does not cough. Sudden total obstruction can occur and may be precipitated by stressful procedures such as intravenous cannulation, performing lateral radiographs of the neck to confirm the diagnosis or simply lying the child supine.

TREATMENT

Ampicillin or chloramphenicol were until recently the antibiotics of choice, but because of the emergence of resistant strains of *Haemophilus*, cefotaxime (200 mg/kg/day) is being used more frequently. Airway obstruction should be relieved by nasotracheal intubation. Usually the child can be allowed to breathe spontaneously without sedation (Butt *et al.*, 1988). Criteria for extubation include resolution of fever, passage of time (12–16 h) and improvement in the child's general appearance. Pre-extubation laryngoscopy is unnecessary. Most can be extubated within 24 hours.

Cardiogenic pulmonary oedema (see also Chapters 2 and 4) (**Fig. 6.5**)

TREATMENT

Immediate management of acute left ventricular failure involves sitting the patient up and administering high-flow oxygen, intravenous opiates (e.g. morphine 2.5–10 mg) and intravenous diuretics (e.g. frusemide 40–120 mg). Vasodilators can be used to reduce pre-load (e.g. isosorbide dinitrate), after-load (e.g. hydralazine) or both (e.g. nitroprusside) (see Chapter 4). Inotropic support or intra-aortic balloon counterpulsation may be required (see Chapter 4). When pulmonary oedema is resistant to these measures, ultrafiltration or haemofil-

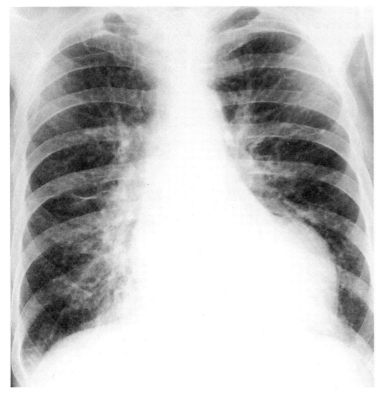

(a)

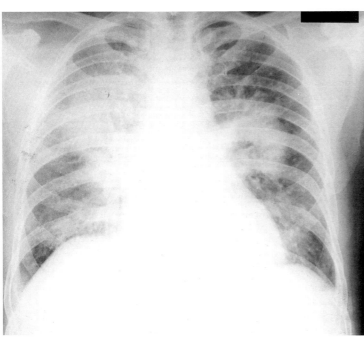

(b)

Fig. 6.5 (a) Cardiogenic pulmonary oedema in a patient with a left ventricular aneurysm. Notice the prominent upper lobe vessels, peribronchial cuffing and Kerley 'B' lines. (b) 'Batswing' pulmonary oedema in a patient with left ventricular failure.

tration (see Chapter 12) should be considered. Some patients may be suitable candidates for heart transplantation.

Unless pulmonary capillary pressure falls to less than 10 mm Hg, hydrostatic oedema resolves slowly by lymphatic drainage, not by the more rapid process of reversal of fluid flux.

Patients with severe respiratory distress and exhaustion due to unresponsive cardiogenic pulmonary oedema may benefit from a period of *mechanical ventilation*. This is particularly the case in those scheduled for corrective cardiac surgery (e.g. closure of a ventricular septal defect or replacement of a leaking mitral valve). The low cardiac output and hypotension often found in these patients need not be a deterrent to mechanical ventilation since hypoxaemia is usually very responsive to IPPV and the application of PEEP, the net effect often being to increase Do_2 (see also Chapter 7).

Adult respiratory distress syndrome/severe acute lung injury (Wiener-Kronish *et al.*, 1990)

In 1967, Ashbaugh *et al.* described a syndrome of acute respiratory distress in adults characterized by:

- severe dyspnoea;
- tachypnoea;
- cyanosis refractory to oxygen therapy;
- a reduction in lung compliance;
- diffuse alveolar infiltrates seen on the chest radiograph.

They remarked on the similarity between this 'adult respiratory distress syndrome' (ARDS) and that seen in neonates (Ashbaugh *et al.*, 1967). Before this description the same clinical syndrome had been given a variety of names such as shock lung, Da Nang lung (during the Vietnam war), septic lung, post-traumatic pulmonary insufficiency, respiratory lung and pump lung (associated with cardiopulmonary bypass).

DEFINITION

ARDS can be defined as *'diffuse pulmonary infiltrates, refractory hypoxaemia, stiff lungs and respiratory distress following a recognized precipitating cause'*. In an attempt to exclude cardiogenic causes a *PAOP < 16 mm Hg* is included in the definition. It should be recognized, however, that in cardiogenic pulmonary oedema, previously elevated left ventricular filling pressures may have been normalized by treatment before pulmonary artery catheterization and that radiological changes may take 24–48 hours to resolve.

Because the term ARDS defined in this way can be applied to such a diverse range of disorders it has been criticized for being too non-specific and some go so far as to question whether it can be considered to be a discrete entity. There is also concern that some patients with uncomplicated acute respiratory failure due to an obvious cause such as pneumonia, may be wrongly labelled as having ARDS. Most, however, accept the value of ARDS as a descriptive term, provided it is used discriminatingly, since the clinical findings, pathological features and approach to management are similar whatever the underlying cause.

CAUSES

The development of ARDS may follow a wide variety of direct and indirect pulmonary insults (**Table 6.2**) including:

- shock, sepsis, trauma, massive blood transfusion (see Chapters 4 and 9);
- fat embolism, lung contusion, inhalation of smoke and/or toxic gases (see Chapter 9);
- pancreatitis (see Chapter 15);
- amniotic fluid embolism (see Chapter 17);
- cardiopulmonary bypass (rarely);

Table 6.2 Disorders associated with adult respiratory distress syndrome.

Shock	
Trauma	Lung contusion Fat embolism Blast injury Severe non-thoracic trauma
Infection	Sepsis Pneumonia
Pulmonary aspiration	Gastric contents Near drowning
Inhalation injury	Smoke Corrosive gases
Haematological	Massive blood transfusion Disseminated intravascular coagulation
Obstetric	Amniotic fluid embolism Eclampsia
Drug overdose	Heroin Barbiturates
Miscellaneous	Cardiopulmonary bypass Pancreatitis High altitude

- pneumonia;
- aspiration of gastric contents.

Hypotension alone is not an important cause of ARDS. By far the commonest predisposing factor is sepsis, and 20–40% of patients with sepsis syndrome will develop ARDS. The second most frequent cause of ARDS is aspiration of gastric contents (see later). Trauma patients may develop ARDS either early as a result of a direct insult or later in association with sepsis. The risk of developing ARDS increases with the number of predisposing disorders and is magnified by the presence of disseminated intravascular coagulation (DIC).

INCIDENCE

The true incidence of ARDS is difficult to determine and is influenced by variations in the diagnostic criteria used, but the widely quoted North American estimate of 150,000 cases/year (about 75 cases/100,000 of the population) is likely to be an overestimate. Recent studies from the Canary Islands (Villar & Slutsky, 1989) and the UK (Webster et al., 1988) suggest an incidence of 1.5–4.5 cases/100,000 of the population.

PATHOGENESIS AND PATHOPHYSIOLOGY

ARDS can be considered to be the earliest manifestation of a generalized inflammatory reaction, the non-cardiogenic pulmonary oedema which is the cardinal feature of the early stages of the disease being the first and clinically most evident sign of a generalized increase in vascular permeability. ARDS is therefore an early complication of systemic inflammatory response syndrome (SIRS) and not surprisingly is therefore frequently complicated by the development of multiple organ dysfunction syndrome (MODS) (Bone et al., 1992). Alternatively ARDS may be precipitated by a direct insult and may or may not be complicated later by SIRS and/or MODS (see Chapter 4).

In the early phase of ARDS, the increased vascular permeability is associated with *endothelial injury*. In sheep with respiratory failure induced by *Escherichia coli* endotoxin, for example, lung lymph flow was markedly increased and, although initially its protein content was low, suggesting that oedema was due to elevated microvascular pressures associated with pulmonary hypertension, later there was a rise in protein content, indicating an increase in vascular permeability (Esbenshade, 1982). In addition, fluid obtained from the airways of patients with ARDS contains a higher concentration of protein than that obtained from patients with cardiogenic pulmonary oedema (Snapper, 1981). The *pulmonary epithelium is also damaged* in the early stages of ARDS, reducing surfactant production by Type II pneumocytes (thereby promoting atelectasis) and lowering the threshold for alveolar flooding. One consequence of epithelial injury is loss of size selectivity and this has been demonstrated by finding much higher concentrations of the large proteins IgM and $\alpha 2$ macroglobulin in bronchoalveolar lavage (BAL) fluid from patients with ARDS than in that obtained from patients with cardiogenic pulmonary oedema (Holter et al., 1986). Another consequence of the loss of integrity of the pulmonary epithelial barrier may be an inability to clear alveolar oedema (Wiener-Kronish et al., 1990), although in the first few hours after an insult approximately 20–25% of high permeability pulmonary oedema fluid is cleared by lymphatics.

As mentioned above, ARDS can be considered to be the pulmonary manifestation of a generalized or, in the case of direct lung injury, a localized, inflammatory response, the components and effects of which have been discussed in Chapter 4. The early phase of pulmonary oedema in ARDS is associated with the presence of large numbers of inflammatory cells, predominantly neutrophils, in the extravascular spaces, and there is evidence that damage to the alveolar–capillary barrier is in part mediated by *granulocytes* (Heflin & Brigham, 1981) stimulated by *activated complement* (e.g. C_{5a} (Jacob, 1981). Elevated levels of C_{5a} seem to accurately predict the development of ARDS in humans (Hammerschmidt et al., 1980) and C_3 and C_{5a} have been found in BAL fluid obtained from patients with ARDS (Robbins et al., 1987). The activated neutrophils are sequestered in the pulmonary capillaries where they attach to endothelium and release a variety of injurious mediators including *toxic oxygen radicals*, *proteolytic enzymes* (trypsin, collagenase and elastase) and *products of arachidonic acid* (Matthay et al., 1984). As discussed in Chapter 4, *adhesion molecules* play a crucial role in leucocyte-endothelial interactions. Interestingly, a recent study demonstrated that initial plasma levels of soluble L-selectin were reduced in patients who subsequently developed ARDS and found a significant correlation between low levels of soluble L-selectin, the severity of lung injury and mortality (Donnelly et al., 1994).

Mononuclear cells such as alveolar and intravascular macrophages also contribute to pulmonary damage, especially in cases of direct lung injury, by releasing *collagenase* and by triggering *coagulation/fibrinolysis*. They also release *cytokines*, but their precise role in the pathogenesis of ARDS requires further investigation, although the presence of tumour necrosis factor (TNF) in the bronchopulmonary secretions of patients with ARDS, but not in controls (Millar et al., 1989) suggests that they are likely to be as involved in the sequence of events leading to lung injury as they are in the systemic inflammatory response.

Toxic oxygen radicals

The theory that *toxic oxygen radicals* derived from activated neutrophils play a key role in the pathogenesis of ARDS is supported by finding higher levels of oxidant activity in the expired breath of mechanically ventilated patients who developed ARDS than in those who did not (Baldwin *et al.*, 1986). In a later study, however, Sznajder *et al.* (1989) found that increased hydrogen peroxide concentrations were present in the expired breath not only of patients with ARDS, but also in those with acute respiratory failure associated with focal pulmonary infiltrates, suggesting that oxygen metabolites participate in the pathogenesis of other forms of acute lung injury as well as ARDS. The lung is protected by a number of specific intracellular and extracellular systems for inactivating oxygen radicals, for example:

- cytochrome oxidase within the mitochondria, which reduces oxygen to water and acts as a sink for free radicals;
- the enzymes superoxide dismutase, catalase and gluta-thione peroxidase;
- the antioxidant activity found in vitamins A, E and C.

These defensive mechanisms can, however, be overwhelmed in those who develop ARDS. In a recent study, elevated serum levels of superoxide dismutase and catalase were shown to be predictive for the subsequent development of ARDS (Leff *et al.*, 1993).

Proteolytic activity

McGuire *et al.* (1982) have found *increased proteolytic activity* attributable to neutrophil elastase in lavage fluid from the lungs of patients with ARDS, supporting the concept that proteases are involved in its pathogenesis. Numerous proteolytic enzymes may be implicated, derived not only from activated white cells, but also from the coagulation and complement cascades, and from other failing organs such as the pancreas, especially in those with sepsis and MODS. Not only may the antiproteinases then be overwhelmed by the amount of proteolytic activity, but it seems likely that neutrophils can generate both hypochlorous acid (HOCl) and *N*-chloramines, which then oxidize the surrounding α1 proteinase inhibitor and perhaps other antiproteinases. This could then allow proteolytic enzymes, such as *neutrophil-derived elastase*, to solubilize the extracellular matrix. The ensuing loss of structural integrity and disruption of the surface anionic charge might contribute to the increase in vascular permeability. It has, however, been shown that there is a considerable excess of antiproteinase activity in patients with ARDS (Wewers *et al.*, 1988), and it has therefore been suggested that protease-induced injury may not be par-

ticularly important in the pathogenesis of acute lung injury.

Coagulation disorders

Thrombocytopenia and microthrombosis are frequently associated with the development of ARDS and activation of the clotting system is likely to be important in its pathogenesis. Platelet and fibrin thrombi have been found at post-mortem in the lungs of patients dying with ARDS, and these can release vasoactive substances such as serotonins and prostaglandins. Fibrinolysis releases fibrin/fibrinogen degradation products (FDPs), which may injure the pulmonary microvasculature, while localized vascular obstruction might be associated with episodes of ischaemia followed by reperfusion injury. These disorders do, however, also occur in patients with sepsis and major tissue injury who do not develop ARDS.

Intra-alveolar exudate

The haemorrhagic intra-alveolar exudate seen in ARDS is rich in platelets, fibrin, fibrinogen and clotting factors; fibrin and fibronectin are deposited along the alveolar ducts, with the incorporation of cellular debris. This exudate may inactivate surfactant and stimulate inflammation, as well as promote hyaline membrane formation and the migration of fibroblasts into the airspaces. Not only does BAL fluid from patients with ARDS contain enhanced procoagulant activity (Idell *et al.*, 1987) and antiplasmins, but urokinase activity is depressed, possibly because it is complexed to plasminogen activator inhibitor type 1 (Bertozzi *et al.*, 1990). The resulting deficiency in fibrin clearance may contribute to the formation or delayed resolution of hyaline membranes and therefore to intra-alveolar fibrosis.

Changes in the subacute phase

Approximately 5–10 days after the onset of ARDS, proliferation of Type II alveolar cells provides a new epithelial lining while activated fibroblasts accumulate in the interstitial spaces. There is collagen deposition and some patients develop an accelerated fibrosing alveolitis. Fibroblast and epithelial cell growth factors, released by macrophages and other cells in the lung, may be involved in this process. Subsequently interstitial fibrosis progresses with loss of elastic tissue and obliteration of the pulmonary vasculature, together with lung destruction and emphysema. In this phase oxygenation may improve, but the increased V_D and reduced lung compliance (secondary to fibrosis and reduced surfactant) persist.

Physiological changes

Physiological changes include an increased shunt and $P_{A-a}O_2$, associated with a reduced FRC and compliance. V_D/V_T rises, especially in the most severe cases in which pulmonary vascular resistance is also increased. As well as the reduction in compliance, airflow resistance is markedly increased in ARDS (Wright & Bernard, 1989), possibly related to the reduction in lung volume, to obliteration of the conducting airways or to airway inflammation and hyperreactivity. The depletion and inactivation of surfactant may contribute to atelectasis.

Pulmonary vascular resistance is often elevated in patients with ARDS (Zapol & Snider, 1977). High right-sided filling pressures are then required to maintain cardiac output, and the right ventricle dilates, increasing myocardial wall tension and jeopardizing coronary perfusion. In severe cases, the interventricular septum may be distorted so that it impinges on the left ventricular cavity, causing a rise in LAP. Left ventricular end-diastolic volume (LVEDV) and stroke index therefore remain low, while PAOP is paradoxically high (Sibbald & Prewitt, 1983).

There are a number of causes of pulmonary hypertension in ARDS. Initially, mechanical obstruction of the pulmonary circulation may occur as a result of vascular compression by interstitial fluid, oedema of the vessel wall and the weight of the oedematous lung. Later, constriction of the pulmonary vasculature may occur in response to increased autonomic activity and circulating substances such as catecholamines, serotonin, $PGF_2\alpha$, thromboxane, FDPs, and complement. Vessels supplying poorly oxygenated alveoli constrict (hypoxic vasoconstrictor response) in an attempt to improve V/Q matching. This response may be enhanced by local acidosis and hypercarbia, but may in some cases be inhibited by vasodilator products of arachidonic acid breakdown.

In some patients with ARDS and pulmonary hypertension, angiography will reveal 'beading' of the arterioles and peripheral pruning of the pulmonary vasculature. This suggests fibrin deposition and is associated with a marked increase in V_D and a poor prognosis. In these cases, subpleural lung segments may be infarcted and liable to rupture. In others both pulmonary vascular resistance and angiography are normal, and the 'wet lung' is more likely to respond to dehydration and respiratory support.

Although the lungs in ARDS are diffusely injured, the pulmonary lesions (when identified as densities on the CT scan) are not homogeneously distributed, being predominantly located in dependent regions (Gattinoni *et*

al., 1991). The likely explanation for this phenomenon is that the distribution of extravascular lung water and areas of lung collapse is influenced by gravitational increases in capillary pressure and air space compression in the lower lung regions. It has been suggested that the lung in ARDS can be considered to consist of three zones:

- apparently healthy;
- recruitable;
- clearly abnormal.

This concept is consistent with the observation that the abnormality of gas exchange is largely due to true shunt, combined with areas of normal or high V/Q ratios. In the 'healthy' zone, which may represent only 20–30% of the normal lung volume, compliance and gas exchange are near normal; this *'baby lung'* has to be ventilated with a high minute volume and F_IO_2 in order to achieve adequate oxygenation and carbon dioxide removal. It is therefore exposed to the potentially damaging effects of high inflation pressures, PEEP and increased oxygen concentrations.

At post-mortem the lungs of patients who die with ARDS are heavy and congested, with atelectasis, hyaline membranes and end-stage fibrosis.

CLINICAL PRESENTATION AND DIAGNOSIS

ARDS usually develops insidiously 12–72 hours after the precipitating event, but in 80% of patients acute lung injury is evident within 24 hours and many of those with sepsis develop signs and symptoms within six hours. Clinically the first sign of ARDS is often an unexplained tachypnoea, followed by increasing hypoxia, dyspnoea and respiratory distress. Fine crepitations are heard throughout both lung fields. Later the chest radiograph shows bilateral, diffuse pulmonary infiltrates, interstitial at first, but subsequently with an alveolar pattern; air bronchograms may be seen (**Fig. 6.6**).

The *diagnosis of ARDS* is therefore based on:

- identifying an antecedent history of a precipitating condition such as sepsis or trauma;
- refractory hypoxaemia (P_aO_2 <8 kPa, $F_IO_2 > 0.4$, $P_aO_2/P_AO_2 < 0.25$);
- radiological evidence of bilateral diffuse pulmonary infiltrates;
- a PAOP < 15–18 mm Hg (with normal oncotic pressure);
- a total thoracic compliance < 30 ml/cm H_2O.

Other disorders such as fibrosing alveolitis and left ventricular failure should be excluded. As V_D rises, minute volume has to be increased to maintain a normal P_aCO_2.

The diagnosis of ARDS is mainly clinical and criteria

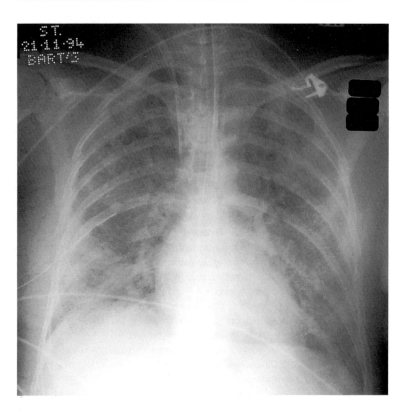

Fig. 6.6 Chest radiograph appearances in adult respiratory distress syndrome. Bilateral diffuse alveolar shadowing with air bronchograms and without cardiac enlargement.

vary between centres. In order to define ARDS more precisely, as well as allow more accurate assessments and comparisons of outcome, an expanded three-part definition has been proposed in which the severity of the lung injury is quantified by assessing chest radiographic appearances, the degree of hypoxaemia, the extent of the reduction in compliance and the requirement for PEEP. On the basis of this score the patient can be categorized as having no lung injury, mild to moderate lung injury or a severe acute lung injury. Only the latter warrants the term ARDS. Additionally the clinical disorder(s) responsible for or associated with the development of acute lung injury are identified and the condition is classified as acute or chronic (Murray *et al.*, 1988).

Nosocomial pneumonia is a common complication of ARDS, especially during the subacute phase. The particular susceptibility of ARDS lungs to superimposed infection may be related to:

- impaired blood supply;
- poor lymphatic drainage;
- the presence of plasma/cellular debris in the air spaces;
- impaired mucociliary transport;
- retention of secretions.

MANAGEMENT (MacNaughton & Evans, 1992)

Management is based on treatment of the underlying condition, especially the eradication and control of sepsis, combined with supportive measures. Enteral nutrition should, if possible, be commenced early, and patients should receive prophylactic subcutaneous heparin. CT scanning of the lungs may reveal occult pneumothoraces, lung abscess, or empyema, as well as 'traction bronchiectasis' and barotrauma; it may also be possible to distinguish between chronic inflammation and fibrosis.

Respiratory support

Conventional methods of mechanical ventilation expose the lung to high airway pressures, especially when combined with high levels of PEEP, and may exacerbate pulmonary injury (see Chapter 7). New approaches to ventilation in ARDS therefore aim to maintain a mean airway pressure just sufficient to recruit unstable alveoli and improve gas exchange whilst avoiding high peak inflation pressures (PIPs) (preferably PIP < 30-35 cm H_2O, certainly < 50 cm H_2O).

Low-volume pressure-limited mechanical ventilation (see Chapter 7). This technique minimizes peak airway pressures and can be combined with *inverse ratio ventilation* and *low levels of PEEP* to achieve optimal improvement in oxygenation. In a retrospective analysis of 50 patients with ARDS managed using this technique, with synchronized intermittent mandatory ventilation (SIMV) and permissive hypercarbia, mortality was impressively low (Hickling *et al.*, 1990).

High-frequency jet ventilation (HFJV). This technique is associated with effective gas exchange at lower peak airway pressures than conventional mechanical ventilation and may thereby reduce the incidence of barotrauma and ventilator-induced lung injury (see Chapter 7). Significant improvement in oxygenation can, however, only be achieved by increasing mean airway pressures. Jet ventilation at frequencies close to the natural resonant frequency of the lung (5–7 Hz) with high mean airway pressures may promote alveolar recruitment, thereby improving gas exchange when conventional ventilation has failed (Lin *et al.*, 1990; MacNaughton & Evans, 1992). A prospective controlled trial has demonstrated that although HFJV can be used safely in acute respiratory failure, outcome was no better than with standard techniques (Carlon *et al.*, 1983).

Low-frequency positive pressure ventilation with extracorporeal carbon dioxide removal (LFPPV-ECCO$_2$-R) (see Chapter 7). The results of uncontrolled trials of LFPPV-ECCO$_2$-R in ARDS were encouraging (Gattinoni *et al.*, 1986), but in a recent randomized trial there was no significant difference in survival between patients treated with ECCO$_2$-R and those supported with pressure-controlled inverse ratio ventilation (Morris *et al.*, 1994). Since the ability to maintain gas exchange with ECCO$_2$-R is well established some continue to use the technique in selected patients with intractable hypoxaemia and hypercarbia. Others feel that extracorporeal support for ARDS should be confined to controlled clinical trials (Morris *et al.*, 1994).

Intravascular oxygenation device (IVOX) (see Chapter 7). Clinical experience with this technique is limited. Although it is safe (Kallis *et al.*, 1991) and its use may allow a reduction in ventilation with a fall in peak and mean airway pressures (Mira *et al.*, 1995), its efficacy has yet to be demonstrated in controlled trials.

Although the concept of 'resting' the lung to promote recovery is theoretically attractive these techniques are invasive, costly, can be associated with significant complications and have not yet been shown to improve outcome in controlled trials (Sim & Evans, 1993).

Reduction of pulmonary oedema

Left ventricular filling pressures should be minimized by fluid restriction, the use of diuretics and, if these measures fail to prevent fluid overload, by haemofiltration. The aim should be to achieve a consistently negative fluid balance. If possible plasma oncotic pressure should be maintained close to the normal range by administering colloidal solutions with a long half-life. In patients with ARDS, however, colloids are unlikely to be retained within the vascular compartment; once they enter the interstitial space, the intravascular oncotic gradient is lost and the main determinants of oedema formation become the microvascular hydrostatic pressure and the efficiency of lymphatic drainage. There is, therefore, some controversy about the relative merits of colloids or crystalloids for volume replacement in patients likely to develop ARDS or in whom the condition is established (see also Chapter 4). Blood should be transfused to maintain the haemoglobin concentration around 12 g/dl.

Body position changes

Both lateral and prone positions have been shown to improve gas exchange. In the lateral position, with the less injured lung down, gravity increases blood flow to the good lung and *V/Q* matching is improved. When the patient is changed from the supine to the prone position lung densities in the dependent regions are redistributed; in some patients this is associated with improved gas exchange (Gattinoni *et al.*, 1991). Failure to respond to position changes may suggest that the initial lung injury was not diffuse, that the patient does not have ARDS (e.g. the problem may be focal consolidation) or that the original microvascular injury has resolved.

Physiotherapy

During the acute phase of ARDS, when large volumes of pulmonary oedema are being produced continuously, chest physiotherapy, manual inflations and endotracheal suction are unlikely to be of any benefit. Later removal of secretions and re-expansion of collapsed lung segments is essential. Hypoxia due to discontinuation of PEEP and loss of supplemental oxygen during endotracheal suction can be avoided by using endotracheal tube adaptors with self-sealing diaphragms.

Inhaled nitric oxide

In patients with ARDS inhaled nitric oxide (NO) can reduce pulmonary artery pressure and increase P_aO_2 by improving V/Q matching without causing systemic vaso-dilatation (Rossaint *et al.*, 1993). The effects of NO are, however, variable and the influence of such treatment on outcome remains to be determined.

Aerosolized prostacyclin

Aerosolized prostacyclin (PGI_2) appears to have similar effects to inhaled NO in patients with ARDS. In one small study pulmonary vascular resistance fell, the P_aO_2/F_IO_2 ratio increased and systemic blood pressure fell only slightly (Walmrath *et al.*, 1993). Again, however, the response to inhaled prostacyclin is variable and its effects on outcome unknown.

Aerosolized surfactant

Surfactant replacement therapy reduces morbidity and mortality in neonatal respiratory distress syndrome and can improve lung function and survival in animal models of ARDS. It might be expected, therefore, that surfactant treatment would benefit adult humans with ARDS. In a recent prospective randomized double-blind placebo-controlled pilot study, however, administration of aero-solized surfactant ('*Exosurf*', Burroughs Wellcome Co.) was not associated with any changes in measured physiological variables and in particular there was no improvement in oxygenation, nor any reduction in com-pliance. Although there appeared to be a dose-dependent reduction in mortality rate, this did not achieve stat-istical significance (Weg *et al.*, 1994). Since there was no improvement in lung function it was suggested that other mechanisms such as the anti-inflammatory action of surfactant might have accounted for this trend towards improved survival. The lack of physiological effect of *Exosurf* might be explained by the choice of an inappropriate synthetic surfactant or the use of aerosol delivery or most likely, to too small a dose. It is also possible that surfactant dysfunction was not an im- port-ant component of the lung injury in these patients.

Perfluorocarbon-associated gas exchange

This technique, in which the functional residual capacity is filled with perfluorocarbon liquid eliminates air/fluid interfaces in the lungs and thereby reduces alveolar surface tension. In a porcine model of gastric aspiration, perfluorocarbon-associated gas exchange improved oxygenation and may have prevented pro-gression to ARDS (Nesti *et al.*, 1994).

Cardiovascular support

Although patients with ARDS are usually hyperdynamic, cardiac output may be compromised by a variety of fac-tors including low filling pressures due to fluid restric-tion, high levels of PEEP, increased pulmonary vascular resistance and the myocardial effects of sepsis. More-over, as many as 20% of patients with ARDS have con-comitant heart disease.

Tissue Do_2 should be optimized (see Chapter 4) by ensuring that the haemoglobin concentration is adequate, cautious expansion of the circulating volume, the use of inotropic support when required, and pos-sibly the administration of specific agents such as prosta-glandin E_1 (PGE_1) to reduce pulmonary hypertension. Because administration of large volumes of fluid in an effort to maintain pre-load is likely to exacerbate· pul-monary oedema there should be no hesitation in using inotropes and vasoconstrictors to achieve an adequate cardiac output and blood pressure in the face of relative hypovolaemia. It should be remembered that the phenomenon of supply dependency has been described in patients with ARDS who may therefore benefit from measures to enhance Do_2 and Vo_2 (see Chapter 4).

Administration of PGE_1 to patients with ARDS reduces systemic and pulmonary vascular resistances; this is accompanied by increases in stroke volume, heart rate and cardiac output (Bone *et al.*, 1989; Silverman *et al.*, 1990). Despite these apparently beneficial physiological effects, PGE_1 failed to improve outcome in a mixed group of medical and surgical patients with ARDS (Bone *et al.*, 1989), although 30-day survival was improved in an earlier study in surgical patients, many of whom were trauma victims (Holcroft *et al.*, 1986). Administration of PGE_1 may be complicated by hypotension, a deteri-oration in gas exchange (Melot *et al.*, 1989) and an increased incidence of diarrhoea (Bone *et al.*, 1989).

Anti-inflammatory agents

Previous administration of corticosteroids to sheep given endotoxin prevents the subsequent increase in lung vascular permeability (Brigham *et al.*, 1981) and the early administration of high-dose corticosteroids to patients with septic ARDS may in some cases reduce alveolar–capillary permeability (Sibbald *et al.*, 1981). High-dose corticosteroids have not, however, been shown to improve outcome in the acute stages of ARDS in humans (Bernard *et al.*, 1987), although they may be beneficial when administered during the late fibroprol-iferative phase (Meduri *et al.*, 1991). Ibuprofen may reduce pulmonary hypertension and improve oxygen-ation in ARDS. The value of other agents that might limit pulmonary damage such as pentoxifylline, antioxidants/oxygen radical scavengers (e.g. catalase, superoxide dismutase, *N*-acetylcysteine) and immuno-therapy is uncertain (see also Chapter 4).

OUTCOME

The mortality of ARDS remains depressingly high at more than 50% overall. Prognosis is, however, very dependent on aetiology. For example, when ARDS occurs in association with septic shock and persistent sepsis, mortality rates may be as high as 90%. In addition, the development of ARDS significantly worsens the prognosis in sepsis and is an independent predictor of outcome. Patients with ARDS due to fat embolism, on the other hand, have a much better prognosis with survival rates of around 90%. ARDS developing after cardiopulmonary bypass also has a relatively good prognosis, while medical patients tend to have a higher mortality than trauma patients.

Acute renal failure is common in patients with ARDS and adversely affects the prognosis, while the development of liver failure is associated with a particularly poor outlook.

Although it is often said that the prognosis of ARDS has not improved since its original description, a number of the patients described by Ashbaugh *et al.* (1967) were probably suffering predominantly from fluid overload and would have been expected to do well. Also there is some evidence to suggest that mortality rates have fallen over the last decade (Suchyta *et al.*, 1991).

Death is rarely due to irreversible respiratory failure (Montgomery *et al.*, 1985), and more than 75% of patients who die with ARDS now do so as a result of MODS and haemodynamic instability rather than impaired gas exchange. Most early deaths are attributable to the underlying illness or injury, while late deaths are usually related to sepsis (Montgomery *et al.*, 1985).

Lung function of patients who recover from ARDS often returns virtually to normal, particularly in young non-smokers (Lakshminarayan *et al.*, 1976), and residual radiographic changes are usually limited to a few linear scars. A more recent study concluded that spirometry and lung mechanics are restored to normal within six months of extubation, but that gas exchange remains impaired. Exercise tolerance may be limited, perhaps due to a reduction in pulmonary capillary blood volume (Buchser *et al.*, 1985).

Aspiration pneumonia

Factors predisposing to pulmonary aspiration include obtundation, impaired laryngo-pharyngeal reflexes and a propensity to vomiting or regurgitation (**Table 6.3**). Nasogastric tubes, especially if wide bore, predispose

Table 6.3 Factors predisposing to pulmonary aspiration.

Reduced consciousness	Overdose Metabolic coma General anaesthesia Head injury Cerebrovascular accident Epilepsy
Impaired cough and gag	Motor or sensory bulbar dysfunction Recent extubation of larynx Elderly patients Severe illness
Increased susceptibility to regurgitation/vomiting	Hiatus hernia Oesophageal obstruction Oesophagectomy Bowel obstruction Pregnancy Presence of nasogastric tube

to aspiration by preventing closure of the oesophageal sphincter and interfering with coughing and clearing of the pharynx. Although the presence of an endotracheal or tracheostomy tube protects against large-volume aspiration, the vocal cords and epiglottis are held open, allowing fluids to accumulate above the cuff. Small amounts may then trickle past the cuff into the lungs.

The consequences of pulmonary aspiration depend on the nature of the aspirate, but overall about a one-third of patients with clearly documented aspiration will subsequently develop ARDS.

TYPES OF ASPIRATION

Aspiration of sterile acidic gastric contents

Aspiration of sterile acidic gastric contents causes severe damage within minutes. The alveolar–capillary barrier loses its integrity, high-permeability oedema develops rapidly and acid denaturation of surfactant leads to atelectasis. Within a few hours there is degeneration of the bronchial epithelium, destruction of Type II alveolar lining cells and an inflammatory cell infiltrate. In those who survive, the inflammatory response resolves, the bronchial epithelium regenerates and the fibroproliferative phase supervenes.

Clinically there is sudden onset of severe dyspnoea, cyanosis and wheeze, often associated with hypovolaemia and hypotension (Mendelson's syndrome, see Chapter 17). Chest radiographic appearances are those of ARDS.

Aspiration of infected fluids

The stomach and oropharynx of patients who have been ill or hospitalized for some time, especially those patients with gastrointestinal pathology and those receiving antacids, are frequently colonized by pathogenic bacteria. Under these circumstances aspiration can result in severe pneumonia, often caused by Gram-negative or anaerobic organisms normally resident only in the lower gastrointestinal tract. Pathological changes are similar to, but generally less severe than those of pure acid aspiration except that they may be complicated later by infection.

Aspiration of particulate matter

Aspiration of particulate matter (e.g. food) may cause acute large airways obstruction or if smaller irritant particles such as meat or vegetables are inhaled may precipitate an inflammatory response followed by a granulomatous reaction with minimal fibrosis. Uncleared particles may lead to persistent infection, necrotizing pneumonia, abscess formation or empyema. Chest radiography may show focal collapse or consolidation.
. The consequences of aspirating large quantities of fine particles in neutral gastric contents, as may occur some time after a meal, are similar, but less severe than those of pure acid aspiration.

Aspiration of inert fluids

Inert fluids free of particulate matter or bacteria produce minimal pulmonary damage. The immediate clinical consequences depend solely on the volume aspirated, and resolution is usually rapid.

DIAGNOSING ASPIRATION

The diagnosis of aspiration is largely clinical, but can often be confirmed by examining an endotracheal aspir-

ate or by bronchoscopy. A sample of aspirate should always be sent for microscopy, culture and sensitivities.

MANAGEMENT

The patient should be positioned head down on his or her right-hand side, the airway secured, the oropharynx suctioned and oxygen given. Those with a depressed conscious level and/or impaired airway protection will require endotracheal intubation. A nasogastric tube should be passed to empty the stomach.

When particulate aspiration has occurred and when focal collapse or foreign bodies are visible on the chest radiograph, *bronchoscopy* may be indicated. *Rigid bronchoscopy* is usually most effective, but a general anaesthetic is required and it may be difficult to maintain acceptable oxygenation. Also access to the upper lobes and more distal airways is limited. *Fibre-optic bronchoscopy* may therefore be preferred, especially in those with more distal airways occlusion and when attempting to remove solid foreign particles such as teeth or amalgam. Bronchial lavage is probably of no value, but *chest physiotherapy* is essential. *Bronchodilators* may be required.

The use of *antibiotics* is controversial. Even when sick hospitalized patients aspirate, the role of infection in the ensuing lung damage is unclear, but many believe that the immediate administration of antibiotics active against intestinal flora, such as cefuroxime and metronidazole, is beneficial. It is even less certain that the prophylactic administration of penicillin, to which the anaerobes that predominate in normal mouth flora are usually sensitive, is indicated when previously well patients aspirate outside hospital. Some therefore adopt an expectant approach and only administer antibiotics for proven infection.

The administration of *corticosteroids* is also controversial. The majority of studies suggest that they are of no benefit (Wynne *et al.*, 1981) and there is a danger that they increase the incidence of superimposed infection and impair the ability of fibroblasts to wall off aspirated foodstuffs.

REFERENCES

Ashbaugh DG, Bigelow DB, Petty TL & Levine BE (1967) Acute respiratory distress in adults. *Lancet* ii: 319-323.

Aubier M, Trippenbach T & Roussos C (1981) Respiratory muscle fatigue during cardiogenic shock. *Journal of Applied Physiology* **51**: 499-508.

Aubier M, Viires N, Syllie G, Mozes R & Roussos C (1982) Respiratory muscle contribution to lactic acidosis in low cardiac output. *American Review of Respiratory Disease* **126**: 648-652.

Aubier M, Murciano D, Lecocgui Y *et al.* (1985) Effect of hypo-

phosphatemia on diaphragmatic contractility in patients with acute respiratory failure. *New England Journal of Medicine* **313**: 420-424.

Baldwin SR, Simon RH, Grum CM, Ketai LH, Boxer LA & Devall LJ (1986) Oxidant activity in expired breath of patients with adult respiratory distress syndrome. *Lancet* i: 11-14.

Barber RE, Lee J & Hamilton WK (1970) Oxygen toxicity in man. A prospective study in patients with irreversible brain damage. *New England Journal of Medicine* **283**: 1478-1484.

Bernard GR, Luce JM, Sprung Cl *et al.* (1987) High-dose corticosteroids in patients with the adult respiratory distress syndrome. *New England Journal of Medicine* **317**: 1565-1570.

Bertozzi P, Astedt B, Zenzuis L *et al.* (1990) Depressed bronchoalveolar urokinase activity in patients with adult respiratory distress syndrome. *New England Journal of Medicine* **322**: 890-897.

Bone RC, Slotman G, Maunder R *et al.* & The Prostaglandin E₁ Study Group (1989) Randomized double-blind, multicenter study of prostaglandin E₁ in patients with the adult respiratory distress syndrome. *Chest* **96**: 114-119.

Bone RC, Balk R, Slotman G *et al.* (1992) Adult respiratory distress syndrome. Sequence and importance of development of multiple organ failure. *Chest* **101**: 320-326.

Bott J, Carroll MP, Conway JH *et al.* (1993) Randomised controlled trial of nasal ventilation in acute ventilatory failure due to chronic obstructive airways disease. *Lancet* **341**: 1555-1557.

Brigham KL, Bowers RE & McKeen CR (1981) Methylprednisolone prevention of increased lung vascular permeability following endotoxemia in sheep. *Journal of Clinical Investigation* **67**: 1103-1110.

Buchser E, Leuenberger Ph, Chiolero R, Perret C & Freeman J (1985) Reduced pulmonary capillary blood volume as a long-term sequel of ARDS. *Chest* **87**: 608-611.

Butt W, Stann F, Walker C, Williams J, Duncan A & Phelan P (1988) Acute epiglottitis: a different approach to management. *Critical Care Medicine* **16**: 43-47.

Caldwell PRB, Lee WL Jr, Schildkraut HS & Archibald ER (1966) Changes in lung volume, diffusing capacity, and blood gases in men breathing oxygen. *Journal of Applied Physiology* **21**: 1477-1483.

Campbell EJM (1960a) A method of controlled oxygen administration which reduces the risk of carbon-dioxide retention. *Lancet* **ii**: 12-14.

Campbell EJM (1960b) Respiratory failure. The relation between oxygen concentrations of inspired air and arterial blood. *Lancet* **ii**: 10-11.

Campbell EJM (1982) How to use the Venturi mask. *Lancet* **ii**: 1206.

Carlon GC, Howland WS, Ray C, Miodownik S, Griffin JP & Groeger JS (1983) High-frequency jet ventilation: a prospective randomized evaluation. *Chest* **84**: 551-559.

Coakley JH, Nagendran K, Honavar M & Hinds CJ (1993) Preliminary observations on the neuromuscular abnormalities in patients with organ failure and sepsis. *Intensive Care Medicine* **19**: 323-328.

Comroe JH Jr, Dripps RD, Dumke PR & Deming M (1945) Oxygen toxicity. The effect of inhalation of high concentrations of oxygen for twenty-four hours on normal men at sea level and at a simulated altitude of 18,000 feet. *Journal of the American Medical Association* **128**: 710-717.

Crompton GK (1990) Nebulized or intravenous beta₂ adrenoreceptor agonist therapy in acute asthma? *European Respiratory Journal* **3**: 125-126.

Deneke SM & Fanburg BL (1982) Oxygen toxicity of the lung: an update. *British Journal of Anaesthesia* **54**: 737-749.

Djukanovic R, Roche WR, Wilson JW *et al.* (1990) Mucosal inflammation in asthma. *American Review of Respiratory Disease* **142**: 434-457.

Donnelly SC, Haslett C, Dransfield I *et al.* (1994) Role of selectins in development of adult respiratory distress syndrome. *Lancet* **344**: 215-219.

Eason J & Markowe HLJ (1987) Controlled investigation of deaths from asthma in hospitals in the North East Thames region. *British Medical Journal* **294**: 1255-1258.

Efthimiou J, Fleming J & Spiro SG (1987) Sternomastoid muscle function and fatigue in breathless patients with severe respiratory disease. *American Review of Respiratory Disease* **136**: 1099-1105.

Esbenshade AM, Newman JH, Lams PM, Jolles H & Brigham KL (1982) Respiratory failure after endotoxin infusion in sheep: lung mechanics and lung fluid balance. *Journal of Applied Physiology* **53**: 967-976.

Gattinoni L, Pesenti A, Mascheroni D *et al.* (1986) Low-frequency positive-pressure ventilation with extracorporeal CO₂ removal in severe acute respiratory failure. *Journal of the American Medical Association* **256**: 881-886.

Gattinoni L, Pelosi P, Vitale G, Pesenti A, D'Andrea L & Mascheroni D (1991) Body position changes redistribute lung computed, tomographic density in patients with acute respiratory failure. *Anesthesiology* **74**: 15-23.

Goldstein RS, Young J & Rebuck AS (1982) Effect of breathing pattern on oxygen concentration received from standard face masks. *Lancet* **ii**: 1188-1190.

Hammerschmidt DE, Weaver LJ, Hudson LD, Craddock PR & Jacob HS (1980) Association of complement activation and elevated plasma-C5a with adult respiratory distress syndrome. Pathophysiological relevance and possible prognostic value. *Lancet* **i**: 947-949.

Heflin AC Jr & Brigham KL (1981) Prevention by granulocyte depletion of increased vascular permeability of sheep lung following endotoxemia. *Journal of Clinical Investigation* **68**: 1253-1260.

Hickling KG, Henderson SJ & Jackson R (1990) Low mortality associated with low volume pressure limited ventilation with permissive hypercapnia in severe adult respiratory distress syndrome. *Intensive Care Medicine* **16**: 372-377.

Holcroft JW, Vassar MJ & Weber CJ (1986) Prostaglandin E₁ and survival in patients with the adult respiratory distress syndrome. A prospective trial. *Annals of Surgery* **203**: 371-378.

Holter JF, Weiland JE, Pacht ER, Gadek JE & Davis WB (1986) Protein permeability in the adult respiratory distress syndrome. Loss of size selectivity of the alveolar epithelium. *Journal of Clinical Investigation* **78**: 1513-1522.

Hussain SNA, Simkus G & Roussos C (1985) Respiratory muscle fatigue: a cause of ventilatory failure in septic shock. *Journal of Applied Physiology* **58**: 2033-2040.

Idell S, Gonzalez K, Bradford H *et al.* (1987) Procoagulant activity in bronchoalveolar lavage in the adult respiratory distress syndrome. Contribution of tissue factor associated with factor vii. *American Review of Respiratory Disease* **136**: 1466-1474.

Jacob HS (1981) The role of activated complement and granulocytes in shock states and myocardial infarction. *Journal of Laboratory and Clinical Medicine* **98**: 645-653.

James OF, Mills RM & Allen KM (1977) Severe bronchial asthma: factors influencing intensive care management and outcome. *Anaesthesia and Intensive Care* **5**: 11-18.

Jansen JE, Sorensen AI, Naesh O, Erichsen CJ & Pedersen A (1990) Effect of doxapram on postoperative pulmonary complications after upper abdominal surgery in high-risk patients. *Lancet* **335**: 936-938.

Jones JG, Sapsford DJ & Wheatley RG (1990) Postoperative hypoxaemia: mechanisms and time course. *Anaesthesia* **45**: 566-573.

Kallis P, al-Saady NM, Bennett D & Treasure T (1991) Clinical use of intravascular oxygenation. *Lancet* **337**: 549 (letter).

Kapanci Y, Weibel ER, Kaplan HP & Robinson FR (1969) Pathogenesis and reversibility of the pulmonary lesions of oxygen toxicity in monkeys. 11. Ultrastructural and morphometric studies. *Laboratory Investigation* **20**: 101-118.

Kikuchi Y, Okabe S, Tamura G et al. (1994) Chemosensitivity and perception of dyspnea in patients with a history of near-fatal asthma. *New England Journal of Medicine* **330**: 1329-1334.

Laaban J-P, Grateau G, Psychoyos I, Laromiguiere M, Vuong TU-K & Rochemaure, J (1989) Hypophosphatemia induced by mechanical ventilation in patients with chronic obstructive pulmonary disease. *Critical Care Medicine* **17**: 1115-1120.

Lakshminarayan S, Stanford RE & Petty TL (1976) Prognosis after recovery from adult respiratory distress syndrome. *American Review of Respiratory Disease* **113**: 7-16.

Leff JA, Parsons PE, Day CE et al. (1993) Serum antioxidants as predictors of adult respiratory distress syndrome in patients with sepsis. *Lancet* **341**: 777-780.

Lin ES, Jones MJ, Mottram SD, Smith BE & Smith G (1990) Relationship between resonance and gas exchange during high frequency jet ventilation. *British Journal of Anaesthesia* **64**: 453-459.

MacDonnell SPJ, Timmins AC & Watson JD (1995) Adrenaline administered via a nebulizer in adult patients with upper airway obstruction. *Anaesthesia* **50**: 35-36.

McFadden ERJ (1991) Fatal or near-fatal asthma. *New England Journal of Medicine* **324**: 409-411.

McGuire WW, Spragg RG, Cohen AB & Cochrane CG (1982) Studies on the pathogenesis of the adult respiratory distress syndrome. *Journal of Clinical Investigation* **69**: 543-553.

MacNaughton PD & Evans TW (1992) Management of adult respiratory distress syndrome. *Lancet* **339**: 469-472.

Marini JJ (1989) Should PEEP be used in airflow obstruction? *American Review of Respiratory Disease* **140**: 1-3.

Matthay MA, Eschenbacher WL & Goetzl EJ (1984) Elevated concentrations of leukotriene D4 in pulmonary edema fluid of patients with the adult respiratory distress syndrome. *Journal of Clinical Immunology* **4**: 479-483.

Meduri GU, Belenchia JM, Estes RJ et al. (1991) Fibroproliferative phase of ARDS; clinical findings and effects of corticosteroids. *Chest* **100**: 943-952.

Melot C, Lejeune P, Leeman M, Moraine J-J & Nacije R (1989) Prostaglandin E$_1$ in the adult respiratory distress syndrome. *American Review of Respiratory Disease* **139**: 106-110.

Millar AB, Foley NM, Singer M, Johnson NMcI, Meager A & Rook GAW (1989) Tumour necrosis factor in bronchopulmonary secretions of patients with adult respiratory distress syndrome. *Lancet* **ii**: 712-714.

Mira JP, Brunet F & Belghith M et al. (1995) Reduction of ventilator settings allowed by intravenous oxygenator (IVOX) in ARDS patients. *Intensive Care Medicine* **21**: 11-17.

Mitchell JP, Schuller D, Calandrino FS & Schuster DP (1992) Improved outcome based on fluid management in critically

ill patients requiring pulmonary artery catheterization. *American Review of Respiratory Disease* **145**: 990-998.

Montgomery AB, Stager MA, Carrio CJ & Hudson LD (1985) Causes of mortality in patients with the adult respiratory distress syndrome. *American Review of Respiratory Disease* **132**: 485-489.

Morris AH, Wallace CJ, Menlove RL et al. (1994) Randomized clinical trial of pressure-controlled inverse ratio ventilation and extracorporeal CO_2 removal for adult respiratory distress syndrome. *American Journal of Respiratory Critical Care Medicine* **149**: 295-305.

Moxham J (1990) Respiratory muscle fatigue: mechanisms, evaluation and therapy. *British Journal of Anaesthesia* **65**: 43-53.

Murray JF, Matthay MA, Luce JM & Flick MR (1988) An expanded definition of the adult respiratory distress syndrome. *American Review of Respiratory Disease* **138**: 720-723.

Nesti FD, Fuhrman BP, Steinhorn DM et al. (1994) Perfluorocarbon-associated gas exchange in gastric aspiration. *Critical Care Medicine* **22**: 1445-1452.

Oswalt CE, Gates GA & Holmstrom FMG (1977) Pulmonary edema as a complication of acute airway obstruction. *Journal of the American Medical Association* **238**: 1833-1835.

Power I (1993) Aspirin-induced asthma. *British Journal of Anaesthesia* **71**: 619-621 (Editorial).

Puri VK, Weil MH, Michaels S & Carlson RW (1980) Pulmonary edema associated with reduction in plasma oncotic pressure. *Surgery, Gynecology and Obstetrics* **151**: 344-348.

Robbins RA, Russ WD, Rasmussen JK & Clayton MM (1987) Activation of the complement system in the adult respiratory distress syndrome. *American Review of Respiratory Disease* **135**: 651-658.

Robertson CE, Steedman D, Sinclair CJ, Brown D & Malcolm-Smith N (1985) Use of ether in life-threatening acute severe asthma. *Lancet* **i**: 187-188.

Rochester DF (1991) The diaphragm in COPD. *New England Journal of Medicine* **325**: 961-962.

Rossaint R, Falke KJ, Lopez F, Slarra K, Pison U & Zapol WM (1993) Inhaled nitric oxide for the adult respiratory distress syndrome. *New England Journal of Medicine* **328**: 399-405.

Selsby D & Jones JG (1990) Some physiological and clinical aspects of chest physiotherapy. *British Journal of Anaesthesia* **64**: 621-631.

Shenfield GM, Hodson ME, Clarke SW & Paterson JW (1975) Interaction of corticosteroids and catecholamines in the treatment of asthma. *Thorax* **30**: 430-435.

Sibbald WJ & Prewitt RM (1983) Right ventricular function. *Critical Care Medicine* **11**: 321-322.

Sibbald WJ, Anderson RR, Reid B, Holliday RL & Driedger AA (1981) Alveolar-capillary permeability in human septic ARDS. Effect of high-dose corticosteroid therapy. *Chest* **79**: 133-142.

Silverman JH, Slotman G, Bone RC et al. & The Prostaglandin E$_1$ Study Group (1990) Effects of prostaglandin E$_1$ on oxygen delivery and consumption in patients with the adult respiratory distress syndrome. *Chest* **98**: 405-410.

Sim KM & Evans TW (1993) Supporting the injured lung. *British Medical Journal* **307**: 1293-1294.

Similouski T, Yan S, Gauthier AP, Macklem PT & Bellemare F (1991) Contractile properties of the human diaphragm during chronic hyperinflation. *New England Journal of Medicine* **325**: 917-923.

Singer MM, Wright F, Stanley LK, Roe BB & Hamilton WK (1970) Oxygen toxicity in man. A prospective study in patients after open-heart surgery. *New England Journal of Medicine* **283**: 1473-1478.

Skatrud JB & Dempsey JA (1983) Relative effectiveness of acetazolamide versus medoxyprogesterone acetate in correction of chronic carbon dioxide retention. *American Review of Respiratory Disease* **127**: 405-412.

Snapper JR (1981) Septic pulmonary edema. *Seminars in Respiratory Medicine* **3**: 92-96.

Suchyta MR, Clemmer TP, Orme JF Jr, Morris AH & Elliott CG (1991) Increased survival of ARDS patients with severe hypoxemia (ECMO criteria). *Chest* **99**: 951-955.

Sznajder JI, Fraiman A, Hall JB et al. (1989) Increased hydrogen peroxide in the expired breath of patients with acute hypoxemic respiratory failure. *Chest* **96**: 606-612.

Tisi GM (1979) Pre-operative evaluation of pulmonary function. Validity, indications and benefits. *American Review of Respiratory Disease* **119**: 293-310.

Tuxen DV (1989) Detrimental effects of positive end-expiratory pressure during controlled mechanical ventilation of patients with severe airflow obstruction. *American Review of Respiratory Disease* **140**: 5-9.

Tuxen DV & Lane S (1987) The effects of ventilatory pattern on hyperinflation, airway pressures and circulation in mechanical ventilation of patients with severe air-flow obstruction. *American Review of Respiratory Disease* **136**: 872-879.

Villar J & Slutsky AS (1989) The incidence of the Adult Respiratory Distress Syndrome. *American Review of Respiratory Disease* **140**: 814-816.

Walmrath D, Schneider T, Pilch J, Grimminger F & Seeger W (1993) Aerosolised prostacyclin in adult respiratory distress syndrome. *Lancet* **342**: 961-962.

Webster NR, Cohen AT & Nunn JF (1988) Adult respiratory distress syndrome—how many cases in the UK? *Anaesthesia* **43**: 923-926.

Weg JG, Balk RA, Tharratt S, Jenkinson SG, Shah JB, Zaccardelli D, Horton J & Pattishall EN (1994) Safety and potential efficacy of an aerosolized surfactant in human sepsis-induced adult respiratory distress syndrome. *Journal of the American Medical Association* **272**: 1433-1438.

Wewers MD, Herzyk DJ & Gadek JE (1988) Alveolar fluid neutrophil elastase activity in the adult respiratory distress syndrome is complexed to alpha-2-macroglobulin. *Journal of Clinical Investigation* **82**: 1260-1267.

Wiener-Kronish JP, Gropper MA & Matthay MA (1990) The adult respiratory distress syndrome: definition and prognosis, pathogenesis and treatment. *British Journal of Anaesthesia* **65**: 107-129.

Williams MH (1989) Increasing severity of asthma from 1960 to 1987. *New England Journal Medicine* **320**: 1015-1016.

Williams S & Seaton A (1977) Intravenous or inhaled salbutamol in severe acute asthma? *Thorax* **32**: 555-558.

Wright PE & Bernard GR (1989) The role of airflow resistance in patients with the adult respiratory distress syndrome. *American Review of Respiratory Disease* **139**: 1169-1174.

Wynne JW, DeMarco FJ & Hood CI (1981) Physiological effects of corticosteroids in foodstuff aspiration. *Archives of Surgery* **116**: 46-49.

Zapol WM & Snider MT (1977) Pulmonary hypertension in severe acute respiratory failure. *New England Journal of Medicine* **296**: 476-480.

7 Respiratory Support

Although orotracheal intubation was first used to facilitate anaesthesia by MacEwen, a Glasgow surgeon, as long ago as 1878, it only became a routine procedure following the work of Magill, Rowbotham and others in the 1920s. Using endotracheal intubation, anaesthetists were able to control their patient's ventilation and, in the 1940s, neuromuscular blockade with intermittent positive pressure ventilation (IPPV), usually performed manually, became a standard anaesthetic technique. Nevertheless, mechanical ventilation for therapeutic purposes was initially performed using negative pressure devices. Not only were morbidity and mortality high with this technique, but it was much less successful in those with abnormal lungs. It was therefore used infrequently except in the treatment of ventilatory failure due to poliomyelitis; when polio became a rare disease, its use declined further. During the polio epidemic in Copenhagen in 1952 the advantages of positive pressure ventilation had been clearly demonstrated (Lassen, 1953) and in 1955 the use of IPPV for the treatment of acute exacerbations of chronic obstructive pulmonary disease (COPD) was described (Bjorneboe et al., 1955). Subsequently, clinicians increasingly accepted that IPPV could be used to treat patients with a variety of diseases affecting the lung parenchyma, as well as those with neuromuscular problems.

The various techniques of respiratory support currently available are shown in **Table 7.1**.

NEGATIVE PRESSURE VENTILATION

'Tank' ventilators ('iron lungs')

At one time, 'tank' ventilators (**Fig. 7.1**) were widely used for the treatment of ventilatory failure complicating polio. They are still occasionally used for nocturnal ventilation of patients with chronic respiratory failure due to neuromuscular disease, skeletal deformity or sleep-related respiratory disturbances since they avoid the complications and constraints of a permanent tracheostomy.

The patient's body is enclosed in an airtight 'tank' within which a negative pressure is created intermittently by a separate pump. During the negative pressure phase, the patient's thorax expands, drawing air into the lungs. Expiration then occurs passively. Although patients who are conscious can speak and swallow in time with the ventilator, this technique has a number of disadvantages. Firstly, the ventilator itself is very bulky and access to the patient is restricted, making it difficult to perform nursing and medical procedures. Secondly, the patient's airway is unprotected and there is no route for endotracheal suction. This technique is therefore only suitable for those with competent swallowing, laryngeal and cough reflexes, and even under

Table 7.1 Techniques for respiratory support.

Negative pressure ventilation	Tank ventilators Cuirass ventilators
Intermittent positive pressure ventilation (IPPV)	ZEEP NEEP PEEP (CPPV)
Intermittent mandatory ventilation (IMV) **Mandatory minute volume** (MMV)	ZEEP PEEP
Continuous positive airway pressure (CPAP)	Endotracheal tube Mask
Pressure limited ventilation	Inverse ratio 'Permissive hypercarbia'
Pressure support ventilation	
Assisted mechanical ventilation (AMV)	
Independent lung ventilation	
High-frequency jet ventilation (HFJV)	
Extracorporeal techniques	ECMO ECCO$_2$-R

ZEEP, zero end-expiratory pressure; NEEP, negative end-expiratory pressure; PEEP, positive end-expiratory pressure; CPPV, continuous positive pressure ventilation; ECMO, extracorporeal membrane oxygenation; ECCO$_2$-R, extracorporeal CO$_2$ removal

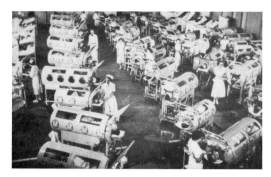

Fig. 7.1 'Tank' ventilators in use during an epidemic of poliomyelitis.

these circumstances pulmonary aspiration can be a problem. Lastly, because the negative pressure is applied to the whole body, the normal inspiratory pressure gradient is lost, venous return is reduced and cardiac output may fall.

Cuirass ventilators

Cuirass ventilators, which encase only the thorax, were originally most frequently used during the recovery phase of poliomyelitis. They are inefficient and difficult to use, a particular problem being the creation of an airtight seal around the lower thorax and abdomen, especially in those with musculoskeletal deformity. Skin chafing may therefore be a problem. Nevertheless, such devices can be useful in those with borderline respiratory function when used to assist ventilation, particularly during sleep. The *Tunnicliffe jacket* or its alternative, the *'pneumosuit'*, is a more efficient alternative.

Rocking beds

Rocking beds can be used for those patients with neuromuscular disease whose respiratory reserve is limited, but who only develop significant hypercapnia when they fall asleep. The rocking motion of the bed causes the abdominal contents to push the diaphragm in and out of the thorax, thereby assisting tidal exchange.

POSITIVE PRESSURE VENTILATION

Adequate pulmonary gas exchange can be achieved by intermittently inflating the lungs with a positive pressure applied via an endotracheal tube or a tracheostomy. As mentioned above, IPPV has a number of important advantages over negative pressure ventilation. In particular:

- the airway is secured and protected;
- secretions can be aspirated more easily;
- it can be used more successfully in those with diseases involving the lung parenchyma;
- access to and movement of the patient is relatively unrestricted.

IPPV has therefore largely superseded the use of negative pressure devices in clinical practice.

In recent years, a number of refinements and modifications of IPPV have been described, and will be discussed later in this chapter. They include:

- synchronized intermittent mandatory ventilation (SIMV);
- mandatory minute volume (MMV);
- IPPV with positive end-expiratory pressure (PEEP) (sometimes known as continuous positive pressure ventilation, CPPV);
- pressure support ventilation;
- pressure-limited ventilation (sometimes with 'permissive hypercarbia' and/or an inverse ratio);
- airway pressure release ventilation.

Classification of positive pressure ventilators

A mechanical ventilator has to perform four operations during each respiratory cycle:

- Inflate the lungs.
- Cycle from inspiration to expiration.
- Allow expiration to take place.
- Cycle from expiration to inspiration.

Mechanical ventilators can therefore be classified according to the method used to inflate the lungs (the 'driving mechanism') and the means by which they change from one phase of the respiratory cycle to the other ('cycling') (**Table 7.2**).

PRESSURE PRE-SET VENTILATION

Either a pre-set pressure is generated or cycling from inspiration to expiration occurs when a designated airway pressure is reached. The magnitude and shape of the inspiratory pressure wave-form produced is therefore uninfluenced by changes in lung mechanics, whereas the pattern of flow during inflation depends on the interaction between the generated pressure pattern and the mechanical properties of the lung and chest wall. Therefore, if pulmonary compliance falls or resistance increases, there will be a reduction in the delivered tidal volume (V_T) unless the operator increases the inflation pressure. Pressure pre-set ventilation compensates for small leaks in the circuit.

Table 7.2 Classification of mechanical ventilators according to the driving mechanism and mode of cycling.

Driving mechanism	Pressure generator
	Flow generator
	Both

Mode of cycling	*Expiration to inspiration*
	Time
	Volume
	Pressure
	Flow
	Mixed
	Other
	Patient triggered (assist)
	Inspiration to expiration
	Time
	Volume
	Pressure
	Flow
	Mixed
	Other

VOLUME PRE-SET VENTILATION

A fixed V_T is delivered to the ventilator circuit regardless of alterations in lung mechanics; if, for example, the lungs become stiffer, there will be a compensatory increase in inflation pressure and there will be only a small reduction in V_T due to the increased volume of gas compressed within the ventilator circuit. This type of ventilation does not compensate for leaks in the circuit.

MINUTE VOLUME DIVIDERS

In addition to being classified as outlined above, some ventilators can be considered as minute volume dividers. With these devices the minute volume depends on the total flow delivered by the gas source, while the ventilation rate is determined by the preset V_T and inflation pressure.

CYCLING

The change from inspiration to expiration is usually time-cycled, while inspiration is nearly always time-cycled and/or patient-triggered. A few ventilators have been designed that are volume-cycled from inspiration to expiration and others are pressure-cycled or flow-cycled. Most sophisticated modern electronic ventilators are time-cycled flow generators.

With volume-cycled ventilators the inspiration : ex-

piration (I : E) ratio is indirectly determined by regulating V_T, frequency and inspiratory flow rate. Direct adjustment of the I : E ratio is possible with some time-cycled ventilators.

Selecting positive pressure ventilators for use in the intensive care unit

A large number of positive pressure ventilators are now available, many of which are very sophisticated and, consequently, extremely expensive. *Cost* and *'user-friendliness'* are therefore important considerations.

There is some advantage in restricting the number of different types of ventilator available on a particular unit since familiarity with the equipment generates confidence and reduces the incidence of mishaps. The provision of *comprehensive monitoring, a high-pressure relief valve* and *suitable alarms* are other important aspects of safety. The alarms should be activated in the event of disconnection or obstruction and if the gas or power supply fails, although the ventilator should in any case continue to function in either of these latter eventualities.

The danger of cross-infection can be minimized by using *autoclavable patient circuits* and these are now an essential feature of ventilators intended for use in an intensive care unit. Some ventilators also incorporate *heated bacterial filters* on both the inspiratory and expiratory limbs of the circuit, although the value of these is uncertain. It should be possible to provide safe, effective *humidification* and to *nebulize* drugs.

It should also be possible to produce *optimal patterns of ventilation* for all clinical circumstances and age groups. The ability to adjust the duration of both the inspiratory and expiratory phases, as well as the ratio of one to the other, and the inspiratory flow rate are fundamental requirements. The ventilator should deliver an accurate stable *inspired oxygen concentration (F_IO_2)* from 30 to 100%. In addition, it should be possible to *apply PEEP* (see later).

Sophisticated ventilators should have facilities for *SIMV* both with and without PEEP. Other features that are often incorporated, but not of proven benefit, include *sigh functions* and a *selection of inspiratory wave forms*. Ventilators should be *robust, reliable* and *easy to maintain*.

These criteria are adequately fulfilled by most modern electronic ventilators. With the increasing use of SIMV as a routine mode of ventilation, one of the most important considerations when selecting a ventilator is that it should allow spontaneous respiration without a significant increase in the work of breathing (Cox & Niblett, 1984).

Humidification

Inspired gas is normally warmed, filtered and moistened during its passage through the upper airways, a process which is prevented by endotracheal intubation and tracheostomy. Exposing the lungs and airways to dry cold gas has a number of adverse effects including:

- an increase in mucus viscosity;
- depressed ciliary activity;
- obstruction of the airways by tenacious secretions.

Artificial humidification of inspired gases is therefore essential when the upper respiratory tract is bypassed.

Humidifiers should be simple to use and service. Their performance should be unaffected by variations in gas flow and they must ensure that gas delivered to the trachea is at a temperature of 32–36°C with a water content of 33–43 g/m^3. The temperature of the humidifier should be constantly controlled at the set value and the humidifier should incorporate alarms and safety mechanisms to prevent overheating, overhydration and electrocution. Ideally humidifiers should be suitable for use during spontaneous as well as controlled ventilation and therefore their dead space, resistance and compliance should all be as low as possible.

CONDENSER HUMIDIFIERS, HEAT AND MOISTURE EXCHANGERS, 'SWEDISH NOSE'

These small, lightweight devices contain various hygroscopic materials and chemicals arranged as pleated or corrugated sheets or sponges. When placed in the breathing circuit close to the airway they retain by condensation the heat and moisture in expired gas. Inspired gas is then warmed and humidified as it passes through the filter. These devices provide up to 30 mg H_2O/l of ventilation at 27–30°C and are suitable for most patients undergoing long-term ventilation, although a heated humidifier may be preferred for those with viscid secretions. Many heat and moisture exchangers (HMEs) also act as efficient bacterial filters, avoiding the need to sterilize breathing systems or decontaminate ventilators, and they offer substantial advantages as regards cost, ease of use and patient safety (Gallagher *et al.*, 1987).

COLD WATER BUBBLE HUMIDIFIERS

Cold water bubble humidifiers are inefficient and there is a risk of bacterial contamination. They are often used to humidify supplemental oxygen administered via a face mask, although some consider that humidification is usually unnecessary under these circumstances.

WARM WATER BATH

The fresh gas is passed over or through a water reservoir heated to 45–60°C so that it leaves the humidifier with a water content of more than 43 g/m^3. Although at this stage it is not fully saturated, cooling in the ventilator tubing causes the relative humidity to approach 100%. The heater is thermostatically controlled to ensure that the temperature of the fully saturated inspired gas is close to 37°C. These devices are efficient, but have the following disadvantages.

- They cause condensation in the ventilator tubing. Water traps are therefore required, although condensation can be minimized by lagging or heating the tubing.
- There is a risk of infection from bacteria, especially *Pseudomonas*, contaminating the water reservoir. They multiply rapidly at 45°C, but infection can be controlled by operating the device at 60°C or by adding 0.02% chlorhexidine gluconate.
- If the thermostat fails and the temperature of the inspired gas exceeds 41°C, damage to the tracheal mucosa is likely. Close observation is therefore essential.
- Their performance depends on the fresh gas flow, the water temperature and the surface area available for vaporization.

NEBULIZERS

Nebulizers produce an aerosol of variously sized microdroplets suspended in the inspired gas. Droplets smaller than 1 μm are thought to reach the alveoli, those of about 5 μm are deposited in the bronchi and larger particles of 7–10 μm are deposited in the nose or oropharynx.

Ultrasonic nebulizers are the most efficient and can produce supersaturation of inspired gas with the risk of overhydration, especially in children. There is a danger of bacterial contamination and infection with these devices. Sterile water should be used to fill the reservoir and the nebulizer should be replaced and sterilized daily. Nebulizers are now rarely used in clinical practice.

BENEFICIAL EFFECTS OF IPPV

Improved carbon dioxide elimination

Using mechanical ventilation, the carbon dioxide that accumulates in some patients with respiratory failure can be removed and the arterial carbon dioxide tension ($P_a co_2$) returned to within normal limits. Because of the operation of the alveolar air equation (see Chapter 2), the reduction in alveolar carbon dioxide tension ($P_A CO_2$) inevitably leads to a rise in alveolar oxygen tension ($P_A O_2$) and improved arterial oxygenation. By adjusting the delivered minute volume, it is possible to compensate for changes in the patient's dead space (V_D) and/or carbon dioxide production. Under certain circumstances, improved distribution of inspired gases may lead to a fall in V_D and further benefit may accrue from abolishing the work of breathing, thereby reducing carbon dioxide production.

Improved oxygenation

The percentage of venous admixture, whether due to alveolar collapse or ventilation/perfusion (V/Q) mismatch generally falls slightly when IPPV is instituted, but this effect is variable and therefore usually of only marginal benefit. Indeed, prolonged mechanical ventilation with small tidal volumes may be associated with an increase in venous admixture and a deterioration in lung function (see later). More importantly, mechanical ventilation decreases or abolishes the work of breathing, relieves exhaustion and rests the respiratory muscles. In those with severe pulmonary parenchymal disease, the lungs may be very stiff and the work of breathing is therefore greatly increased; institution of artificial ventilation may then significantly reduce oxygen consumption ($\dot{V}O_2$). This reduction in oxygen requirements allows mixed venous oxygen tension ($P_v O_2$), and consequently arterial oxygen tension ($P_a O_2$), to rise. Finally, because ventilated patients are connected to a leak-free circuit it is possible to administer high concentrations of oxygen (up to 100%) accurately, and to apply PEEP. In selected patients, the latter may reduce shunt and increase $P_a O_2$ (see later).

INDICATIONS FOR MECHANICAL VENTILATION

Respiratory failure

Mechanical ventilation is most clearly indicated in the treatment of patients with severe respiratory failure who fail to respond to conventional medical treatment (see Chapter 6), including those with left ventricular failure.

Prophylactic mechanical ventilation

Mechanical ventilation can also be used to prevent a deterioration to respiratory failure in susceptible patients. For example, prophylactic *postoperative ventilation* is now a well-established practice in poor-risk patients in whom some degree of respiratory failure might otherwise be anticipated. Ventilatory support may also be used prophylactically in patients with *neuromuscular or skeletal abnormalities*. In these patients, a fall in vital capacity (VC) impairs the ability to cough, sigh and take deep breaths; consequently, retention of secretions and progressive alveolar collapse eventually lead to respiratory failure, often in association with secondary infection. This sequence of events can be prevented by instituting IPPV when the VC has fallen to approximately one-quarter of the predicted value (see Chapter 6).

Mechanical ventilation may also be instituted to prevent deterioration in those with *severe thoracic or upper abdominal injuries*, especially when associated with a *head injury* (see Chapters 9 and 14).

By no means all patients with respiratory failure and/or a reduced VC require ventilation, however, and clinical assessment of each individual case is of paramount importance. Factors such as the patient's general condition, degree of exhaustion and level of consciousness are at least as important as blood gas values.

Raised intracranial pressure, cerebral ischaemia, cerebrovascular accident

In patients with intracranial hypertension (e.g. following severe head injury), it is most important to avoid hypercarbia and/or hypoxia, since both will increase intracranial blood volume and exacerbate cerebral oedema. Furthermore, elective hyperventilation, even in those not in respiratory failure, can temporarily decrease cerebral blood flow and, secondarily, intracranial pressure, although the value of such treatment remains uncertain (see Chapter 14). Mechanical ventilation may also be indicated in some patients following an episode of cerebral ischaemia (see Chapter 8) or a cerebrovascular accident.

DANGERS OF MECHANICAL VENTILATION (Table 7.3)

General

Mechanically ventilated patients are exposed to the dangers and complications inherent in *endotracheal intubation or tracheostomy* (see below). In addition, *disconnection* from the ventilator is an ever-present danger. *Failure of gas or power supplies* and *mechanical faults* are unusual, but equally dangerous, and a suitable means of manually ventilating the patient with oxygen must always be available by the bedside.

Table 7.3 Dangers of intermittent positive pressure ventilation.

General	Endotracheal intubation/ tracheostomy Disconnection Failure of gas or power supply Mechanical faults
Cardiovascular depression	
Ileus	
Hepatic dysfunction	
Water retention	
Respiratory changes and ventilator-induced lung injury	Maldistribution of inspired gases Collapse of distal lung units Decreased surfactant activity Damage to alveolar/capillary membrane Barotrauma Bronchopulmonary dysplasia Bronchiolectasis Nosocomial pneumonia

Cardiovascular

The application of positive pressure to the lungs and thoracic wall *reduces venous return* and distends alveoli, thereby 'stretching' the pulmonary capillaries and causing a *rise in pulmonary vascular resistance*. Both these mechanisms can produce a *fall in cardiac output* in patients on IPPV. It has been suggested that this may be exacerbated by reflex mechanisms, impaired coronary perfusion and reductions in P_{CO_2} (Editorial, 1981).

In *normal subjects*, the fall in cardiac output is limited by constriction of capacitance vessels, which restores venous return. *Hypovolaemia, pre-existing pulmonary hypertension, right ventricular failure* and *autonomic dysfunction* (e.g. in Guillain–Barré syndrome, acute spinal cord injury and diabetes) will exacerbate the haemodynamic disturbance. Expansion of the circulating volume, on the other hand, can often restore cardiac output. In some cases, inotropic support is required in addition to volume expansion.

In patients with *heart failure*, a paradoxical rise in blood pressure and cardiac output may occur in response to both IPPV and IPPV with PEEP. This may be due to reversal of hypoxia and a reduction in $\dot{V}_{O_2}$, both of which will reduce the burden on a failing heart. Moreover, after-load falls as a result of the increased pressure gradient between the intra- and extrathoracic vascular beds and this is associated with an increase in

stroke volume. The reduction in after-load and pre-load reduces ventricular wall tension, allowing increased coronary blood flow and improved myocardial function. Finally, when the ventricular function curve is flat, the reduction in pre-load has little effect on stroke volume, while stiff lungs limit the transmission of high inflation pressures to the great veins and pulmonary capillaries. One should therefore not hesitate to institute IPPV in patients with cardiogenic pulmonary oedema who have severe respiratory distress and exhaustion (see also Chapter 6).

Respiratory changes and ventilator-induced lung injury (Parker *et al.*, 1993)

During spontaneous breathing, ventilation is preferentially distributed to the lower lung zones and is matched by a similar pattern of blood flow (see Chapter 2). During IPPV, however, there is *maldistribution of inspired gas*, with ventilation being more evenly distributed throughout the lungs, leading to an increase in the overall V/Q ratio. This effect is enhanced when high intra-alveolar pressure (high inflation pressures, PEEP) and/or a reduced pulmonary artery pressure (PAP) divert blood flow away from apical lung zones. IPPV therefore normally increases V_D/V_T, but this effect is variable and usually of little clinical significance. Patients ventilated with small tidal volumes become progressively more hypoxic, with a reduction in functional residual capacity (FRC) and compliance. This is probably due to *collapse of distal lung units* and can be largely prevented by using greater tidal volumes (10–15 ml/kg) and reducing the respiratory rate to avoid hypocarbia, or by the application of PEEP. Some ventilators incorporate a 'sigh' mechanism, which regularly hyperinflates the lungs in an attempt to re-expand distal lung segments and prevent hypoxia. The benefits of 'sigh functions' have not, however, been established and they may damage the lung parenchyma.

There is evidence that *high peak inspiratory pressures* (e.g. > 50 cm H_2O), or perhaps more importantly plateau pressures with *overdistension* of compliant alveoli may lead to progressive impairment of pulmonary mechanics and lung function associated with reduced surfactant activity (Kolobow *et al.*, 1987). Oedema formation is probably enhanced by an increase in both microvascular permeability and the filtration pressure across the pulmonary vasculature (due to the rise in PAP), especially when the inspiratory phase is prolonged or as PEEP is applied. High airway pressures and overdistension may also disrupt the alveolar epithelium, lowering the threshold for alveolar flooding. This damage to the alveolar-capillary membrane seems to be related to both circumferential stress (vascular pressures) and longitudinal stress (lung volume). Large tidal volumes and overdistension ('volutrauma') are probably more important than high inflation pressures. On the other hand, lung injury may be exacerbated if lung volume, which is largely dependent on mean airway pressure and PEEP, is allowed to fall below a critical point (Dreyfuss *et al.*, 1988).

BAROTRAUMA

Overdistension of the lungs may also be associated with alveolar rupture, causing air to dissect centrally along the perivascular sheaths. This *pulmonary interstitial air* is difficult to detect, but can sometimes be seen on a good quality chest radiograph as linear or circular perivascular collections or, most specifically, subpleural blebs (Rohfling *et al.*, 1976). In some cases, this progresses to produce pneumomediastinum, pneumoperitoneum, air in the retroperitoneal space, subcutaneous emphysema and pneumothorax (when gas under pressure in the pulmonary ligament penetrates the thin visceral pleura or a subpleural bleb ruptures) (**Fig. 7.2**). Each of these may occur in isolation or in combination with any of the others. Pneumomediastinum, pneumoperitoneum and subcutaneous emphysema can all precede the appearance of a pneumothorax and their presence should alert the clinician to an increased risk of this complication. Intra-abdominal air originating in the lungs is probably always associated with pneumomediastinum; this can help distinguish pneumoperitoneum due to barotrauma from a ruptured viscus. In infants and neonates, air may rupture into the pericardial space, causing cardiac tamponade.

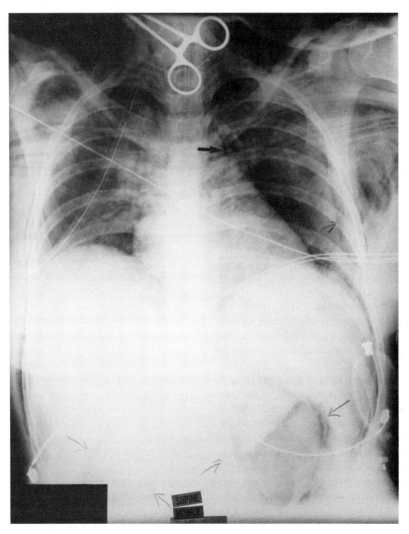

Fig. 7.2 Pulmonary barotrauma. Note subcutaneous air, left pneumothorax, right pleural drain, pneumomediastinum (air outlining aortic arch) and retroperitoneal air outlining left and right kidneys. (Courtesy of Dr KM Hillman.)

The incidence of barotrauma is greatest in those patients who require high inflation pressures, with or without PEEP (**Fig. 7.3**), and the risk of pneumothorax is increased in those with destructive lung disease (e.g. necrotizing pneumonia, acid aspiration, emphysema, asthma or fractured ribs) (**Fig. 7.4**). Barotrauma may also be the result of endotracheal tube obstruction, intubation of a main bronchus or overvigorous manual ventilation.

PNEUMOTHORAX

Because a life-threatening *tension pneumothorax* (see **Fig. 7.4**) can develop extremely quickly in mechanically ventilated patients and may be rapidly fatal, facilities for chest drain insertion should be immediately available at the bedside of all such high-risk cases. In addition, intensive care personnel must always be alert to the possibility of this complication. Suggestive signs include:

- the sudden development or worsening, of hypoxia;
- cyanosis;
- fighting the ventilator;
- an unexplained increase in inflation pressure;
- hypotension and tachycardia;
- a rising CVP.

Examination may reveal reduced expansion on one side of the chest, mediastinal shift (deviated trachea, displaced apex beat) and hyperresonance of one hemithorax. Although breath sounds are traditionally diminished over the pneumothorax, this sign can be extremely misleading in ventilated patients. If there is time, the diagnosis can be confirmed by chest radiography.

Treatment. In an extreme emergency, the tension can be relieved by inserting a large-bore intravenous cannula anteriorly through the second intercostal space in the midclavicular line. Otherwise a chest drain should be inserted.

For *chest drain insertion* (**Fig. 7.5**) some recommend the second or third intercostal space in the midclavicular line as the safest site for emergency insertion of chest drains by the inexperienced. Generally, however, it is preferable to place the drain through the sixth or seventh intercostal space in the mid-axillary line. In this position both fluid and air can be removed, and it is cosmetically more acceptable. The drain should not be inserted posteriorly since in this position it is very uncomfortable and easily kinked. If the patient is conscious, the procedure should be explained and, when possible, consent should be obtained. Additional sedation and analgesia may be required.

Technique

- The patient is positioned supine, with the affected side slightly elevated and the arm flexed over the head.
- The chest wall is prepared and draped as a sterile field; a gown, mask and gloves should be worn if time allows.
- Chest drain insertion can be a very painful procedure and generous amounts of local anaesthetic should be used (20 ml 1% lignocaine).
- A skin incision should be made over the proposed site of insertion.
- A 'purse string' suture should be placed around, and a retaining suture adjacent to this incision.
- The pleural space should be entered using blunt dissection with, for example, a large artery clip close to the top of the rib to avoid the neurovascular bundle on the underside of the rib above.
- The chest drain (with introducer tip withdrawn) is then guided into position with an index finger, which has gently explored the pleural space.
- The chest tube is passed up to the apex of the chest wall to drain a pneumothorax, while the lowest side hole is positioned only 1–2 cm into the chest to drain fluid.
- The drain is then secured with the retaining suture and connected to the underwater seal.
- A sterile dressing is applied and the tubing taped to the skin.
- A chest radiograph is obtained to check the position of the drain and the adequacy of drainage.
- When the drain is removed, the purse string suture is pulled tight to close the wound.

An air leak that persists for more than 24 hours following insertion of a chest drain suggests the development of a *bronchopleural fistula*. This will be associated with loss of V_T and PEEP, as well as failure of lung re-expansion and a risk of pleural infection. Management involves reducing or discontinuing mechanical ventilation and PEEP (e.g. by using SIMV). Independent lung ventilation or high-frequency ventilation may be useful (see later). The presence of a persistent bronchopleural fistula is an ominous sign with a mortality rate of about 60–70%.

Bronchopulmonary dysplasia

In neonates with respiratory distress syndrome, pulmonary interstitial air is a harbinger of bronchopulmonary dysplasia in which individual small areas of emphysema distend and compromise the expansion of remaining areas of lung. In those who survive, the lung damage persists with interstitial fibrosis, microscopic emphys-

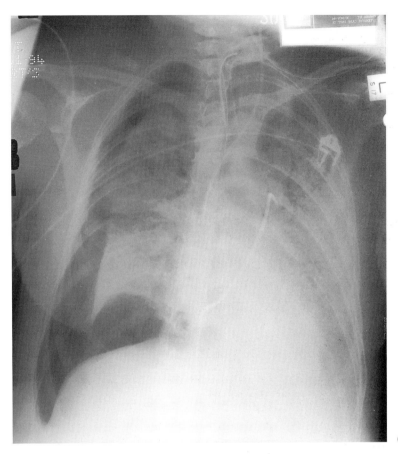

(a)

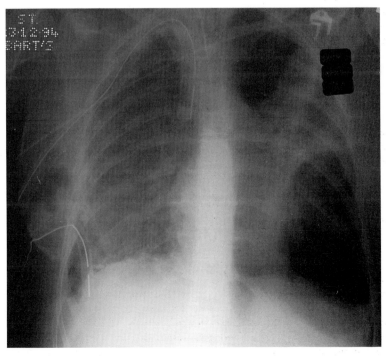

(b)

Fig. 7.3 (a) and (b) Recurrent pneumo-thoraces in a patient with adult respiratory distress syndrome.

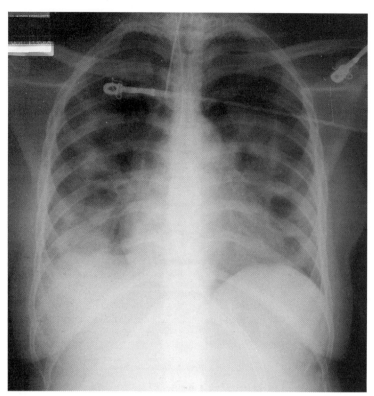

(a)

Fig. 7.4 (a) Bilateral consolidation with multiple cavities. (b) The same patient has developed a right tension pneumothorax, displacing the right hemidiaphragm inferiorly and the mediastinum to the left.

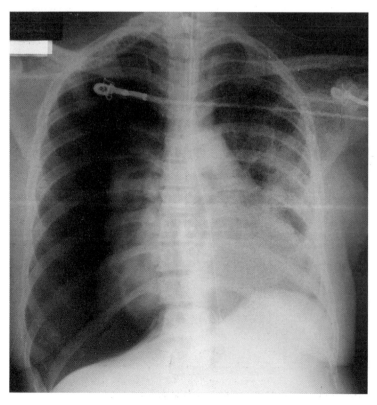

(b)

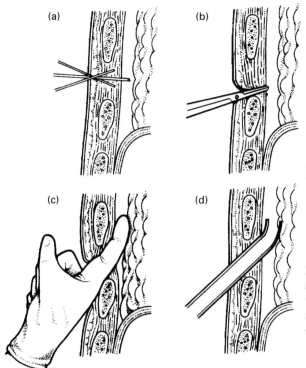

(a)   (b)

(c)   (d)

Fig. 7.5 Chest drain insertion. (a) Infiltration of skin, muscle and periosteum of upper border of rib below with local anaesthetic. Pleura may be punctured with needle. (b) Blunt dissection. (c) Digital exploration of pleural cavity. (d) Chest drain, with introducer withdrawn, guided into position.

ema and mucosal destruction. This gradually recovers over the next few years and pulmonary function is usually clinically normal by the time the child reaches school age. The aetiology of bronchopulmonary dysplasia is unknown, but as well as increased airway pressures, high F_1O_2 levels are thought to contribute to its development.

Bronchiolectasis

Bronchiolectasis is the term that has been applied to the pronounced dilatation of terminal and respiratory bronchioles that has been described in adults who die following a period of positive pressure ventilation with sustained high levels of PEEP (Slavin *et al.*, 1982). These changes were associated with an increased V_D/V_T ratio. The authors felt that oxygen toxicity was unlikely to be important in the pathogenesis of the lung lesions, and a subsequent study suggests that the changes are reversible in those who survive (Navaratnarajah *et al.*, 1984).

NOSOCOMIAL PNEUMONIA

Pulmonary infection is a common complication of mechanical ventilation, being present in about 28% of patients ventilated for 30 days (Fagon *et al.*, 1989) and is associated with a significantly worse prognosis (Fagon *et al.*, 1989; Torres *et al.*, 1990). Risk factors include intubation on more than one occasion, previous aspiration of gastric contents, ventilation for more than three days, the presence of COPD and the use of PEEP (Torres *et al.*, 1990). This topic is discussed further in Chapter 11.

Gastrointestinal

Initially, many artificially ventilated patients will develop an *ileus* and abdominal distension. The cause is unknown, although the use of non-depolarizing neuromuscular blocking agents and the administration of opiates may be partly responsible.

Hepatic dysfunction

Hepatic dysfunction is usually related to the underlying disease, but the reduction in splanchnic flow combined with the effects of raised intra-abdominal pressure on portal vein pressure, hepatic venous flow and biliary drainage may contribute to liver impairment.

Water retention

Positive pressure ventilation, particularly with PEEP, is associated with a reduction in renal blood flow, glomerular filtration rate, urinary output and sodium excretion. These changes are probably largely related to the reduction in cardiac output and systemic blood pressure combined with increased sympathetic activity and renin release (Payen *et al.*, 1987). The role of increased antidiuretic hormone levels and decreased release of atrial natriuretic peptide in ventilation-induced salt and water retention is unclear (Leithner *et al.*, 1987; Payen *et al.*, 1987; Teba *et al.*, 1990).

For reasons outlined above, this fluid retention is often particularly noticeable in the lungs, and may cause a deterioration in pulmonary function. It is therefore advisable to restrict the total amount of salt and water administered to ventilated patients; approximately 20 ml/kg/day of 5% dextrose or dextrose saline intravenously is usual in the first instance.

INSTITUTION OF INTERMITTENT POSITIVE PRESSURE VENTILATION

Intubating patients in severe respiratory failure is potentially dangerous and should only be performed by experienced staff. The patient is usually hypoxic and may be hypercarbic, with increased sympathetic activity, and the oxygen mask has to be removed to allow intubation, although nasal cannulae can be left *in situ*. Under these circumstances, the stimulus of laryngoscopy followed by intubation can precipitate dangerous arrhythmias and even cardiac arrest.

Except in an extreme emergency, therefore, the *ECG and oxygen saturation should be monitored throughout*. Many patients are hypotensive and most are hypovolaemic. If time allows the *circulating volume should be optimized* and, if necessary, *inotropes* commenced before attempting intubation. In some cases it may be appropriate to establish *intra-arterial and central venous pressure monitoring* before instituting mechanical ventilation, although many patients will not tolerate the supine or head-down position. Occasionally a *pulmonary artery catheter* may be required.

The patient should be *pre-oxygenated* or *ventilated* with added *oxygen* using a face mask and a self-inflating bag before laryngoscopy. In some deeply comatose patients, no sedation will be required, although when there is a possibility of intracranial hypertension, an *intravenous anaesthetic agent* should be administered to prevent surges in intracranial pressure. In the majority of patients, a short-acting intravenous anaesthetic agent followed by *muscle relaxation* will be necessary. In those at risk of regurgitation and aspiration of stomach contents, pre-oxygenation should be followed by administration of an intravenous anaesthetic agent and a rapidly acting muscle relaxant (usually suxamethonium). *Cricoid pressure* should be applied as soon as the patient loses consciousness and should not be released until the endotracheal tube is in place with the cuff inflated. It must be remembered that there is a risk of precipitating dangerous hyperkalaemia when suxamethonium is used in those with burns, renal failure, spinal injury or neuromuscular disease. Some institutions favour *awake intubation*.

Following endotracheal intubation, it is important to avoid the temptation to hyperventilate the patient, since this can lead to overinflation of the lungs and a fall in cardiac output, particularly in those with airway obstruction.

MANAGEMENT OF PATIENTS ON VENTILATORS

General

Because the upper respiratory tract has been bypassed, the inspired gases must be artificially warmed, humidified and filtered. Patients on ventilators are unable to cough, sigh or take deep breaths and therefore regular physiotherapy, manual hyperinflation of the lungs and endotracheal suction are normally employed. (For further discussion of the general aspects of managing these patients, see Chapters 6 and 10.)

Settling the patient on the ventilator

It is most important that patients receiving controlled mechanical ventilation (CMV) do not 'fight the ventilator.' Not only does this increase $\dot{V}o_2$ and carbon dioxide production, but the rise in mean intrathoracic pressure can reduce cardiac output. It is also distressing for the patient, relatives and staff.

Frequent explanation, reassurance and encouragement are essential for all alert patients. Manual hyperventilation with 100% oxygen will often assist initial synchronization with the ventilator by ensuring adequate oxygenation and a degree of hypocarbia. Most ventilated patients will require sedation. In the majority, the drug of first choice is a *parenteral narcotic*, which also provides analgesia and some respiratory depression. Many patients will also need an anxiolytic agent and usually a *benzodiazepine* is administered in combination with the opiate (see Chapter 10). In most cases—provided large tidal volumes are used, the P_aO_2 is within normal limits, there is moderate hypocarbia and sedation/analgesia is adequate—the patient will not fight the ventilator. If, despite these measures, the patient continues to make spontaneous respiratory efforts, synchronization may be achieved by using larger tidal volumes bearing in mind the dangers of lung injury discussed above. This is thought to increase afferent impulses from stretch receptors in the lungs and inhibit the inspiratory neurones. Undue hypocarbia can be avoided by decreasing the respiratory rate and/or adding an extra dead space.

Causes of persistent failure to synchronize with the ventilator include:

- hypoxia/hypercarbia;
- obstructed ventilation;
- severe pulmonary parenchymal disease (e.g. adult respiratory distress syndrome—ARDS);
- bladder distension;
- metabolic acidosis;
- raised intracranial pressure.

If specific treatment is not possible, heavy sedation with opiates and benzodiazepines, and occasionally *muscle relaxation*, may be required. Muscle relaxants should, however, only be used as a last resort, or in certain special situations (e.g. in those with severe hypoxia or airway obstruction). The administration of muscle relaxants must always be accompanied by sedative/analgesic drugs to avoid the intolerable situation of a patient who is aware and possibly in pain, but unable to move.

Clearly, bolus administration of sedatives and analgesics produces wide fluctuations in conscious level and often precipitates hypotension. Moreover, the administration of nitrous oxide in oxygen to critically ill patients has been implicated in the development of megaloblastic bone marrow change (Amos *et al.*, 1982) and can no longer be recommended as a means of providing continuous analgesia and sedation for ventilated patients. More recently, therefore, *continuous infusions of intravenous anaesthetic agents* such as propofol, or a benzodiazepine such as midazolam, usually combined with opiates, are used to provide a consistent level of sedation and analgesia (see Chapter 10). It is, however, questionable whether it is desirable to anaesthetize ventilated patients for long periods, except in certain specific situations such as traumatic coma. In addition, by using SIMV (see later) the requirements for sedatives and muscle relaxants can be dramatically reduced.

Selecting the pattern of ventilation

The aim is to achieve optimal gas exchange while minimizing the adverse effects of positive pressure ventilation on haemodynamics, the respiratory system and vital organ function as outlined above.

IPPV WITH NEGATIVE END-EXPIRATORY PRESSURE (NEEP)

To minimize the fall in cardiac output that occurs with IPPV, it was at one time suggested that the application of a NEEP might increase venous return and restore cardiac output. Although this is in fact the case, NEEP is no longer used because it also causes progressive alveolar collapse.

IPPV WITH ZERO END-EXPIRATORY PRESSURE (ZEEP)

As discussed above, IPPV alone may improve oxygenation by re-expanding collapsed alveoli, improving gas distribution and reducing oxygen requirements. To prevent progressive alveolar collapse, tidal volumes of 10–15 ml/kg are normally used (see above). The length of the *inspiratory phase* should be sufficient to allow filling of all distal lung segments. Since an alveolus will be 95% filled in three time constants (i.e. on average within 1.8 seconds in a normal lung), inspiration is conventionally timed to last for 1.5–2.0 seconds (see Chapter 2). In order to minimize the fall in cardiac output, the

expiratory phase should be at least twice as long as inspiration (I : E ratio of 1 : 2) and both inflation and deflation should be relatively rapid. In those with severe lung disease, however, there is an increased 'scatter' of time constants and it may therefore be beneficial to further prolong the inspiratory phase (see below). In some cases, *extending inspiration* so that the I : E ratio is reversed, sometimes to as much as 4 : 1, can improve gas distribution, recruit or stabilize alveoli and increase P_aO_2 (Cole *et al.*, 1984). The obvious danger of reversing the I : E ratio is that it could lead to air trapping with 'auto-PEEP' and severe cardiovascular depression; in this respect the same considerations apply as during CPPV (see below). In addition, inverse ratio ventilation is uncomfortable and the use of heavy sedation and paralysis is often necessary (Duncan *et al.*, 1987).

The influence of the *shape of the inspiratory wave-form* on the efficiency of gas exchange is less certain and probably of little clinical relevance (**Fig. 7.6**). A decelerating inspiratory flow wave-form is produced when a constant pressure is applied to the airway. This pattern of ventilation may lower airway resistance and peak pressure, as well as produce optimal distribution of inspired gas and improving oxygenation (Al-Saddy &

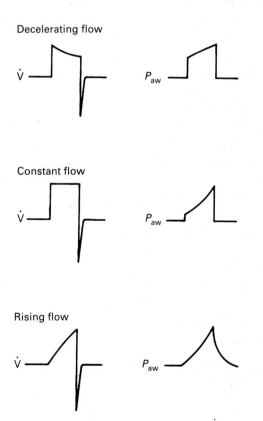

Decelerating flow

Constant flow

Rising flow

Fig. 7.6 Inspiratory wave-forms (see text). ($\dot{V}$, flow; P_{aw}, airway pressure.)

Bennett, 1985). It is also thought to be the most effective for re-expanding collapsed lung. Mean intrathoracic pressure is, however, highest with this 'square wave' pattern of positive pressure ventilation and it therefore causes the greatest reduction in cardiac output. In contrast, the pressure wave required to produce a constant flow pattern is associated with a relatively low mean intrathoracic pressure and minimal cardiovascular depression. An accelerating flow pattern appears to offer little clinical advantage and may increase V_D.

Neonates and infants should be ventilated at a higher respiratory rate (25–30 breaths/minute) than older children and adults. They will normally require a minute volume of 100–200 ml/kg.

IPPV WITH PEEP (ALSO REFERRED TO AS CONTINUOUS POSITIVE PRESSURE VENTILATION—CPPV)

If it proves impossible to achieve adequate oxygenation of arterial blood (e.g. > 90% saturation of haemoglobin with oxygen) without raising the F_IO_2 to potentially dangerous levels (conventionally, $F_IO_2 > 0.5$, see Chapter 6), then the application of PEEP should be considered. PEEP is not, however, a panacea for all patients who are hypoxic and indeed can be detrimental, not least because the use of high levels is associated with an increased risk of ventilator-induced lung injury and barotrauma. Furthermore, it is by no means certain that the application of PEEP influences the outcome of acute respiratory failure (Petty, 1981a). Although at one time it was suggested that the early or prophylactic use of PEEP in those at risk of developing ARDS could decrease the incidence and severity of subsequent pulmonary complications (Weigelt et al., 1979), a later controlled study demonstrated that the early application of PEEP had no effect on the incidence of ARDS or other associated complications (Pepe et al., 1984).

The rational use of PEEP is based on a knowledge of its physiological effects and of the pathophysiology of the patient's pulmonary disease.

Respiratory effects of PEEP

The application of PEEP expands underventilated lung units and *increases FRC*. Provided that shunting is due to alveolar collapse, this will *reduce venous admixture* and improve arterial oxygenation (Ashbaugh & Petty, 1973). It has also been suggested that the improvement in oxygenation with PEEP may be partly related to an increase in the alveolar surface available for gas exchange and layering of oedema fluid in the expanded alveoli. Provided the rise in arterial oxygen content (C_aO_2) is not offset by a fall in cardiac output (see

below), oxygen delivery (DO_2) also improves. In general, the worse the shunt, the greater the response to PEEP. It seems unlikely that PEEP primarily decreases extravascular lung water (Miller et al., 1981); indeed, the associated rise in PAP may enhance oedema formation by increasing filtration pressure across the pulmonary vasculature. On the other hand, there is some evidence that moderate levels of PEEP (e.g. 10 cm H_2O) may protect the lung from ventilator-induced lung damage (Dreyfuss et al., 1988), perhaps by preventing collapse of distal airways during expiration and thereby avoiding high shear stresses when they reopen during inspiration. In some cases, the application of PEEP may be associated with an increased V_D/V_T ratio.

Haemodynamic effects of PEEP

Unfortunately, the inevitable rise in mean intrathoracic pressure that follows the application of PEEP may further *reduce venous return and increase pulmonary vascular resistance* and therefore *reduce cardiac output* (Ashbaugh & Petty, 1973; Qvist et al., 1975; Editorial, 1981). This effect may be proportional to lung compliance (i.e. the stiffer the lungs, the less the fall in cardiac output), although some studies do not support this contention (Beyer et al., 1982). At levels of PEEP higher than 10 cm H_2O the rise in pulmonary vascular resistance and therefore right ventricular after-load, may be associated with *dilatation of the right ventricle*. Because lateral expansion is restricted by the pericardium, the interventricular septum is displaced and encroaches on the left ventricular cavity. This is thought to restrict left ventricular filling and reduce stroke volume, despite a slight increase in myocardial contractility (Editorial, 1981; Jardin et al., 1981). Left ventricular expansion may be further limited by compression from the distended lungs.

The fall in cardiac output can be ameliorated by *volume loading* (Qvist et al., 1975), although when PEEP is removed, relative hypervolaemia may precipitate pulmonary oedema (Qvist et al., 1975), and in some cases *inotropic support* may be required. As mentioned above CPPV may be beneficial in patients with cardiac failure and low cardiac output since the reduction in pre-load and after-load can decrease ventricular wall tension, improve the balance between myocardial oxygen supply and demand, and increase stroke volume.

Although arterial oxygenation is often improved by the application of PEEP, a simultaneous fall in cardiac output can lead to a reduction in DO_2. This reduction in cardiac output is associated with a redistribution of blood flow to vital organs such as the brain, heart and kidneys, which may precipitate ischaemia of other organs such as stomach, pancreas and liver. In one study, CPPV produced a *fall in hepatic flow*, which was related to the level of PEEP and proportional to the reduction in cardiac output; hepatic Do_2 fell to an even greater extent, mainly due to a decrease in portal venous oxygen content (Sha *et al.*, 1987). Although total renal blood flow is preserved, oliguria with salt and water retention is often observed and may be due to *intrarenal redistribution of blood flow* (Beyer *et al.*, 1982) exacerbated by increased sympathetic activity and renin release. The application of PEEP may also be associated with reductions in bronchial blood flow (Baile *et al.*, 1984), and this may limit the delivery of oxygen and nutrients to the lung parenchyma.

Clinical implications

The net effect of PEEP in an individual patient is therefore unpredictable and dependent on a balance of many factors, including left ventricular pre-load and right ventricular function (Schulman *et al.*, 1988). It is clear, however, that the most beneficial effects are likely to occur in those patients with low FRCs, large shunts, stiff lungs and good cardiovascular function. This is exemplified by the young fit patient with ARDS (see Chapter 6). On the other hand, in those with normal or high FRCs, compliant lungs and only a modest degree of shunting, any improvement in P_aO_2 is likely to be negated by the fall in cardiac output, particularly in those with impaired cardiovascular function. Therefore, PEEP is usually of limited value in those with fibrotic lung disease or bacterial pneumonia (Ashbaugh & Petty, 1973), and is potentially dangerous in those with emphysema, asthma or COPD. There is, however, evidence that low levels of PEEP may reduce expiratory resistance and the work of breathing in patients with severe airflow obstruction without substantially increasing the hazards of hyperinflation (Smith & Marini, 1988) (see also Chapter 6).

In patients with only localized areas of diseased lung (e.g. unilateral aspiration pneumonia), PEEP may adversely affect oxygenation by overexpanding normal lung tissue and diverting blood to underventilated lung units. On the other hand, the use of low-level PEEP (e.g. 5–10 cm H_2O) is often an extremely effective and safe means of improving oxygenation in hypoxic postoperative patients with basal atelectasis and it could be argued that most mechanically ventilated patients benefit from the application of about 5 cm H_2O PEEP. Children under six years of age have low FRCs that are less than their closing volume and should therefore always be ventilated with 5 cm H_2O PEEP unless this is specifically contraindicated.

If PEEP is removed, P_aO_2 falls almost immediately, while following its reapplication P_aO_2 may take up to 60 minutes to return to previous levels (Kumar *et al.*, 1970).

Obviously, careful monitoring of the effects of PEEP is essential. It should now be clear that simply measuring P_aO_2 is often not sufficient and that it is important to select the level of PEEP at which Do_2 is maximal; so-called 'best PEEP'. By measuring P_aO_2, P_vO_2 and cardiac output, as well as calculating venous admixture, Do_2 and $\dot{V}o_2$, the effect of PEEP can be accurately assessed. In difficult cases, it is therefore necessary to catheterize the pulmonary artery, although oesophageal Doppler ultrasonography may be a satisfactory non-invasive technique for optimizing PEEP (Singer & Bennett, 1989). A few centres optimize PEEP by measuring the changes in FRC.

CONTINUOUS POSITIVE AIRWAY PRESSURE (CPAP)

Cardiorespiratory effects of CPAP

CPAP achieves for the spontaneously breathing patient what PEEP does for the ventilated patient. Not only can it *improve oxygenation* by the same mechanism, but *lung mechanics improve, breathing becomes easier, respiratory rate falls, V_T increases* and both *VC* and *inspiratory force* have been shown to improve (Feeley *et al.*, 1975; Venus *et al.*, 1979; Katz & Marks, 1985).

The cause of the increased compliance can be appreciated by referring to **Fig. 2.21** (Chapter 2), which shows the compliance curve for the lung and chest wall combined. Normally, tidal exchange takes place from the resting expiratory position at which the propensity for the lungs to collapse is exactly counterbalanced by the tendency of the chest wall to expand. It can be seen that this is also the steepest point on the curve, where relatively small changes in pressure produce a large change in volume (i.e. compliance is greatest and the work of breathing minimal). As lung volume falls, however, the curve becomes flatter (i.e. the lungs become stiffer and the work of breathing increases). The application of positive airway pressure re-expands the lungs and compliance increases. If the lungs are overexpanded, compliance will again fall.

Because mean intrathoracic pressure is lower with CPAP than with IPPV plus PEEP, haemodynamic depression is minimized (Venus *et al.*, 1979; Simonneau *et al.*, 1982), renal perfusion is maintained and the incidence of barotrauma may be reduced. Furthermore, heavy sedation is unnecessary. A circuit suitable for applying CPAP is shown in **Fig. 7.7a**.

Clinical use of CPAP

CPAP can be used as the primary treatment in patients with acute hypoxaemic respiratory failure who are not

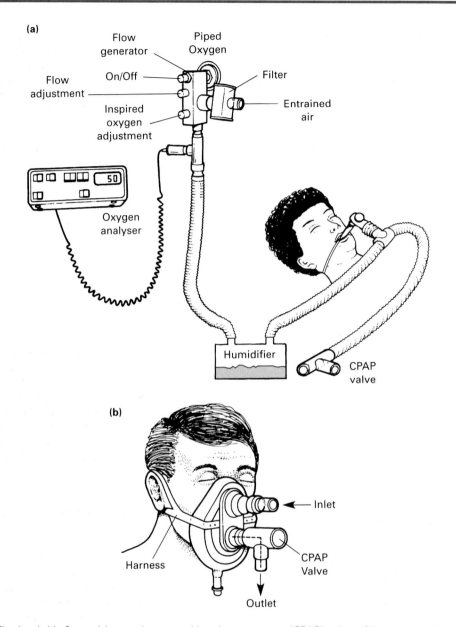

(a)

Flow generator

Piped Oxygen

Flow adjustment

On/Off

Filter

Inspired oxygen adjustment

Entrained air

Oxygen analyser

Humidifier

CPAP valve

(b)

Inlet

Harness

CPAP Valve

Outlet

Fig. 7.7 (a) Circuit suitable for applying continuous positive airway pressure (CPAP) using a flow generator in a patient with an endotracheal tube in place. (b) CPAP can be applied using a tight-fitting face mask.

exhausted and in whom alveolar ventilation is adequate (Venus *et al.*, 1979). The use of a *tight-fitting face mask* (**Fig 7.7b**) allows the application of CPAP without the need for endotracheal intubation or tracheostomy (Greenbaum *et al.*, 1976), and mask CPAP has been shown to produce early physiological improvement as well as reduce the need for intubation and mechanical ventilation in patients with severe cardiogenic pulmonary oedema (Bersten *et al.*, 1991).

Such masks are, however, uncomfortable to wear for prolonged periods and the technique is only suitable for those who are alert, able to clear secretions and protect their airway. Gastric distension, vomiting and aspiration are a potential risk and a nasogastric tube should be inserted in most patients receiving mask CPAP.

Nasal masks may be better tolerated and safer, but mouth breathing renders them less effective. They may be useful when applied at night in patients with obstructive sleep apnoea and nocturnal hypoventilation.

CPAP is also useful for weaning patients who have required PEEP while being ventilated since it prevents the alveolar collapse and hypoxia that may otherwise occur (Feeley *et al.*, 1975). In general, therefore, patients who have required CPAP should not be allowed to breathe spontaneously through an endotracheal tube with ZEEP, but rather should be extubated directly from 5 cm H_2O PEEP. Once extubated, patients probably provide their own 'PEEP' using, for example, pursed lip breathing.

Infants are obligate nose breathers and thereby produce their own CPAP. Therefore, when breathing spontaneously through an endotracheal tube, they should always receive CPAP. Positive pressure can also be applied via 'nasal prongs' or, in neonates, using a head box.

INDEPENDENT LUNG VENTILATION (Hillman & Barber, 1980)

Occasionally, a patient with predominantly unilateral lung disease (e.g. following aspiration of gastric contents) will require positive pressure ventilation. Under these circumstances, conventional IPPV may fail to achieve satisfactory gas exchange. The normal 'compliant' lung tends to become overinflated, while the stiff, diseased lung collapses progressively, causing further mechanical deterioration. Furthermore, pulmonary blood flow is diverted away from normal alveoli to underventilated areas of lung and shunt is increased. The application of PEEP in an attempt to re-expand the diseased lung simply exacerbates the situation. Finally, the 'good' lung is exposed to the high concentrations of oxygen required to combat hypoxia, as well as high airway pressures and overdistension and as a result may itself be damaged.

In such cases, it is possible to ventilate each lung independently, using separate ventilators, through a double-lumen endotracheal tube (**Fig. 7.8**). The diseased lung can then be ventilated using high inflation pressures, an increased F_1O_2 and, if indicated, PEEP or a reversed I : E ratio. The good lung is ventilated conventionally and is therefore protected from the adverse effects of exposure to high airway pressures and potentially toxic concentrations of oxygen. Initially, it was thought that to avoid marked reductions in cardiac output, both lungs should inflate and deflate synchronously. It is possible to achieve this by linking two ventilators electronically, but it is not, in fact, necessary to do so (Hillman & Barber, 1980). Numerous variations of the technique have been described, including the application of CPAP or high-frequency jet ventilation (see below) to the diseased lung.

ASSISTED MECHANICAL VENTILATION (AMV)

Also known as *assist-control ventilation*, this technique in which the patient's own respiratory efforts trigger a

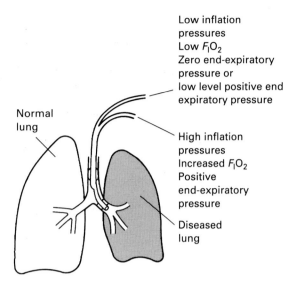

Low inflation pressures
Low F_1O_2
Zero end-expiratory pressure or low level positive end expiratory pressure

Normal lung

High inflation pressures
Increased F_1O_2
Positive end-expiratory pressure

Diseased lung

Fig. 7.8 Independent lung ventilation.

positive pressure inflation, has been used in some centres, particularly in North America, as an alternative to controlled mechanical ventilation (CMV). Using AMV, it is not necessary to abolish the patient's respiratory efforts, and the use of heavy sedation and paralysis can in some cases be avoided. If a spontaneous respiratory effort does not occur within a pre-set period, the ventilator will deliver an untriggered V_T. Hyperventilation is common with this technique, and the work of breathing can be considerable.

INTERMITTENT MANDATORY VENTILATION (IMV)

Originally introduced as a technique for weaning patients from mechanical ventilation (Downs *et al.*, 1973), IMV is now frequently used in preference to conventional IPPV (either CMV or AMV). IMV allows the patient to breathe spontaneously between the 'mandatory' tidal volumes delivered by the ventilator. It is important that the mandatory breaths are timed to coincide with the patient's own inspiratory effort (*synchronized IMV, SIMV*), and IMV can be used with or without PEEP/CPAP and pressure support ventilation (see below).

When used to wean patients from IPPV, the frequency of the mandatory breaths is progressively reduced so that spontaneous respiration accounts for an increasing proportion of the total minute volume (see below).

As a technique for providing ventilatory support, IMV has a number of potential advantages when compared with CMV (Weisman *et al.*, 1983). Firstly, because it is unnecessary to abolish all respiratory efforts, heavy sedation and muscle relaxation can be avoided. This, combined with the reduction in mean intrathoracic pressure means there is less cardiovascular depression and renal function is preserved (Steinhoff *et al.*, 1984). It has also been suggested that the risk of barotrauma is reduced (Mathru *et al.*, 1983). Respiratory alkalosis may be avoided and intrapulmonary gas distribution may be more uniform. Finally, because patients continue to breathe, the strength and coordination of respiratory muscles is relatively well maintained.

Disadvantages of IMV include an increase in the work of breathing with respiratory muscle fatigue and a risk of carbon dioxide retention; most patients with acute respiratory failure should therefore have a rest period of at least 24–48 hours before commencing SIMV. In addition, the potential advantages of IMV are less clear when compared with AMV rather than CMV.

MANDATORY MINUTE VOLUME (MMV) (Hewlett *et al.*, 1977)

This modification of IMV ensures that the patient always receives the preset minute volume despite moment-to-moment variations in the level of spontaneous ventilation. Although MMV is inherently safer than SIMV, it is in fact rarely used in clinical practice.

PRESSURE SUPPORT VENTILATION (PSV) (Brochard *et al.*, 1987)

With this technique spontaneous breaths are augmented by a constant pre-set positive pressure (usually between 5 and 20 cm H_2O) triggered by the patient's spontaneous inspiratory effort and applied for a given fraction of inspiratory time or until inspiratory flow decreases below a specified level. Respiratory frequency, inspiratory time and inspiratory flow rate are controlled by the patient, while V_T is determined by the level of PSV, patient effort and lung mechanics. Patients may find this form of respiratory support particularly easy to tolerate. PSV can reduce the work of breathing, in part by counteracting the load imposed by the endotracheal tube and ventilator circuit. The technique can be used with SIMV and, by gradually reducing the level of pressure support, for weaning (see later in this chapter).

AIRWAY PRESSURE RELEASE VENTILATION (APRV)

Alveolar ventilation is achieved by the periodical release of PEEP, following which there is a marked reduction in airway pressure and expiration occurs passively. Peak airway pressures are minimized and theoretically the

risk of barotrauma is reduced. It can be combined with IMV (intermittent mandatory pressure release ventilation—IMPRV) by releasing PEEP every two, three, four, five or six spontaneous breaths. This technique is not widely used in clinical practice.

LOW VOLUME PRESSURE-LIMITED MECHANICAL VENTILATION

A constant pre-set inspiratory pressure is delivered for a prescribed time, generating low tidal and minute volumes and reducing peak inspiratory pressures. When combined with *inverse ratio ventilation* and *low levels of PEEP* this may provide optimal improvement in oxygenation while minimizing peak airway pressures, although mean airway pressure may be unchanged or even increase (Tharratt *et al.*, 1988). An alternative is to use volume-controlled ventilation with low V_T (e.g. 5–6 ml/kg). Both techniques can be used with SIMV. Although respiratory rate can be increased to limit the rise in P_aCO_2, hypercarbia is inevitable; this is generally well tolerated and should be accepted ('permissive hypercarbia') (see Chapter 6).

HIGH-FREQUENCY VENTILATION (Editorial, 1991)

Surprisingly, it is possible to achieve adequate oxygenation and carbon dioxide elimination by injecting gas into the trachea at rates of between 60 and several thousand breaths per minute with tidal volumes of only 1–5 ml/kg.

High-frequency jet ventilation (HFJV)

In clinical practice, HFJV through a small bore cannula at 100–200 breaths/min, with tidal volumes of 2–5 ml/kg, is usually used.

Although it is known that adequate oxygenation can be produced by 'apnoeic diffusion', it is unclear how carbon dioxide elimination is achieved with this technique. Some consider that this can be explained by the reduction in V_D that is known to occur as V_T falls (see Chapter 2). Others feel that conventional physiology cannot account for the removal of carbon dioxide, particularly at higher frequencies, and attribute the gas exchange produced with this technique to *'augmented' or 'facilitated' diffusion and gas dispersion*. These are thought to be more important than convection.

HFJV can be applied via an intravenous cannula incorporated into a T-shaped connector and positioned centrally in an endotracheal tube. Alternatively, a modified endotracheal tube with a small additional lumen opening distally can be used. With these arrangements, the

T-piece provides both a route for expiration and a source of fresh gas for entrainment. It has been suggested that HFJV via the cricothyroid membrane may be a useful approach in emergencies (e.g. when endotracheal intubation proves impossible). This technique may, however, be dangerous in the presence of upper airway obstruction, when overinflation of the lungs may cause serious barotrauma, and correct positioning of the cannula is clearly essential, particularly in view of the high pressure at which gas is being delivered. Aspiration will be prevented as long as 'jetting' continues (Klain *et al.*, 1983), but most clinicians inflate the cuff on the endotracheal tube to protect the airway in the event of a technical mishap or disconnection. The main practical difficulties are the provision of adequate humidification and satisfactory monitoring of V_T and airway pressures, although techniques have recently been introduced to monitor end-expiratory pressure and minute volume.

Potential advantages of HFJV are largely related to the low peak airway pressures and possibly a reduction in mean airway pressure; therefore, venous return is preserved, changes in pulmonary vascular resistance are minimal and cardiac output is well maintained. Furthermore, the risk of barotrauma in patients with stiff lungs may be reduced and it is possible that ventilator-induced lung injury is minimized. Another possible advantage is that HFJV appears to suppress respiratory drive and unobstructed spontaneous respiration can take place via the T-piece circuit. Many alert patients therefore find this form of artificial ventilation particularly easy to tolerate, and weaning from ventilatory support can normally be achieved relatively smoothly.

Although it is clear that this technique is valuable in the management of patients with large air leaks (e.g. those with bronchopleural fistulae or lung lacerations) who require ventilatory support (Derderian *et al.*, 1982), the place of HFJV in the management of patients with acute respiratory failure is less certain (Schuster *et al.*, 1982). Although it is possible to apply PEEP to the expiratory limb of the circuit (and also to achieve a PEEP effect by increasing the respiratory rate to higher than 200/min), the institution of HFJV may be associated with a temporary increase in shunt (Sladen *et al.*, 1984), and this justifies the initial administration of a high F_IO_2 (0.8–1.0) until oxygenation can be assessed. In general, however, it appears that at the same F_IO_2 and level of PEEP, arterial oxygenation is either unchanged (Schuster *et al.*, 1982) or improved (Vincken & Cosio, 1984) when HFJV is compared with IPPV. HFJV has therefore been recommended for patients with stiff lungs who require very high inflation pressures during IPPV, and in those in whom conventional IPPV produces severe cardiovascular depression (Vincken & Cosio, 1984). Prospective randomized evaluations, however, suggest that neither HFJV nor high-frequency percussive ventilation (Hurst *et al.*, 1990) offer tangible advantages compared

to CMV (see also Chapter 6). In patients with airflow limitation HFJV may rapidly precipitate extreme hyperinflation with barotrauma and cardiovascular collapse.

High-frequency oscillation (HFO)

With HFO there is no bulk flow of gas; rather it oscillates to and fro at rates of 60–3000 cycles/min with a V_T of 1–3 ml/kg. Both inspiration and expiration are actively controlled with a sine wave pump. The mechanism of gas exchange with HFO is still not clearly defined, but is probably largely related to *augmented dispersion*.

High-frequency positive pressure ventilation (HFPPV)

Gas from a high-pressure source is delivered via an endotracheal tube at a frequency of around 60–120 breaths/min with a V_T of approximately 3–5 ml/kg and an I : E ratio less than 0.3. This technique is used mainly during laryngoscopy and bronchoscopy when a narrow-bore endotracheal tube is used, but may have advantages in patients with non-compliant lungs.

NON-INVASIVE MECHANICAL VENTILATION

Non-invasive IPPV delivered via a close-fitting nasal mask can relieve chronic respiratory failure and control nocturnal hypoventilation. It may also be a useful technique in selected patients with acute exacerbations of chronic respiratory failure, especially those in whom endotracheal intubation is considered inappropriate or difficulties with weaning are anticipated. Non-invasive ventilatory support:

- avoids many of the complications of mechanical ventilation, including those related to endotracheal intubation/tracheostomy;
- permits early mobilization;
- facilitates provision of adequate nutrition;
- maintains morale;
- allows the patient to participate in discussions about future management.

Disadvantages include the absence of a route for endotracheal suction and the lack of airway protection. Correction of abnormal blood gas tensions is also less complete and achieved more slowly than with conventional positive pressure ventilation; combined with the avoidance of sedation this may minimize the incidence of hypotension (Elliott *et al.*, 1990). Non-invasive mechanical ventilation has also been applied via a face mask in acute hypercapnic respiratory failure (Meduri *et al.*, 1991), and inspiratory assistance via a face mask has been used to avoid mechanical ventilation in patients with acute exacerbations of COPD (Brochard *et al.*, 1990).

EXTRACORPOREAL RESPIRATORY ASSISTANCE

Extracorporeal membrane oxygenation (ECMO)

The technique of ECMO using veno-arterial bypass has been used in an attempt to save the lives of some patients who would otherwise inevitably have died from severe progressive acute respiratory failure. It was based on the premise that the lungs of such patients would eventually recover provided death from hypoxia could be avoided. This proved not to be the case since in the majority of cases the lung lesion continued to progress, culminating in irreversible pulmonary fibrosis. When a prospective randomized study demonstrated that the mortality of patients with severe ARF was similar whether or not ECMO was used (Zapol *et al.*, 1979), its use was largely abandoned.

Low-frequency positive pressure ventilation with extracorporeal carbon dioxide removal (Gattinoni *et al.*, 1980)

There has been renewed interest in using extracorporeal gas exchange to reduce ventilation requirements, avoid ventilator-induced lung injury and 'rest' the lungs. Carbon dioxide is removed using a veno–venous bypass with low flows of only 20–30% of the cardiac output. The lungs are ventilated at a very low frequency and oxygenation is maintained by applying a positive pressure to the airways and adjusting the F_IO_2. Although alveolar oxygen concentrations may be high, the combination of normal pulmonary perfusion and minimum ventilation may minimize barotrauma and provide optimal conditions for lung healing.

The major complication of this technique is bleeding associated with thrombocytopenia, altered platelet function, abnormal fibrinogen and anti-thrombin III concentrations and the need for systemic heparinization. The incidence of bleeding can be reduced by using surface heparinized extracorporeal circuits or by the simultaneous administration of aprotinin with heparin. In general, however, extracorporeal techniques are contraindicated in patients at risk of haemorrhage. In contrast to the use of ECMO, thromboembolic complications have not been reported and the technique is simplified by the use of percutaneous venous cannulation.

Intravascular oxygenation device (IVOX) (Skoyles and Pepperman, 1993)

The IVOX device is inserted percutaneously via the femoral vein and is positioned in the vena cava. Gas exchange takes place across a bundle of microbore tubes coated with heparin. It can be used to augment oxygenation temporarily and reduce requirements for supplemental oxygen and PEEP, although its effects on gas exchange are often disappointing.

Weaning (Feeley & Hedley-Whyte, 1975; Marini, 1991)

As discussed above, mechanical ventilation can be complicated by collapse of distal lung units, impaired surfactant activity, damage to the alveolar–capillary membrane, barotrauma and nosocomial pneumonia. Moreover, cardiac output and renal blood flow are compromised. It is therefore important to discontinue mechanical ventilation, and, if possible, to extubate the patient, as soon as possible. On the other hand, premature attempts at weaning may be deleterious and can adversely affect the morale of conscious patients; during weaning a fine balance must be drawn between proceeding too quickly and unnecessarily prolonging the process. Because mechanical ventilation reduces or abolishes the work of breathing, the respiratory muscles eventually become weak and discoordinated. Ventilatory function may be further compromised by:

- critical illness neuropathy (see Chapter 14);
- a neurogenic weakness;
- pathological changes in muscle, including corticosteroid myopathy;
- chest wall instability;
- hyperinflation of the lungs (see Chapter 6);
- operative or traumatic damage to the phrenic nerves.

Critical illness neuropathy may be responsible for severe respiratory weakness and a predominantly motor neuropathy has been described in patients who had been mechanically ventilated for severe airways obstruction (Coakley *et al.*, 1992) and acute respiratory failure (Gorson & Ropper, 1993). Abnormalities of muscle, including fibre atrophy, myopathic changes (Douglas *et al.*, 1992) and fibre necrosis, may also contribute to the development of weakness. Although some investigators attribute many of these neuromuscular disorders to drug therapy, in particular muscle relaxants and corticosteroids, this is almost certainly an oversimplification, and the aetiology is probably multifactorial.

In addition, there is usually some persisting abnormality of lung function. In patients who have been ventilated for any length of time, therefore, spontaneous respiration normally has to be resumed gradually.

CRITERIA FOR WEANING PATIENTS FROM MECHANICAL VENTILATION

Clinical criteria

Clinical assessment is of paramount importance when deciding whether a patient is ready to be weaned from the ventilator. The patient's conscious level, psychological state, metabolic function, the effects of drugs, cardiovascular performance, lung mechanics, pulmonary gas exchange and ventilatory function must all be taken into account.

An altered *level of consciousness* does not necessarily prevent weaning, but patients should not be extubated until they can cough, cooperate with physiotherapy and protect their own airway. Weaning will, however, often prove difficult in those who are *restless, confused* and *uncooperative*. In such cases, it is sometimes preferable to continue mechanical ventilation while instituting measures to improve the patient's mental state. Some patients who have undergone a prolonged period of respiratory support become *psychologically dependent* on the ventilator (see Chapter 10) and will require particular care and continual reassurance throughout the weaning period.

Malnourished patients may have difficulty in sustaining adequate alveolar ventilation. For this, and many other reasons (see Chapter 10), malnutrition should if possible be prevented or corrected by providing an adequate protein and energy intake during the patient's hospitalization and by correcting any specific deficiencies, in particular *hypophosphataemia, hypocalcaemia* and *hypokalaemia*. On the other hand, some patients with borderline respiratory function may be unable to excrete the large quantities of carbon dioxide produced by the metabolism of high-energy carbohydrate feeds, although it remains unclear whether the use of high-fat feeds can facilitate weaning in difficult cases (Al-Saady, 1994). Similarly, *increased oxygen demands* (e.g. in response to fever or shivering) can prevent successful weaning.

It is also important to correct any significant abnormalities of *acid–base balance*; although a metabolic alkalosis increases muscle strength, it can blunt the respiratory drive and cause carbon dioxide retention, while metabolic acidosis decreases muscle strength and stimulates respiration.

Anaemia should be corrected.

The possibility that the residual *effects of drugs* are impairing respiration must also be considered. Of most importance in this respect are the opiates and the non-depolarizing muscle relaxants; both are a particular problem in the presence of renal failure. In particular, morphine metabolites such as morphine-6-glucuronide can accumulate in patients with renal impairment, and the long-term administration of vecuronium may be especially likely to cause persistent paralysis, perhaps due to the accumulation of a metabolite (Segredo *et al.*, 1992).

Cardiovascular stability is another important prerequisite for successful weaning. In particular, weaning is likely to be difficult in those with left ventricular failure and a low cardiac output. This is partly because when cardiac output is low there is a reduction in pulmonary artery pressures, which increases the number of relatively underperfused alveoli; V_D/V_T ratio therefore rises. Also Do_2 is limited and may be insufficient for the increase in Vo_2 associated with resumption of respiratory efforts. Venous return and after-load both increase and catecholamine release may exacerbate the situation by causing vasoconstriction and tachycardia. In difficult cases a pulmonary artery catheter may be required to guide haemodynamic support during and after the weaning period. Life-threatening arrhythmias and bleeding likely to require surgical intervention (e.g. after cardiac surgery) are other contraindications to discontinuing ventilation. On the other hand, provided the patient is stable, dependence on inotropic support and/or intra-aortic balloon counterpulsation is not a contraindication to commencing cautious weaning.

Finally, *mechanical factors* likely to impair ventilation, such as residual pulmonary oedema, abdominal distension and pleural effusions should, if possible, be corrected. A subjective evaluation of the patient's response to a short period of spontaneous respiration by an experienced clinician remains the most reliable predictor of weaning success or failure. Asynchronous or paradoxical respiration, respiratory alternans, use of accessory muscles, tachypnoea and low tidal volumes all suggest incipient decompensation.

Objective criteria

Although many objective criteria for predicting the ability to wean have been suggested (Skillman *et al.*, 1971; Sahn & Lakshminarayan, 1973; Feeley & Hedley-Whyte, 1975), these often prove misleading (Kreiger *et al.*, 1989). In most cases, a clinical assessment as outlined above, together with blood gas analysis (considered in conjunction with the F_1O_2 and the minute volume) and an assessment of the mechanical state of the patient's lungs, will be sufficient to make the correct decision. The various quantitative criteria that have been recommended for predicting the outcome of weaning are best used as adjuncts to clinical assessment in difficult cases.

The gas exchanging properties of the lungs may be considered adequate for weaning if the P_aO_2 is >10 kPa (80 mm Hg) with an $F_1O_2 < 0.5$ (some suggest a $P_aO_2 > 8$ kPa (60 mm Hg) with an F_1O_2 of 0.4), if the $P_{A-a}O_2$ is < 40–47 kPa (300–350 mm Hg) with an $F_1O_2 =$

Table 7.4 Objective criteria for weaning
Gas exchange
$P_aO_2 > 10$ kPa (80 mm Hg) with an $F_iO_2 < 0.5$
or
$P_aO_2 > 8$ kPa (60 mm Hg) with an $F_iO_2 = 0.4$
$P_{A-a}O_2 < 40–47$ kPa (300–350 mm Hg) with an $F_iO_2 = 1.0$
Percentage venous admixture $< 15\%$
V_D/V_T ratio $< 0.58–0.60$
Patient should not require > 15 cm H_2O PEEP
Mechanical
Vital capacity $> 10–15$ ml/kg
Maximum inspiratory force > -20 cm H_2O
f/V_T ratio ≤ 105 breaths/min/litre
CROP index ≥ 13 ml/breath/min

1.0, if the percentage venous admixture is $< 15\%$ and if the V_D/V_T ratio is $< 0.58-0.6$ (Skillman *et al.*, 1971: Feeley & Hedley-Whyte, 1975). The patient should not require >15 cm H_2O PEEP (**Table 7.4**).

The strength of the respiratory muscles in relation to the mechanical properties of the lungs can be assessed by measuring VC, which should be higher than 10–15 ml/kg to commence weaning, and the maximum inspiratory force (P_{imax}), which should be more than -20 cm H_2O, although these tests are dependent on the ability of the patient to cooperate. In one study, all those patients who were able to produce a peak negative pressure of more than -30 cm H_2O weaned successfully, while a resting minute volume of less than 10 l/min and the ability to double this voluntarily correlated well with the ability to wean (Sahn & Lakshminarayan, 1973). If the cardiac index can be measured, it should be higher than 2 l/min/m^2 at least and preferably within the normal range. Finally, the pH should be 7.3-7.5.

A recent study conducted in medical patients (Yang & Tobin, 1991) demonstrated that the most accurate predictor of failure to wean was rapid shallow breathing, as reflected by the f/V_T ratio. P_{imax} and expired minute volume, ($\dot{V}_E$) were poor predictors, whereas an index that integrated thoracic compliance, respiratory rate, arterial oxygenation and P_{imax} (called CROP) was considerably more accurate. Of the primary indices, V_T was the most accurate predictor of weaning outcome.

Measuring the airway occlusion pressure 0.1 secs after the onset of inspiration ($P_{0.1}$), and its response to a hypercapnic challenge may also prove to be a useful means of predicting the likely outcome of weaning attempts (Montgomery *et al.*, 1987).

TECHNIQUES FOR WEANING

Patients who have undergone artificial ventilation for less than 24 hours (e.g. elective IPPV after major surgery) can usually resume spontaneous respiration immediately and no weaning process is required. They should be connected to a T-piece circuit and provided with humidified fresh gas of an appropriate F_iO_2 (**Fig. 7.9**). This procedure can also be adopted for those who have been ventilated for longer periods, but who clearly fulfil the criteria for weaning outlined above.

The *traditional method of weaning* in difficult cases is to allow patients to breathe entirely spontaneously for a short time, following which they are reconnected to the ventilator. The periods of spontaneous breathing are gradually increased and periods of IPPV are reduced. Initially, it is usually advisable to ventilate the patient throughout the night. This method has several practical disadvantages: during the periods of spontaneous respiration, the patient may develop progressive hypoxia and/or hypercarbia as well as increasing sympathetic drive with tachycardia and hypertension. After a predetermined period, or earlier if tachypnoea and exhaustion develop, the patient is reconnected to IPPV. At this time, respiratory drive is high, synchronization with the ventilator is difficult and heavy sedation may be required. It is then necessary to wait until the effects of these drugs have worn off before trying another period of spontaneous respiration. This method is stressful and tiring for both patients and staff, but may prove successful when other methods have failed, and is especially useful in patients with COPD. It is now usual to rest the patient on SIMV, pressure support and CPAP between periods of increased respiratory work using CPAP and lower levels of pressure support.

These disadvantages may be overcome by using *SIMV*. As described above, this technique provides a smoother, more controlled method of weaning, and may enable weaning to commence at an earlier stage than is possible using the traditional method. The performance of the SIMV circuits on some ventilators is unsatisfactory (Cox & Niblett, 1984) and this may actually hinder weaning in those with borderline respiratory function. The application of *inspiratory pressure support* has been shown to prevent diaphragmatic fatigue and limit hyperinflation during weaning from mechanical ventilation (Brochard *et al.*, 1989) and is becoming an increasingly popular technique, often used in combination with SIMV/CPAP. Recently, weaning by gradually reducing the level of pressure support ventilation (by 2-4 cm H_2O twice a day) with no mandatory breaths has been shown to be superior to withdrawing ventilatory support using T-piece trials or SIMV (Brochard *et al.*, 1994).

The *application of CPAP* can prevent the alveolar col-

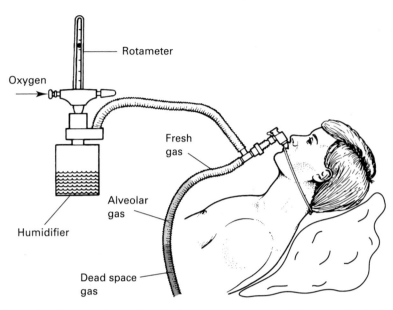

Fig. 7.9 A T-piece circuit: situation at end-expiration. Expired gases are prevented from entering the inspiratory limb by the flow of fresh gas. During the end-expiratory pause fresh gas enters the expiratory limb, pushing the expired gases distally. At peak-inspiration, when the fresh gas flow may be insufficient, fresh gas can be entrained from the expiratory limb of the T-piece. In order to prevent rebreathing of alveolar gas, the fresh gas flow must exceed 2½ times the patient's minute volume. In order to prevent entrainment of air, the volume of the expiratory limb must be greater than the patient's tidal volume.

lapse, hypoxaemia and fall in compliance that may otherwise occur when patients start to breathe spontaneously (Feeley & Hedley-Whyte, 1975; Feeley *et al.*, 1975). It is therefore often used during weaning with SIMV/pressure support ventilation and in spontaneously breathing patients before extubation, particularly when the patient was previously receiving CPPV. CPAP may also assist weaning in patients with severe airflow obstruction by decreasing the work of breathing and sensation of breathlessness (Petrof *et al.*, 1990), and there are good arguments for using at least 3–5 cm H_2O PEEP during weaning in all bedridden patients receiving mechanical ventilation. It is also important to provide sufficient inspiratory pressure support during spontaneous breaths to overcome the resistance of the ventilator circuit and endotracheal tube (about 5 cm H_2O). It is important to extubate such patients from PEEP rather than following a period of spontaneous ventilation at ZEEP.

To discourage atelectasis during weaning, patients should remain as upright and mobile as possible, and should be encouraged to take deep breaths periodically. It is important to avoid overtaxing the respiratory muscles because recovery from fatigue may take 24 hours or more and sufficient ventilatory support should be provided at night to allow the patient to sleep. The value of *training the respiratory muscles* remains in doubt, but reconditioning of respiratory muscles, the return of coordinated muscular activity and the match-

ing of ventilation to requirements are important adjustments during successful weaning. Indeed, weaning time can be reduced by using V_T and relaxation biofeedback techniques (Holliday & Hyers, 1990). In difficult cases the use of mask CPAP, intermittent non-invasive ventilatory support and augmentation of gas exchange by tracheal catheterization may assist the transition to independence.

EXTUBATION

Extubation should not be considered until patients can cough, swallow, protect their own airway and are sufficiently alert to be cooperative. Patients who fulfil these criteria can be extubated provided their respiratory function has improved sufficiently to sustain spontaneous ventilation indefinitely. This is often difficult to assess and is usually largely based on the patient's ability to breathe spontaneously via the endotracheal tube over a period of time. In those who have undergone prolonged mechanical ventilation, this period may be for 24–48 hours, or even longer, while patients ventilated for less than 12–24 hours can often be extubated within 10–15 minutes. During this *trial of spontaneous respiration*, the patient should be closely observed for any signs of respiratory distress (tachypnoea, use of accessory muscles, 'gasping' respirations, tachycardia, sweating) and the V_T and respiratory rate should be recorded frequently. Some suggested quantitative criteria for extubation include:

- a respiratory rate of less than 35/min;
- a VC higher than 10–15 ml/kg;
- an inspiratory force of more than – 25 cm H_2O.

The criteria relating to oxygenation are similar to those for weaning mentioned above, except that the patient should not require more than 5 cm H_2O CPAP.

In patients with upper airway obstruction it is generally accepted that the safety of extubation is best determined by demonstrating a leak around the endotracheal tube when the cuff is deflated. Although the presence of such a leak suggests that extubation is likely to be successful, a failed cuff-leak test does not preclude uneventful extubation and if used in isolation may prolong the period of intubation or lead to unnecessary tracheostomy (Fisher & Raper, 1992).

ENDOTRACHEAL INTUBATION

Indications

Apart from providing a route for mechanical ventilation and the application of CPAP, endotracheal intubation may be required to secure and maintain a clear airway, protect the lungs from aspiration and to allow control of bronchial secretions with tracheal suction.

Complications

EARLY

All the common immediate hazards of endotracheal intubation cause difficulty with inflation of one or both lungs. It is therefore essential to ensure that both sides of the chest are expanding equally and adequately at all times and that the inflation pressure is not excessive.

A common mistake is *intubation of one or other bronchus*, usually the right since this is most directly in line with the trachea, and in one series this occurred in 9% of all endotracheal intubations (Stauffer *et al.*, 1981). As a result, the left lung, and often the right upper lobe, collapse and the patient becomes hypoxic. Therefore, the length of an endotracheal tube must always be checked on the chest radiograph and if the tip is close to or beyond the carina, the tube should be withdrawn. Some recommend that a mark should be made a few cm proximal to the cuff and that the tube should be positioned so that this mark lies between the vocal cords.

Accidental *intubation of the oesophagus* can occasionally be surprisingly difficult to recognize. Hypoxia with gaseous distension of the stomach may then develop rapidly. Endotracheal tubes can *migrate*

out of the trachea so that they come to lie in the pharynx; this process is often accelerated by overinflation of the cuff in an attempt to abolish the leak that inevitably develops when the cuff herniates between the vocal cords. A leak around the tube is usually clearly audible and will also develop if the *cuff ruptures*.

Obstruction may be due to inspissated secretions, kinking, biting on the tube, cuff herniation, compression of the tube by an overinflated cuff or the bevel of the tube impinging on the tracheal wall or carina.

All these acute complications are potentially extremely dangerous; they must be recognized promptly and dealt with appropriately. If at any time the tube becomes obstructed—indicated by the patient becoming distressed and/or cyanosed with inadequate or absent expansion of one or both sides of the chest, accompanied by a rise in inflation pressures and activation of the ventilator alarm—the following procedure should be adopted:

- Attempt manual inflation with 100% oxygen.
- Check and adjust position of tube.
- If position of tube is correct carry out endotracheal suction may confirm or relieve obstruction.
- Check that the tube is not kinked in the oropharynx.
- Deflate cuff (relieves obstruction if due to cuff herniation or tube compression).
- Change endotracheal tube (the tube can be changed over a bougie).

If a significant leak develops that cannot be abolished by reinflating the cuff, either the endotracheal tube has dislodged into the oropharynx or the cuff has ruptured. If the tube has become misplaced, it should be removed and the patient ventilated using a face mask and rebreathing bag before reintubation. If the cuff is leaking, the endotracheal tube should be replaced electively.

LATE

Prolonged pressure on the structures of the upper respiratory tract, caused either by the tube itself or the cuff, causes *mucosal oedema*, which may then progress to *ulceration*. This later heals by *granulation* with the development of *fibrotic scar* tissue and tracheal narrowing. The points at which excessive pressure may occur are shown in **Fig. 7.10**. At the level of the glottis, the posterior aspect of the vocal cords, the arytenoid cartilages and the cricoarytenoid joints may be damaged, while in some patients the lesions extend down into the subglottic space (Stauffer *et al.*, 1981). Damage may also occur at the level of the cuff, often anteriorly; this may be extensive with complete loss of mucosa and exposure of underlying tracheal cartilage. Granuloma formation is unusual (Stauffer *et al.*, 1981). The ways in which this damage may be minimized are as follows:

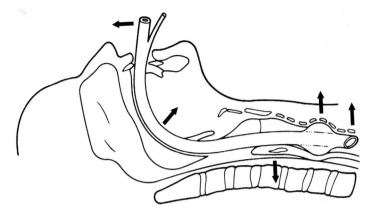

Fig. 7.10 Points at which excessive pressure is exerted by an endotracheal tube. From Lindholm & Grenvik (1977), with permission.

- *Tube size.* To avoid the risk of circular subglottic stenosis, a tube with an external diameter well below the internal diameter of the cricoid ring should be used. This is particularly important in children in whom an uncuffed tube small enough to allow an audible leak should be used (see below).
- *Tube material.* It is important that the endotracheal tube is made of thermolabile material so that once in place it conforms to the shape of the airway. Otherwise undue force is exerted, particularly on the medial aspects of the arytenoid cartilages and on both sides of the midline at the cricoid plate (see **Fig. 7.10**). Only tubes made of non-irritant (implant tested—IT) material should be used.
- *Movements of the larynx.* Coughing and straining on the tube is thought to increase the risk of mucosal damage; the arytenoid cartilages are again particularly vulnerable.
- *Tube cuff.* High pressures were required to inflate the cuffs of red rubber endotracheal tubes and because their shape did not conform to that of the trachea, this high pressure was concentrated on a small area of the tracheal wall, impairing capillary blood flow in the underlying tracheal mucosa. In addition, prolonged high cuff pressures may lead to distension of the trachea, with eventual erosion of the cartilaginous rings. It has been shown that by using *high-volume preshaped low-pressure cuffs* made of *non-irritant material*, the severity of the tracheal injury can be minimized (Grillo *et al.*, 1971). It is important that these cuffs are not overinflated since once a seal has been created further inflation causes a steep rise in intracuff pressure. Inflation of the cuff beyond this point can be avoided by monitoring the intracuff pressure or by using a pressure-limiting valve, and this may reduce the incidence of cuff-related complications. Theoretically the pressure exerted by the cuff on the tracheal mucosa should not exceed the capillary perfusion pressure (i.e. about 30 mm Hg).

Nevertheless, severe laryngotracheal injury may still occur (Stauffer *et al.*, 1981) and progressive, but temporary, tracheal dilatation, mainly affecting the muscles of the posterior wall, has been described following the prolonged use of low-pressure cuffs (Leverment *et al.*, 1975). This may partly account for the observation that low-pressure cuffs are not an entirely reliable barrier to the aspiration of liquid such as acidic gastric secretions. Intermittent deflation of the cuff is no longer practised since it is unnecessary and may precipitate aspiration of pooled infected material from the oropharynx. It should be remembered that nitrous oxide will diffuse into an air-filled cuff and that this may be responsible for a significant rise in intracuff pressure during a general anaesthetic.

Other factors thought to increase the risk of mucosal damage include:

- prolonged intubation;
- episodes of hypotension during which mucosal blood flow is further compromised;
- the administration of corticosteroids;
- tracheitis due to pooling of infected material above the cuff.

Despite the relatively high incidence of laryngeal injury detected at autopsy, including posterior glottic ulceration and laryngeal haematoma, late laryngeal sequelae of prolonged endotracheal intubation are rare in survivors. Subglottic stenosis is more common, and in one series was detected in 19% of cases following endotracheal intubation. The incidence was even higher after tracheostomy (65%), but in most of these patients tracheal narrowing occurred at stomal, rather than cuff, level. However, only one patient with tracheal stenosis had symptoms of upper airway obstruction (Stauffer *et al.*, 1981).

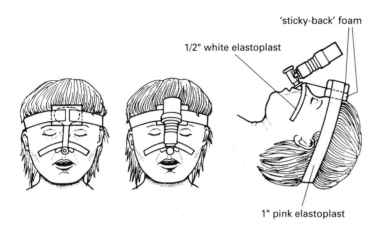

'sticky-back' foam

1/2" white elastoplast

Fig. 7.11 A suitable method of fixation for paediatric endotracheal tubes using a Tunstall connector.

1" pink elastoplast

Oral or nasal endotracheal intubation?

Many patients find it difficult to tolerate oral endotracheal tubes. This applies particularly to those who are fully conscious and require prolonged intubation. In these cases, the nasal route may be preferred since it is more comfortable and secure fixation of the tube is more easily achieved. Furthermore, damage to, or occlusion of, the tube by the teeth is avoided. Nasal endotracheal intubation does, however, have a number of disadvantages, including:

● epistaxis;
● damage to the nasopharyngeal mucosa (including submucosal insertion of the tube);
● erosion of the alar cartilages;
● necrosis of the nasal septum;
● difficulty with bronchial suction (due to the greater length and increased angle of curvature);
● increased resistance to gas flow, which may delay or prevent weaning.

Nasal intubation is contraindicated in patients with adjacent facial or skull fractures and may be associated with bacteraemia secondary to sinus infection (Bach *et al.*, 1992) or otitis media (Stauffer *et al.*, 1981). On the other hand, ulceration of the corners of the mouth and superadded fungal infection may complicate the use of oral tubes. Also laryngeal injury may be more common with oral, as opposed to nasal, intubation (Stauffer *et al.*, 1981). The choice of route in an individual patient often depends largely on the experience and preference of a particular unit, but each undoubtedly has its place.

Endotracheal intubation in paediatric practice

Secure fixation of the endotracheal tube is particularly important in paediatric practice since displacement is a constant danger in these small patients. This is best achieved using the nasal route, which has the additional

advantages of reducing the risk of kinking in the oropharynx and avoiding the danger of palatal ulceration. Moreover, in neonates, infants and young children, as large a tube can be passed via the nasal route as can be inserted orally. Uncuffed tubes should always be used in prepubertal patients and, because of the risk of stenosis at the level of the cricoid cartilage, which is extremely difficult to treat, there should be as large a leak around the tube as is compatible with efficient positive pressure ventilation. An approximate guide to suitable tube sizes in relation to age is shown in **Table 7.5**. If long-term ventilation is envisaged, the smaller of the two sizes should be used and, if there is any doubt, one-half size smaller than that. A Tunstall connector is preferred for tube sizes smaller than 6.0 mm, and a suitable method of fixation is shown in **Fig. 7.11**.

It is always safest to first control the airway with an oral tube. If this is the correct size, it can then be replaced by a nasal tube of the same size, measured and cut to length under direct vision. The cut end of the tube should be taped to the bed so that its diameter can be easily checked and a tube of the same size should be immediately available.

Table 7.5 Recommended sizes of endotracheal tubes in relation to age.

Age	Tube size (internal diameter) in mm
< 2 months	2.5–3.0
3–5 months	3.0–3.5
6–9 months	3.5–4.0
10–12 months	4.0–4.5
2–4 years	4.5–5.0
5 years	5.0–5.5
6–7 years	5.5–6.0
8–9 years	6.0–6.5
10 years	6.5–7.0
11–12 years	7.0–7.5

CARE OF THE INTUBATED CHILD

A daily check should be made for the presence or absence of a leak around the tube. If the leak disappears and the tube was originally a loose fit, it is not necessary to change down to a smaller size, but if there was any doubt about its size initially, it is prudent to change down one-half size. Otherwise, it is generally recommended that endotracheal tubes be changed weekly unless extubation is imminent.

The risk of obstruction of small-diameter endotracheal tubes with encrusted secretions must be minimized by ensuring adequate humidification and by regular tracheobronchial suction. It is important to use suction catheters of the correct size to avoid large negative intrathoracic pressures on the one hand or inefficient suction on the other. Recommended sizes of suction catheters are shown in **Table 7.6**.

To reduce the possibility of aspiration of gastric contents, a nasogastric tube should always be passed and left on free drainage. This also helps to avoid gastric distension, which may compromise respiration in those breathing spontaneously. Slight head-up tilt can also be used if the circulation permits. An oropharyngeal pack is irritant and unnecessary unless there is a particular likelihood of regurgitation or if the leak around the endotracheal tube is too great to allow effective IPPV.

TRACHEOSTOMY

Indications

There is a small, but significant, mortality (up to 3%) associated with tracheostomy and the morbidity is greater than that of prolonged endotracheal intubation (Stauffer *et al.*, 1981). Although tracheostomy is therefore performed less often than in the past, there are a number of situations in which it remains invaluable. Furthermore, the long-term laryngeal dysfunction that may occur following prolonged intubation, although rare, is difficult to treat.

The only indication for immediate tracheostomy is a life-threatening obstruction of the upper respiratory tract that cannot be bypassed with an endotracheal tube. Tracheostomy performed under these circumstances can be extremely hazardous, mainly because of engorgement of the blood vessels in the neck. An emergency tracheostomy may also be necessary to secure the airway in patients with head and neck injuries, including burns to the face and upper airway.

Tracheostomy may be required for the long-term control of excessive bronchial secretions, particularly in those with a reduced conscious level, and/or to maintain an airway and protect the lungs in those with impaired pharyngeal and laryngeal reflexes. Because endotracheal tubes can now remain safely in place for several weeks (Stauffer *et al.*, 1981), tracheostomy is less often performed simply for prolonged control of the airway. However, many patients require sedation to tolerate endotracheal intubation and when patients are extubated following an extended period of intubation, their vocal cords are oedematous and rigid, impairing their ability to cough. This may influence the decision to perform a tracheostomy, particularly in those who continue to produce excessive secretions and/or are unable to cooperate fully with physiotherapy. The reduction in V_D that occurs when tracheostomy is performed is not considered to offer any significant advantage.

Techniques

SURGICAL

It is important to avoid damaging the cricoid cartilage or first tracheal ring since this renders the larynx unstable. On the other hand, a low tracheostomy increases the risk of erosion of the innominate artery. The trachea should therefore be opened through the second, third and fourth tracheal rings. Ligation and division of the thyroid isthmus is not usually necessary. Duke's modification of the *Bjork flap*, in which an inverted U incision is made in the trachea and the flap is sutured to the lower skin edge, remains a popular technique. It has the advantages of supporting the tracheostomy tube, thereby minimizing erosion of the lower border of the trachea and facilitating reinsertion. Alternatively, a simple *'window'* of tracheal wall can be removed. Both these methods weaken the tracheal wall and a *vertical slit* is now preferred, the edges of which are held apart with hooks while the tracheostomy tube is inserted. Some use a *T-shaped incision*. Strong stay sutures should be left in place to assist re-insertion. Certainly in neonates and infants a vertical slit should always be used. In general, however, there are a large number of surgical approaches and there is little information concerning the influence of these various techniques on the incidence of long-term complications.

Table 7.6 Recommended size of suction catheters in relation to internal diameter of endotracheal tube.	
Tube size (mm)	Suction catheter (French gauge)
2.5	6
3.0–4.5	8
> 4.5	10

PERCUTANEOUS TRACHEOSTOMY (Bodenham *et al.*, 1991)

Percutaneous tracheostomy involves introducing a cannula into the trachea via a small (1.5–2.0 cm) transverse skin incision midway between the cricoid cartilage and the sternal notch, through which a 'J tipped' guide wire is passed. A dilator is introduced into the trachea over the guide wire, the jaws of which are then opened to allow insertion of the tracheostomy tube. Alternatively, a guiding catheter can be advanced over the guide wire, followed by serial dilatation of the stoma with dilators of increasing size. Finally the tracheostomy tube, pre-loaded onto a dilator of the appropriate size, is advanced over the guide wire and guiding catheter into the tracheal lumen.

This approach has a number of potential advantages. The skin incision is small, disruption of deeper tissues is minimized and there is no tracheal resection. The risk of bleeding and the incidence of infection and scar formation may therefore be reduced. Percutaneous tracheostomy is generally safe and avoids the hazards associated with moving critically ill patients, although much of the information regarding the complications associated with surgical tracheostomies is out of date and the relative risks of the different approaches requires re-assessment. In particular, the incidence of long-term complications following percutaneous tracheostomy has not been documented. The use of dilatational techniques for reformation of healed tracheostomies, where distorted anatomy increases the risk of bleeding from major vessels is controversial. Percutaneous tracheostomy may also be a useful means of rapidly securing the airway in an emergency.

CRICOTHYROIDOTOMY

The technique of cricothyroidotomy is generally only performed in an emergency. A large-bore needle and cannula (e.g. 14G) can be inserted percutaneously via the cricothyroid membrane to provide a temporary route for oxygenation, although ventilation is inefficient and a surgical tracheostomy will normally be required within 30–45 minutes to avoid hypercarbia.

Needle cricothyroidotomy is preferred in infants and young children because the cricoid cartilage is essential to the stability of their upper airway. In adults, however, a surgical approach via a transverse skin incision allows insertion of a size 6 or 7F tracheostomy or endotracheal tube under direct vision.

Alternatively, the guide-wire technique described above or the Penlon cricothyrotomy cannula can be used. The latter technique involves extending the patient's head, making a small skin incision and pushing the cannula blade through the cricothyroid membrane into the trachea. The blade is then retracted and the integral metal dilators advanced and opened, allowing insertion of a tracheostomy tube.

Minitracheostomy (Ryan, 1990)

A small diameter (e.g. 4.0 mm) uncuffed tube can be inserted percutaneously via the cricothyroid membrane following infiltration with local anaesthetic. A Seldinger technique in which the minitracheostomy and a dilator are inserted over a guide wire is probably safer and less traumatic. This provides a route for repeated tracheo-bronchial suction using a 10 FG catheter and for the administration of oxygen, while being comfortable and allowing the patient to speak and eat. This technique has also been used in the emergency management of upper airway obstruction, to administer HFJV and in obstructive sleep apnoea.

Complications include haemorrhage, misplacement in the mediastinum, displacement and surgical emphysema. Minitracheostomy should not be used in patients who are unable to protect their airway or in those with coagulopathy.

Tracheostomy tubes

During mechanical ventilation, and for protection against aspiration, a cuffed tracheostomy tube is clearly required. As with endotracheal tubes for long-term use, these should be constructed of non-irritant material and have low-pressure, high-volume cuffs. The tip is normally cut square, rather than bevelled, to decrease the risk of obstruction.

When the patient's condition has improved, it is usual to change to an uncuffed tube. Traditionally, these are made of silver, which is non-irritant and bactericidal. They have an inner tube which can be removed for cleaning at regular intervals. They can also be modified with a fenestration at the angle of the tube and a one-way flap valve to allow the patient to speak. Alternatively, the patient can simply use a finger to temporarily occlude the tracheostomy. Plastic uncuffed tubes are now available, some with disposable inner cannulae, both with and without 'fenestrations'. In some cases a cuffed fenestrated tube with inner cannula may be preferred as a means of protecting the airway while allowing the patient to speak intermittently. Various tracheal 'buttons' are also available to maintain patency of the tracheostomy and provide a route for endotracheal suction. In an attempt to enable mechanically ventilated patients to phonate with the cuff inflated, tracheostomy tubes are available that incorporate an additional small lumen, which allows a separate gas flow to be diverted through the larynx.

Management

Tracheostomy tubes must be securely fixed, a dry dressing is used and the wound cleaned with saline. Wound swabs should be cultured regularly. The tube is left in place for 7 days and then changed every 4–7 days, depending on local policy. Emergency equipment must always be available at the bedside and should include a tracheostomy tube of the same size and one size smaller as well as a tracheal dilator.

Complications

Because a tracheostomy tube is merely a short endotracheal tube inserted via the neck, the complications of intubation occurring below the level of the glottis are common to both. There are, however, certain additional complications peculiar to tracheostomy.

EARLY

The tracheostomy tube is easily *misplaced* in the pretracheal subcutaneous tissue, particularly during emergency reinsertion in the early postoperative period. This danger may be minimized by using a Bjork flap. The tube may *obstruct* if tilted, and *leaks* around the cuff can give rise to *surgical emphysema. Pneumothorax, pneumomediastinum* and *perioperative haemorrhage* are other well-recognized complications (Stauffer *et al.*, 1981).

INTERMEDIATE

As with endotracheal intubation, ulceration of the tracheal mucosa may occur at the level of the cuff and because a tracheostomy tube is prone to tilting, the mucosa may also be damaged by the tip of the tube. Erosion of the tracheal cartilages and neighbouring structures may lead to fatal *haemorrhage* from the innominate artery or to a *tracheo-oesophageal fistula*.

Tracheostomy wounds are usually colonized with resident bacteria which are often resistant to the commonly used antibiotics. Sometimes these are responsible for serious *infection*, particularly of sternotomy wounds in those who have undergone cardiac surgery.

LATE

Tracheal *stenosis* may occur at the level of the stoma, the cuff or the tip of the tube; sometimes, the *tracheal rings collapse* at stomal level, a tracheal granuloma may develop or there may be a *persistent sinus* at the tracheostomy stoma. The incidence of these complications may be decreased by preserving as much tracheal cartilage as possible at operation, correct positioning of the tube and minimizing movement of the tube relative to the trachea.

These complications are particularly serious in paediatric patients in whom tracheostomy should be avoided if possible. Uncuffed tracheostomy tubes must always be used before puberty.

DECANNULATION

Following removal of the tracheostomy tube the stoma should be covered by a dry occlusive dressing and allowed to heal spontaneously. This usually occurs rapidly and within one or two days re-insertion of a similar-sized tracheostomy tube is likely to be extremely difficult.

REFERENCES

Al-Saady NM (1994) Does dietary manipulation influence weaning from artificial ventilation? *Intensive Care Medicine* **20**: 463–465.

Al-Saady N & Bennett ED (1985) Decelerating inspiratory flow waveform improves lung mechanics and gas exchange in patients on intermittent positive-pressure ventilation. *Intensive Care Medicine* **11**: 68–75.

Amos RJ, Amess JAL, Hinds CJ & Mollin DL (1982) Incidence and pathogenesis of acute megaloblastic bone marrow change in patients receiving intensive care. *Lancet* **ii**: 835–838.

Ashbaugh DG & Petty TL (1973) Positive end-expiratory pressure. Physiology indications and contraindications. *Journal of Thoracic and Cardiovascular Surgery* **65**: 165–170.

Bach A, Boehrer H, Schmidt H & Geiss HK (1992) Nosocomial sinusitis in ventilated patients. Nasotracheal versus orotracheal intubation. *Anaesthesia* **47**: 335–339.

Baile EM, Albert RK, Kirk W, Lakshaminarayan S, Wiggs BJR & Pare PD (1984) Positive end-expiratory pressure decreases bronchial blood flow in the dog. *Journal of Applied Physiology* **56**: 1289–1293.

Bersten AD, Holt AW, Vedig AE, Skowronski GA & Baggoley CJ (1991) Treatment of severe cardiogenic pulmonary edema with continuous positive airway pressure delivered by face mask. *New England Journal of Medicine* **325**: 1825–1830.

Beyer J, Beckenlechner P & Messmer K (1982) The influence of PEEP ventilation on organ blood flow and peripheral oxygen delivery. *Intensive Care Medicine* **8**: 75–80.

Bjorneboe M, Ibsen B, Astrup P *et al.* (1955) Active ventilation in treatment of respiratory acidosis in chronic diseases of the lungs. *Lancet* **ii**: 901–903.

Bodenham A, Diament R, Cohen A & Webster H (1991) Percutaneous dilatational tracheostomy. A bedside procedure on the intensive care unit. *Anaesthesia* **46**: 570–572.

Brochard L, Pluskwa F & Lemaire F (1987) Improved efficacy of spontaneous breathing with inspiratory pressure support. *American Review of Respiratory Disease* **136**: 411–415.

Brochard L, Harf A, Lorino H & Lemaire F (1989) Inspiratory pressure support prevents diaphragmatic fatigue during weaning from mechanical ventilation. *American Review of Respiratory Disease* **139**: 513–521.

Brochard L, Isabey D, Piquet J et al. (1990) Reversal of acute exacerbations of chronic obstructive lung disease by inspiratory assistance with face mask. *New England Journal of Medicine* **323**: 1523–1530.

Brochard L, Rauss A, Benito S et al. (1994) Comparison of three methods of gradual withdrawal from ventilatory support during weaning from mechanical ventilation. *American Journal of Respiratory Critical Care Medicine* **150**: 896–903.

Coakley JH, Nagendran K, Honavar M & Hinds CJ (1993) Preliminary observations on the neuromuscular abnormalities in patients with organ failure and sepsis. *Intensive Care Medicine* **19**: 323–328.

Cole AGH, Weller SF & Sykes MK (1984) Inverse ratio ventilation compared with PEEP in adult respiratory failure. *Intensive Care Medicine* **10**: 227–232.

Cox D & Niblett DJ (1984) Studies on continuous positive airway pressure breathing systems. *British Journal of Anaesthesia* **56**: 905–911.

Derderian SS, Rajagopal KR & Abbrecht PH et al. (1982) High frequency positive pressure jet ventilation in bilateral bronchopleural fistulae. *Critical Care Medicine* **10**: 119–121.

Douglass JA, Tuxen DV, Horne M, Scheinkestel CD, Weinmann M, Czarny D & Bowes G (1992) Myopathy in severe asthma. *American Review of Respiratory Disease* **146**: 517–519.

Downs JB, Klein EF Jr, Desautels D, Modell JH & Kirby RR (1973) Intermittent mandatory ventilation: a new approach to weaning patients from mechanical ventilators. *Chest* **64**: 331–335.

Dreyfuss D, Soler P, Basset G & Saumon G (1988) High inflation pressure pulmonary edema. Respective effects of high airway pressure, high tidal volume, and positive end-expiratory pressure. *American Review of Respiratory Disease* **137**: 1159–1164.

Duncan SR, Rizk NW & Raffin TA (1987) Inverse ratio ventilation. PEEP in disguise? *Chest* **92**: 390–391 (Editorial).

Editorial (1981) Artificial ventilation and the heart. *British Medical Journal* **283**: 397–398.

Editorial (1991) High-frequency ventilation. *Lancet* **337**: 706–708.

Elliott MW, Steven MH, Phillips GD & Branthwaite MA (1990) Non-invasive mechanical ventilation for acute respiratory failure. *British Medical Journal* **300**: 358–360.

Fagon J-Y, Chastre J, Domart Y et al. (1989) Nosocomial pneumonia in patients receiving continuous mechanical ventilation. *American Review of Respiratory Disease* **139**: 877–884.

Feeley TW & Hedley-Whyte J (1975) Weaning from controlled ventilation and supplemental oxygen. *New England Journal of Medicine* **292**: 903–906.

Feeley TW, Saumarez R, Klick JM, McNabb TG & Skillman JJ (1975) Positive end-expiratory pressure in weaning patients from controlled ventilation. A prospective randomised trial. *Lancet* **ii**: 725–729.

Fisher MMcD & Raper RF (1992) The 'cuff-leak' test for extubation. *Anaesthesia* **47**: 10–12.

Gallagher J, Strangeways JEM & Ault-Graham J (1987) Contamination control in long-term ventilation. A clinical study using a heat and moisture exchanging filter. *Anaesthesia* **42**: 476–481.

Gattinoni L, Agostoni, A, Pesenti A, et al. (1980) Treatment of acute respiratory failure with low-frequency positive-pressure ventilation and extracorporeal removal of CO_2. *Lancet* **ii**: 292–294.

Gorson KC & Ropper AH (1993) Acute respiratory failure neuropathy: a variant of critical illness neuropathy. *Critical Care Medicine* **21**: 267–271.

Greenbaum DM, Millen JE, Eross B et al. (1976) Continuous positive airway pressure without tracheal intubation in spontaneously breathing patients. *Chest* **69**: 615–620.

Grillo HC, Cooper JD, Geffin B & Pontoppidan H (1971) A low-pressure cuff for tracheostomy tubes to minimize tracheal injury. A comparative clinical trial. *Journal of Thoracic and Cardiovascular Surgery* **62**: 898–907.

Hewlett AM, Platt AS & Terry VG (1977) Mandatory minute volume. A new concept in weaning from mechanical ventilation. *Anaesthesia* **32**: 163–169.

Hillman KM & Barber JD (1980) Asynchronous independent lung ventilation (AILV). *Critical Care Medicine* **8**: 390–395.

Holliday JE & Hyers TM (1990) The reduction of weaning time from mechanical ventilation using tidal volume and relaxation biofeedback. *American Review of Respiratory Disease* **141**: 1214–1220.

Hurst JM, Branson RD, Davis K Jr, Barrette RR & Adams KS (1990) Comparison of conventional mechanical ventilation and high-frequency ventilation. *Annals of Surgery* **211**: 486–491.

Jardin F, Farcot J-C, Boisante L et al. (1981) Influence of positive end-expiratory pressure on left ventricular performance. *New England Journal of Medicine* **304**: 387–392.

Katz JA & Marks JD (1985) Inspiratory work with and without continuous positive airway pressure in patients with acute respiratory failure. *Anesthesiology* **63**: 598–607.

Klain M, Keszler H & Stool S (1983) Transtracheal high frequency jet ventilation prevents aspiration. *Critical Care Medicine* **11**: 170–172.

Kolobow T, Moretti MP, Fumagalli R et al. (1987) Severe impairment in lung function induced by high peak airway pressure during mechanical ventilation. An experimental study. *American Review of Respiratory Disease* **135**: 312–315.

Kreiger BP, Ershowsky PF, Becker DA & Gazeroglu HB (1989) Evaluation of conventional criteria for predicting successful weaning from mechanical ventilatory support in elderly patients. *Critical Care Medicine* **17**: 858–861.

Kumar A, Falke KJ, Geffin B et al. (1970) Continuous positive-pressure ventilation in acute respiratory failure: effects on hemodynamics and lung function. *New England Journal of Medicine* **283**: 1430–1436.

Lassen HCA (1953) A preliminary report on the 1952 epidemic of poliomyelitis in Copenhagen with special reference to the treatment of acute respiratory insufficiency. *Lancet* **i**: 37–41.

Leithner C, Frass M, Pacher R, Hartter E, Pesl H & Woloszczuk W (1987) Mechanical ventilation with positive end-expiratory pressure decreases release of alpha-arterial natriuretic peptide. *Critical Care Medicine* **15**: 484-488.

Leverment JN, Pearson FG & Rae S (1975) Tracheal size following tracheostomy with cuffed tracheostomy tubes: an experimental study. *Thorax* **30**: 271-277.

Lindholm CE & Grenwick A (1977) Flexible fibreoptic bronchoscopy and intubation in intensive care. In Ledingham IMCA (ed.) *Recent Advances in Intensive Therapy 1*, Edinburgh: Churchill Livingstone, pp. 47-66.

Marini JJ (1991) Weaning from mechanical ventilation. *New England Journal of Medicine* **324**: 1496-1498 (Editorial).

Mathru M, Rao TLK & Venus B (1983) Ventilator-induced barotrauma in controlled mechanical ventilation versus intermittent mandatory ventilation. *Critical Care Medicine* **11**: 359-361.

Meduri GU, Abou-Shala N, Fox RC, Jones CB, Leeper KV & Wunderink RG (1991) Noninvasive face mask mechanical ventilation in patients with acute hypercapnic respiratory failure. *Chest* **100**: 445-454.

Miller WC, Rice DL, Unger KM & Bradley BL (1981) Effect of PEEP on lung water content in experimental noncardiogenic pulmonary edema. *Critical Care Medicine* **9**: 7-9.

Montgomery AB, Holle RH, Neagley SR, Pierson DJ & Schoene RB (1987) Prediction of successful ventilator weaning using airway occlusion pressure and hypercapnic challenge. *Chest* **91**: 496-499.

Navaratnarajah M, Nunn JF, Lyons D & Milledge JS (1984) Bronchiolectasis caused by positive end-expiratory pressure. *Critical Care Medicine* **12**: 1036-1038.

Parker JC, Hernandez LA & Peevy KJ (1993) Mechanisms of ventilator-induced lung injury. *Critical Care Medicine* **21**: 131-143.

Payen DM, Farge D, Beloucif S, Leisel F, De La Coussaye JE, Carli P & Wirquin V (1987) Involvement of antidiuretic hormone in acute antidiuresis during PEEP ventilation in humans. *Anaesthesiology* **66**: 17-23.

Pepe PE, Hudson LD & Carrico CJ (1984) Early application of positive end-expiratory pressure in patients at risk for the adult respiratory distress syndrome. *New England Journal of Medicine* **311**: 281-286.

Petrof BJ, Legare M, Goldberg P, Milic-Emili J & Gottfried SB (1990) Continuous positive airway pressure reduces work of breathing and dyspnea during weaning from mechanical ventilation in severe chronic obstructive pulmonary disease. *American Review of Respiratory Disease* **141**: 281-289.

Petty TL (1981) Why (not) try PEEP? *Critical Care Medicine* **9**: 67-68 (Editorial).

Qvist J, Pontoppidan H, Wilson RS, Lowenstein E & Laver MB (1975) Hemodynamic responses to mechanical ventilation with PEEP: the effect of hypervolemia. *Anesthesiology* **42**: 45-55.

Rohfling BM, Webb WR & Schlobohm RM (1976) Ventilator-related extra-alveolar air in adults. *Radiology* **121**: 25-31.

Ryan DW (1990) Minitracheostomy. *British Medical Journal* **300**: 958-959.

Sahn SA & Lakshminarayan S (1973) Bedside criteria for discontinuation of mechanical ventilation. *Chest* **63**: 1002-1005.

Schulman DS, Biondi JW, Matthay RA, Barash PG, Zaret B & Soufer R (1988) Effect of positive end-expiratory pressure on right ventricular performance. Importance of baseline right ventricular function. *American Journal of Medicine* **84**: 57-67.

Schuster DP, Klain M & Snyder JV (1982) Comparison of high frequency jet ventilation to conventional ventilation during severe acute respiratory failure in humans. *Critical Care Medicine* **10**: 625-630.

Segredo V, Caldwell JE, Matthay MA, Sharma ML, Gruenke LD & Miller RD (1992) Persistent paralysis in critically ill patients after long-term administration of vecuronium. *New England Journal of Medicine* **327**: 524-528.

Sha M, Saito Y, Yokoyama K, Sawa T & Amaha K (1987) Effects of continuous positive-pressure ventilation on hepatic blood flow and intrahepatic oxygen delivery in dogs. *Critical Care Medicine* **15**: 1040-1043.

Simonneau G, Lemaire F, Harf A, Carlet J & Teisseire B (1982) A comparative study of the cardiorespiratory effects of continuous positive airway pressure breathing and continuous positive pressure ventilation in acute respiratory failure. *Intensive Care Medicine* **8**: 61-67.

Singer M & Bennett D (1989) Optimisation of positive end expiratory pressure for maximal delivery of oxygen to tissues using oesophageal Doppler ultrasonography. *British Medical Journal* **298**: 1350-1353.

Skillman JJ, Malhotra IV, Pallotta JA & Bushnell LS (1971) Determinants of weaning from controlled ventilation. *Surgical Forum* **22**: 198-200.

Skoyles J & Pepperman M (1993) IVOX. *British Journal of Anaesthesia* **70**: 603-604.

Sladen A, Guntupalli K & Klain M (1984) High-frequency jet ventilation versus intermittent positive-pressure ventilation. *Critical Care Medicine* **12**: 788-790.

Slavin G, Nunn JF, Crow J & Dore CJ (1982) Bronchiolectasis— a complication of artificial ventilation. *British Medical Journal* **285**: 931-934.

Smith TC & Marini JJ (1988) Impact of PEEP on lung mechanics and work of breathing in severe airflow obstruction. *Journal of Applied Physiology* **65**: 1488-1499.

Stauffer JL, Olson DE & Petty TL (1981) Complications and consequences of endotracheal intubation and tracheotomy. *American Journal of Medicine* **70**: 65-76.

Steinhoff HH, Kohlhoff RJ & Falke KJ (1984) Facilitation of renal function by intermittent mandatory ventilation. *Intensive Care Medicine* **10**: 59-65.

Teba L, Dedhia H, Schiebel FG, Blehschmidt NG & Linder WJ (1990) Postive-pressure ventilation with positive end-expiratory pressure and atrial natriuretic peptide release. *Critical Care Medicine* **18**: 831-835.

Tharrat RS, Allen RP & Albertson TE (1988) Pressure controlled inverse ratio ventilation in severe adult respiratory failure. *Chest* **94**: 755-762.

Torres A, Aznar R, Gatell JM, Jimenez P, Gonzalez J, Ferrer A, Celis R & Rodriguez-Rosin R (1990) Incidence, risk and prognosis factors of nosocomial pneumonia in mechanically ventilated patients. *American Review of Respiratory Disease* **142**: 523-528.

Venus B, Jacobs HK & Lim L (1979) Treatment of the adult respiratory distress syndrome with continuous positive airway pressure. *Chest* **76**: 257-261.

Vincken W & Cosio MG (1984) Clinical applications of high-frequency jet ventilation. *Intensive Care Medicine* **10**: 275-280.

Weigelt JA, Mitchell RA & Snyder WH 3rd (1979) Early positive end-expiratory pressure in the adult respiratory distress syndrome. *Archives of Surgery* **114**: 497-501.

Weisman LM, Rinaldo JE, Rogers RM & Sanders MH (1983) Intermittent mandatory ventilation. *American Review of Respiratory Disease* **127**: 641-647.

Yang KL & Tobin MJ (1991) A prospective study of indexes predicting the outcome of trials of weaning from mechanical ventilation. *New England Journal of Medicine* **324**: 1445-1450.

Zapol WM, Snider MT, Hill JD *et al.* (1979) Extracorporeal membrane oxygenation in severe acute respiratory failure. A randomized prospective study. *Journal of the American Medical Association* **242**: 2193-2196.

8 Cardiopulmonary Resuscitation and Management of Arrhythmias

The commonest cause of cardiac arrest and life-threatening arrhythmias is ischaemic heart disease; in the UK approximately 160,000 deaths occur each year as a result of coronary artery disease while in the United States the annual mortality from this condition is in excess of 650,000. Recognized risk factors include increasing age, smoking, hypertension, high serum lipid levels, diabetes and familial predisposition. Men are affected three to four times more frequently than women, and coronary disease seems to be more common among lower social classes.

CARDIORESPIRATORY ARREST

Diagnosis

Cardiorespiratory arrest is diagnosed clinically. The patient rapidly loses consciousness, becoming unresponsive and lifeless with absent pulsation in the major vessels (carotid and femoral arteries). Heart sounds cannot be heard and respiratory efforts are absent or gasping. The pupils soon dilate and become unresponsive to light. It may be difficult to determine whether the primary event was a respiratory or a cardiac arrest, although if a history can be obtained, this may suggest the likely sequence of events. When the primary aetiology is respiratory, profound bradycardia and cyanosis often precede cardiac arrest.

Treatment (Chamberlain, 1989; Niemann, 1992; Wardrope & Morris, 1993)

Having established the diagnosis it is vital to *call for assistance* since it is virtually impossible to perform adequate resuscitation unaided. *Basic cardiac life support* (European Resuscitation Council, 1993a) should start at once. When the collapse is witnessed in hospital, however, and provided a defibrillator is readily available a *precordial thump* (Robertson, 1992) can be delivered; this can be followed by defibrillation if unsuccessful. The pulse should then be checked again before starting basic life support with chest compressions and assisted ventilation. The rationale for this recommendation is that immediately following collapse due to unheralded ventricular fibrillation the lungs and arterial blood are likely to contain a sufficient reservoir of oxygen and the most urgent priority is therefore to restore the circulation.

AIRWAY AND RESPIRATION

The first priority is to establish a *clear airway*. The oropharynx must be cleared of false teeth, vomit, blood and other debris before flexing the neck, extending the head and inserting an oropharyngeal airway. The patient should then be *ventilated* with added *oxygen* at a rate of approximately 12 breaths/min using a face mask and a self-inflating bag. A pocket mask, such as that manufactured by Laerdal, with expired air respiration (**Fig. 8.1**) may be easier to use than the more familiar bag-and-mask technique, especially for one-person resuscitation.

Whichever method is used, it is important to ensure that the chest expands with each insufflation. If it proves impossible to achieve adequate ventilation using any of these methods, then *endotracheal intubation* may be required, although this should normally only be attempted by those experienced in the technique. Prolonged attempts at intubation by unskilled personnel waste valuable time, may exacerbate hypoxia and hypercarbia and can cause structural damage. Nevertheless, the trachea should be intubated as soon as skilled assistance arrives since this secures the airway, ensures effective positive pressure ventilation and protects the lungs from aspiration of stomach contents.

Despite immediate vigorous manual ventilation, *respiratory acidosis* is common during cardiopulmonary resuscitation (CPR) and this may be compounded by the administration of sodium bicarbonate, which generates carbon dioxide. This impairs cerebral autoregulation and may exacerbate ischaemic brain injury. *Hypoxia* is also common during CPR and is probably largely a result of collapse of distal lung units caused by chest compression, combined with reduced lung perfusion. Arterial hypoxaemia is further exacerbated by the fall in mixed venous arterial oxygen tension ($P_v O_2$) caused by

(a)   **(b)**

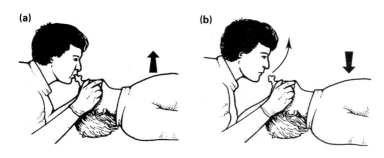

Fig. 8.1 Mask–mouth ventilation. (a) open airway, blow slowly into mouth piece observing chest inflation; (b) allow patient to exhale passively.

poor tissue perfusion (Weil *et al.*, 1986). Finally, lung function may be further compromised during CPR by pre-existing cardiac failure or lung disease and by aspiration of gastric contents. In some circumstances, the application of positive end-expiratory pressure (PEEP) during CPR might be expected to improve oxygenation, and although often associated with a reduction in cardiac output (see Chapter 7), could actually enhance forward flow by further augmenting the overall rise in intrathoracic pressure.

CARDIAC MASSAGE

External cardiac massage

Effective external cardiac massage (ECM) can only be performed on a *hard surface*. This may be provided by an intensive care or coronary care unit bed, a board placed under the mattress or, failing either of these, by placing the patient on the floor. *Chest compression* must be achieved using a vertical force in the midline. A downward pressure should be delivered with a rhythmic rather than a jerky action using straight arms, with the heel of the hand placed on the lower half of the patient's sternum. The sternum should be depressed to a depth of 1.5–2 in. keeping the fingers away from the chest wall. There should be *15 compressions for every two inflations for a single attendant* or *five compressions to one inflation where two rescuers are present*.

Once effective cardiac massage and artificial ventilation have been established, the patient's colour should improve, the pupils may return to normal size, there will be a palpable pulse (although this does not necessarily indicate adequate flow, merely that the pressure wave has been transmitted along a patent fluid-filled vessel), and the conscious level may improve (head shaking, grimacing). At this stage, an *ECG monitor* should be attached to the patient if one is not already in place, and more specific treatment should be instituted.

Mechanisms by which ECM produces forward flow (Robertson & Holmberg, 1992). It was originally suggested that forward flow through the aortic and pulmonary valves was produced by direct compression of the heart between sternum and spine, which elevated intraventricular pressures above those in the great vessels. Cyclical release of sternal pressure allowed chest recoil, reducing intrathoracic pressure and encouraging venous return, while reflux of blood into the aorta and pulmonary artery was prevented by the one-way valves. Later, however, measurement of intravascular pressures in dogs receiving CPR demonstrated, as some had already suspected, that ECM produced simultaneous and equal pressure increases in both central venous and arterial vessels (Rudikoff *et al.*, 1980). Moreover, the rises in intrathoracic pressure were transmitted fully to the carotid artery, but only minimally to the jugular vein, creating a peripheral arteriovenous pressure gradient and antegrade flow. Angiographic studies have shown that aortic flow is produced initially by direct compression of this vessel, and that this is followed by delayed, but simultaneous, opening of the mitral and aortic valves. Flow through the heart persists throughout the period of cardiac compression, and for this reason, ECM is most effective when sternal depression is sustained. In fact, lung inflation alone can produce some forward flow, and simultaneous external cardiac compression and positive pressure ventilation produces greater rises in aortic systolic pressure, thereby enhancing forward flow (Rudikoff *et al.*, 1980). During ECM, backward flow is prevented by competent aortic, mitral, pulmonary and tricuspid valves, while transmission of the pressure wave to the venous system is minimized by collapse of the great veins and by valves situated at the thoracic inlet (Rudikoff *et al.*, 1980; Mair *et al.*, 1993). The latter probably close when intrathoracic pressure increases rapidly (e.g. during coughing), but remain patent when the increase in pressure is more gradual (e.g. in cardiac failure).

Therefore, the whole thorax performs as a pump during ECM with flow from intra- to extrathoracic vessels, the heart and lungs acting as a single one-way reservoir of blood. During chest compression, blood is expelled from the thorax into patent arteries and during this phase retrograde venous flow is minimized by the presence of valves and by venous collapse at high intrathoracic pressures. Venous return occurs during chest recoil and may be augmented by newer methods of cardiopulmonary resuscitation that provide active decompression, using a hand-held suction device (Cohen *et al.*, 1992). Other recent developments include the use of a pneumatic vest to achieve circumferential chest compression; this technique augments aortic and coronary perfusion pressures and may increase the likelihood of the return of spontaneous circulation (Halperin *et al.*, 1993). The cardiac output achieved in this way is, however, probably still only a fraction of normal values.

Although clinical assessment of the efficacy of CPR is extremely difficult it has been suggested that measurement of the *end-tidal carbon dioxide concentration* may be a suitable means of monitoring blood flow generated by precordial compression (Falk *et al.*, 1988; Higgins *et al.*, 1990).

Complications of external cardiac massage include:

- traumatic injury to the abdominal viscera (in particular rupture of the liver and spleen);
- damage to the myocardium;
- chest wall injury;
- pulmonary aspiration;
- impaired lung function.

In one study, *rib fractures* were seen in 34% of those who had received CPR, while *myocardial contusion* occurred in 1.3% and *haemopericardium* in 8.1%. *Aspiration pneumonia* was seen in 1.3% (Nagel *et al.*, 1981).

Internal cardiac massage

Open chest cardiac compression produces a radically different haemodynamic response to ECM since antegrade blood flow is achieved by direct ventricular compression. Between 1950 and 1960 open chest cardiac compression became a routine procedure, access to the heart being gained through a standard left thoracotomy, by a subdiaphragmatic approach or via a median sternotomy. Following the description of closed chest cardiac compression, internal cardiac massage was rapidly and almost completely abandoned (except following cardiac surgery) even though various studies (Del Guercio *et al.*, 1965; Bircher & Safer, 1984; Sanders *et al.*, 1984) have demonstrated that the open technique is associated with better forward flow, improved coronary perfusion and well-maintained cerebral blood flow. In addition, in cases of suspected intrathoracic trauma, thoracotomy can facilitate the diagnosis and treatment of some of the

common reversible causes for cardiac arrest such as pericardial tamponade, tension pneumothorax and hidden intrathoracic bleeding.

Despite these advantages, open chest cardiac compression is currently rarely used outside the operating theatre. It may, however, still be preferred in those with profound hypothermia following drowning or in the younger patient with cardiac arrest complicating status asthmaticus. It may also be useful when ECM is ineffective.

INTRAVENOUS ACCESS ISOFORMS OF (Hapnes & Robertson, 1992)

Expansion of the circulating volume is generally not required during CPR, but powerful vasoconstrictors must be given into a large vein to ensure rapid delivery to the myocardium. The peripheral veins may be collapsed and difficult to cannulate and it may be necessary to use the *internal jugular vein. Intratracheal instillation* of drugs has been recommended as an alternative when venous cannulation proves difficult, and even as an immediate measure before intravascular access is established. Some, however, consider this route to be unreliable (McCrirrick & Monk, 1994).

In children an *intraosseus infusion device* inserted into the tibia may also prove life-saving (Glaeser *et al.*, 1993).

Management of life-threatening arrhythmias and electromechanical dissociation (European Resuscitation Council, 1993b)

VENTRICULAR FIBRILLATION AND PULSELESS VENTRICULAR TACHYCARDIA

Ventricular fibrillation (VF) and pulseless ventricular tachycardia (VT) (**Fig. 8.2**) are most easily terminated

(a)

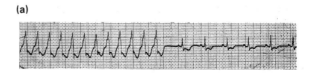

(b)

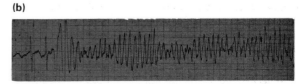

Fig. 8.2 (a) Ventricular tachycardia terminating spontaneously. (b) Ventricular fibrillation.

by delivering a *DC shock* with minimal delay (**Fig. 8.3**). The paddles of the defibrillator should be positioned so as to enclose as much ventricular muscle as possible, but should avoid contact with monitoring electrodes, the nipples, glyceryl trinitrate (GTN) patches and permanent pacemaker generators. The first three shocks should be delivered as quickly as possible, with an intervening pause sufficient only to confirm that the rhythm is still VF or pulseless VT, and to recharge; then reapply the defibrillator. It is recommended that the energy delivered by the first two shocks should be 200 J since if the first shock fails to terminate VF the reduction in tissue impedance will allow a greater current flow for the same delivered energy during the second shock.

If three promptly administered DC shocks (the third at 360 J) fail to restore a coordinated rhythm, prolonged CPR is likely to be required. At this stage the patient's trachea should be intubated, positive pressure ventilation should commence, intravenous access should be secured and emergency drugs should be prepared.

The drug of first choice is *adrenaline* 1 mg (Lindner & Koster, 1992) given into the central circulation if possible. Ten sequences of five compressions to one ventilation are then completed before a further set of three DC shocks, all at 360 J. If VF remains refractory, the loop is repeated, each time including intravenous adrenaline 1 mg or, alternatively adrenaline 2 mg via the endotracheal tube.

After every three loops the administration of an *alkalizing agent* (e.g. 8.4% sodium bicarbonate 50 ml intravenously) is considered, as is the use of *antiarrhythmic agents* (lignocaine, bretylium or amiodarone).

Traditionally, a bolus dose of 100 mg *lignocaine* is administered intravenously, followed if necessary by a continuous infusion at a rate of 1-3 mg/min. If necessary, the bolus can be repeated, provided that a total dose of 3 mg/kg is not exceeded. The main value of lignocaine lies in its ability to prevent ventricular arrhythmias; its role in assisting defibrillation is less clear. Some authorities therefore recommend the use of intravenous *bretylium tosylate* in refractory VF since this raises the fibrillation threshold. It should be administered as a bolus of 5-10 mg/kg, which can be repeated after 30-60 minutes and continued as an infusion. Bretylium can produce hypotension and vasodilatation, but does not appear to depress myocardial contractility (Bexton & Camm, 1982). In some cases, *β-blockade*, which also raises the fibrillation threshold, or *mexiletine*, which has a profile similar to lignocaine, but is less negatively inotropic, may be indicated. *Amiodarone* is a very powerful antiarrhythmic, useful against both supraventricular and ventricular tachycardias, and can be used to prevent recurrence of VT or VF (Bexton & Camm, 1982). Although intravenous administration may precipitate hypotension, many now prefer amiodarone

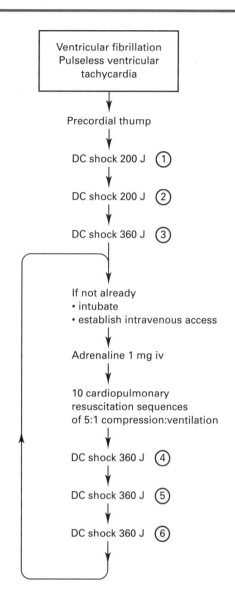

Notes: (i) The interval between shocks 3 and 4 should not be more than two mins.
(ii) Adrenaline given during the loop approximately every 2 – 3 mins.
(iii) Continue loops for as long as defibrillation is indicated.
(iv) After three loops consider:
   ● an alkalizing agent
   ● an antiarrhythmic agent.

Fig. 8.3 Treatment algorithm for ventricular fibrillation and pulseless ventricular tachycardia. Reproduced with the kind permission of the European Resuscitation Council. Originally published in the *BMJ* (1993) **306**, 1587–1589, 1589–1593, ©1993 BMJ Publishing

to bretylium for the treatment of refractory VF/VT. A bolus dose of 300 mg can be followed by a continuous infusion of 1200 mg/24 hours.

Persistent ventricular arrhythmias may be related to:

- hypokalaemia;
- hypoxia;
- acidosis or alkalosis;
- hyperosmolar syndrome;
- alterations in plasma levels of magnesium or calcium;
- myocardial failure.

ASYSTOLE

Electrical activity is absent in association with clinical cardiac arrest. Malfunction of the ECG monitor must be excluded. It is also important to consider whether the apparent asystole is in fact VF. If this possibility cannot be excluded, then the VF treatment algorithm (see **Fig. 8.3**) should be followed.

For confirmed asystole immediate *tracheal intubation* and *manual ventilation with oxygen* are mandatory since in a few cases this may prove sufficient to restart the heart. Otherwise drug therapy (**Fig. 8.4**) comprises first, *adrenaline* 1 mg intravenously (or 2 mg via the endotracheal tube) and then a single dose of *atropine* 3 mg intravenously (or 6 mg via the endotracheal tube). *Transthoracic external pacing* is very occasionally effective in those with some residual electrical activity and can be used while a transvenous pacing system is established. In the absence of electrical activity, further loops of 1 mg adrenaline and continued CPR are recommended.

ELECTROMECHANICAL DISSOCIATION

Electromechanical dissociation (EMD) is a clinical condition in which there is no cardiac output in spite of ordered ventricular electrical activity. This may be *primary* when the myocardium fails to contract adequately in response to electrical stimulation, or *secondary* when the loss of forward flow is due to mechanical problems such as:

- hypovolaemia;
- pneumothorax;
- cardiac tamponade or acute rupture of the heart;
- pulmonary embolism.

Hypothermia, profound electrolyte disturbance and *drug overdose* may also be associated with EMD.

Specific therapies must be considered from the outset (**Fig. 8.5**), especially volume replacement for hypovolaemia, pericardial aspiration for tamponade and urgent drainage of a tension pneumothorax.

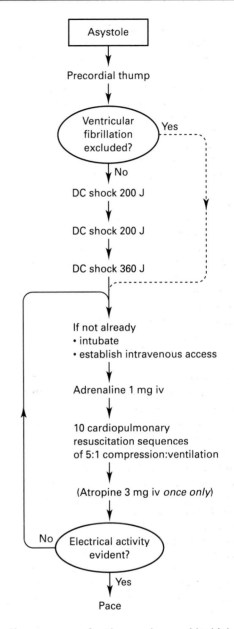

Note: If no response after three cycles consider high dose adrenaline: 5 mg iv.

Fig. 8.4 Treatment algorithm for asystole. Reproduced with the kind permission of the European Resuscitation Council. Originally published in the *BMJ* (1993) **306**, 1587–1589, 1589–1593, ©1993 BMJ Publishing

When there is no immediately obvious remediable cause, the drug of first choice is *adrenaline*. The dose is 1 mg given centrally if possible. A 5 mg dose of adrenaline may be considered if the arrest is prolonged. *Calcium chloride* is now only recommended for the treatment of EMD due to hyperkalaemia, hypocalcaemia

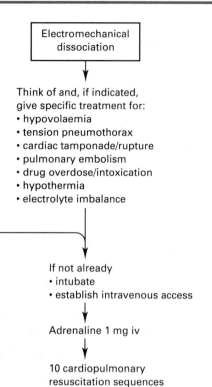

Think of and, if indicated, give specific treatment for:
• hypovolaemia
• tension pneumothorax
• cardiac tamponade/rupture
• pulmonary embolism
• drug overdose/intoxication
• hypothermia
• electrolyte imbalance

If not already
• intubate
• establish intravenous access

Adrenaline 1 mg iv

10 cardiopulmonary resuscitation sequences of 5:1 compression:ventilation

Consider: • Pressor agents
• Calcium
• Alkalizing agents
• Adrenaline 5 mg iv

Fig. 8.5 Treatment algorithm for electromechanical dissociation. Reproduced with the kind permission of the European Resuscitation Council. Originally published in the *BMJ* (1993) **306**, 1587–1589, 1589–1593, ©1993 BMJ Publishing

or an overdose of calcium-channel blocking drugs (Vincent, 1987).

CORRECTION OF ELECTROLYTE DISTURBANCES

Hyperkalaemia is relatively common during CPR, partly due to the release of potassium into the circulation from injured and/or hypoxic tissues. It should be treated with *calcium chloride, glucose and insulin mixtures,* and diuretics such as *frusemide*.

In some cases (e.g. following cardiac surgery) ventricular fibrillation or tachycardia may have been precipitated by *hypokalaemia or hypomagnesaemia* and this will require treatment with intravenous potassium chloride.

CORRECTION OF ACIDOSIS (Niemann, 1992)

Anaerobic metabolism during the period of poor tissue perfusion is associated with increased lactic acid production. Furthermore, metabolism of lactic acid by the liver is impaired by the reduction in hepatic blood flow, and during extreme ischaemia the liver itself contributes to lactate production. Nevertheless, since metabolic acidosis is only deleterious when extremely severe, the routine administration of large quantities of sodium bicarbonate during CPR is unnecessary, particularly following short periods of cardiorespiratory arrest, and may be dangerous. Potential adverse effects of excessive sodium bicarbonate administration include:

• hypernatraemia with an increased plasma osmolality;
• hypokalaemia;
• increased cardiac irritability;
• impaired myocardial performance;
• exacerbation of respiratory acidosis;
• increased affinity of haemoglobin for oxygen.

In addition, sympathomimetic agents may be inactivated when mixed with sodium bicarbonate.

As an approximation, about 0.5 mmol of sodium bicarbonate per litre of extracellular fluid (ECF) is required for each minute of CPR in order to neutralize the acidosis. It is therefore not necessary to administer sodium bicarbonate immediately unless the patient is known to have had a pre-existing acidosis (e.g. due to cardiogenic shock). Ideally, subsequent administration of alkali should be guided by frequent acid–base determinations (see Chapter 4).

POSTRESUSCITATION MANAGEMENT

A minority of patients will be resuscitated easily and quickly. They rapidly regain consciousness and resume spontaneous ventilation. They can be extubated immediately and further treatment is aimed at preventing a recurrence. Many of those who are successfully resuscitated, however, will initially remain unconscious, often with absent or inadequate spontaneous respiratory efforts and hypotension. In these cases, subsequent management is aimed at restoring cardiovascular and respiratory function and minimizing cerebral damage.

Respiratory function

The tracheal tube must be left in place until the patient is conscious and has effective cough, gag and swallowing reflexes. Later, some patients may require a tracheostomy. Mechanical ventilation is clearly indicated when respiratory function is impaired (e.g. in those with pulmonary oedema, aspiration pneumonitis or a significant flail segment). Furthermore, hyperventilation may improve cerebral autoregulation as well as reduce cerebral acidosis (see Chapter 14). Nevertheless, although it is universally accepted that *hypoxaemia and hypercarbia must be avoided* at all costs, the role of deliberate hyperventilation, and of prolonged (> 48 hours) controlled ventilation when respiratory function is adequate, remains unclear (Gisvold *et al.*, 1984a (see also Chapter 14)). A reasonable approach is to initiate controlled ventilation in all patients who have suffered a global ischaemic insult and to reassess the situation 4–6 hours later. Selected patients can then be allowed to breathe spontaneously.

Cardiovascular function

It is vital to ensure that cerebral and coronary blood flow are adequate following resuscitation and it is therefore essential to *restore the systemic blood pressure*. This requires manipulation of the circulating volume, guided by the central venous pressure (CVP) or pulmonary artery occlusion pressure (PAOP) as indicated and, if necessary, the administration of inotropic or vasopressor agents. Metabolic derangements and fluid and electrolyte disturbances must also be corrected. Intra-aortic balloon counterpulsation (IABCP) may be indicated in selected patients with cardiogenic shock or persistent myocardial ischaemia (see Chapter 4).

Cerebral function

Provided there is no pre-existing intracranial pathology (e.g. cerebrovascular disease) and cardiac arrest was not preceded by hypoxia, ischaemic brain damage can probably be prevented by maintaining a cerebral blood flow as low as one-seventh of normal. This can usually be achieved if CPR is correctly performed. Nevertheless, cerebral perfusion is not usually sufficient to sustain normal brain activity during CPR and patients may remain unconscious, sometimes with fixed dilated pupils, and yet recover normal cerebral function. Sometimes, signs of cerebral activity such as frowning, head shaking, struggling and an eyelash reflex may be present during CPR and these suggest that the brain is being adequately oxygenated.

If, however, resuscitation is protracted, cerebral function usually deteriorates progressively due to a gradual reduction in cerebral blood flow and persistent relative ischaemia. Furthermore, cerebral lactic acidosis, which is not corrected by the systemic administration of sodium bicarbonate, impairs autoregulation (the mean perfusion pressure during CPR is less than 50 mm Hg and is therefore below the lower limit for autoregulation) and depresses cerebral function.

The ultimate outcome for those patients who are successfully resuscitated could be considerably improved if it were possible to ameliorate the cerebral damage caused by cardiorespiratory arrest and protracted CPR. Clearly, this could be achieved if improved techniques of CPR were developed that maintained normal cerebral perfusion. It is also possible that events occurring during or after *reperfusion* may initiate or exacerbate cell damage (see Chapter 4) and that appropriate interventions might therefore limit the degree of brain damage.

CONTROL OF SEIZURES

Seizure discharges may exacerbate post-ischaemic cerebral damage by increasing metabolic demands and precipitating neuronal hypoxia in areas of marginally perfused brain. Moreover, sympathetic nervous activity is increased and this places an extra demand on the patient's limited cardiorespiratory reserve. It is therefore accepted that prophylactic administration of anticonvulsants and aggressive treatment of seizures, both of which are associated with minimal risks, is normally justified (Shapiro, 1984; Hinds, 1985) (see Chapter 14).

CEREBRAL PERFUSION

There is evidence that the degree of cerebral damage is influenced by the adequacy of cerebral perfusion following restoration of cardiac activity. Thus, it appears that the brain can recover from quite prolonged periods of normothermic relative ischaemia (up to 20 minutes) provided that cerebral blood flow is subsequently adequate.

Initially, systemic hypertension combined with the loss of autoregulation may cause cerebral hyperperfusion with oedema formation and disruption of the blood–brain barrier. Subsequently, however, hypoperfusion is nearly always the dominant abnormality. This is associated with prolonged severe depression of cerebral cortical blood flow and an increased cerebrovascular resistance. Possible explanations have included cellular swelling with raised intracranial pressure, intravascular coagulation, increases in viscosity, microvascular endothelial swelling and release of vasoactive metabolites of arachidonic acid such as thromboxane (see Chapter 4). It has also been suggested that cerebrovascular spasm may be caused by an influx of calcium ions into anoxic vascular smooth muscle (White *et al.*, 1983).

Based on these observations, suggested therapeutic interventions have included:

- anticoagulation;
- haemodilution with dextrans or oxygen-carrying blood substitutes;
- calcium antagonists;
- prostacyclin;
- diuretics;
- steroids;
- manipulation of the arachidonic acid cascade.

There is little evidence to support the use of steroids, diuretics or anticoagulants in this situation, and it appears that cerebral oedema is unusual following global brain ischaemia except in those who have sustained extensive neuronal damage incompatible with survival (Gisvold *et al.*, 1984a). Because autoregulation is impaired, the aim should be to achieve normotension or slight hypertension during the post-arrest period (Shapiro, 1984); extreme hypertension, which might exacerbate oedema formation and intracranial hypertension, should be avoided. The value of other measures remains uncertain.

METABOLIC FACTORS

It has been suggested that elevated brain glucose levels predispose to cerebral oedema and enhance lactic acid production by increasing the supply of substrate, thereby exacerbating neuronal damage. A number of experimental studies have in fact demonstrated that high blood glucose levels prior to cardiac arrest are associated with a worse neurological outcome (Pulsinelli *et al.*, 1982). The clinical implications of these findings are unclear, although it would seem sensible to avoid hyperglycaemia in high-risk situations.

BIOCHEMICAL ABNORMALITIES

The rapid depletion of cellular energy stores that follows sudden complete ischaemia leads to failure of the ionic pump, membrane depolarization and cellular swelling. There is also an accumulation of calcium ions within the cells. This may initiate a number of harmful reactions, including the release of free fatty acids, particularly arachidonic acid, and the production of free radicals of oxygen, and could be the 'final common pathway' leading to cell death.

The potential of *calcium entry blocking drugs* as cerebral protective agents has therefore been extensively investigated (White *et al.*, 1983). It was postulated that these agents might prevent cerebrovascular spasm and maintain cerebral blood flow as well as reduce the calcium-induced liberation of free fatty acids and radicals of oxygen. In a recent randomized clinical trial, however, the calcium channel blocker lidoflazine was

ineffective in reducing either mortality or brain damage after cardiac arrest (Brain Resuscitation Clinical Trial II Study Group 1991).

It has also been suggested that *barbiturates* might protect the brain from ischaemic damage by virtue of their 'free radical scavenging' activity. These agents also suppress brain metabolism, as well as reduce cerebral blood flow and intracranial pressure and may improve the cerebral oxygen supply/demand ratio. A number of early experimental studies suggested that barbiturate pretreatment and possibly early post-insult therapy might be beneficial in focal ischaemia. Later studies, however, have failed to confirm earlier work, which had indicated that barbiturates might be of value in experimental global brain ischaemia (Gisvold *et al.*, 1984b), and in a randomized clinical trial of thiopentone loading in comatose survivors of cardiac arrest there were no significant differences in outcome between treatment and control groups (Brain Resuscitation Clinical Trial I Study Group, 1986).

At present, therefore, the clinical use of barbiturates, other intravenous anaesthetic agents or calcium antagonists to ameliorate post-ischaemic cerebral damage cannot be justified. The role of other specific agents remains unclear. Although it seems likely that multiple therapeutic interventions will ultimately be required to achieve a significant beneficial effect, there is a danger that some treatments will counteract the effects of others (Shapiro, 1984). Furthermore, the timing of each intervention in relation to the episode of cardiorespiratory arrest will probably prove to be crucial.

Current management of patients following CPR is therefore based on supporting cardiorespiratory function to ensure optimum conditions for brain recovery (Saltuari & Marosi, 1994), and the only undisputed therapeutic principles are to:

- restore systemic blood pressure;
- ensure adequate oxygenation;
- avoid hypercapnia;
- abolish seizures.

Thrombolytic therapy

Thrombolysis should be considered for those in whom cardiac arrest was precipitated by myocardial infarction provided there are no contraindications **(Table 8.1)**. The safety of thrombolysis following CPR seems to depend on the duration of the resuscitation attempt, and successful resuscitation immediately following early defibrillation should not normally preclude thrombolytic therapy. On the other hand, it is generally accepted that thrombolysis is contraindicated if vigorous resuscitation has taken place, particularly when prolonged energetic ECM has been performed and when central venous or arterial cannulation has been necessary.

Table 8.1 Contraindications to thrombolysis.

Absolute contraindications

Active peptic ulceration or intestinal bleeding
Known bleeding diathesis
Pregnancy
Suspected aortic dissection
Diabetic haemorrhagic retinopathy
Recent head injury or known intracranial neoplasm
Recent trauma or surgery (within 1 week)
Cerebrovascular accident within 3 months
Patient unconscious

Relative contraindications

Significant liver dysfunction
Prolonged or traumatic cardiopulmonary resuscitation
Severe hypertension (blood pressure > 200/120 mm Hg)

CARDIORESPIRATORY ARREST ASSOCIATED WITH SPECIAL CIRCUMSTANCES

A number of conditions other than major cardiac arrhythmias can present with life-threatening disturbances of circulatory or respiratory function. This can often be suspected from the patient's immediate history or surroundings, but sometimes the underlying pathology is obscure. Airway protection, ventilation and circulatory support as previously described remain central to their treatment.

Primary respiratory arrest

In adults primary respiratory arrest is uncommon and is usually the result of:

- acute severe intracerebral event (e.g. intracranial haemorrhage);
- the effect of depressant drugs (e.g. opioids or tricyclic antidepressants);
- profound metabolic derangements;
- acute upper airway obstruction (e.g. asphyxiation in an eating place—'cafe coronary').

Initially cardiac output is maintained, but in the face of progressive hypoxaemia heart rate falls and myocardial contractility is impaired, culminating in asystole.

The diagnosis usually rests on the observation of an apnoeic and cyanosed patient with a palpable pulse. The essential requirement is to establish an airway and restore oxygenation, if necessary with tracheal intubation and assisted ventilation. If the patient is treated promptly, recovery of a satisfactory circulation may follow restoration of the airway and ventilatory support alone; in such cases the eventual outcome is usually determined by the underlying diagnosis. Chest compression and adrenaline administration will be required for the patient who remains pulseless.

Asthma and severe bronchospasm (see Chapter 6)

Asthmatic patients are vulnerable to episodes of severe lower airway narrowing and in the most serious cases profound hypoxia and exhaustion can lead to marked bradycardia followed by asystole. Support of ventilatory function is of paramount importance. Patients should be intubated and ventilated with 100% oxygen. Bilateral air entry should be confirmed clinically and the possibility of a complicating tension pneumothorax excluded. Profound bronchospasm and air trapping may necessitate external chest compression to reduce hyperinflation. In the younger patient, internal cardiac massage should be considered for cardiac arrest complicating life-threatening asthma.

Pulmonary embolism (see also Chapter 14) (see Chapter 4)

Massive pulmonary embolism characteristically causes circulatory arrest with a markedly elevated jugular venous pressure, deep cyanosis and an initial tachypnoea before spontaneous respiration ceases. Adrenaline should be administered early to reverse bradycardia, maintain systemic venous return and coronary perfusion, and augment right ventricular contraction. When pulmonary obstruction is severe, cardiac compression is ineffective and the patient remains suffused, pulseless and deeply cyanosed. If resuscitation fails to restore the circulation within a few minutes, continued CPR is futile. In successful cases the embolus is dispersed into distal vessels and as oxygenation improves pulmonary arterial pressure falls.

Anaphylaxis (see Chapter 4)

The airway should be opened, cleared and maintained. 100% oxygen should be administered using assisted ventilation if necessary. If an effective airway cannot be established and laryngeal oedema prevents orotracheal intubation, emergency cricothyroidotomy may prove necessary. If there is no detectable cardiac output, chest compressions should commence together with rapid volume expansion and administration of *adrenaline* (a slow intravenous injection of 0.1 mg every 1–3 minutes, the dose titrated against the response). *Antihistamines* (H$_1$-receptor antagonists) are commonly given by slow intravenous injection (e.g. chlorpheniramine 10 mg) together with intravenous *aminophylline* (250 mg over five minutes). *Hydrocortisone*, 200 mg, should also be administered intravenously.

Electrocution

Casualties may be struck by lightning or injured by domestic or industrial electricity. Lightning consists of direct current of an extremely high voltage. It may cause immediate asystole or VF, as well as inflict a severe primary injury on the central nervous system.

VF is the commonest initial arrhythmia and should be promptly treated by defibrillation. For other arrhythmias, standard protocols should be followed. After successful resuscitation, myoglobinuria may result from muscle damage. Intravenous fluid therapy and mannitol administration may maintain adequate urinary output (see Chapter 9). Electrical burns, compartment syndromes and other traumatic lesions may require later specialist surgical attention.

Resuscitation in late pregnancy (see also Chapter 17)

Circulatory arrest from a variety of acute conditions remains an important cause of maternal mortality. The causes of maternal cardiac arrest include:

- massive haemorrhage;
- pulmonary embolism;
- amniotic fluid embolism;
- placental abruption;
- eclampsia.

An obstetrician and a paediatrician should be involved at an early stage.

After clearing and opening the airway, early endotracheal intubation is recommended since gastric emptying is prolonged in pregnant women and there is an increased risk of regurgitation and pulmonary aspiration. In the later stages of pregnancy the diaphragm will be splinted by the large uterus and high inflation pressures may be required. To improve venous return and cardiac output it is vital that pressure on the inferior vena cava from the gravid uterus is relieved by placing sandbags, pillows or a purpose-made wedge under the patient's right side. Alternatively, the uterus can be moved to the left by manual displacement or the patient's right hip can be raised. Arrhythmias should be treated according to standard protocols. During epidural anaesthesia high levels of local anaesthetic may be present in the blood and lignocaine administration should therefore be avoided.

After five minutes of unsuccessful in-hospital resuscitation, emergency caesarean section is indicated to save the fetus and improve the mother's chances of survival. Surgery must be accompanied by uninterrupted CPR.

Miscellaneous causes of cardiac arrest

Collapse following drug overdose and poisoning is dealt with in Chapter 18. Cardiopulmonary arrest following near-drowning is discussed in Chapter 9 and hypothermia in Chapter 19.

PROGNOSIS OF CARDIORESPIRATORY ARREST

Not surprisingly, the results of CPR initiated in the community are inferior to those achieved within the hospital environment (Weaver, 1991), probably largely because of delays in initiating resuscitation combined with lack of skill and interruptions in CPR while the patient is moved. In particular, coma is more frequent in those who suffer a cardiorespiratory arrest outside hospital and the prognosis for cerebral recovery is closely related to the duration of unconsciousness.

Even within hospitals, organizational deficiencies and absent or malfunctioning equipment may significantly delay the institution of effective CPR, and the outcome for those who arrest on general wards is poor (only 3% of patients are discharged). The outlook for those who arrest in the coronary or intensive care unit or emergency department is, however, considerably better (Tunstall-Pedoe *et al.*, 1992). This disparity between survival rates in the two locations appears not to be attributable to differences in the immediate response to CPR since in one series 58% of cases on general wards and 60% of those in the intensive care unit or emergency department were initially successfully resuscitated. Rather, it seems to reflect the severity of the underlying illness in those receiving CPR on the general wards, for many of whom attempted resuscitation is clearly inappropriate (Hershey & Fisher, 1982).

Good prognostic features include a previously normal heart, prompt initiation of effective CPR and cardiac arrest due to primary VF. Conversely, when cardiac arrest occurs in a patient with progressive myocardial failure, often in asystole, the outlook is grave.

Assessment of neurological prognosis in comatose survivors of cardiac arrest

Early accurate prediction of neurological outcome in comatose survivors of cardiac arrest would encourage the clinician to continue aggressive supportive treatment in those with a favourable prognosis while avoiding the futile prolongation of costly therapy when the situation is hopeless. Unfortunately, reliable and widely accepted prognostic indicators are not yet available. Analysis of outcome in 262 comatose survivors of cardiac arrest followed for up to one year (Edgren *et al.*, 1994) demonstrated the unreliability of early (within the first few hours) prognostications, but raised the possibility that accurate prediction might be possible within a few days. Thus the best predictor of poor outcome was therefore the absence of motor responses to painful stimuli on day three. The suggestion that in patients with hypoxic/ischaemic coma a permanent vegetative state can be accurately predicted after three days of intensive care is, however, extremely contentious and others have suggested that in view of the uncertainty, unlimited care should be maintained in such cases for at least a month (Shewmon & De Giorgio, 1989). Others have reached a similar conclusion having apparently observed recovery from persistent vegetative state after four or more months (Andrews, 1993).

Abandoning CPR and 'do not resuscitate' orders (Gray *et al.*, 1991; Niemann, 1992)

It is not possible to diagnose brain stem death with confidence during CPR and therefore attempts at resuscitation should only be abandoned when it proves impossible to restore effective myocardial activity. Time should not be a major factor in reaching this decision, which is the responsibility of the leader of the resuscitation team. The size of the pupils or their lack of response to light should not be taken as a guide to the activity of the central nervous system or the likelihood of recovery. CPR should continue for longer in those who are hypothermic or the victims of near-drowning and when cardiac arrest is associated with drug overdose (see Chapters 9, 18 and 19).

In some patients with terminal disease, CPR is started inappropriately (Hershey & Fisher, 1982) and should then be abandoned as soon as the circumstances are clear. This situation can usually be avoided by establishing beforehand that resuscitation would be inappropriate as soon as the nature and extent of the underlying disease have been determined (Florin, 1994). Many hospitals have instituted formal 'Do not resuscitate' policies (Doyal & Wilsher, 1993). Once a decision not to resuscitate has been made it must be reviewed regularly and changed if circumstances alter. All such decisions should be discussed with the next of kin and must be communicated to the medical and nursing staff involved in the patient's care, as well as being recorded clearly in the patient's notes and dated and signed by the most senior available medical member of the team caring for that patient. Each case must be considered on its own merit (Blackhall, 1987). The patient's quality of life and perception of the situation are important. Age alone should not be a bar to resuscitation. It is usually appropriate to discuss the decision with patients who are both conscious and mentally competent (see also Chapter 1).

GUIDELINES FOR PAEDIATRIC LIFE SUPPORT (Paediatric Life Support Working Party of the European Resuscitation Council, 1994)

Causes of cardiorespiratory arrest in children

Whereas in adults the commonest cause of cardiac arrest is heart disease, in children *respiratory failure* is the most frequent aetiology. This may be due to:

- pulmonary disease (e.g. croup, bronchiolitis, asthma, pneumonia);
- injury (e.g. birth asphyxia, inhalation of a foreign body, pneumothorax);
- respiratory depression caused by prolonged convulsions, raised intracranial pressure, neuromuscular problems or poisoning.

The poor long-term outlook from many cardiac arrests in childhood is related to the severity of the preceding cellular anoxia.

The second commonest cause of cardiac arrest in children is *circulatory failure* usually due to *loss of blood, dehydration* or *sepsis*. Cardiac arrests of primarily cardiac origin are uncommon and are seen most often in children in the paediatric cardiothoracic intensive care unit.

The likely cause of cardiac arrest depends on the age of the child. At birth, asphyxia is the commonest cause, while sudden infant death syndrome and respiratory illness account for the majority of cases in infancy; in later childhood, trauma predominates.

Prevention of injury and earlier recognition of cardiorespiratory disease are clearly the most effective means of reducing the incidence of cardiac collapse in children.

Paediatric basic life support

Establishing a *clear airway* and *oxygenation* are the most important actions in paediatric resuscitation (**Fig. 8.6**). If aspiration of a foreign body is strongly suspected because of a sudden onset of severe upper airway obstruction the steps outlined in **Fig. 8.7** should be taken immediately. *Blind finger sweeps of the pharynx should never be performed in children* as these can impact a foreign body in the larynx below the vocal cords. Measures that create a sharp increase in pressure are intended to simulate coughing.

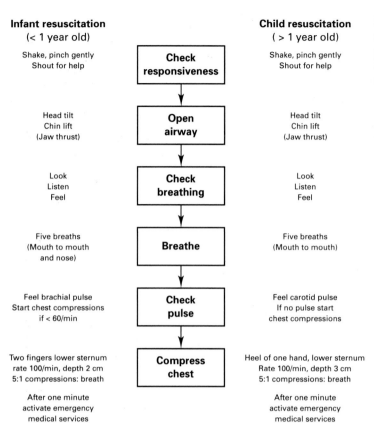

Infant resuscitation
(< 1 year old)

Shake, pinch gently
Shout for help

Head tilt
Chin lift
(Jaw thrust)

Look
Listen
Feel

Five breaths
(Mouth to mouth
and nose)

Feel brachial pulse
Start chest compressions
if < 60/min

Two fingers lower sternum
rate 100/min, depth 2 cm
5:1 compressions: breath

After one minute
activate emergency
medical services

Check responsiveness

Open airway

Check breathing

Breathe

Check pulse

Compress chest

Child resuscitation
(> 1 year old)

Shake, pinch gently
Shout for help

Head tilt
Chin lift
(Jaw thrust)

Look
Listen
Feel

Five breaths
(Mouth to mouth)

Feel carotid pulse
If no pulse start
chest compressions

Heel of one hand, lower sternum
Rate 100/min, depth 3 cm
5:1 compressions: breath

After one minute
activate emergency
medical services

Fig. 8.6 Paediatric basic life support. Reproduced with the kind permission of the European Resuscitation Council. Originally published in the *BMJ* (1994) **308**, 1350–1355, ©1994 BMJ Publishing.

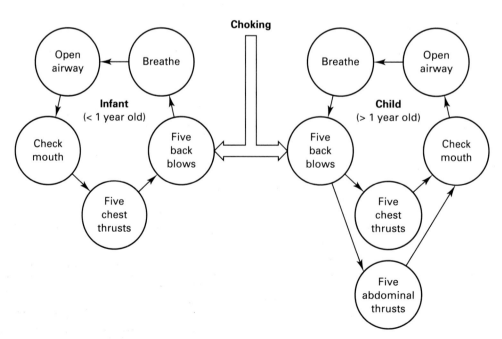

Choking

Infant
(< 1 year old)

Open airway — Breathe — Check mouth — Five back blows — Five chest thrusts

Child
(> 1 year old)

Breathe — Open airway — Check mouth — Five back blows — Five chest thrusts — Five abdominal thrusts

Fig. 8.7 Management of choking in infants and children. Reproduced with the kind permission of the European Resuscitation Council. Originally published in the *BMJ* (1994) **308**, 1350–1355, ©1994 BMJ Publishing.

Paediatric advanced life support

AIRWAY AND VENTILATION

Tracheal intubation is the most effective method of securing the airway and facilitating oxygenation and ventilation. A child's larynx is narrower and shorter than that of an adult; the epiglottis is relatively longer and more 'U-shaped'. Uncuffed tubes should be used until puberty to minimize damage to the cricoid ring, which is narrower in children than in adults (see Chapter 7).

The appropriate size and length of the tracheal tube for the age, weight and length of the child can be assessed using a standard reference chart (**Fig. 8.8**) (Oakley *et al.*, 1993). Appropriate drug doses converted to volumes in standard concentrations can also be obtained from this age, weight and length nomogram. Alternatively a specifically designed tape measure (Luten *et al.*, 1992) can be used to measure the child's height and derive appropriate drug and fluid doses as well as equipment sizes.

ROUTES OF DRUG AND FLUID ADMINISTRATION

While speed is vital when giving drugs and fluid, peripheral venous cannulation in small ill children is notoriously difficult. If venous access is not gained within 90 seconds, intraosseous administration is recommended. If circulatory access cannot be gained within two or three minutes some drugs, including adrenaline, atropine and lignocaine can be administered via the endotracheal tube using a fine cannula or suction catheter. The agent should be flushed in with an equal volume of normal saline. Several manual ventilations should then follow.

ASYSTOLE (Fig. 8.9)

Because VF is unusual it is considered inappropriate to include a blind precordial thump or DC shock in the management of cardiorespiratory collapse in infancy and childhood. Asystole is usually preceded by an agonal bradycardia. The initial dose of *adrenaline* recommended in paediatric cardiac arrest is 10 µg/kg, but for second and subsequent doses a tenfold increase is suggested. The situation in an asystolic child who does not respond to the first or second dose of adrenaline is

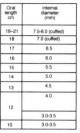
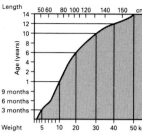

Endotracheal tube					
Oral length cm	Internal diameter (mm)				
18–21	7.5-8.0 (cuffed)				
18	7.0 (cuffed)				
17	6.5				
16	6.0				
15	5.5				
14	5.0				
13	4.5				
	4.0				
12					
	3.0-3.5				
10	3.0-3.5				

Weight	5	10	20	30	40	50 kg
Adrenaline (ml of 1 in 10 000) initial intravenous or intraosseous	0.5	1	2	3	4	5
Adrenaline (ml of 1 in 1000) subsequent intravenous or intraosseous (or initial endotracheal)	0.5	1	2	3	4	5
* **Atropine** (ml of 100 µg/ml) Intravenous or intraosseous (or double if endotracheal)	1	2	4	6	6	6
Atropine (ml of 600 µg/ml)	-	0.3	0.7	1	1	1
Bicarbonate (ml of 8.4%) intravenous or intraosseous (dilute to 4.2% in infants)	5	10	20	30	40	50
** **Calcium chloride** (ml of 10%) Intravenous or intraosseous	0.5	1	2	3	4	5
Diazepam (ml of 5 mg/ml emulsion) intravenous or rectal	0.4	0.8	1.6	2	2	2
Diazepam (mg rectal tube solution) rectal	2.5	5	10	10	10	10
Glucose (ml of 50%) intravenous or intraosseous (dilute to 25% in infants)	5	10	20	30	40	50
*** **Lignocaine** (ml of 1%) intravenous or intraosseous	0.5	1	2	3	4	5
Naloxone neonatal (ml of 20 µg/ml) intravenous or intraosseous	2.5	5	-	-	-	-
Naloxone adult (ml of 400 µg/ml)	-	0.25	0.5	0.75	1	1.25
+ **Salbutamol** (mg nebulizer solution) by nebulizer (dilute to 2.5–5 ml in physiological saline)	-	2.5	5	5	5	5
Initial DC defibrillation (J) for ventricular fibrillation or pulseless ventricular tachycardia	10	20	40	60	80	100
Initial DC defibrillation (J) for supraventricular tachycardia with shock (synchronous) or ventricular tachycardia with shock (non-synchronous)	5	5	10	15	20	25
Initial fluid bolus in shock (ml) crystalloid or colloid	100	200	400	600	800	1000

* **Caution!** Non-standard drug concentrations may be available:
Use atropine 100 µg/ml or prepare by diluting 1 mg to 10ml or 600 µg to 6ml in physiological saline.
**Note that 1 ml of calcium chloride 10% is equivalent to 3ml of calcium gluconate 10%.
***Use lignocaine (without adrenaline) 1% or give twice the volume of 0.5%; give half the volume of 2% or dilute appropriately.
+Salbutamol may also be given by slow intravenous injection (5 µg/kg), but beware the different concentrations available (eg, 50 and 500 µg/ml).

Fig. 8.8 Modified paediatric resuscitation chart. Reproduced with the kind permission of the European Resuscitation Council. Originally published in the *BMJ* (1993) **306**, 1613, ©1993 BMJ Publishing.

Asystole in children

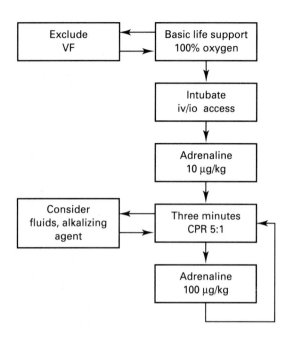

Note:
ETT Adrenaline dose at 10 times the iv dose if iv/io not established within 90 seconds

Fig. 8.9 Management of asystole in children. Reproduced with the kind permission of the European Resuscitation Council. Originally published in the *BMJ* (1993) **306**, 1613, ©1993 BMJ Publishing.

desperate. Although there is evidence that the use of large doses of adrenaline improves neurological outcome in children (Goetting & Paradis, 1991), prospective trials have not confirmed this observation in adults (Brown *et al.*, 1992).

Because hypoxia is the most important cause of bradycardia and asystole in infancy and childhood, adequate ventilation and oxygenation should be achieved before *atropine* is considered.

VENTRICULAR FIBRILLATION AND PULSELESS VENTRICULAR TACHYCARDIA

VF may be encountered:

- in the cardiothoracic intensive care unit;
- in those with congenital heart disease;
- complicating hypothermia;
- following poisoning with tricyclic antidepressants;
- in those with electrolyte disturbances such as hypokalaemia.

A *precordial thump* can be given if the onset of ventricular fibrillation is witnessed (**Fig. 8.10**). Paediatric defibrillator paddles should be used in children weigh-

Ventricular fibrillation in children

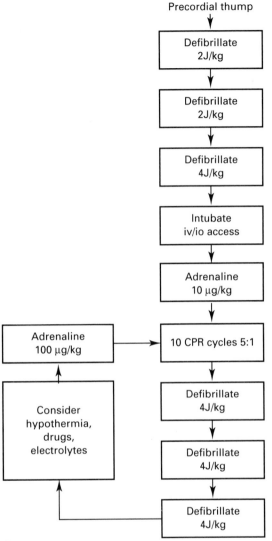

Note:
1. ETT Adrenaline at 10 times the iv dose if iv/io not established within 90 seconds
2. After 3 loops consider alkalizing and/or antiarrhythmic agents

Fig. 8.10 Management of ventricular fibrillation in children. Reproduced with the kind permission of the European Resuscitation Council. Originally published in the *BMJ* (1994) **308**, 1350–1355, ©1994 BMJ Publishing.

ing less than 10 kg. In larger children, the adult paddles can be used provided the child's thorax is broad enough to permit skin contact over the entire paddle surface when one is placed over the apex of the heart and the other is positioned beneath the right clavicle.

If there is no response after three sets of three sequential shocks at 4 J/kg combined with chest compression, ventilation, oxygenation and adrenaline, different paddle positions (e.g. front to back) or an alternative defibrillator can be tried. The use of antiarrhythmics such as *lignocaine* (1 mg/kg) has recently been questioned since although they may prevent VF, there is no evidence that they reverse it (Chamberlain, 1991). There is little experience with bretylium in children. Phenytoin has a specific place in the management of VT induced by tricyclic depressants (see Chapter 18).

ELECTROMECHANICAL DISSOCIATION

In children the most likely cause for apparent EMD is profound hypovolaemic shock. Other causes to consider, especially in trauma, are tension pneumothorax and cardiac tamponade. Metabolic abnormalities such as hypothermia, electrolyte imbalance and drug overdose should also be considered. Occasionally air trapping in a ventilated baby with bronchiolitis may be sufficiently severe to obstruct venous return and dramatically reduce cardiac output.

Management (**Fig. 8.11**) is similar to that for asystole, but in view of the likelihood of correctable hypovolaemia an *early rapid infusion of 20 ml/kg intravenous fluid* is indicated. If fluid resuscitation is initially unsuccessful, cerebral and coronary perfusion should be sustained by ventilation, chest compression and *adrenaline* 100 μg/kg every three minutes while trying to identify and correct any precipitating cause.

MANAGEMENT OF ARRHYTHMIAS

Arrhythmias occurring in critically ill patients are frequently secondary to associated abnormalities such as:

- hypoxia;
- electrolyte disturbances (particularly hypokalaemia or hypomagnesaemia);
- sudden alterations in arterial carbon dioxide tension (P_aCO_2);
- increased circulating catecholamine levels;
- sepsis.

In some cases, pre-existing *cardiac disease* or *myocardial contusion* (see Chapter 9) may contribute to the development of rhythm disturbances.

Because of the dangers associated with the use of antiarrhythmic agents (see below), these abnormalities must be identified and if possible corrected before resorting to specific therapy. Subsequent definitive treatment is then only indicated when the arrhythmia persists and is associated with a significant haemodynamic disturbance. Specific therapy may also be required when persistence of the abnormality is likely to impair cardiac performance (e.g. when the ventricular rate is very rapid) or if the arrhythmia is of a type conven-

Electromechanical dissociation in children

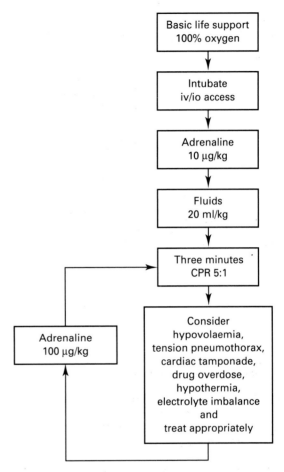

Note:
ETT Adrenaline dose at 10 times the iv dose if iv/io not established within 90 seconds

Fig. 8.11 Management of electromechanical dissociation in children. Reproduced with the kind permission of the European Resuscitation Council. Originally published in the *BMJ* (1994) **308**, 1350–1355, ©1994 BMJ Publishing.

tionally considered to predispose to more serious rhythm disturbances (e.g. 'R on T' ventricular premature contractions—VPCs). Furthermore, if it is not possible to correct the underlying abnormality immediately (e.g. a patient with atrial fibrillation secondary to pneumonia and sepsis), it is often futile to attempt to restore sinus rhythm since even if this is achieved the arrhythmia will almost certainly recur. Under these circumstances, the ventricular rate should be controlled and any haemodynamic disturbance minimized (Sanai *et al.*, 1993).

Critically ill patients are generally intolerant of antiarrhythmics, almost all of which are negatively inotropic, and in general these agents should be avoided. If this is not possible, they should be administered cautiously in reduced dosage. *Direct current cardioversion* does not impair myocardial function unless excessively high energy shocks (> 300 J) are used or administered repeatedly (Doherty *et al.*, 1979), and this is therefore often the most appropriate initial treatment when restoration of sinus rhythm is essential. Similarly, *digoxin* does not depress the myocardium and may have a positive inotropic effect (see Chapter 4) and remains a valuable agent for use in seriously ill patients.

The choice of the most appropriate antiarrhythmic for a particular patient is often difficult and the various classifications of the available agents are unlikely to be of much practical help to the intensive care clinician (Aronson, 1985).

When complex arrhythmias are encountered and/or the abnormality fails to respond to simple measures, a cardiologist should be consulted if possible.

Treatment of specific arrhythmias

Treatment of asystole, VF and pulseless VT is discussed earlier in this chapter.

ATRIAL PREMATURE CONTRACTIONS (APCS)

APCs (**Fig. 8.12**) are *usually benign* and do not therefore normally warrant intervention. Treatment may be indicated, however:

- in a patient who has reverted to sinus rhythm following an episode of atrial fibrillation as in this situation closely coupled APCs may precipitate further atrial fibrillation;
- when APCs are not conducted (this may lead to a very slow effective ventricular rate);
- in those in whom APCs are known to precipitate a re-entry tachycardia.

APCs are usually treated with either *disopyramide* or *quinidine*.

VENTRICULAR PREMATURE CONTRACTIONS

The significance of VPCs (**Fig. 8.13**) is uncertain, particularly in the absence of ischaemic heart disease. They may be idiopathic and benign or related to associated abnormalities, most commonly hypokalaemia. Specific treatment is usually instituted because of concern that they may precipitate VF/VT. Traditionally 'warning arrythmias,' which may degenerate into VF/VT and therefore require treatment, are considered to include:

- a bigeminal rhythm;
- VPCs occurring more frequently than five/minute or in runs of two or more;
- multifocal VPCs;
- those in which the R wave is superimposed on the T wave.

The value of prophylactic treatment has, however, been questioned since although it is possible to reduce the incidence of these warning arrhythmias and possibly the occurrence of VF/VT, it is uncertain whether this influences the ultimate outcome. Nevertheless most would recommend prophylactic treatment in those with sinister VPCs that persist after correction of associated abnormalities, and certainly it is usual to institute such therapy after a recurrence of VF/VT.

Lignocaine probably remains the drug of first choice in this situation since it is well tried and generally effective (see ventricular tachycardia). Side-effects include dizziness, drowsiness, speech disturbances, tremor and agitation. It is metabolized by the liver and the dose should therefore be reduced in those with hepatic failure or a low cardiac output. In overdose, lignocaine can produce hypotension, fits and conduction disturbances. Alterna-

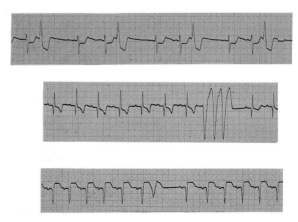

Fig. 8.13 Ventricular premature contractions (VPCs): (top) unifocal trigeminy; (middle) salvo of VPCs; (bottom) R on T VPC.

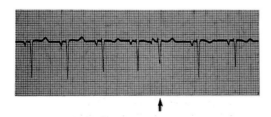

Fig. 8.12 Atrial premature contraction associated with an inferior myocardial infarction.

tives to lignocaine include *amiodarone* or occasionally, *bretylium* or *procainamide* (see ventricular tachycardia).

TACHYCARDIAS

Ventricular tachycardia

VT (see **Fig. 8.2**) usually originates in a small group of abnormal myocardial cells and may be associated with an area of infarction or ischaemia. It may also arise in ventricular muscle that is hypertrophied or myopathic.

Hypokalaemia, reduced tissue magnesium concentrations, raised catecholamine levels and a slow sinus rate all predispose to its development. Established VT may be preceded by warning arrhythmias such as R on T or multiform ectopics and brief runs of VT.

Therapy for ventricular tachycardia is directed at conversion to sinus rhythm and the prevention of recurrence. The priorities for treatment (**Fig. 8.14**) depend on the rate and the haemodynamic consequences of the arrhythmia. Pulseless VT, VT with poor or deteriorating haemodynamics or sustained VT in symptomatic patients require *DC cardioversion*. Normally this should be synchronized to the R wave to avoid a 'shock on T'

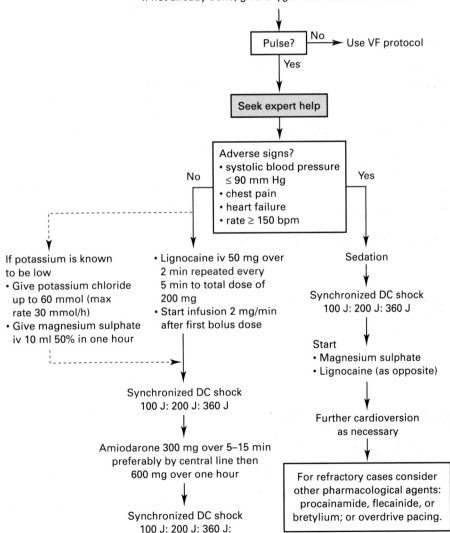

Sustained ventricular tachycardia
If not already done, give oxygen and establish iv access

Fig. 8.14 Treatment algorithm for sustained ventricular tachycardia (doses based on adult of average body weight). Modified with the kind permission of the European Resuscitation Council. Originally published in *Resuscitation* (1994) **28**, 151–159

tients require *DC cardioversion*. Normally this should be synchronized to the R wave to avoid a 'shock on T' phenomenon, although if VT is truly pulseless or is very rapid the ventricles may be 'fluttering', in which case synchronization is unnecessary. Previous intravenous sedation may be required. For VT at rates less than 150/min with acceptable haemodynamics or when VT is paroxysmal and recurrent rather than sustained, pharmacological treatment is indicated once other predisposing conditions such as slow atrial rate or hypokalaemia have been corrected. Hypokalaemia may be associated with hypomagnesaemia, especially in those who were receiving diuretic treatment before admission; an intravenous magnesium infusion can be considered in such cases as well as in those with underlying conduction defects. Many anti-tachycardia drugs exacerbate torsade de pointes (an unusual rhythm characterized by changing wave fronts of ventricular activation, which is often related to a long Q–T interval). This disorder should if possible be treated by correcting electrolyte disorders, especially hypocalcaemia, and by attempting to increase the underlying heart rate if it is slow. β-blockers or phenytoin may be useful.

Lignocaine is the agent of first choice for the conversion of VT and for prophylaxis against recurrent attacks. An initial loading dose of 50 mg is given intravenously over 2 minutes, repeated at 5-minute intervals to a total of four doses provided there are no serious adverse responses. Simultaneously an infusion is started at a rate of 2 mg/min. After 3 hours the infusion rate is reduced to 1.5 mg/minute and continued for the next 24 hours. The dose should be reduced in the elderly, in those with hepatic impairment and when treatment is complicated by bradycardia or hypotension.

Agents that can be used if lignocaine fails include the following.

- *Amiodarone*, 300 mg intravenously, preferably via a central venous catheter, over 5–15 minutes in urgent cases, followed by 600 mg over 1 hour and an infusion of 1200 mg over 24 hours.
- *Flecainide*, 50–100 mg slowly intravenously. Because of its arrhythmogenicity this agent is reserved for life-threatening ventricular arrhythmias.
- *Procainamide*, 100 mg intravenously given over 5 minutes, followed by one or two further boluses before commencing an infusion at 3 mg/minute.
- *Mexiletine*, 100–250 mg intravenously at a rate of 25 mg/min followed by an infusion of 250 mg over 1 hour, 125 mg/hour for 2 hours and then 500 μg/min.
- *Bretylium tosylate*, 400–500 mg diluted in dextrose 5% solution and infused over 10 minutes.
- *Propranolol*, 0.5–1 mg intravenously and repeated if necessary; should only be used when the underlying pathology is myocardial infarction or ischaemia.
- *Sotalol*, 100 mg intravenously over 5 minutes. Recently this agent was shown to be superior to lignocaine for the acute termination of sustained VT (Ho *et al.*, 1994).

Single or dual chamber pacing can suppress VT by increasing the heart rate.

The presence of an implanted automatic defibrillator should not influence the conduct of the recommended emergency measures for treating ventricular fibrillation and tachycardia.

Supraventricular tachycardias

The term supraventricular tachycardia (SVT) encompasses all tachycardias originating above the division of the His bundle and includes atrial flutter and fibrillation, atrial ectopic tachycardia, multifocal atrial tachycardia and ectopic junctional rhythms.

In all forms of supraventricular tachycardia the QRS complexes are narrow (**Fig. 8.15**) unless there is a pre-existing antegradely conducting accessory pathway,

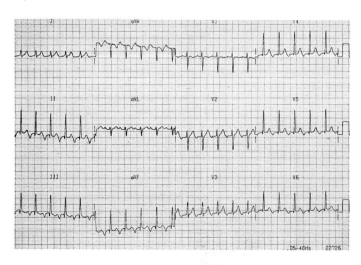

Fig. 8.15 Supraventricular tachycardia.

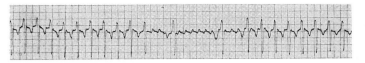

Fig. 8.16 Carotid sinus massage reveals atrial flutter.

bundle branch block or the increased heart rate precipitates aberrant conduction. It must be emphasized, however, that it can be extremely difficult to distinguish between an SVT with abnormal conduction and VT on the ECG (**Table 8.2**) and *broad complex tachycardias must therefore be treated as VT unless proved to be otherwise.*

It is uncommon for SVT to cause profound circulatory collapse, but the circulation may be compromised if the attack is prolonged and if unusually high ventricular rates are superimposed on underlying coronary, valvular or myocardial disease. Particularly high ventricular rates may be seen when the speed of atrioventricular (AV) conduction is enhanced by an abnormal pathway that bypasses the AV node. Occasionally *carotid sinus massage* restores AV block enabling atrial and junctional tachycardias to be distinguished from each other and from atrial flutter (**Fig. 8.16**).

Patients with circulatory collapse require immediate *synchronized DC cardioversion* following intravenous sedation (**Fig. 8.17**). In less urgent cases, the shock may be preceded by an intravenous infusion of 300 mg *amiodarone* given over 5–15 minutes. When an SVT is thought to have been precipitated by digitalis toxicity, *phenytoin* (50–100 mg intravenously every 5 minutes, not exceeding a total dose of 1 g) is a particularly effective antiarrhythmic. Recently *adenosine* has become popular for the management of SVT (Garratt *et al.*, 1992). This agent is a naturally occurring compound that has profound short-lived electrophysiological actions when administered intravenously. It depresses AV nodal conduction with a half-life of 2–10 seconds and often converts paroxysmal SVT to sinus rhythm, particularly where AV nodal re-entry is the underlying mechanism. Adenosine is administered as a rapid intravenous bolus injection over 2 seconds followed by a saline flush. An initial 3 mg injection may be followed

if required by a second dose of 6 mg and a third dose of 12 mg at 1–2-minute intervals. Care should be taken with asthmatic patients since adenosine is a broncho-constrictor. Other side-effects include flushing and headache.

Verapamil, a calcium channel blocker predominantly affecting the AV node, is likely to slow the ventricular rate and may restore sinus rhythm in paroxysmal SVT (Heng *et al.*, 1975) (**Fig. 8.18**). It should be administered slowly intravenously in a dose of up to 5 mg, repeated if necessary at approximately 5-minute intervals up to a total dose of 15 mg. Verapamil can, however, produce marked myocardial depression with profound hypotension, and should be used extremely cautiously in the critically ill. In addition, it should never be given with intravenous β-blockade since the combination is known to cause extreme bradycardia, hypotension (Packer *et al.*, 1982) and even asystole.

Provided the patient is not digitalized, and there is no possibility of digitalis toxicity, *digoxin* (500 μg intravenously over 45 minutes) can be used as a safer alternative to verapamil to slow the ventricular rate.

β-blocking agents are sometimes used to slow the ventricular rate in SVTs, and may occasionally restore sinus rhythm in those with a junctional tachycardia. They must be given cautiously when myocardial function is impaired. β-blockade may also be used to prevent recurrence and *esmolol*, 80 mg over 15 seconds, followed by an infusion of 12 mg/min, has proved particularly effective in this respect.

If it proves impossible to restore sinus rhythm or if the above measures fail to prevent a recurrence, *atrial 'overdrive' pacing* may effectively terminate the arrhythmia.

Atrial flutter. Synchronized direct current *cardioversion* is nearly always the treatment of choice, particularly since this arrhythmia usually responds poorly to drug therapy. Intravenous *verapamil* may slow the ventricular rate and rarely restores sinus rhythm (Heng *et al.*, 1975), while *atrial 'overdrive' pacing* is sometimes effective. Digoxin is not generally recommended since very large, potentially toxic doses are often required to control the ventricular rate.

Atrial fibrillation (**Fig. 8.19**). This arrhythmia may present with a wide variety of ventricular rates and treatment depends on the likely underlying cause, as well as the degree of any haemodynamic disturbance (Sanai *et al.*, 1993). Treatment is usually unnecessary when the

---

Table 8.2 ECG distinction between supraventricular tachycardia with bundle branch block and ventricular tachycardia.

VT is the more likely diagnosis when there is:

A very broad QRS (> 0.14 secs)
Atrioventricular dissociation
A bifid upright QRS with a taller first peak in V_1
A deep S wave in V_6
A concordant (same polarity) QRS direction in all chest leads (V_1–V_6)

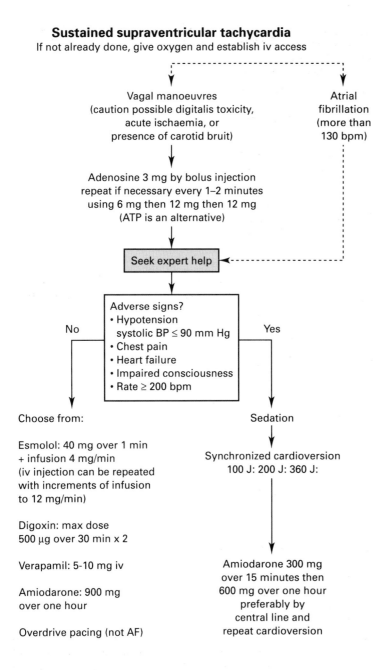

Sustained supraventricular tachycardia
If not already done, give oxygen and establish iv access

Vagal manoeuvres
(caution possible digitalis toxicity,
acute ischaemia, or
presence of carotid bruit)

Atrial
fibrillation
(more than
130 bpm)

Adenosine 3 mg by bolus injection
repeat if necessary every 1–2 minutes
using 6 mg then 12 mg then 12 mg
(ATP is an alternative)

Seek expert help

Adverse signs?
• Hypotension
  systolic BP ≤ 90 mm Hg
• Chest pain
• Heart failure
• Impaired consciousness
• Rate ≥ 200 bpm

No

Yes

Choose from:

Esmolol: 40 mg over 1 min
+ infusion 4 mg/min
(iv injection can be repeated
with increments of infusion
to 12 mg/min)

Digoxin: max dose
500 μg over 30 min x 2

Verapamil: 5-10 mg iv

Amiodarone: 900 mg
over one hour

Overdrive pacing (not AF)

Sedation

Synchronized cardioversion
100 J: 200 J: 360 J:

Amiodarone 300 mg
over 15 minutes then
600 mg over one hour
preferably by
central line and
repeat cardioversion

Fig. 8.17 Treatment algorithm for sustained supraventricular tachycardia (doses based on adult of average body weight). Modified with the kind permission of the European Resuscitation Council. Originally published in *Resuscitation* (1994) **28**, 151–159

impairment normally respond to intravenous *digoxin*. If rapid treatment is needed, the regimen can be digoxin, 500 μg in 100 ml 5% dextrose given over 30 minutes, and repeated over 1 hour. In those with heart failure or thyrotoxicosis and postoperatively, the increased sympathetic drive may make it extremely difficult to control the ventricular rate with digoxin and there is a danger of digoxin toxicity. There is no evidence that digoxin influences the likelihood of reversion to sinus rhythm (Falk *et al.*, 1987). In those with haemodynamic compromise, recent unstable cardiac ischaemia or myo-

cardial infarction, synchronized DC *cardioversion* is indicated.

It should be remembered that if atrial fibrillation has been present for more than a few hours, restoration of sinus rhythm occasionally results in arterial embolization. In some such cases, digoxin (to control the ventricular rate) and anticoagulation may be appropriate. Alternatively *verapamil* can be used to control the ventricular rate and provided there is no coronary artery disease and ventricular function is not impaired, subsequent administration of *flecainide*, 50–100 mg slowly

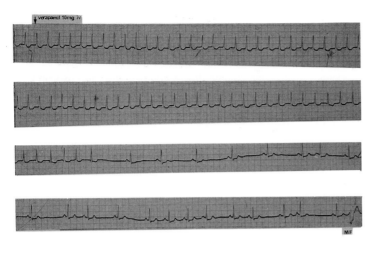

Fig. 8.18 Supraventricular tachycardia terminated by intravenous verapamil 10 mg.

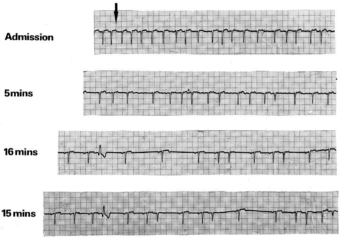

Fig. 8.19 Atrial fibrillation. The ventricular rate is slowed by the administration of a β-blocker.

intravenously, may then restore sinus rhythm. This agent should only be used when the arrhythmia is life-threatening (e.g. extreme hypotension) or causing disabling symptoms. Intravenous *amiodarone* may also restore sinus rhythm. *β-blockade* is sometimes used to control the ventricular rate, although in patients with increased sympathetic drive (e.g. heart failure or thyrotoxicosis) this may precipitate heart failure.

Paroxysmal atrial fibrillation associated with critical illness can often be controlled by an *amiodarone* infusion. Its use is particularly recommended where digoxin and/or β-blockers cannot be used or where the underlying condition is self-limiting (e.g. pericarditis after cardiac surgery or myocardial infarction).

Sinus tachycardia

Sinus tachycardia is nearly always a secondary phenomenon related to one or more of the following:

- hypovolaemia;
- pyrexia;
- hypoxaemia;
- hypercarbia;
- anaemia;
- pain;
- anxiety.

These abnormalities must be identified and, when possible, corrected. Specific treatment is therefore not usually required, and because a reduction in heart rate may be associated with a fall in cardiac output, it may actually be deleterious. Nevertheless, because tachycardia markedly increases myocardial oxygen requirements, it is sometimes prudent to control the heart rate, usually with a β-blocker. This applies particularly to patients with ischaemic heart disease, although β-blockers must be used cautiously, if at all, in those with impaired ventricular performance.

BRADYCARDIA

A pathological bradycardia may be the result of conducting system disease, inferior myocardial infarction or both. Bradycardia may be exacerbated by β-blockade, calcium channel blockers and other depressant agents. In acute ischaemic syndromes a modest bradycardia is advantageous in reducing myocardial oxygen consumption, but more serious slowing predisposes to arrhythmias and reduces cardiac output. The management of brachycardia is outlined in **Fig. 8.20**.

Profound bradycardia and asystole may also follow severe hypoxia or hypothermia or the massive parasympathetic outflow of facial injury or near-drowning. Treatment in these cases should initially be directed at the underlying pathology.

Sinus bradycardia

As heart rate falls, cardiac output is maintained by an increase in stroke volume, due largely to a rise in end-diastolic volume. If this compensatory mechanism fails, blood pressure falls, ventricular filling pressures rise and coronary perfusion is jeopardized. Sometimes nodal or ventricular *'escape' rhythms* are seen. The heart rate should be increased, initially by administering *atropine* intravenously. In persistent cases, repeated administration of atropine up to a maximum of 3 mg may be required. Alternatively, a continuous intravenous infusion of a *β-stimulant* such as isoprenaline or salbutamol can be instituted. Provided there is no abnormality of AV conduction, *atrial pacing* is occasionally indicated, but a temporary ventricular electrode should also

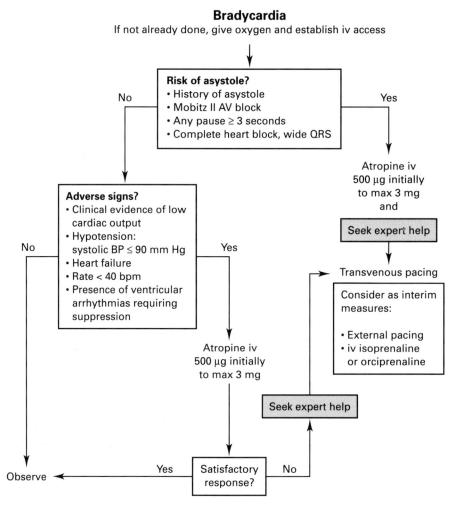

Bradycardia
If not already done, give oxygen and establish iv access

Risk of asystole?
• History of asystole
• Mobitz II AV block
• Any pause ≥ 3 seconds
• Complete heart block, wide QRS

No — Yes

Atropine iv
500 μg initially
to max 3 mg
and

Seek expert help

Transvenous pacing

Consider as interim measures:

• External pacing
• iv isoprenaline
  or orciprenaline

Adverse signs?
• Clinical evidence of low cardiac output
• Hypotension:
  systolic BP ≤ 90 mm Hg
• Heart failure
• Rate < 40 bpm
• Presence of ventricular arrhythmias requiring suppression

No — Yes

Atropine iv
500 μg initially
to max 3 mg

Seek expert help

Observe ← Yes — Satisfactory response? — No

Fig. 8.20 Treatment algorithm for bradycardia (doses based on adult of average body weight). Modified with the kind permission of the European Resuscitation Council. Originally published in *Resuscitation* (1994) **28**, 151–159

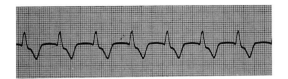

Fig. 8.21 Idioventricular rhythm associated with inferior myocardial infarction.

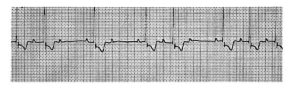

Fig. 8.23 Second degree atrioventricular block—Mobitz Type I.

be inserted in case the atrial system fails or an AV conduction abnormality supervenes. As well as producing haemodynamic improvement, increasing the heart rate may abolish escape rhythms.

Idioventricular rhythm

A reduction in the sinus rate, sinus arrest or sino-atrial block may be associated with an idioventricular escape rhythm (**Fig. 8.21**). Often, the ventricular rate is increased above the expected 40-60 beats/minute by the effects of the underlying disease (e.g. a myocardial infarction). This rhythm can be benign, but if associated with a haemodynamic disturbance can usually be abolished by increasing the sinus rate.

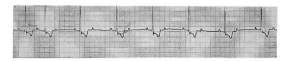

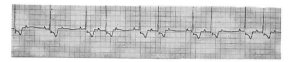

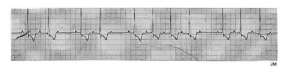

Fig. 8.24 Second degree atrioventricular block—Mobitz Type II.

Disturbances of conduction

First-degree AV block (**Fig. 8.22**). This is generally benign, but may progress to second-degree block, in which case the Wenckebach phenomenon (Mobitz Type I) usually develops.

Second-degree AV block—Mobitz Type I (Wenckebach) (**Fig. 8.23**). This is commonly associated with an inferior myocardial infarction and is almost always self-limiting. The Wenckebach phenomenon does not usually therefore require treatment, although if a 2 : 1 cycle

develops it may be associated with haemodynamic deterioration.

Mobitz Type II (**Fig. 8.24**). This infranodal conduction disorder often progresses to complete heart block and some authorities therefore recommend prophylactic insertion of a temporary transvenous pacing wire.

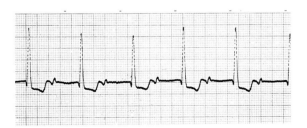

Fig. 8.22 First degree atrioventricular block.

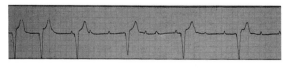

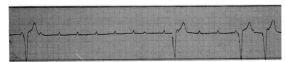

Fig. 8.25 Third degree atrioventricular block.

Third-degree AV block (**Fig. 8.25**). When associated with inferior myocardial infarction, this is caused by ischaemia of the AV node and the conduction disturbance is usually transient. When complete heart block accompanies anterior myocardial infarction, however, it is indicative of a large infarct sufficient to damage the His–Purkinje system. This implies a poor prognosis.

Treatment involves the administration of drugs to increase the ventricular rate (e.g. *atropine*, if the ventricular complexes are narrow, or *isoprenaline*), followed by insertion of a temporary transvenous wire. β-stimulants should only be used if the patient is hypotensive since they may increase infarct size and precipitate arrhythmias.

Fascicular block. Prophylactic pacemaker insertion has been recommended for patients with right bundle branch block and left anterior or posterior hemiblock, as well as for those with bifascicular block and a prolonged P–R interval. This is most often indicated in the context of evolving acute myocardial infarction.

In patients with impaired ventricular function, the loss of atrial transport may be poorly tolerated and in these cases *atrioventricular sequential pacing* may produce haemodynamic improvement.

REFERENCES

Andrews K (1993) Recovery of patients after four months or more in the persistent vegetative state. *British Medical Journal* **306**: 1597–1600.

Aronson JK (1985) Cardiac arrhythmias: theory and practice. *British Medical Journal* **290**: 487–488.

Bexton RS & Camm AJ (1982) Drugs with a class III antiarrhythmic action. *Pharmacology and Therapeutics* **17**: 315–355.

Bircher N & Safar P (1984) Manual open-chest cardiopulmonary resuscitation. *Annals of Emergency Medicine* **13**: 770–773.

Blackhall LJ (1987) Must we always use CPR? *New England Journal of Medicine* **317**: 1281–1285.

Brain Resuscitation Clinical Trial I Study Group (1986) Randomized clinical study of thiopental loading in comatose survivors of cardiac arrest. *New England Journal of Medicine* **314**: 397–403.

Brain Resuscitation Clinical Trial II Study Group (1991) A randomized clinical study of a calcium-entry blocker (lidoflazine) in the treatment of comatosed survivors of cardiac arrest. *New England Journal of Medicine* **324**: 1225–1231.

Brown CG, Martin DR, Pepe PE, *et al.* and The Multicenter High-Dose Epinephrine Study Group (1992) A comparison of standard-dose and high-dose epinephrine in cardiac arrest outside the hospital. *New England Journal of Medicine* **327**: 1051–1055.

Chamberlain DA (1989) Guidelines for cardiopulmonary resuscitation. Advanced life support. *British Medical Journal* **299**: 446–448.

Chamberlain DA (1991) Lignocaine and bretylium as adjuncts to electrical defibrillation. *Resuscitation* **22**: 153–157.

Cohen TJ, Tucker KJ, Lurie KG, *et al.* (1992) Active compression–decompression. A new method of cardiopulmonary resuscitation. *Journal of the American Medical Association* **267**: 2916–2923.

Del Guercio LRM, Feins NR, Cohn JD, Coomaraswarmy RP, Wollman SB & State D (1965) Comparison of blood flow during external and internal cardiac massage in man. *Circulation* **31/32** Suppl. I: I-171–I-180.

Doherty PW, McLaughlin PR, Billingham M *et al.* (1979) Cardiac damage produced by direct current countershock applied to the heart. *American Journal of Cardiology* **43**: 225–232.

Doyal L & Wilsher D (1993) Withholding cardiopulmonary resuscitation: proposals for formal guidelines. *British Medical Journal* **306**: 1593–1596.

Edgren E, Hedstrand U, Kelsey S, Sutton-Tyrrell K & Safar P (1994) Assessment of neurological prognosis in comatose survivors of cardiac arrest. *Lancet* **343**: 1055–1059.

European Resuscitation Council Basic Life Support Working Group (1993a) Guidelines for basic life support. *British Medical Journal* **306**: 1587–1589.

European Resuscitation Council Working Party (1993b) Adult advanced cardiac life support. *British Medical Journal* **306**: 1589–1593.

European Resuscitation Council Advanced Cardiac Life Support Committee (1994) Peri-arrest arrhythmias. *Resuscitation* **28**: 151–159.

Falk JL, Rackow EC & Weil MH (1988) End-tidal carbon dioxide concentration during cardiopulmonary resuscitation. *New England Journal of Medicine* **318**: 607–611.

Falk RH, Knowlton AA, Bernard SA, Gotlieb ME & Battinelli NJ (1987) Digoxin for converting recent-onset atrial fibrillation to sinus rhythm. A randomized, double blinded trial. *Annals of Internal Medicine* **106**: 503–506.

Florin D (1994) Decisions about cardiopulmonary resuscitation. *British Medical Journal* **308**: 1653–1654.

Garratt C, Malcolm AD & Camm AJ (1992) Adenosine and cardiac arrhythmias. The preferred treatment for supraventricular tachycardia. *British Medical Journal* **305**: 3–4.

Gisvold SE, Safar P, Rao G *et al.* (1984a) Prolonged immobilization and controlled ventilation do not improve outcome after global brain ischemia in monkeys. *Critical Care Medicine* **12**: 171–179.

Gisvold SE, Safar P, Hendrickx HHL *et al.* (1984b) Thiopental treatment after global brain ischemia in pigtailed monkeys. *Anesthesiology* **60**: 88–96.

Glaeser PW, Hellmich TR, Szewczuga D, Losek JD & Smith DS (1993) Five year experience in prehospital intraosseous infusions in children and adults. *Annals of Emergency Medicine* **22**: 1119–1124.

Goetting MG & Paradis NA (1991) High-dose epinephrine improves outcome from paediatric cardiac arrest. *Annals of Emergency Medicine* **20**: 22–26.

Gray WA, Capone RJ & Most AS (1991) Unsuccessful emergency medical resuscitation—are continued efforts in the emergency department justified? *New England Journal of Medicine* **325**: 1393–1398.

Halperin HR, Tsitlik JE, Gelfand M *et al.* (1993) A preliminary study of cardiopulmonary resuscitation by circumferential compression of the chest with use of a pneumatic vest. *New England Journal of Medicine* **329**: 762-768.

Hapnes SA & Robertson C (1992) CPR: drug delivery routes and systems. *Resuscitation* **24**: 137-142.

Heng MK, Singh BN, Roche AHG, Norris RM & Mercer CJ (1975) Effects of intravenous verapamil on cardiac arrhythmias and on the electrocardiogram. *American Heart Journal* **90**: 487-498.

Hershey CO & Fisher L (1982) Why outcome of cardiopulmonary resuscitation in general wards is poor. *Lancet* **i**: 31-34.

Higgins D, Hayes M, Denman W & Wilkinson DJ (1990) Effectiveness of using end tidal carbon dioxide concentration to monitor cardiopulmonary resuscitation. *British Medical Journal* **330**: 581.

Hinds CJ (1985) Prevention and treatment of brain ischaemia. *British Medical Journal* **291**: 758-760.

Ho DSW, Zecchin RP, Richards DAB, Uther JB & Ross DL (1994) Double-blind trial of lignocaine versus sotalol for acute termination of spontaneous sustained ventricular tachycardia. *Lancet* **344**: 18-23.

Lindner KH & Koster R (1992) Vasopressor drugs during cardiopulmonary resuscitation. *Resuscitation* **24**: 147-153.

Luten RC, Wears RL, Broselow J et al. (1992) Length-based endotracheal tube and emergency equipment selection in pediatrics. *Annals of Emergency Medicine* **21**: 900-904.

McCrirrick A & Monk CR (1994) Comparison of iv and intratracheal administration of adrenaline. *British Journal of Anaesthesia* **72**: 529-532.

Mair P, Furtwaengler W & Baubin M (1993) Aortic valve function during cardiopulmonary resuscitation. *New England Journal of Medicine* **329**: 1965-1966.

Nagel EL, Fine EG, Krischer JP & Davis JH (1981) Complications of CPR. *Critical Care Medicine* **9**: 424.

Niemann JT (1992) Cardiopulmonary resuscitation. *New England Journal of Medicine* **327**: 1075-1080.

Oakley P, Phillips B, Molyneux E & Mackway-Jones K (1993) Updated standard reference chart. *British Medical Journal* **306**: 1613.

Packer M, Meller J, Medina N et al. (1982) Hemodynamic consequences of combined beta-adrenergic and slow calcium channel blockade in man. *Circulation* **65**: 660-668.

Paediatric Life Support Working Party of the European Resuscitation Council (1994) Guidelines for paediatric life support. *British Medical Journal* **308**: 1349-1355.

Pulsinelli WA, Waldman S, Rawlinson D & Plum F (1982) Moderate hyperglycaemia augments ischemic brain damage: a neuropathologic study in the rat. *Neurology* **32**: 1239-1246.

Robertson C (1992) The precordial thump and cough techniques in advanced life support. *Resuscitation* **24**: 133-135.

Robertson C & Holmberg S (1992) Compression techniques and blood flow during cardiopulmonary resuscitation. *Resuscitation* **24**: 123-132.

Rudikoff MT, Maughan WL, Effron M, Freund P & Weisfeldt ML (1980) Mechanisms of blood flow during cardiopulmonary resuscitation. *Circulation* **61**: 345-352.

Saltuari L & Marosi M (1994) Coma after cardiac arrest: will he recover all right? *Lancet* **343**: 1052-1053.

Sanai L, Armstrong IR & Grant IS (1993) Supraventricular tachydysrhythmias in the critically ill: a review of antidysrhythmic therapy in patients with SVT. *British Journal of Intensive Care* **3**: 358-364.

Sanders AB, Kern KB, Ewy GA, Atlas M & Bailey L (1984) Improved resuscitation from cardiac arrest with open-chest massage. *Annals of Emergency Medicine* **13**: 672-675.

Shapiro HM (1984) Brain resuscitation: the chicken should come before the egg. *Anesthesiology* **60**: 85-87.

Shewmon DA & De Giorgio CM (1989) Early prognosis in anoxic coma. Reliability and rationale. *Neurology Clinics* **7**: 823-843.

Tunstall-Pedoe H, Bailey L, Chamberlain DA, Marsden AK, Ward ME & Zidemann DA (1992) Survey of 3765 cardiopulmonary resuscitations in British hospitals (the BRESUS study): methods and overall results. *British Medical Journal* **304**: 1347-1351.

Vincent JL (1987) Should we still administer calcium during cardiopulmonary resuscitation? *Intensive Care Medicine* **13**: 369-370.

Wardrope J & Morris F (1993) European guidelines on resuscitation. *British Medical Journal* **306**: 1555-1556.

Weaver WD (1991) Resuscitation outside the hospital—What's lacking? *New England Journal of Medicine* **325**: 1437-1439.

Weil MH, Rackow EC, Trevino R, Grundler W, Falk JL & Griffel MI (1986) Difference in acid-base state between venous and arterial blood during cardiopulmonary resuscitation. *New England Journal of Medicine* **315**: 153-156.

White BC, Winegar CD, Wilson RF, Hoehner PJ & Trombley JH Jr (1983) Possible role of calcium blockers in cerebral resuscitation: a review of the literature and synthesis for future studies. *Critical Care Medicine* **11**: 202-207.

9 Trauma

Death following civilian trauma has a trimodal distribution. (Trunkey, 1983).

- The *first peak* comprises the 50% or so of individuals who die within 30 minutes of the event, in these cases death being due to injuries which are so complex and severe that survival is almost certainly impossible within the constraints of our current knowledge and technology. Typical examples would be deaths resulting from major cerebral or brain-stem lacerations or massive vascular disruption within the thorax.
- The *second peak*, accounting for about 30% of all trauma deaths occurs within four hours of injury. These deaths are characterized by major losses of circulating blood volume and are frequently compounded by a failure to provide and maintain an adequate airway and ventilation.
- The *third peak*, accounting for the remaining 20% of trauma deaths includes those patients who die days or weeks following trauma. This is commonly a result of multiple organ failure and sepsis, or pulmonary embolism (see Chapter 4). There is evidence that with rapid, aggressive resuscitation and competent early surgical intervention this third peak of mortality can be significantly reduced.

The principles of respiratory support are discussed in Chapter 7, the management of shock in Chapter 4, and head trauma in Chapter 14.

ADVANCED TRAUMA LIFE SUPPORT AND TRAUMA RESUSCITATION

Three fundamental principles underpinned the development of the Advanced Trauma Life Support (ATLS) programme by the American College of Surgeons.

- The greatest threat to life should be treated first.
- The lack of a definitive diagnosis should never hinder the application of an indicated treatment.
- A detailed history is not an essential prerequisite for the evaluation of an acutely injured patient.

The result was the development of the 'ABCs' (Airway, Breathing and Circulation) approach to the assessment and treatment of the victim of trauma.

The ATLS programme emphasizes that life-threatening injuries kill and maim in certain reproducible time frames. Obstruction of the airway kills more quickly than impaired respiration, and the latter is more rapidly lethal than loss of the circulating volume. An expanding intracranial mass lesion is the next most dangerous problem. The letters 'ABCDE' define a specific, ordered, prioritized sequence of evaluations and treatments, which should be followed in all injured patients. It provides one acceptable method for the safe, immediate management of trauma (Driscoll & Skinner, 1990a, b; Trunkey, 1991) (**Table 9.1**).

Airway with cervical spine control
(Watson, 1990)

All severely injured patients are to a greater or lesser extent hypoxaemic. Immediate administration of supplementary *oxygen* to the *unobstructed airway* is of paramount importance. Simultaneously the *neck* must at all times be kept *immobilized* without traction (for example using a spine board, sandbags, and a hard collar or manual in-line immobilization) until the possibility of neck injury is excluded.

In an unconscious patient foreign bodies obstructing the airway must be removed under direct vision. The laryngeal and pharyngeal reflexes should then be assessed and respiratory performance evaluated. If protective reflexes are adequate retracting the tongue forward by employing the chin lift/jaw thrust manoeuvre or by inserting an *oropharyngeal* or *nasopharyngeal airway* may suffice. If the reflexes are depressed or absent (i.e. there is no gag reflex when oropharyngeal suction is attempted) the airway must be secured at the earliest opportunity by intubation with an appropriately sized *endotracheal tube*. Many patients will require ventilation with oxygen before intubation is attempted.

Table 9.1 Immediate management of trauma.

A	Airway with cervical spine control
B	Breathing
C	Circulation
D	Disability or neurological status
E	Exposure (undress) with temperature control

During these manoeuvres the neck must be kept immobilized (**Fig. 9.1**) (Criswell *et al.*, 1994).

A large-bore *gastric tube* should also be passed. Nasal passage of a gastric tube is contraindicated in patients with suspected basal skull fractures or injury to the soft palate.

Tracheostomy is rarely necessary as an emergency procedure. Severe distorting injury to the structures above or at the level of the larynx can render endotracheal intubation impossible, but *cricothyroidotomy* is preferred to emergency tracheostomy in such circumstances (see Chapter 7).

Breathing (Westaby & Brayley, 1990a)

Hypoxic patients often decompensate rapidly and unpredictably. Once a secure airway has been established adequate ventilation must be ensured, although it is important to remember that positive pressure ventilation may precipitate circulatory collapse, especially if the patient is hypovolaemic. Moreover raised intrathoracic pressure during positive pressure ventilation is associated with an increased risk of pneumothorax in patients with chest injuries and may induce 'tension' in existing pneumothoraces. This complication must be anticipated and chest drains should be inserted in all patients with a pneumothorax who require positive pressure ventilation (see Chapter 7). Because hypercapnia and hypoxia from asphyxia or inadequate ventilation can cause considerable deterioration in cerebral function, especially when combined with fluctuations in arterial blood pressure, mechanical ventilation must always be considered when there is coincidental head injury, even in those without overt respiratory failure.

Six life-threatening injuries may be identified in relation to the airway and breathing.

- Airway obstruction.
- Tension pneumothorax.
- Open pneumothorax (sucking chest wound).
- Massive haemothorax.
- Flail chest.
- Cardiac tamponade.

A further *six potentially lethal chest injuries* may be identified in a secondary examination after primary resuscitation.

- Pulmonary contusion.
- Myocardial contusion.
- Aortic disruption.
- Traumatic diaphragmatic rupture.
- Tracheobronchial disruption.
- Oesophageal disruption.

Circulation

The classical sign of shock, namely hypotension, is not observed in previously fit young patients until they have lost 30% or more of their circulating volume (**Table 9.2**). Intravenous *volume replacement* should ideally

Table 9.2 Classification of severity of haemorrhage in previously fit young patients.	
Class 1	Loss of up to 15% of the circulating volume (up to 750 ml in a 70 kg patient) No change in vital signs
Class 2	Loss of 15–30% (up to 1500 ml) of circulating volume Fall in pulse pressure Sweating restless patient with moderate tachycardia
Class 3	Loss of 30–40% (up to 2000 ml) of circulating volume Marked tachycardia (> 120/min) Systolic blood pressure falls to 90 mm Hg Patient very restless, agitated, sweating
Class 4	Loss of greater than 40% (> 2000 ml) of circulating volume Patient is drowsy, the pulse is thready and tachycardia (> 140/min) or preterminal Bradycardia may be present The blood pressure is less than 90 mm Hg and may be unrecordable by non-invasive means

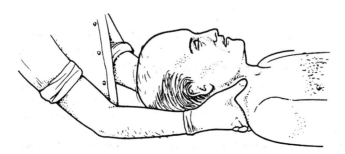

Fig. 9.1 Manual immobilization of the neck.

be instituted before blood pressure falls to minimize the duration of tissue ischaemia and reduce the risk of subsequent multiple organ dysfunction (see Chapter 4). If the signs of shock do not rapidly improve, blood transfusion will be required and a surgical opinion must be obtained. The possibility of concealed intra-abdominal bleeding should be considered (Cope & Stebbings, 1990) and major thoracic injuries may require immediate thoracotomy.

In contrast to traditional teaching there is some controversial evidence to suggest that in hypotensive patients with penetrating torso injuries outcome is improved if aggressive fluid resuscitation is delayed until operative intervention. It is suggested that fluids given before surgery may accentuate ongoing bleeding or disrupt effective thrombus, leading to fatal secondary haemorrhage. Bleeding may be further exacerbated by dilution of coagulation factors and a reduction in viscosity (Bickell *et al.*, 1994).

Disability or neurological status (Bullock & Teasdale, 1990a, b)

The patient's *conscious level* should be recorded using the Glasgow coma scale or AVPU system (A, alert; V, responsive to verbal stimuli; P, responsive only to painful stimuli; U, unresponsive). The *pupillary response to light* must also be examined. Any deterioration in conscious state should prompt re-evaluation of airway control, adequacy of ventilation and volume replacement.

Exposure and control of the environment

The patient should be completely undressed to allow a thorough examination and assessment, but it is imperative to *prevent hypothermia*. Warm blankets are useful, intravenous fluids should be warmed and a warm environment should be maintained.

Although *limb injuries* are not generally immediately lethal in themselves (Willett *et al.*, 1990), except when associated with life-threatening haemorrhage, it is particularly important to identify those injuries that may threaten the survival of a limb, as well as fractures, the acute management of which may influence overall mortality and morbidity. *Compartment syndrome, crush syndrome*, and *fat embolism syndrome* can all cause multiple organ dysfunction in the early post-injury phase.

At the earliest opportunity following the immediate resuscitative procedures the patient's *back and perineum must be carefully inspected*. This will usually involve log-rolling the patient, during which it is important to maintain in-line cervical spine immobiliza-

tion. While the patient is on his or her side the spine should be palpated along its entire length for tenderness and any 'gaps' indicating spinal injury. In males, *rectal examination* will identify the position of the prostate, which may be displaced upwards or feel *boggy* in those with urethral injury. Rectal examination will also detect blood in the rectum indicating bowel injury. The anal reflex should be observed and sensation in the perineum tested and recorded (see Spinal injuries below).

Radiological assessment

Although radiological investigations have an important role in the initial management of trauma patients, it is important not to allow these procedures to compromise treatment and continued monitoring of the patient.

Three radiographs are of prime importance.

- *The chest radiograph*: it is important to appreciate that pneumo- or haemothorax and widening of the mediastinum are less easily detected on supine, antero-posterior chest radiographs.
- *A lateral cervical spine* film: this must include all vertebrae from C1 to T1.
- *Pelvic radiograph*: in particular the sacro-iliac regions must be closely inspected as major disruptions can often lead to significant concealed haemorrhage.

Further radiographs, particularly of the limbs, should not be performed until cardiovascular stability has been achieved. A *lateral skull film* and a *lateral view of the thoracolumbar spine* may then be obtained (Perry & Lewars, 1990).

Other investigations

Once intravenous access has been established, blood should be taken for cross-matching, full blood count, haematocrit, and urea and electrolyte estimation. Regular and repeated estimations of arterial blood gas tensions and acid–base state should be performed, particularly if the admission values are abnormal and following any intervention involving the airway or ventilation.

PERITONEAL LAVAGE

Peritoneal lavage can be invaluable when assessing the injured abdomen. The technique should be performed in the following categories of patient.

- Patients in whom blunt or penetrating trauma is suspected and in whom clinical examination is difficult or impossible because of altered consciousness (e.g. due to head injury or substance abuse).
- Multiple-trauma patients requiring general anaesthesia

for other injuries or those already intubated and sedated/paralysed.

- Trauma patients with unexplained hypotension or those with equivocal findings on clinical examination of the abdomen, lower chest or pelvis.

Peritoneal lavage involves the aseptic insertion of a dialysis catheter into the peritoneal cavity at a point one-third of the distance from the umbilicus to the symphysis pubis in the midline. If gross blood or enteric contents are not aspirated then 10 ml/kg body weight of warmed Ringer's lactate/0.9% saline (up to 1 litre) is instilled into the peritoneum through intravenous tubing attached to the dialysis catheter. If peritoneal lavage fluid drains via a chest tube or an indwelling urinary catheter, or if the fluid is heavily blood-stained, urgent laparotomy is indicated. Otherwise lavage fluid should be drained off by gravity and after 5 minutes a sample should be sent to the laboratory for erythrocyte and leucocyte counts. More than 100,000 erythrocytes/ml or more than 500 leucocytes/ml indicate a positive result and the need for exploratory laparotomy.

CHEST INJURIES (Westaby & Brayley, 1990a, b)

In Europe and Australasia, most cases of chest trauma involve *non-penetrating* injuries, usually as a result of road traffic accidents (RTAs). *Penetrating* injuries caused by knife or gunshot wounds are also seen, but are much more common in the USA.

Less than 15% of patients with chest injuries require surgical intervention. Multiple rib fractures with pulmonary contusion, haemothorax or pneumothorax can be dealt with simply and effectively by insertion of a chest drain, administration of analgesics, fluid restriction and physiotherapy. When ignored, underestimated or inadequately treated, however, such injuries may ultimately prove fatal. The necessity for surgical intervention is based on the rate of bleeding or leakage of air from the intercostal drain. If 1500 ml of blood is immediately evacuated or the hourly drainage exceeds 200 ml then it is highly likely the patient will require early thoracotomy. Definite indications for thoracotomy include:

- cardiac tamponade;
- transmediastinal missile track;
- injury to the major airways or oesophagus.

Specific injuries

LUNGS AND AIRWAYS

Tears or *punctures* of lung tissue, often involving small airways, are relatively common following penetrating injuries and chest wall trauma with rib fractures. They are associated with pneumo- or haemopneumothoraces, and the presence of surgical emphysema will often alert the clinician to the diagnosis. *Rupture of a large bronchus* may cause:

- haemoptysis;
- complete atelectasis of the affected lung;
- mediastinal emphysema;
- pneumothorax.

Less commonly, the *trachea* itself may be either partially or totally *disrupted*. If there is a wide separation of the two ends, the patient usually dies rapidly from asphyxia. Lesser degrees of separation are, however, compatible with survival.

Lung contusion may be diffuse and bilateral (e.g. following a blast injury, Haywood & Skinner, 1990), or relatively localized (e.g. underlying a limited area of chest wall trauma). Occasionally, an *isolated intrapulmonary haematoma* is seen. Severe respiratory failure usually ensues in those with extensive contusion, especially when associated with chest wall instability, but oedema formation and chest radiograph changes are often delayed for about 24 hours.

Management

Although, in those breathing spontaneously, a small *pneumothorax* can be allowed to resolve spontaneously (provided it is not enlarging and not compromising respiratory function), larger collections of air, haemopneumothoraces and those under tension will require insertion of an underwater seal drain. A chest drain should always be inserted when a patient with a pneumothorax requires intermittent positive pressure ventilation (IPPV). Some authorities recommend prophylactic insertion of chest drains in those with multiple rib fractures who need controlled ventilation, even in the absence of a pneumothorax. This practice is, however, associated with a risk of damaging the underlying lung. It may be preferable simply to be alert to the possibility of this complication and to have the facilities for immediate chest drain insertion available at the bedside.

In order to ensure satisfactory drainage of blood and fluid, the drain should be inserted through the sixth or seventh intercostal space in the midaxillary line (see Chapter 7). If the pneumothorax fails to re-expand, and the air leak persists, it may be necessary to apply a negative pressure (e.g. – 5 cm H_2O) using a high-volume, low-pressure suction device. Patients with a persistent pneumothorax associated with a large air leak may require surgical repair or resection of the damaged lung, and may benefit from high-frequency jet ventilation (see Chapter 7).

As with other causes of non-cardiogenic pulmonary oedema, treatment of *lung contusion* consists of:

● supplemental oxygen;
● continuous positive airway pressure (CPAP); or
● controlled ventilation with positive end expiratory pressure (PEEP) (see Chapter 7);
● fluid restriction;
● diuretics.

Prophylactic antibiotics should not be used, except possibly in those with pre-existing chronic obstructive pulmonary disease (COPD). In the past some authorities suggested that corticosteroids might limit the degree of pulmonary abnormality (Trinkle *et al.*, 1975), particularly in those with blast injuries, but this is not currently recommended.

CHEST WALL

Major chest wall injuries produce *instability of the thoracic cage* and *lung contusion.*

If several ribs are fractured in more than one place, or if broken ribs are combined with fracture dislocations of the costochondral junctions or sternum, the negative intrapleural pressure generated on inspiration causes the isolated segment of chest wall to collapse inwards (*'flail segment'*), compromising ventilation. These mechanical problems, exacerbated by severe pain, can cause significant hypoventilation, as well as impair the patient's ability to cough and maintain lung expansion. There is, then, a risk of atelectasis, sputum retention and secondary infection.

Flail segments can be classified according to their anatomical location (**Fig. 9.2**). An associated fractured clavicle exacerbates chest wall instability, and raises the possibility that ventilation may be further compromised by phrenic nerve injury. Sternal fractures can be particularly unstable.

Associated *pulmonary contusion* (see above) causes hypoxaemia and a progressive fall in lung compliance. The latter exacerbates chest wall instability; as lung compliance falls, increasingly negative intrapleural pressures are generated in order to sustain ventilation and the flail segment becomes progressively more obvious. Indeed, in some cases paradoxical chest wall movement is only noticed when lung mechanics have deteriorated 12–24 hours after the injury.

Management

The most appropriate management for a particular patient depends not only on the severity and nature of the chest injury, but is also influenced by the presence of pre-existing obesity or lung disease, the nature of any associated injuries and the patient's age.

Associated injuries to the head, face, abdomen or extremities can significantly complicate the management of chest trauma. In particular, comatose patients should always be intubated and ventilated, while painful laparotomy wounds can further embarrass ventilation. The prognosis following chest wall injury is significantly worse in:

● the obese;
● the elderly;
● those with pre-existing COPD;
● patients suffering pre-existing hypertension;
● those with myocardial ischaemia.

Patients with diseases such as ankylosing spondylitis that interfere with normal chest wall expansion will be particularly seriously compromised by chest wall injuries.

Following initial assessment and treatment, the patient must be closely observed for several days, since deterioration is almost inevitable over the first 24–48 hours. As well as *clinical evaluation* and *blood gas analysis*, serial measurements of *vital capacity* provide a useful means of assessing the patient's progress.

As a guide to the most appropriate management for a particular patient, chest injuries can be categorized into one of *three grades of severity.*

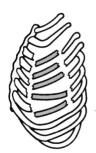 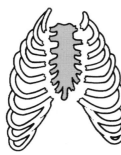 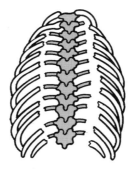

Lateral   Anterior   Posterior

Fig. 9.2 Types of flail chest. A lateral injury is the most common. Anterior injuries are caused by frontal impact and may be associated with damage to the heart. Posterior injuries are unusual and strong muscular support prevents serious paradoxical movement. From Webb (1978), with permission.

Grade I (mild). These patients are able to maintain adequate alveolar ventilation and can cough. They may have a small flail segment, but underlying pulmonary damage is minimal and there is no pre-existing lung disease. Associated trauma is limited to moderate peripheral injuries and there is no head or intra-abdominal injury.

Grade I injuries can be treated with:

- analgesia;
- oxygen if required;
- physiotherapy;
- early mobilization.

The success of this regimen depends on the provision of adequate analgesia. In some cases, simple *oral anti-inflammatory agents* such as aspirin, indomethacin or diclofenac may be sufficient. Others will require *narcotics*. *Intercostal blocks* may be useful, but they usually have to be repeated at approximately 12-hourly intervals. This may be facilitated by using a catheter technique. Premixed 50% nitrous oxide in oxygen *(Entonox)* can be used to provide supplementary analgesia during painful procedures.

Although this regimen is often referred to as 'conservative management,' this is a misleading term since, to be successful, it requires a particularly active approach to all aspects of patient care and is very demanding of both the patient and staff. If possible, therefore, even patients with grade I injuries should be admitted to a high dependency or intensive care unit.

Grade II (moderate). Although these patients can ventilate adequately, their ability to cough is seriously impaired. They may have an obvious flail segment and associated lung contusion. As compliance falls and intrapulmonary shunt increases during the first 24–48 hours, these patients can deteriorate sufficiently to be reclassified as grade III. Patients with associated extensive limb injuries, a mild head injury, pre-existing lung disease, obesity or old age are also classified as grade II.

Treatment consists of:

- analgesia;
- physiotherapy;
- supplemental oxygen;
- early mobilization.

Some patients may also require *endotracheal intubation* or *tracheostomy* to protect their airway and control secretions. Pulmonary contusion should be treated as outlined above with *fluid restriction* and *diuretics*. It is especially important to control pain in this category of patient in order to permit coughing and adequate physiotherapy. *Thoracic epidurals* are particularly effective and can increase functional residual capacity (FRC), compliance, vital capacity and P_aO_2, as well as decrease paradoxical movement of the chest wall (Dittmann *et al.*, 1978).

Intercostal blocks are generally less satisfactory, but *opiates* can be very effective if administered as a continuous intravenous infusion. Some authorities recommend the application of *CPAP by face mask* (see Chapter 7) for 20–30 minutes each hour in order to increase FRC (Dittmann *et al.*, 1982). With this regimen, it may be possible to avoid mechanical ventilation, even in those with a large flail segment. This may, however, be at the expense of a degree of permanent chest wall deformity and some consider this to be unacceptable, especially in young patients.

Grade III (severe). These patients have severe chest wall instability with extensive pulmonary contusion. They are extremely hypoxaemic, cannot cough and are often unable to sustain adequate alveolar ventilation. They rapidly become exhausted. Patients with associated visceral injuries requiring laparotomy and/or a severe head injury, as well as those with moderate chest injury, but who are elderly, obese or who have pre-existing lung disease may be categorized as grade III.

Patients in grade III require *controlled ventilation*. PEEP can be used to improve oxygenation (see Chapter 7). Although traditionally patients have been prevented from making spontaneous respiratory efforts because of concern that this could perpetuate chest wall instability, most now recommend the use of *synchronized intermittent mandatory ventilation (SIMV)* with PEEP. Patients with severe unilateral pulmonary abnormalities may require *independent lung ventilation* (see Chapter 7). An alternative is to nurse the patient in the lateral position with the damaged lung uppermost. This diverts pulmonary blood flow away from the damaged lung and limits preferential ventilation of the good lung. In those with a large and persistent air leak, *high frequency jet ventilation* may prove useful (Chapter 7). Weaning should commence as soon as the lung lesion has resolved and can be facilitated by *thoracic epidural analgesia*.

Although secondary chest infection is common, especially in the presence of lung contusion, *antibiotics* should be withheld until infection is obvious and preferably until the responsible organism has been identified, although some administer prophylactic antibiotics to those with pre-existing COPD.

Early mobilization is recommended, even for these severely injured patients, and it is certainly possible for ventilated patients to stand and sit out of bed.

HEART

Penetrating injury

Surprisingly, a number of patients with penetrating cardiac injuries make a complete recovery, although high-velocity gunshot wounds of the heart are invariably fatal.

In those who remain shocked despite apparently adequate volume replacement, with signs of cardiac tamponade (see Chapter 4), *pericardiocentesis* (**Fig. 9.3**) must be performed. The pericardial sac can be aspirated using an intravenous cannula or continuously drained using a soft, flexible catheter. Improvement is often dramatic following removal of relatively small amounts of blood. Relief of tamponade may, however, simply encourage further haemorrhage and some patients may be more stable if a degree of cardiac compression is allowed to persist. *Emergency stematory or thoracotomy* is required in the majority of cases. If possible, this should be performed by a competent cardiothoracic surgeon because once the pericardium is opened, haemorrhage can be catastrophic and is most likely to be controlled quickly by those with experience of cardiac surgery. Ideally, the facilities for cardiopulmonary bypass should be available.

Blunt injury

Myocardial contusion is a common, but often unrecognized, complication of non-penetrating chest injury and may occur in up to 17% of such cases (Macdonald *et al.*, 1981). The diagnosis is suggested by ST segment and T wave changes on the ECG, sinus tachycardia, arrhythmias and elevated plasma levels of cardiac enzymes, although the latter, with the possible exception of increases in creatine kinase muscle–brain isoenzyme, is a non-specific finding in traumatized patients. Early, and transient, prolongation of the Q–T interval may be a sensitive indicator of myocardial contusion.

Management is as for myocardial infarction. When contusion is severe, myocardial function may be significantly impaired (Torres-Mirabal *et al.*, 1982) in which case catheterization of the pulmonary artery may be indicated to guide volume replacement. Some patients will require inotropic support (Macdonald *et al.*, 1981).

Complications are common and may include sudden unexpected cardiac arrest, as well as supraventricular and ventricular arrhythmias. The prophylactic use of antiarrhythmics, however, remains controversial. *Cardiac rupture* may occur either at the time of impact or later as a delayed consequence of myocardial contusions. Intracardiac lesions, such as *disruption of a valve* or *rupture of the interventricular septum*, may also occur and are often fatal. These complications are, however, uncommon (Macdonald *et al.*, 1981). *Intrapericardial haemorrhage* following blunt injuries originates from torn pericardial and epicardial vessels or, occasionally, small myocardial tears. If cardiac tamponade develops it should be relieved by pericardiocentesis. In some cases, bleeding will stop spontaneously while others will require surgical intervention.

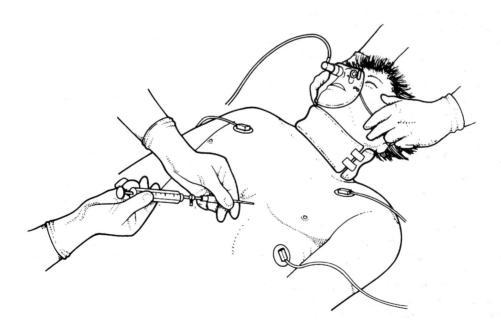

Fig. 9.3 Needle pericardiocentesis. With the patient supine, the skin is punctured slightly to the left of the xiphisternum and the cannula is directed upwards, backwards and to the left until the pericardial sac is entered. ECG monitoring is essential in order to detect arrhythmias or myocardial injury.

Pericardium

The pericardium may be torn by a blunt injury, usually in association with rupture of the diaphragm (see later in this chapter). More often, however, pericardial damage is the result of a penetrating injury. The main danger of a pericardial tear is that the heart will herniate through the defect, severely compromising cardiac function. If this happens, immediate surgery is indicated.

AORTA

The aorta can be disrupted, usually as a result of a rapid deceleration injury, at the junction between the fixed and mobile portions of the aortic arch (i.e. most frequently just distal to the origin of the left subclavian artery). This is usually rapidly fatal in the elderly in whom the aorta is rigid, but young patients may suffer partial rupture and survive for long enough to be investigated and undergo definitive surgery. Disruption of the aorta just above the aortic valve may also occur, but is usually fatal.

Diagnosis

Aortic rupture should be suspected when widening of the superior mediastinum, sometimes in association with some fluid in the pleural cavity, is seen on the chest radiograph of a patient who has suffered an injury compatible with this complication. Other features suggestive of aortic rupture include depression of the left main bronchus, blurred outline of the arch or descending aorta, fractured first rib or left apical haematoma and displacement of the mid-oesophagus to the right. On examination, there may be a discrepancy between the blood pressure in each arm and femoral pulses may be diminished or absent. The significance of mediastinal widening is, however, notoriously difficult to assess in trauma patients and, except in the rare cases when the diagnosis is obvious on the plain radiograph, confirmatory evidence should be obtained using echocardiography, CT scan, MRI scan or angiography (**Fig. 9.4**). Recent evidence suggests that transoesophageal echocardiography is a highly sensitive and specific method for detecting injury to the thoracic aorta (Smith *et al.*, 1995).

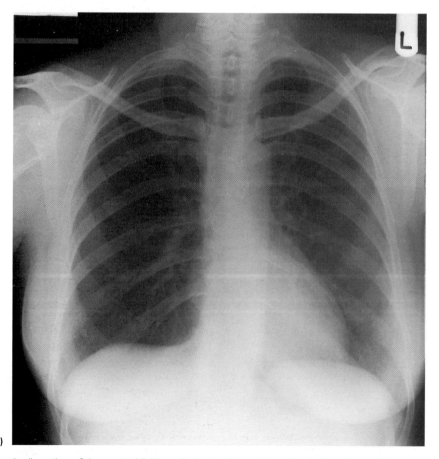

(a)

Fig. 9.4 Traumatic disruption of the aorta. (a) Normal chest radiograph ten days before the accident.

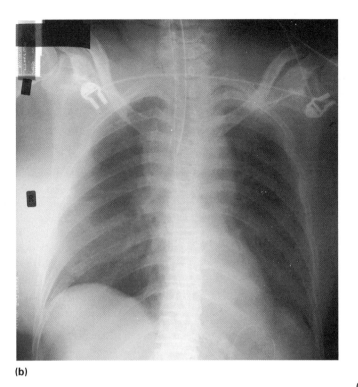

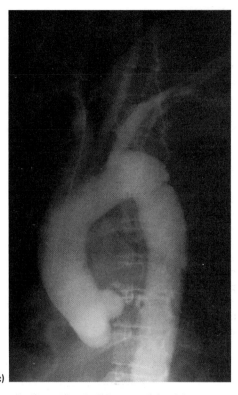

(b)

(c)

Fig. 9.4 Traumatic dissruption of the aorta. (b) Obvious widening of the mediastinum with displacement of the right paratracheal stripe. There is a left-sided pleural effusion overlying the apex of the lung in this supine film. (c) Aortagram showing a complete tear of the aorta at the level of the isthmus, with an aneurysm extending to the origin of the left subclavian artery.

DIAPHRAGMATIC RUPTURE

Diaphragmatic rupture is rare and usually follows trauma to the anterior abdominal wall. It may also be associated with acetabular fractures, when the force of the impact is transmitted along the length of the femur and through the abdomen. It is a relatively benign injury and may not be recognized until many years after the accident when the patient presents with abdominal contents within the left hemithorax. If the right hemidiaphragm is ruptured, the liver usually prevents herniation.

OESOPHAGEAL TRAUMA

Oesophageal trauma should be considered in any patient who has a left haemothorax or pneumothorax without a rib fracture and when there is particulate matter in the chest drain. The presence of mediastinal air also suggests oesophageal rupture. The diagnosis can be confirmed by contrast studies and endoscopy.

Drainage of the pleural space and mediastinum with direct repair of the injury is the definitive surgical option. Occasionally more extensive procedures have to

be undertaken to prevent continued soiling of the mediastinum and pleura by gastric and oesophageal contents.

Prognosis

Reported overall mortality rates for those with chest injuries vary considerably depending on the patient population studied, but death solely attributable to an isolated chest injury is rare. Most often, death is related to associated extrathoracic injuries, particularly head injury, or pre-existing morbidity, such as COPD and old age.

BURNS (Muller & Herndon, 1994)

The majority of burn injuries occur in the home and frequently involve children aged 1–5 years who are scalded by hot liquids or whose clothing is ignited. Among teenagers and adults, men aged 17–30 years are the most frequent victims, usually as a result of accidents with inflammable liquids. Bedding and house fires most frequently affect the elderly and infirm, while about 25% of burns admissions are due to industrial accidents. Major structural fires account for only a small proportion of those admitted to hospital with thermal injury.

Although improved fire-fighting techniques and emergency medical services, as well as the increased use of smoke detectors, may have made some contribution to a reduction in burn-related deaths, in general preventive measures have had only limited success. In contrast, major advances in the resuscitation and subsequent care of burns patients have been responsible for an improved overall survival rate and reduced hospital stay among those admitted to specialized burn centres. Therefore, high-risk patients must always be admitted to such units following initial resuscitation.

Assessment

The severity of a thermal injury depends on the area damaged and the depth of the burn. The percentage surface area burned can be estimated using the 'rule of nine' (**Fig. 9.5**), modified in children to take into account the greater proportion of the body represented by the head and neck and the lesser contribution of the legs. In those with extensive burns, it may be easier to assess the area of undamaged skin and subtract this from 100. The depth of the burn can be classified as:

- erythema only;
- partial thickness;
- full thickness.

Erythematous changes, without blistering, will usually resolve spontaneously within a few days and should not be included in the calculation of the surface area burned. In areas of partial thickness involvement, some viable deep epithelial elements remain from which regeneration of skin is possible. This occurs beneath the eschar of dead dermis within 1–4 weeks. Because nerve endings are exposed and remain intact, partial thickness burns are extremely painful. In contrast, epithelial structures and nerve endings are virtually completely destroyed following a full thickness burn. Healing can therefore only occur by ingrowth of skin from surrounding structures or by contraction, and pain sensation is absent. Full thickness burns may also involve underlying structures. In some cases, the distribution of the burn suggests the possibility of child abuse.

It is also important to identify *associated trauma* to other organs and vital structures.

Patients with burns involving more than 15% of their body surface area (BSA), as well as those with pulmonary or electrical injuries, must be referred to a specialist unit. Children with a burn of more than 6% of their BSA have a small, but definite risk of dying and should always be admitted to hospital for observation. Burns involving the face, hands or perineum in a child need specialist care and should be referred to a burns unit, even when less than 6% of the BSA is affected.

Management

VOLUME REPLACEMENT AND CARDIOVASCULAR SUPPORT

Thermal injury increases microvascular permeability, in part because of the release of vasoactive substances (Demling & LaLonde, 1990), and plasma is lost both externally (into blisters and as an exudate on the surface of the burn) and into the interstitial spaces. There is also intracellular swelling due to a generalized cell membrane defect. Increases in the osmotic pressure within the interstitium of both burned and adjacent non-burned tissue also appear to be important in the genesis of oedema and may be related to the release of osmotically active cellular elements (Demling, 1985). It has been suggested, however that although there is an early transient generalized increase in microvascular permeability, the oedema that occurs in non-burned tissues is largely related to severe hypoproteinaemia rather than capillary endothelial injury (Demling, 1985). These changes, combined with evaporation of salt and water from the exposed surfaces, cause a considerable reduction in

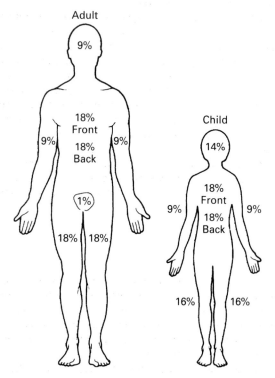

Fig. 9.5 The 'rule of nine' for estimating the percentage surface area burned in an adult and a child.

circulating volume and haemoconcentration. Without aggressive volume replacement, hypovolaemic shock supervenes and, if this is allowed to persist, acute renal failure may follow.

Assessing fluid requirements

Because fluid losses are not obvious, and the patient may at first appear well, the extent of the volume deficit is often underestimated. Significant reductions in plasma volume follow burns involving more than 15% BSA in adults and more than 10% BSA in children. Although the magnitude of the losses is variable (e.g. partial thickness scalds may be associated with massive reductions in plasma volume while deep flame burns are often charred and relatively dry), the volume of intravenous fluid required can be estimated using one of a number of formulae. For example, *the Mount Vernon formula* (Muir, 1981) recommends:

Volume of plasma to be given in each period =

$$\frac{\% \ area \ burned \times weight \ (kg)}{2}.$$

Provided the patient's condition remains satisfactory, the calculated volume of plasma is infused in successive periods of 4, 4, 4, 6, 6 and 12 hours.

Others favour resuscitation with Ringer's lactate solution, for example 4 ml/kg of body weight multiplied by the percentage of body surface area burned. Half of the calculated fluid requirements are administered during the first 8 hours after injury. It must be emphasized, however, that frequent clinical assessment of the adequacy of volume replacement is essential and that the rate of transfusion should be adjusted as indicated. This should be guided by the urine output, which must be maintained at more than 0.6 ml/kg/h, and the haematocrit. The latter is influenced by red cell destruction, as well as plasma losses, and in the presence of significant haemolysis the packed cell volume (PCV) should be maintained at 10% below the expected value. When there is obvious haemoglobinuria, a value 20% below normal is thought to be ideal. Retrospectively collected evidence has demonstrated that those with smoke inhalation require a higher than expected fluid input to maintain adequate cardiovascular performance (Navar *et al.*, 1985) and in these patients aggressive volume replacement reduces the incidence of organ dysfunction (Herndon *et al.*, 1988).

Some consider that the central venous pressure (CVP) is an unreliable guide to volume requirements in burns patients and, in view of the high risk of infection and often limited availability of suitable access sites, avoid cannulating central veins. Others recommend CVP monitoring of all patients with serious burns and the

use of a thermodilution pulmonary artery catheter in the most difficult cases (Aikawa *et al.*, 1978).

Choice of fluid for volume replacement

Severely burned patients require replacement of their circulating volume with large quantities of salt-containing solutions, but the type of fluid used for resuscitation is less important than the volume given and the experience of those responsible for its administration. Some authorities suggest that crystalloids alone should be administered during the first 24 hours because accumulated extravascular water can later be mobilized relatively easily (see Chapter 4). Subsequently, colloids and blood are usually given as required to maintain the circulating volume and the PCV respectively. For reasons discussed in Chapter 4, some use colloids even during the early phase of resuscitation while others add colloid to a background crystalloid regimen in order to maintain intravascular volume and the plasma albumin concentration. On the other hand some have cautioned against the addition of colloids to crystalloid fluids for resuscitation in thermal injury (Goodwin *et al.*, 1983). These authors found that, although the volumes of fluid required for successful resuscitation were reduced and the cardiac indices were higher in the early phase, the use of colloids promoted the accumulation of lung water when oedema fluid was mobilized from the burn wound.

Despite this aggressive approach to the restoration and maintenance of an adequate circulating volume, *acute renal failure* or transient episodes of *renal impairment* may complicate thermal injury. These may follow periods of hypoperfusion and hypoxia, and can be exacerbated by haemoglobinuria or myoglobinuria in those with electrical or crush injuries. Established acute renal failure is associated with a particularly high mortality in burns patients and must be avoided at all costs (see Chapter 12).

Congestive cardiac failure may occur during the acute phase, or a few days after the injury when oedema fluid is mobilized. *Myocardial infarction* is a rare complication.

SURGERY

Urgent surgical intervention may be required for patients with circumferential burns of the trunk or the limbs, which can impair respiration, or constrict blood vessels and cause ischaemic damage, respectively. Decompression is achieved by incising the skin and, sometimes, the deep fascia.

Elective surgery is performed to repair areas of full thickness skin loss, and to prevent infection, by excision of eschar and grafting. This is usually first undertaken

2–4 days after burning and can be associated with considerable blood loss.

ANALGESIA

Initially, analgesia is best achieved by administering small incremental doses of an opiate intravenously (e.g. 1 mg increments of morphine up to a total of 10 mg over 10 minutes). Subsequently, a continuous intravenous infusion of morphine can be given at a rate of 1–4 mg/h.

CONTROL OF INFECTION

A number of immunological abnormalities have been identified in burns victims including:

- impaired phagocytic function;
- decreased neutrophil chemotaxis;
- disturbances of the lymphocyte system.

It is not surprising, therefore, that the commonest cause of death following thermal injury is *sepsis* and *multiple organ failure*. Most often, this is related to infection of the burn wound or the lungs, but in some cases urinary tract infections or contamination of intravascular catheters are incriminated. As with other infections occurring in the critically ill, the most common pathogens causing burn wound sepsis have altered from the Gram-positive cocci (e.g. the β-haemolytic streptococcus) to Gram-negative rods, such as *Pseudomonas aeruginosa* and fungi. Recently, however, methicillin-resistant strains of *Staphylococcus aureus* have been responsible for a number of epidemics of infection in burns units and there has been an increase in the incidence of Gram-positive infections.

The burn wound usually becomes colonized within a few days of admission, as a result of either autogenous infection or cross-contamination from another patient. The topical application of antibacterial agents for prophylaxis is controversial, but may delay colonization and reduce the concentration of bacteria. Antibiotics should only be used to treat documented infection. This is usually diagnosed clinically, and can be confirmed by positive blood culture and/or wound biopsy. The risk of cross-contamination can be minimized by barrier nursing in a single cubicle. Antitetanus prophylaxis is routine in most units.

METABOLIC RESPONSE AND NUTRITIONAL SUPPORT

Serious burns are associated with:

- increased basal metabolic rate;
- raised core temperature;
- hyperdynamic circulation;
- protein catabolism;
- lipolysis;
- increased susceptibility to infection;
- poor wound healing.

The two most effective means of controlling hypermetabolism remain a warm ambient environment (32°C) and effective pain relief (Wilmore *et al.*, 1974, 1975).

Provision of adequate nutritional support is also vital. Enteral feeding is preferred because it maintains intestinal mucosal integrity and probably diminishes translocation of bacteria from the gut lumen into the lymphovascular system (Herndon & Ziegler, 1993); it may also reduce the incidence of gastric ulceration. Indeed mortality has been shown to be higher in patients receiving parenteral nutrition than in those given the maximum amount of calories that can be tolerated enterally (Herndon *et al.*, 1989).

Pulmonary embolism is an unusual complication of thermal injury, but some centres use *prophylactic subcutaneous heparin*.

Prognosis

The mortality of thermal injury is related to the depth of the burn, the percentage of BSA involved and the age of the patient. Survival rates have improved significantly over the last decade or so. For example, in 1964, 50% of patients between 10 and 30 years of age with second- and third-degree burns involving 50% of their BSA would have died. Currently, mortality rates of less than 10% are being reported for such cases. Similarly, until recently the mortality rate of 70–80% burns approached 90%, whereas now survival rates of about 50% are being achieved.

Inhalation injury (Kinsella, 1993)

Inhalation injury may occur in as many as 20% of patients admitted to burn centres. Not only does it increase the mortality for a given surface area burn, but it is also associated with an increased risk of death at the scene of the accident.

Patients with inhalation burns may develop *pharyngeal* and *laryngeal oedema*, with *upper airways obstruction*, due to thermal and/or chemical damage. There may also be *pulmonary parenchymal damage*, which can cause acute hypoxaemic respiratory failure.

PATHOPHYSIOLOGY

Few gases, except superheated steam, have sufficient thermal capacity to carry heat beyond the trachea. Pulmonary parenchymal damage is therefore usually chemical and due to water-soluble gaseous products of combustion such as ammonia, chlorine and sulphur dioxide. These react with the water in mucous membranes to produce strong acids and alkalis, which can induce bronchospasm, ulceration of the mucous membranes and oedema. Lipid soluble compounds such as phosgene, nitrous oxide, hydrogen chloride and aldehydes can reach the distal airways on carbon particles that adhere to the mucosa. These damage the cell membrane directly and impair ciliary clearance. Moreover, the inflammation is aggravated by activation of alveolar macrophages (Loke *et al.*, 1984). Smoke inhalation promotes tracheobronchitis and formation of casts (destroyed epithelium and fibrin), and also enhances leucocyte margination in pulmonary capillaries and the release of inflammatory mediators (Herndon *et al.*, 1988).

PRESENTATION AND DIAGNOSIS

Inhalation injury should be suspected in any patient with:

- facial burns;
- stridor;
- erythema of the nasopharyngeal mucosa;
- singed nasal vibrissae;
- soot in expectorated secretions.

Such an injury is most likely following facial flame burns or when the victim has been confined within a small, smoke-filled room. *Elevated carboxyhaemoglobin (COHb) levels* on admission also suggest that there has been significant respiratory involvement provided allowance is made for the time interval between smoke inhalation and admission (**Fig. 9.6**) (Clark *et al.*, 1981). Although there is a significant correlation between carbon monoxide levels and blood cyanide concentrations (Baud *et al.*, 1991), it is not possible to predict with confidence the presence or absence of cyanide poisoning from COHb levels. A recent study has suggested that in fire victims with minor or no cutaneous burns a *high plasma lactate concentration* strongly suggests that the patient is suffering from cyanide poisoning (Baud *et al.*, 1991).

The *chest radiograph* and *blood gas analysis* may be within normal limits initially, but should be repeated at intervals in order to detect subsequent deterioration. In some centres, *indirect laryngoscopy* or *fibre-optic bronchoscopy* is performed early to assess airway obstruction, confirm the diagnosis, define the extent and severity of the airway burn and to perform tracheobronchial toilet.

Early increases in extravascular lung water are rare, but may result from the direct chemical toxicity of

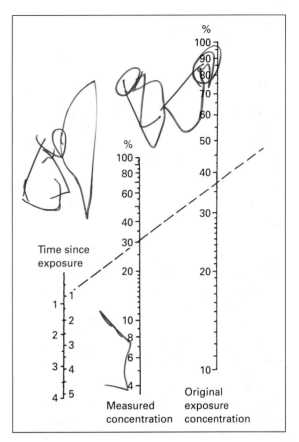

Fig. 9.6 Nomogram for calculating carboxyhaemoglobin concentration at time of exposure. Time since exposure is given in two scales to allow for the effects of previous oxygen administration on the half life of carboxyhaemoglobin. (Left scale assumes a half life of three hours, that on the right assumes a half life of four hours.) Reproduced from Clarke *et al.* (1981) Blood carboxy haemoglobin and cyanide levels in fire survivors *Lancet* **i** 1332–1335. © by the Lancet Ltd with permission.

inhaled gases in the most severe cases of inhalation injury. More often the increase in microvascular permeability leads to *pulmonary oedema* some 2–3 days after injury and to pneumonia some 7–14 days later. Delayed increases in lung water may be related to systemic or pulmonary sepsis (Tranbaugh *et al.*, 1983). *Pulmonary fibrosis* is commonly encountered among survivors. *Bronchorrhoea*, which is usually a response to the inhaled irritants rather than a sign of infection, is common after smoke inhalation.

Presentation is frequently delayed, but *early diagnosis* may be possible using:

- fibre-optic bronchoscopy;
- Xe[133] lung scans;
- ventilation/perfusion scans;
- lung function testing.

MONITORING

The value of pulse oximetry is limited because current instruments do not distinguish between oxyhaemo-globin and COHb. The difficulties of adequately measuring arterial blood pressure indirectly in extensively burned patients and the need to measure arterial blood gases frequently justify arterial cannulation. Controversy exists over the role of central venous and pulmonary artery flotation catheters (see Volume replacement).

MANAGEMENT OF INHALATION INJURY (Deitch 1990; Langford & Armstrong, 1989)

Management should begin as soon as possible with the administration of *supplemental oxygen*. All those with suspected airway burns must be closely observed for the signs of impending airway obstruction and/or respiratory failure. Early *intubation* is preferable to a late *tracheostomy* under unfavourable circumstances. Indeed, tracheostomy should be avoided if possible because it is associated with an increased risk of pulmonary infection in burns injury. Supplemental oxygen should be continued until the COHb concentration has fallen to less than 10%. If hypoxia persists despite supplemental oxygen the application of *CPAP* may be beneficial (Davies *et al.*, 1983), although mask CPAP can be difficult to achieve in those with facial burns and tracheal intubation may then be required. Mechanical ventilation with PEEP is often necessary, but patients with inhalation injury are particularly prone to barotrauma, probably due to air-trapping in small airways obstructed by casts. In a recent study, high-frequency, percussive ventilation decreased airway pressure, the incidence of pneumonia and mortality (Cioffi *et al.*, 1991).

The use of *steroids* is controversial. Several studies have been unable to demonstrate any benefit from their use and there seems to be an increased risk of infection (Neiman *et al.*, 1991). The value of *hyperbaric oxygen therapy* in carbon monoxide poisoning remains uncertain, although in one study it did not appear to be useful in patients who had not lost consciousness or who had sustained only a brief period of unconsciousness (Raphael *et al.*, 1989) (see Chapter 18). Similarly the use of *cyanide antidotes* is controversial and, in view of their potential toxicity, their use is difficult to justify as blind therapy for an already ill patient (see Chapter 18).

SPINAL INJURIES (Swain *et al.*, 1990)

Spinal injuries are a feature of modern mechanized societies, the majority of cases being the result of RTAs. Other causes include falls at work or in the home, sports injuries (mainly diving accidents) and battlefield casu-alties. It is estimated that there are approximately 15–50 new cases of spinal injury/million population/year, although this is probably an underestimate since many immediately fatal cases are unrecognized and many others are inadequately documented.

Pathophysiology

Although spinal cord trauma produces a variable degree of irreversible neuronal destruction and haemorrhage, there is evidence that the ultimate neurological deficit is exacerbated by ischaemia, which may persist for up to 24 hours after injury. This is associated with impaired blood flow, particularly in the grey matter, which may extend beyond the limits of the site of injury (Sandler & Tator, 1976), and oedema formation (cf. Head injuries, Chapter 14).

Immediate management

Patients with isolated spinal injury should be *resuscitated* and, if possible, transferred immediately to a specialized unit (Albin, 1978). Those with serious associated injuries or respiratory failure are usually admitted directly to an intensive care unit. (Chest trauma is common in those with thoracolumbar fracture dislocations, and damage to the cervical spine is frequently associated with head injury. A number of patients will have multiple injuries.)

High thoracic or cervical lesions may produce immediately life-threatening respiratory failure and cardiovascular disturbances (see later in this section). Some patients may therefore require *emergency endotracheal intubation* and *controlled ventilation*, as well as measures to *restore haemodynamic stability*.

Further damage to the spinal cord must be avoided when moving the patient from the site of the accident and during transfer. Patients must therefore be lifted on a spine immobilization device and extricated from wreckage with extreme care; this will usually require several people. Flexion, extension and lateral movements of the spinal column should be prevented by using in line manual immobilization, a cervical collar or sandbags placed on either side of the head, and by positioning pillows to maintain the natural curvatures of the spine. Slight hyperextension at the site of the fracture is preferred and slight traction should be applied to the patient's head and legs.

Diagnosis and assessment

Spinal injury is easily overlooked in the absence of cord damage and in those who are unconscious. If the patient is comatose, a cord lesion should be suspected if deep tendon *reflexes are absent* and in the presence of *urinary retention* or *priapism*. Lesions above T11 produce intercostal paralysis and an *abnormal respiratory pattern*, while cervical cord damage may be associated with *Horner's syndrome*. Nevertheless, all comatose patients should be handled as if a cord injury is present until this possibility has been excluded.

On admission to hospital, a full neurological examination should be performed to determine the level and completeness of the lesion. Subsequently, neurological assessment should be repeated at frequent intervals in order to detect extension of the deficit as cord oedema progresses upwards. It is particularly important to recognize increasing paralysis of respiratory muscles so that controlled ventilation can be instituted without delay. *Neck movements should only be examined in conscious patients and by an expert.*

INVESTIGATIONS

In a patient with multiple trauma it is essential to obtain radiographs of the cervical spine. A *CT scan* or an *MRI* scan may be performed to demonstrate the nature and extent of the cord lesion. *Somatosensory evoked responses* (Chapter 14) can be used to assess the completeness of the cord lesion and to document subsequent recovery or deterioration.

Management

RESPIRATORY SYSTEM

Lesions above T11 interrupt the innervation of respiratory muscles. *Intercostal paralysis* may be partial or complete, and may be asymmetrical. Diaphragmatic breathing in the presence of intercostal paralysis produces a *paradoxical pattern of respiration* with abdominal distension and indrawing of the affected segments of the chest wall during inspiration. Lesions at or above C4 deprive the diaphragm of its major segmental nerve supply and ventilation is grossly impaired. Immediate intubation and ventilation may be life-saving in such cases.

Associated *chest injuries* are common, particularly in those with thoracolumbar injuries, and can further impair respiratory function. These abnormalities may be exacerbated by *aspiration* of gastric contents (the patient is usually nursed supine and often has an impaired ability to cough, a reduced conscious level and paralytic ileus) and *pulmonary oedema* (see later in this section).

It is recommended that *controlled ventilation* is instituted early on the basis of a clinical assessment, assisted by blood gas analysis, in order to avoid a progressive deterioration in respiratory function. Because of the sympathetic denervation, many of these patients are unable to compensate for the increased mean intrathoracic pressure during positive pressure ventilation and become markedly hypotensive. Cautious volume replacement, with or without inotropic support, may then be required to restore perfusion of vital organs.

The treatment of these respiratory abnormalities is complicated by the positioning and immobilization required to treat the spinal injury, which hampers effective physiotherapy. Moreover, vital capacity is reduced (Ohry *et al.*, 1975) and the ability to cough impaired. Diaphragmatic breathing in the presence of intercostal paralysis is, however, most efficient in the supine position. *Intensive physiotherapy* is essential.

CARDIOVASCULAR SUPPORT

There is some experimental evidence to suggest that spinal cord injury can produce *immediate hypertension and bradycardia* lasting for approximately 3–4 minutes (Rawe & Perot, 1979). This may be associated with a *transient rise in intracranial pressure* and an increase in *pulmonary artery pressure* (Albin *et al.*, 1979). These changes can be compared with those described in neurogenic pulmonary oedema (see Chapter 14).

Subsequently, *spinal shock* supervenes, vasomotor tone is lost and both resistance and capacitance vessels dilate. Since the sympathetic innervation of the heart arises from spinal segments T1–T5 it is interrupted by lesions above this level, while parasympathetic fibres remain intact. Patients with high thoracic or cervical injuries are therefore *hypotensive* (systolic blood pressure, commonly 80–90 mm Hg, sometimes as low as 40 mm Hg), but *without an associated tachycardia*. Furthermore, vagal stimulation, for example in response to hypoxia or endotracheal suction, is unopposed and can produce a profound *bradycardia*, or even *asystole* (Welply *et al.*, 1975). This can be prevented by administering atropine regularly or, in resistant cases, by oral sustained-release isoprenaline. Hypoxaemic episodes must be avoided.

Despite the hypotension and relative hypovolaemia, which may or may not be combined with significant blood loss from associated injuries, the circulating volume must be replaced extremely cautiously. Because the CVP is an unreliable guide to volume requirements and cardiovascular function in these patients, pulmonary artery catheterization may be required in the more difficult cases. Patients with high spinal injuries are unable to respond to a volume challenge by increasing heart rate and contractility, and there is therefore a considerable risk of overtransfusion. In some cases, an inotropic agent will be required to improve myocardial performance and restore the systemic blood pressure to an acceptable level. Furthermore, these patients are particularly prone to pulmonary oedema, possibly because pulmonary capillaries are disrupted during the initial hypertensive episode.

Following the period of spinal shock, reflex activity gradually returns and there is some recovery of sympathetic tone. Nevertheless, although the tendency to bradycardia diminishes, a degree of postural hypotension generally persists.

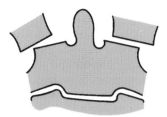

Fig. 9.7 Displaced lateral masses of the atlas. From Johnson (1978), with permission.

MANAGEMENT OF THE SPINAL FRACTURE OR FRACTURE DISLOCATION

The stability of the spinal column depends on the integrity of the posterior ligamentous complex. This consists of the supraspinous and interspinous ligaments, the ligamentum flavum and the capsules of the facet joints. If these are disrupted, the spinal injury will be unstable. In general, controversy continues as to whether operative or non-operative management of spinal fractures and fracture dislocations is preferable.

Cervical spine injuries

In the absence of facet joint dislocation, cervical spine injuries can be managed with a *cervical collar* or *skull traction* to maintain the position and immobilize the site of injury. If one, or both, posterior facet joints are dislocated, *early reduction* is indicated. This can be achieved either by manipulation under a relaxant general anaesthetic, guided by an image intensifier, or by graded traction using skull tongs. Some centres perform *open reduction* in all cases, whereas others only resort to this method when more conservative measures have failed. Subsequently, the position must be maintained with traction. Patients can be nursed in a *Stryker frame*, although this is unsuitable for those with limb fractures requiring traction and the prone position is poorly tolerated by those with associated chest injuries. Moreover, it is dangerous when an endotracheal or tracheostomy tube is in place. In most situations, therefore, the Egerton Stoke Mandeville *tilting and turning bed* is more satisfactory.

Specific types of cervical spine injury. The *atlas* may be fractured where the arch meets the lateral masses. Displacement occurs if the transverse ligament is torn (**Fig. 9.7**). Such an injury is usually caused by a vertical force, such as a fall on the head. Neurological damage is generally minimal and the injury can be treated with a cervical collar worn for three months.

The *odontoid process* may be fractured, usually through the base, most often as a result of an RTA or a severe fall (**Fig. 9.8**). Cord damage is usually mild or

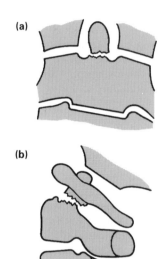

Fig. 9.8 Fractured odontoid process. (a) Anteroposterior view through the mouth of a basal fracture. (b) Lateral view in extension. From Johnson (1978), with permission.

absent, but skull traction is generally indicated and surgery may be necessary if the fracture fails to unite.

Posterior dislocation of the *axis* may occur without a fracture. This causes few neurological signs and is treated with traction followed, if necessary, by fusion.

Burst fractures (**Fig. 9.9**) are very painful, but stable. Unless there is marked bony displacement, cord damage is unusual, but they require support in a collar until fusion is seen radiologically.

Lateral radiographs of the cervical spine may appear normal in patients with *hyperextension injury*, although instability is demonstrable if films are obtained with the neck extended. In some cases, a small fragment of bone may be avulsed from the lower anterior edge of a vertebral body (**Fig. 9.10**). Because the posterior ligaments remain intact, these injuries are stable in the neutral position and can be treated with a cervical collar. The degree of neurological damage is variable.

Anterior dislocations (**Fig. 9.11**) disrupt the posterior ligaments and are therefore unstable unless the

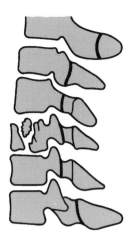

Fig. 9.9 Burst fracture of C5. From Johnson (1978), with permission.

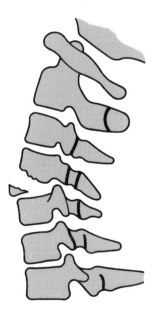

Fig. 9.10 Hyperextension injury of C4/C5: avulsion of fragment from C4. From Johnson (1978), with permission.

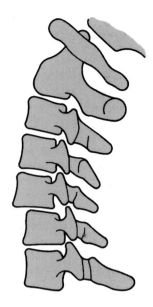

Fig. 9.11 Anterior dislocation: unifacet dislocation of C5 on C6. From Johnson (1978), with permission.

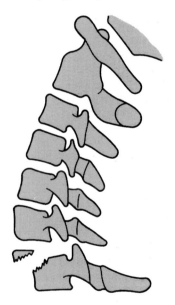

Fig. 9.12 Fracture dislocation of C6/C7: avulsion of fragment of C7. From Johnson (1978), with permission.

facet joints lock. Tetraplegia may occur as a result of this type of injury, but often neurological damage is minimal. Treatment consists of immediate reduction (e.g. using graded skull traction under radiographic control), followed by fusion approximately three weeks later.

The great majority of serious neck injuries involve *fracture dislocations* (**Fig. 9.12**), most often at C5/6 or C6/7. These injuries are very unstable and are associated with the highest incidence of severe neurological damage. The safest treatment is probably continuous skull traction under radiographic control, although some surgeons will manipulate the injury under general anaesthesia. Traction for 4-6 weeks may be followed by

operative fusion in the absence of satisfactory callus formation.

Thoracic spine injuries

Anterior wedge fractures often occur in association with osteoporosis or malignant deposits. They are stable and should be treated symptomatically. On the other hand, fracture dislocations in this region are irreducible and almost invariably cause paraplegia.

Thoracolumbar injuries

Anterior wedge and burst fractures are stable and require only symptomatic treatment. The integrity of the posterior ligaments in this region can be assessed by palpating the midline. If there is a palpable gap between the spinous processes, into which the finger sinks, then the fracture is unstable. These injuries can be treated by postural reduction with the patient extended over a foam bolster positioned at the level of the injury. Some cases will require open reduction and fixation.

TREATMENT OF SPINAL CORD INJURY

It is generally accepted that early immobilization and reduction of fracture dislocations, together with prompt resuscitation to restore oxygen delivery, can minimize neurological damage.

A number of additional measures aimed at preventing or minimizing secondary cord damage have been evaluated, but in general the results have been either inconclusive or discouraging (Albin, 1978). Nevertheless recent evidence suggests that *steroids* may be of value in certain patients with incomplete spinal cord injuries (Bracken *et al.*, 1990). Their use should be determined in consultation with a neurosurgeon.

GASTROINTESTINAL TRACT, FLUID AND ELECTROLYTE BALANCE, NUTRITION

In the acute phase, it can be difficult to exclude significant intra-abdominal trauma since patients with spinal injury are unable to appreciate abdominal pain and up to 20% develop a neurogenic paralytic ileus. *Peritoneal lavage* is a useful diagnostic technique, but interpretation may be complicated by blood leaking into the abdominal cavity from a paravertebral haematoma.

Some patients develop discoordinated bowel activity with progressive *abdominal distension* and *vomiting*, despite the presence of bowel sounds. This is associated with an increased risk of aspiration, fluid and electrolyte disturbances and impaired ventilation. Usually, these abnormalities resolve within 4–7 days and in most cases it is possible to establish enteral nutrition. Occasionally, parenteral nutrition is indicated.

The rectum must be emptied on about the fourth day after injury and this should be followed by regular evacuation on three days of the week. This is achieved with oral aperients, rectal suppositories and, if necessary, manual evacuation. Provided this regimen is started soon after the injury, so that overdistension of the bowel is avoided, a pattern of reflex evacuation can be established and faecal incontinence is prevented.

URINARY TRACT

Initially, patients admitted to the intensive care unit will require urethral or suprapubic catheterization with continuous drainage. Later, a regimen of intermittent catheterization may be instituted to encourage the return of reflex bladder function.

BODY TEMPERATURE

The ability to adjust skin blood flow and sweating is lost below the level of a complete spinal cord lesion. This is a particular problem for tetraplegics who are therefore prone to hypothermia and require air conditioning during hot weather.

GENERAL MEASURES

Finally, prophylactic measures to minimize the risk of gastrointestinal haemorrhage and thromboembolic complications are essential (see Chapter 10), as are first-class nursing care and physiotherapy to prevent pressure sores and fixed deformities.

ANAESTHETIC CONSIDERATIONS

Endotracheal intubation is difficult and hazardous in those with unstable cervical spines. In such cases, the *head and neck should be immobilized* with traction, sandbags or by an assistant before intubation. The usual flexion–extension manoeuvres must be avoided. Because of the dangers of vagal stimulation, the patient must be *preoxygenated* and given *atropine* (Welply *et al.*, 1975). Suxamethonium can precipitate *hyperkalaemia* between three days and six months after the injury (Snow *et al.*, 1973) and should therefore be avoided. In the acute situation, however, patients are at risk of aspiration and some recommend *rapid sequence induction* with suxamethonium and the application of cricoid pressure. Many authorities recommend *awake intubation*, if necessary using a fibre-optic bronchoscope or laryngoscope, as the safest technique. Emergency *cricothyrotomy* or *tracheostomy* is occasionally necessary. Adequate monitoring of cardiovascular and respiratory function is essential throughout.

Prognosis

The outlook for patients with spinal injury has markedly improved since the First World War, when approximately 90% of all cases died within one year; currently the mortality is only 2–3% in the first 12 months. Furthermore, although the life expectancy of a tetraplegic is undoubtedly reduced, on average by about 15 years, paraplegics can generally anticipate a normal lifespan. However, these figures only apply to young patients; the prognosis is considerably worse in the elderly. Nevertheless, since the majority of spinally injured patients are less than 25 years old, they represent a considerable long-term financial commitment. Effective preventive measures are therefore of the utmost importance and must include improvements in safety standards on the roads, at work and in the home.

Approximately 80% of patients with incomplete lesions achieve some form of useful recovery, whereas only 10–15% of those with complete lesions recover any neurological function. Of all cases, 74% eventually become independent, either in or out of a wheelchair, 20% remain partly dependent and only 6% are totally dependent.

NEAR DROWNING (Modell, 1993)

In Great Britain, 1000–1500 people die each year as a result of accidental drowning. The incidence is higher in North America and Australia because of the large number of domestic swimming pools and the popularity of water sports. Almost half of those who drown are less than 20 years old, the highest incidence being in the second decade, and approximately 75% of the victims are male (Modell *et al.*, 1976). Blood alcohol levels are often high. About one-third are competent swimmers and a number of these individuals drown during an attempt at prolonged underwater swimming. In these cases, it is thought that the swimmer hyperventilate before diving in order to lower the arterial carbon dioxide tension and extend the length of time they can remain under water. Unfortunately, they may then lose consciousness due to severe hypoxia before the arterial carbon dioxide tension has reached a level sufficient to stimulate respiration. Subsequently, P_aCO_2 rises and the ensuing inspiratory effort is accompanied by pulmonary aspiration.

Pathophysiology

Drowning can be defined as suffocation by submersion. It occurs without aspiration in only approximately 7–10% of victims; the remaining 90% aspirate liquid, predominantly water (Modell *et al.*, 1976). Although the composition of the water influences the ultimate physiological response, all victims of submersion are hypoxaemic. In those who have not aspirated, hypoxaemia is simply related to a period of apnoea, whereas in those who have inhaled water, there is often primary lung injury. In addition to hypoxaemia, metabolic acidosis is also present in the majority of patients (Modell *et al.*, 1968) and occasionally there are significant fluid and electrolyte abnormalities. Cerebral damage and renal dysfunction may complicate the most serious cases. Delayed deaths following near drowning are usually associated with unrecognized pulmonary insufficiency, secondary chest infection, hypoxic cerebral damage or raised intracranial pressure.

RESPIRATORY ABNORMALITIES

Aspiration of large volumes of fresh water alters the alveolar surface tension (Giammona & Modell, 1967) and even though the water is rapidly absorbed into the circulation this produces hypoxaemia due to *V/Q mismatch* and *alveolar collapse* (Modell *et al.*, 1968). Salt water, on the other hand, remains within the alveoli and draws fluid into the lungs from the intravascular space. Although the total amount of surfactant is reduced, that which remains continues to function normally (Giammona & Modell, 1967). This produces predominantly a large, fixed *right-to-left shunt*. In both instances, a severe *permeability pulmonary oedema* can develop and lung compliance is reduced. Development of non-cardiogenic pulmonary oedema may be delayed for up to 72 hours.

Over-expansion of the lungs with areas resembling *acute emphysema* can frequently be demonstrated at post-mortem in those who have drowned, and are probably the result of violent fluctuations in intrathoracic pressure occurring during the period of airway obstruction. In many, there is also evidence of *aspiration of particulate matter*, such as gastric contents, mud or sand. In those who die later, there may be *bronchopneumonia*, sometimes with multiple *abscess formation* but, in those who survive, recovery of lung function is usually complete.

CARDIOVASCULAR ABNORMALITIES

The most frequent cardiovascular abnormality is *bradycardia*, which is often associated with intense *vasoconstriction*. This response can be elicited by submerging the face in water at less than 20°C, when it is known as the 'diving reflex' (Ramey *et al.*, 1987). The vasoconstriction may divert blood flow to the brain and myocardium and, together with the protective effect of hypothermia, may account for survival following prolonged submersion in cold water. (A 5-year-old Norwegian boy has survived without neurological sequelae after 40 minutes' submersion in iced water, Siebke *et al.*, 1975.) Bradycardia and vasoconstriction can also occur as a response to hypoxaemia and acidosis, while catecholamine release and hypothermia may further contribute to the increased vascular tone.

Theoretically, salt water drowning would be expected to cause hypovolaemia, while aspiration of fresh water should expand the circulating volume. In clinical practice, however, victims of near drowning rarely inhale sufficient quantities to cause significant changes in blood volume (Modell *et al.*, 1976). Nevertheless, *hypovolaemia* may be present because of fluid shifts and loss of circulating volume (e.g. as pulmonary oedema).

A wide variety of *ECG changes* have been described in association with near drowning. These have included:

- absent P waves;
- ST segment elevation;
- increased P–R interval;
- AV dissociation;
- ventricular tachycardia/fibrillation.

Generally, these are secondary changes that revert to normal following correction of hypoxaemia, acidosis, hypothermia and hypovolaemia.

ELECTROLYTE DISTURBANCES

Although plasma levels of sodium and chloride may be elevated following experimental salt water drowning (sea water contains 509 mmol/l of sodium), and low plasma sodium levels have been demonstrated in animal studies of freshwater aspiration, serious electrolyte disturbances are unusual clinically and it is doubtful that they play a significant role in determining survival (Modell *et al.*, 1976). Occasionally, *hyperkalaemia* occurs in association with metabolic acidosis or acute renal failure, and rarely complicates haemolysis caused by absorption of very large volumes of fresh water. *Magnesium* levels may be elevated following sea water drowning.

BODY TEMPERATURE

Hypothermia is a common complication of near drowning and may protect vital organs from hypoxic/ischaemic damage. As body temperature falls below 30°C, however, ventricular fibrillation becomes increasingly likely, and at less than 28°C, established ventricular fibrillation is usually resistant to cardioversion. Rapid rewarming may then be necessary (see Chapter 19).

RENAL DYSFUNCTION

Renal dysfunction is unusual, but may occur in association with hypoxia, metabolic acidosis, severe haemoglobinuria or hypothermia. Established acute renal failure is even more unusual and usually follows an extended period of hypotension.

NEUROLOGICAL DAMAGE

Ischaemic cerebral damage can follow prolonged asphyxia, hypoxaemia or cardiac arrest, while some patients develop *cerebral oedema* and *intracranial hypertension*.

Management

IMMEDIATE CARE

Once the victim has been removed from the water, the first priority is to establish a *clear airway* followed, if necessary, by *mouth-to-mouth resuscitation* and *external cardiac massage*. If it is impossible to reach dry land immediately, expired air ventilation should be attempted in the water since a few breaths may be sufficient to restart spontaneous respiration and cardiac activity. Time should not be wasted in attempting to remove water from the patient's lungs, since the amount recovered, if any, is usually too small to be significant. It is, however, essential to *prevent further heat loss* by wrapping the victim in blankets or warm clothing.

Once experienced personnel arrive at the scene, comatose patients and those requiring continued artificial ventilation must be *intubated* and an *intravenous infusion* should be established. An ECG will allow the detection and treatment of arrhythmias.

HOSPITAL CARE

On admission to hospital it is important to determine the circumstances of the accident (duration of immersion, salt or fresh water, warm or cold, history of alcohol or drug ingestion) as well as the efficacy of any attempts at resuscitation. The patient should be fully examined, and this includes searching for associated injuries, which may significantly complicate the management of near drowning. In particular, cervical spine and head injuries are frequently associated with diving accidents and are easily missed in comatose patients. Analysis of serum electrolyte concentrations should be carried out as necessary. Body temperature should be measured. All patients should be admitted to hospital for observation because of the risk of delayed respiratory failure.

Respiratory management

Hypoxaemia is common following immersion and all patients should receive *supplemental oxygen*. The single most effective means of reversing hypoxaemia is the application of *continuous positive airway pressure (CPAP)* in patients breathing spontaneously or *PEEP* in those receiving controlled ventilation (Modell *et al.*, 1974). Some patients develop irritative bronchospasm requiring *bronchodilator therapy*. The principles of treatment for acute respiratory failure are discussed in Chapter 7.

Cardiovascular support

This will involve the *restoration of sinus rhythm, correction of acidosis and hypoxaemia, volume replacement* and, occasionally, *inotropic support*. In complicated cases, a pulmonary artery catheter may provide useful information, particularly in those with pulmonary oedema. The principles of cardiovascular support are discussed in Chapter 4.

Neurological management

With the improvement in emergency services and intensive pulmonary and cardiovascular care during the last two decades, the prevention and treatment of brain injury has become the main therapeutic challenge in patients who survive near drowning. Unfortunately, the value of aggressive measures aimed at minimizing cerebral damage and controlling intracranial hypertension in comatose victims of near drowning is uncertain; for example, pentobarbital therapy failed to improve outcome in nearly drowned, flaccid and comatose children (Nussbaum & Maggi, 1988). Although many advocate monitoring intracranial pressure, significant intracranial hypertension is unusual after near drowning and when cerebral swelling does occur it does so late in the course of therapy, often after irreversible brain damage has occurred. The value of such monitoring is therefore questionable.

Exposure and environment

Victims of near drowning are frequently hypothermic and their body temperature must be closely monitored. The degree of hypothermia depends not only on the temperature of the water from which patients are retrieved, but also on the amount of insulation provided by their clothing. Several methods of rewarming patients with hypothermia have been advocated (see Chapter 19). It is important to choose a technique that does not produce shivering and increase oxygen demand before the circulation has been restored.

Additional measures

Administration of *steroids* is no longer recommended in near drowning (Modell *et al.*, 1976) since they do not appear to limit the pulmonary abnormality (Calderwood *et al.*, 1975) and may impair lung healing.

Although the use of *prophylactic antibiotics* has been advocated by some authorities, it is generally considered preferable to perform frequent bacteriological investigations and treat only established infections (Modell *et al.*, 1976).

Prognosis

The proportion of victims who survive with normal cerebral function following near drowning varies considerably in retrospective studies. Factors reported to adversely influence outcome include:

- prolonged submersion;
- delay in initiating effective cardiopulmonary resuscitation;
- severe metabolic acidosis (pH < 7.1);
- asystole on arrival in hospital;
- fixed, dilated pupils;
- a low Glasgow Coma Score (< 5).

None of these predictors is infallible, however, and survival with normal cerebral function has been reported even in apparently hopeless cases. For children who are comatose on arrival at the hospital approximately 40% can be expected to survive with normal cerebral function, 30% will die, and the remainder will survive with permanent brain damage. For comatose adults, the mortality is broadly comparable, although survival with impaired brain function is less likely. Since outcome appears to be largely dependent on the extent of irreversible brain damage, prevention of drowning accidents must remain the highest priority.

FAT EMBOLISM SYNDROME (Fabian, 1993)

Fat embolism syndrome (FES) has been recognized since the latter part of the nineteenth century. Classically it presents as a triad of:

- respiratory insufficiency;
- cerebral dysfunction;
- petechial haemorrhages.

In 90% of instances, FES follows blunt trauma complicated by long bone fractures. It has also been described in association with:

- acute pancreatitis;
- diabetes mellitus;
- burns;
- joint reconstruction;
- liposuction;
- cardiopulmonary bypass;
- decompression sickness;
- parenteral infusion of lipids (Levy, 1990).

Paradoxical FES through a patent foramen ovale has also recently been reported (Pell *et al.*, 1993).

Pathophysiology and pathogenesis

Fractures are almost invariably associated with the presence of fat emboli in the lungs and the degree of embolization is generally related to the number and severity of the fractures (Sevitt, 1973). Moreover, subclinical hypoxaemia can be detected in up to 50% of patients with long bone fractures, although a number of factors other than fat embolism, such as the effects of a general anaesthetic, may partly account for this finding (Sevitt, 1973). The majority of cases, however, are asymptomatic, and clinically obvious fat embolism occurs in only 1–5% of those with fractures (Sevitt, 1973). It is not understood why most cases are subclinical while others, with similar or even less severe injuries, develop FES.

The source of the emboli in FES is still disputed, although there is considerable evidence to support the classical *mechanical theory*, which proposes that damage to intramedullary veins allows marrow fat to intravasate and embolize to the lungs (Peltier, 1988). The alternative 'biochemical' hypothesis postulates that the fat emboli are composed of chylomicrons aggregated with very-low-density lipoproteins, which coalesce within the vasculature to form fat macroglobules, perhaps triggered by high levels of plasma C-reactive protein (Hulman, 1988).

The delayed appearance of the petechial rash and neurological dysfunction, and the progressive deterioration in pulmonary dysfunction are consistent with the theory that fat embolism is associated with widespread secondary tissue damage, possibly due to the toxic effects of free fatty acids (FFAs) liberated by the hydrolysis of fat emboli in the lungs (Fonte & Hausberger, 1971) and the release of inflammatory mediators. The possibility that the passage of emboli across a patent foramen ovale is involved in the pathogenesis of the systemic manifestations of the FES has been recognized for some time (Sevitt, 1962) and has recently been demonstrated (Pell *et al.*, 1993). It seems that paradoxical embolism can be precipitated by increased right atrial pressure secondary to the increased pulmonary vascular resistance due to widespread microvascular occlusion.

Pathologically, the lung damage in FES is indistinguishable from that seen in adult respiratory distress syndrome (ARDS) (see Chapter 6). The physiological changes have been described as an initial increase in V_D/V_T ratio caused by embolization, with V/Q mismatch and hypoxaemia (Bruecke *et al.*, 1971). Later, the dead space returns to normal as an interstitial pneumonitis develops.

Massive fat embolism obstructs the pulmonary circulation and rapid deterioration may occur with death from acute right ventricular failure.

Cerebral changes in FES may be due to embolization or hypoxaemia or both.

Clinical features and diagnosis (Fabian *et al.*, 1990)

The onset of the symptoms of FES is usually delayed for up to 48 hours after the injury. Generally, the earliest signs are *dyspnoea* and *tachypnoea*; *hypoxaemia*, most often with a low P_aCO_2, develops later. *Tachycardia*, *hypotension* and *pyrexia* are common. These signs are followed by diffuse shadowing on the chest radiograph.

The syndrome may remain mild and resolve or progress to severe *respiratory failure* with hypoxaemia persisting for up to 14 days. Secondary pulmonary infection is then common. Many fatal cases are fulminating and follow the early onset of coma. Some patients may have associated cerebral involvement manifested as *confusion*, *restlessness* and *drowsiness* following an initial lucid interval. This may progress to *convulsions* and *deep coma*. Some cases present with cerebral involvement without respiratory failure.

A *petechial rash* develops in approximately 50% of patients and appears particularly over the anterior axillary fold, the root of the neck and the conjunctivae. This rash is pathognomonic of FES. Patients with FES may also have retinal exudates and haemorrhages, and occasionally fat droplets can be seen traversing the retinal vessels. *Fat globules* may also be detected in urine and bronchoalveolar lavage specimens (Chastre *et al.*, 1990).

Thrombocytopenia, elevated fibrin/fibrinogen degradation products (FDP), hypocalcaemia and a fall in haematocrit may all be demonstrated, but are nonspecific. Mild jaundice and renal impairment are common. The ECG may show ischaemic ST segment changes and right ventricular strain.

Management

In the absence of specific therapy of proven efficacy, treatment of FES is *supportive*. Respiratory failure is managed according to the principles outlined for ARDS in Chapter 7. Those who are deeply comatose may require treatment aimed at reducing and controlling intracranial pressure (see Chapter 14). Plasma ionized calcium levels occasionally fall sufficiently to cause tetany, in which case calcium should be given intravenously. Platelets should be administered only when indicated for the treatment of severe thrombocytopenia.

Prompt *immobilization of the fracture site* may minimize further embolization (Gossling & Donohue, 1979; Bone *et al.*, 1989) and even if this is not possible initially, surgical stabilization may be required later if embolic episodes persist. However, such surgical intervention may itself be associated with further deterioration. It is therefore often difficult to select the most appropriate course of action for an individual patient.

A variety of *specific agents* have been used in an attempt to reduce the severity of organ damage in FES, but none is of proven clinical efficacy (Gossling & Donohue, 1979). It has, for example, been suggested that heparin might enhance clearance of fat globules by stimulating lipase activity and that this might be beneficial despite the inevitable increase in circulating FFAs. Moreover, heparin can decrease serotonin release from platelets and inhibit disseminated intravascular coagulation (DIC). There is no evidence, however, that heparin administration is of value in FES and its use increases the risk of bleeding into the lungs and from associated injuries. Similarly, the results of administering large doses of alcohol intravenously to inhibit serum lipase activity and minimize FFA production have been unimpressive. Dextran 40 has been used to improve tissue perfusion and inhibit platelet aggregation, but this has the disadvantage that it may leak across the damaged capillary membrane and exacerbate oedema formation. It is unlikely that clofibrate is of any value.

Anecdotal experience has supported the use of pharmacological doses of *steroids* in FES (Fischer *et al.*, 1971) and, as in other circumstances, such treatment is likely to be most effective when given early. Some have suggested that high-dose methylprednisolone can effectively prevent FES when administered prophylactically to patients with isolated long bone fractures (Schonfeld *et al.*, 1983), possibly by preventing complement-induced leucoaggregation.

Prognosis

The mortality of classical FES may approach 10–20%, but a proportion of these deaths are attributable to associated injuries. In one series, there were no deaths in a group of 54 patients with FES who did not have associated life-threatening diseases (Guenter & Braun, 1981). The condition is self-limiting and the majority of survivors will make a full recovery.

CRUSH INJURIES

Traumatic rhabdomyolysis and compartment syndrome

Traumatic rhabdomyolysis or 'crush syndrome' is caused by prolonged continuous pressure on the limbs or torso. Rhabdomyolysis can also be induced by ischaemia, overuse of skeletal muscle, hyperthermia, poisoning, alcohol, infections (e.g. viral myopathies), drugs (e.g. theophyllines) and metabolic disorders (e.g. hypokalaemia).

Pathogenesis (Odeh, 1991)

Crush syndrome is a consequence of the destruction of muscle tissue, leading to an efflux of myoglobin, potassium and phosphate into the circulation. Systemic release of muscle constituents is normally delayed until the limbs have been extricated, decompressed or revascularized. Direct compression of muscle is aetiologically important in almost half the patients with rhabdomyolysis, although a similar situation may arise following temporary interruption of the vascular supply to a limb.

The microvascular damage induced by ischaemia and reperfusion, and the resulting interstitial oedema is thought to have an important role in the pathogenesis of post-ischaemic skeletal muscle injury. Since many muscles are enclosed by a sheath of tight fascia, the development of oedema and swelling is associated with a marked increase in intracompartmental pressure. This may in turn lead to ischaemic necrosis, nerve compression and rhabdomyolysis. This is termed the '*compartment syndrome*'.

The pathogenesis of *renal failure* in rhabdomyolysis and the crush syndrome is still not fully understood. Direct toxic effects of myoglobin, which avidly binds nitric oxide, and tubular obstruction by myoglobin or uric acid crystals have been proposed.

Clinical features

Typically the patient has suffered some form of entrapment or compression injury. Following extrication and decompression, the crush syndrome is characterized by *hypovolaemic shock* and *hyperkalaemia*, and, unless preventive measures are instituted early, usually precipitates *acute renal failure*. Massive rhabdomyolysis may also be associated with *DIC, life-threatening haemorrhage, acute cardiomyopathy* and *multiple organ failure*.

Compartment syndromes usually develop over a period of several hours. They may be initiated by crush injuries, closed or open fractures or sustained compression of an extremity in a comatose patient, or may follow restoration of blood flow to a previously ischaemic extremity.

The signs and symptoms of compartment syndrome are:

- pain, which is typically increased by passively stretching involved muscles;
- decreased sensation within the area of the involved compartment;
- tense swelling of the limb;
- weakness or paralysis of involved muscles.

Diagnosis

The serum creatine phosphokinase level is elevated, there is myoglobinuria and the serum potassium is markedly elevated. Hypocalcaemia may also occur. Intracompartmental pressure can be measured by inserting a hypodermic needle connected to a transduced manometer line. Pressures greater than 30 mm Hg are considered to be abnormal.

Management

Aggressive resuscitation is essential (Better & Stein, 1990). In extensive traumatic rhabdomyolysis, it is quite common to sequester huge volumes of fluid in the damaged muscle (more than 12 litres over a 48-hour period in a 70 kg adult). Inadequate replacement of these losses, which are often compounded by haemorrhage, will increase the risk of acute renal failure. Sometimes bleeding can only be controlled by amputating the affected limb.

The management and prevention of renal insufficiency in patients with rhabdomyolysis is discussed elsewhere (Chapter 12). Regular administration of *mannitol* and *alkalinization of the urine* are the mainstays of treatment.

Prompt recognition of the compartment syndrome is essential. If there are symptoms or a suspicion of a compartment syndrome all potentially constricting circumferential dressings or casts must be removed. If there is not a prompt symptomatic improvement *fasciotomy* must be performed to release tight muscle compartments before necrosis ensues. If capabilities for such procedures are not available locally, immediate orthopaedic consultation should be obtained and early transfer is indicated. Decompressive fasciotomy may have to be combined with excision of necrotic tissue and may not avert amputation of the affected limb.

Outcome

Compartment syndrome may be complicated by permanent paralysis or necrosis, which can lead to a form of Volkmann's ischaemic contracture or gangrene. In a recent study of crush injuries, acute renal failure developed in 16.5% of patients with rhabdomyolysis. The mortality in this subgroup was 42.3% (Ward, 1988).

REFERENCES

Aikawa N, Martyn JAJ & Burke JF (1978) Pulmonary artery catheterization and thermodilution cardiac output determination in the management of critically burned patients. *American Journal of Surgery* **135**: 811-817.

Albin MS (1978) Resuscitation of the spinal cord. *Critical Care Medicine* **6**: 270-276.

Albin MS, Bunegin L, Helsel P, Balrinski M, Marlin AE (1979) Intracraneal pressure and cardiovascular responses to experimental corneal cord transection. *Critical Care Medicine* **7**: 127.

Baud FJ, Barriot P, Toffis V, Riou B, Vicaut E, Lecarpentier Y, Bourdon R, Astier A & Bismuth C (1991) Elevated blood cyanide concentrations in victims of smoke inhalation. *New England Journal of Medicine* **325**: 1761-1766.

Better OS & Stein JH (1990) Early management of shock and prophylaxis of acute renal failure in traumatic rhabdomyolysis. *New England Journal of Medicine* **322**: 825-829.

Bickell WH, Wall MJ Jr, Pepe PE, Martin RR, Ginger VF, Allen MK & Mattox KL (1994) Immediate versus delayed fluid resuscitation for hypotensive patients with penetrating torso injuries. *New England Journal of Medicine* **331**: 1105-1109.

Bone LB, Johnson KD, Weigelt J & Scheinberg R (1989) Early versus delayed stabilization of femoral fractures: a prospective randomized study. *Journal of Bone Surgery (AM)* **71**: 336-340.

Bracken MB, Shepard MJ, Collins WF, *et al.* (1990) A randomized controlled trial of methylprednisolone or naloxone in the treatment of acute spinal cord injury. *New England Journal of Medicine* **322**: 1405-1411.

Bruecke P, Burke JF, Lam KW, Shannon DC & Kazemi H (1971) The pathophysiology of pulmonary fat embolism. *Journal of Thoracic and Cardiovascular Surgery* **61**: 949-955.

Bullock R & Teasdale G (1990a) ABC of major trauma. Head injuries I. *British Medical Journal* **300**: 1515-1518.

Bullock R & Teasdale G (1990b) ABC of major trauma. Head injuries II. *British Medical Journal* **300**: 1576-1579.

Calderwood HW, Modell JH & Ruiz BC (1975) The ineffectiveness of steroid therapy for treatment of fresh-water near-drowning. *Anesthesiology* **43**: 642-650.

Chastre J, Fagon J-Y, Soler P, *et al.* (1990) Bronchoalveolar lavage for rapid diagnosis of the fat embolism syndrome in trauma patients. *Annals of Internal Medicine* **113**: 583–588.

Cioffi WG Jr, Rue LW III, Graves TA, *et al.* (1991) Prophylactic use of high-frequency percussive ventilation in patients with inhalation injury. *Annals of Surgery* **213**: 575–582.

Clark CJ, Campbell D & Reid WH (1981) Blood carboxyhaemoglobin and cyanide levels in fire survivors. *Lancet* **i**: 1332–1335.

Cope A & Stebbings W (1990) ABC of major trauma. Abdominal trauma. *British Medical Journal* **301**: 172–176.

Criswell JC, Parr MJA, Nolan JP (1994) Emergency airway management in patients with cervical spine injuries. *Anaesthesia* **49**: 900–903.

Davies LK, Poulton TJ & Modell JH (1983) Continuous positive airway pressure is beneficial in treatment of smoke inhalation. *Critical Care Medicine* **11**: 726–729.

Deitch EA (1990) The management of burns. *New England Journal of Medicine* **323**: 1249–1253.

Demling RH (1985) Burns. *New England Journal of Medicine* **313**: 1389–1398.

Demling RH & LaLonde C (1990) Identification and modification of the pulmonary and systemic inflammatory and biochemical changes caused by a skin burn. *Journal of Trauma* **30**: 557–562.

Dittmann M, Keller R & Wolff G (1978) A rationale for epidural analgesia in the treatment of multiple rib fractures. *Intensive Care Medicine* **4**: 193–197.

Dittmann M, Steenblock U, Kränzlin M & Wolff G (1982) Epidural analgesia or mechanical ventilation for multiple rib fractures? *Intensive Care Medicine* **8**: 89–92.

Driscoll P & Skinner D (1990a) ABC of major trauma. Initial assessment and management: I. primary survey. *British Medical Journal* **300**: 1265–1267.

Driscoll P & Skinner D (1990b) ABC of major trauma. Initial assessment and management: II. secondary survey. *British Medical Journal* **300**: 1329–1333.

Fabian TC (1993) Unravelling the fat embolism syndrome. *New England Journal of Medicine* **329**: 961–963.

Fabian TC, Hoots AV, Stanford DS, Patterson CR & Mangiante EC (1990) Fat embolism syndrome: prospective evaluation in 92 fracture patients. *Critical Care Medicine* **18**: 42–46.

Fischer JE, Turner RH, Herndon JH & Riseborough EJ (1971) Massive steroid therapy in severe fat embolism. *Surgery, Gynecology and Obstetrics* **132**: 667–672.

Fonte DA & Hausberger FX (1971) Pulmonary free fatty acids in experimental fat embolism. *Journal of Trauma* **11**: 668–672.

Giammona ST & Modell JH (1967) Drowning by total immersion. Effects on pulmonary surfactant of distilled water, isotonic saline, and sea water. *American Journal of Diseases of Children* **114**: 612–616.

Goodwin CW, Dorethy J, Lam V & Pruitt BA Jr (1983) Randomized trial of efficacy of crystalloid and colloid resuscitation on hemodynamic response and lung water following thermal injury. *Annals of Surgery* **197**: 520–531.

Gossling HR & Donohue TA (1979) The fat embolism syndrome. *Journal of the American Medical Association* **241**: 2740–2742.

Guenter CA & Braun TE (1981) Fat embolism syndrome. Changing prognosis. *Chest* **79**: 143–145.

Haywood I & Skinner D (1990) ABC of major trauma. Blast and gunshot injuries. *British Medical Journal* **301**: 1040–1042.

Herndon DN, Barrow RE, Linares HA *et al.* (1988) Inhalation injury in burned patients: effects and treatment. *Burns* **14**: 349–356.

Herndon DN, Barrow RE, Stein M *et al.* (1989) Increased mortality with intravenous supplemental feeding in severely burned patients. *Journal of Burn Care Rehabilitation* **10**: 309–313.

Herndon DN & Zeigler ST (1993) Bacterial translocation after thermal injury. *Critical Care Medicine* **21**: S50–S54.

Hulman G (1988) Pathogenesis of non-traumatic fat embolism. *Lancet* **i**: 1366–1367.

Johnson PG (1978) The management of spinal injuries. In Hanson GC & Wright PL (eds) *The Medical Management of the Critically Ill*. London: Academic Press, pp. 412–429.

Kinsella J (1993) Smoke inhalational injury: diagnosis and treatment. *British Journal of Intensive Care* **3**: 8–14.

Langford RM & Armstrong RF (1989) Algorithm for managing injury from smoke inhalation. *British Medical Journal* **299**: 902–905.

Levy DL (1990) The fat embolism syndrome: a review. *Clinic Orthopaedics* **261**: 281–286.

Loke J, Paul E, Virgulto JA & Smith GJW (1984) Rabbit lung after acute smoke inhalation. Cellular responses and scanning electron microscopy. *Archives of Surgery* **119**: 956–959.

Macdonald RC, O'Neill D, Hanning CD & Ledingham IMcA (1981) Myocardial contusion in blunt chest trauma: a ten-year review. *Intensive Care Medicine* **7**: 265–268.

Modell JH (1993) Drowning. *New England Journal of Medicine* **328**: 253–256.

Modell JH, Moya F, Williams HD & Weibley TC (1968) Changes in blood gases and $A-a_DO_2$ during near-drowning. *Anesthesiology* **29**: 456–465.

Modell JH, Calderwood HW, Ruiz BC, Downs JB & Chapman R Jr (1974) Effects of ventilatory patterns on arterial oxygenation after near-drowning in sea water. *Anesthesiology* **40**: 376–384.

Modell JH, Graves SA & Ketover A (1976) Clinical course of 91 consecutive near-drowning victims. *Chest* **70**: 231–238.

Modell JH, Graves SA and Kuck EJ (1980) Near drowning: correlation of level of consciousness and survival. *Canadian Society of Anaesthetists Journal* **27**: 211–215.

Muir I (1981) The use of the Mount Vernon Formula in the treatment of burn shock. *Intensive Care Medicine* **7**: 49–53.

Muller MJ & Herndon DN (1994) The challenge of burns. *Lancet* **343**: 216–220.

Navar PD, Saffle JR & Warden GD (1985) Effect of inhalational injury on fluid resuscitation requirements after thermal injury. *American Journal of Surgery* **150**: 716–720.

Neiman GF, Clark WR & Hakim T (1991) Methylprednisolone does not protect the lung from inhalation injury. *Burns* **17**: 384–390.

Nussbaum E & Maggi JC (1988) Pentobarbital therapy does not improve neurological outcome in nearly drowning, flaccid-comatose children. *Paediatrics* **81**: 630–634.

Odeh M (1991) The role of reperfusion-induced injury in the pathogenesis of the crush syndrome. *New England Journal of Medicine* **324**: 1417–1422.

Ohry A, Molho M & Rozin R (1975) Alterations of pulmonary

function in spinal cord injured patients. *Paraplegia* **13**: 101-108.

Pell ACH, Hughes D, Keating J, Christie J, Busuttil A & Sutherland GR (1993) Fulminating fat embolism syndrome caused by paradoxical embolism through a patent foramen ovale. *New England Journal of Medicine* **329**: 926-929.

Peltier LF (1988) Fat embolism: a perspective. *Clinical Orthopaedics* **232**: 263-270.

Perry NM & Lewars MD (1990) ABC of major trauma. Radiological assessment I. *British Medical Journal* **301**: 805-809.

Ramey CA, Ramey DN & Hayward JS (1987) Dive response of children in relation to cold-water near-drowning. *Journal of Applied Physiology* **63**: 665-668.

Raphael J-C, Elkharrat D, Jars-Guincestre M-C, Chastang C, Chasles V, Vercken J-B & Gajdos P (1989) Trial of normobaric and hyperbaric oxygen for acute carbon monoxide intoxication. *Lancet* **ii**: 414-419.

Rawe SE & Perot PL Jr (1979) Pressor response resulting from experimental contusion injury to the spinal cord. *Journal of Neurosurgery* **50**: 58-63.

Sandler AN & Tator CH (1976) Effect of acute spinal cord compression injury on regional spinal cord blood flow in primates. *Journal of Neurosurgery* **45**: 660-676.

Schonfeld SA, Ploysongsang Y, DiLisio R *et al.* (1983) Fat embolism prophylaxis with corticosteroids. A prospective study in high-risk patients. *Annals of Internal Medicine* **99**: 433-443.

Sevitt S (1962) Venous thrombosis and pulmonary embolism. Their prevention by oral anticoagulants. *American Journal of Medicine* **33**: 703-716.

Sevitt S (1973) The significance of fat embolism. *British Journal of Hospital Medicine* **9**: 784-793.

Siebke H, Breivik H, Rod T & Link B (1975) Survival after 40 minutes' submersion without cerebral sequelae. *Lancet* **i**: 1275-1277.

Smith MD, Cassidy JM, Souther S *et al.* (1995) Transesophageal echocardiography in the diagnosis of traumatic rupture of the aorta. *New England Journal of Medicine* **332**: 356-362.

Snow JC, Kripke BJ, Sessions GP & Finck AJ (1973) Cardio-vascular collapse following succinylcholine in a paraplegic patient. *Paraplegia* **11**: 199-204.

Swain A, Dove J & Baker H (1990) ABC of major trauma. Trauma of the spine and spinal cord. II. *British Medical Journal* **301**: 110-113.

Torres-Mirabel P, Gruenberg JC, Talbert JG & Brown RS (1982) Ventricular function in myocardial contusion: a preliminary study. *Critical Care Medicine* **10**: 19-24.

Tranbaugh, RF, Elings VB, Christensen JM & Lewis FR (1983) Effect of inhalation injury on lung water accumulation. *Journal of Trauma* **23**: 597-604.

Trinkle JK, Richardson JD, Franz JL *et al.* (1975) Management of flail chest without mechanical ventilation. *Annals of Thoracic Surgery* **19**: 355-363.

Trunkey DD (1983) Trauma. *Scientific American* **249**: 28-35.

Trunkey DD (1991) Initial treatment of patients with extensive trauma. *New England Journal of Medicine* **324**: 1259-1263.

Ward MM (1988) Factors predictive of acute renal failure in rhabdomyolysis. *Archives of Internal Medicine* **148**: 1553-1557.

Watson D (1990) ABC of major trauma. Management of the upper airway. *British Medical Journal* **300**: 1388-1391.

Webb AK (1978) Flail chest: management and complications. *British Journal of Hospital Medicine* **20**: 406-412.

Welply NC, Mathias CJ & Frankel HL (1975) Circulatory reflexes in tetraplegics during artificial ventilation and general anaesthesia. *Paraplegia* **13**: 172-182.

Westaby S & Brayley N (1990a) ABC of major trauma. Thoracic trauma I. *British Medical Journal* **300**: 1639-1643.

Westaby S & Brayley N (1990b) ABC of major trauma. Thoracic trauma II. *British Medical Journal* **300**: 1710-1712.

Willett KM, Dorrell H & Kelly P (1990) Management of limb injuries. *British Medical Journal* **301**: 229-233.

Wilmore DW, Long JM, Mason AD Jr, Skreen RW & Pruitt BA Jr (1974) Catecholamines: mediator of the hypermetabolic response to thermal injury. *Annals of Surgery* **180**: 653-669.

Wilmore DW, Mason AD Jr, Johnson DW & Pruitt BA Jr (1975) Effect of ambient temperature on heat production and heat loss in burn patients. *Journal of Applied Physiology* **38**: 593-597.

10 General Aspects of Managing Critically Ill Patients

FLUID AND ELECTROLYTE BALANCE

Physiological background

Water constitutes 45–80% of body weight, depending on age, sex and body build, the proportion being greater in men and infants and less in the obese. Approximately two-thirds of body water is contained within the *intracellular* compartment, the remainder being extracellular fluid (ECF) distributed between the *interstitial* space (two-thirds) and the *vascular* space (one-third). There is also a fourth '*transcellular*' compartment, which includes water in the gut as well as cerebrospinal, synovial, pericardial and pleural fluid (**Fig. 10.1**). Although in health this compartment is small, it may become important in disease (e.g. in those with bowel obstruction or with a large pleural effusion).

Each of these spaces has a unique function and composition, the distribution of water between the compartments depending on the osmotic equilibrium between them, the osmotic pressure exerted by non-diffusible plasma proteins (the 'oncotic pressure') (see Chapter 2) and the Gibbs–Donnan equilibrium. The latter explains the unequal distribution of diffusible ions on either side of a semipermeable membrane when one side contains a poorly diffusible ion. Allowing for the Gibbs–Donnan distribution and the plasma oncotic pressure, the electrolyte content of plasma and interstitial fluid is essentially the same, whereas the composition of the intracellular fluid (ICF) differs considerably from the other two. Due to the operation of cellular pumps, sodium and chloride ions are largely extracellular, while potassium is the dominant intracellular cation, balanced by phosphate, sulphate and bicarbonate anions, as well as protein (**Table 10.1**).

These differences in the distribution of body water between the four compartments, and of sodium and chloride between the intracellular and extracellular spaces, have important clinical implications. Intravenous infusion of 'normal' (0.9%) or 'isotonic', saline, for example, primarily expands the extracellular compartment and, because it contains 150 mmol sodium/litre there is a small increase in the osmolality of the ECF, which causes a slight shift of fluid into the vascular space. Administration of 0.18% saline in glucose 4%, on the other hand, reduces the osmolality of the ECF, water moves into the cells until a new osmolar equilibrium is established and the increase in ECF volume is considerably less than that achieved with 0.9% saline. When dextrose solutions are administered they are distributed throughout the total body water according to the relative volumes of the various compartments;

Table 10.1 Electrolyte composition of intracellular and extracellular fluids.

	Plasma (mmol/l)	Interstitial fluid (mmol/l)	Intracellular fluid (mmol/l)
Na^+	142	144	10
K^+	4	4	160
Ca^{2+}	2.5	1.25	1.5
Mg^{2+}	1.0	0.5	13
Cl^-	102	114	2
HCO_3^-	26	30	8
PO_4^{2-}	1.0	1.0	57
SO_4^{2-}	0.5	0.5	10
Organic acid	6	5	
Protein	16	0	55

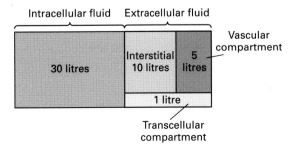

Fig 10.1 Distribution of body water in a 75 kg man.

consequently only about one-tenth of the infused volume remains in the intravascular space. Finally colloidal solutions are normally confined to the intravascular space, at least initially, and are the most effective solutions for expanding the circulating volume, although their distribution can be profoundly influenced by changes in capillary permeability (see Chapters 2 and 4).

General principles of fluid and electrolyte management

The average water requirement for a normal adult is 20–60 ml/kg/day. In most intensive care patients, however, the stress response promotes sodium and water retention, a tendency that is exacerbated by mechanical ventilation (see Chapter 7), while in those breathing humidified gases, insensible losses are approximately half the estimated normal 500–900 ml/day. In many patients there is also a degree of renal dysfunction, which further impairs their ability to excrete a sodium and water load. Finally it must be remembered that normal oxidation of food produces significant volumes of water (0.41, 0.60 and 1.07 ml of water/g of protein, carbohydrate and fat, respectively). Critically ill patients are therefore particularly susceptible to salt and water overload and, especially when combined with an increase in capillary permeability and hypoproteinaemia (see Chapter 2), they are at considerable risk of developing peripheral and pulmonary oedema.

Some degree of fluid restriction with reduced sodium intake is therefore usually necessary, particularly in mechanically ventilated patients (e.g. 20–30 ml/kg of 5% dextrose or 0.18% saline in dextrose 4%/24 hours). Additional sources of fluid and electrolytes, such as the heparinized saline used to flush intravascular catheters, the high sodium content of colloid replacement fluids and the solutions used as vehicles for intravenous drugs, must also be taken into account. Conversely, some patients will be losing abnormally large volumes of fluid and electrolytes (e.g. as diarrhoea or drainage from fistulae). If the patient is pyrexial, sweating or hyperventilating with inadequate humidification, insensible losses will be increased. Urine output may be increased by diuretic therapy or by an osmotic diuresis, as may occur with hyperglycaemia. Sometimes polyuria may be the result of diabetes insipidus (e.g. complicating a head injury, see Chapters 14 and 16).

In some cases, therefore, ill-advised fluid restriction or inadequate replacement of large losses can cause significant dehydration with intravascular volume depletion and a risk of renal impairment, whereas in others excessive administration of fluid and electrolytes may lead to overhydration with 'wet lungs' and peripheral oedema.

An appropriate intravenous fluid regimen must be devised for each individual patient based on clinical assessment and experience, guided by the results of laboratory investigations. Most of the variables routinely monitored in intensive care patients, such as blood pressure, heart rate, central venous pressure (CVP) and pulmonary artery occlusion pressure (PAOP), and even to some extent urine output, are largely a reflection of the volume of the intravascular space. Assessment of the interstitial and intracellular volumes is more difficult and is usually based on chest radiograph appearances and the detection of peripheral oedema on clinical examination. In some units, patients are weighed daily to assist assessment of fluid balance, although this is practically difficult and requires a meticulous technique to be accurate. Plasma urea, creatinine, electrolyte and blood sugar levels should be measured at least once a day, and sometimes more frequently. The total output of fluid as urine, gastric aspirate and from any drains, together with the total intravenous and oral input should be calculated 12-hourly and the overall fluid balance recorded. In difficult cases it may be helpful to measure urinary urea and electrolyte concentrations, as well as plasma and urinary osmolalities and the electrolyte content of the gastric aspirate and any drainage fluid. The total input and output of each individual constituent can then be calculated.

Fortunately, patients are generally surprisingly tolerant of what are inevitably rather crude attempts to control their fluid and electrolyte balance, particularly when the kidneys are functioning normally. Nevertheless, if the basic principles of management are not understood, or careless mistakes are made, serious abnormalities will result. The important constituents to be considered are water, sodium, potassium and magnesium. There may be an excess or deficit of each, either singly or in combination.

Water depletion

CAUSES

Water depletion rarely occurs in isolation since it is usually combined with some degree of sodium loss. Predominant water depletion may occur if:

● intake is inadequate
● there are excessive losses of hypotonic fluid (diarrhoea, sweating, hyperventilation).

DIAGNOSIS

Losses of water are initially distributed evenly throughout the body compartments. Once the deficit is severe enough to cause a decreased circulating volume, aldosterone is released causing renal retention of sodium. Because of the osmotic effect of the increase in plasma sodium concentration, water then leaves the cells and there is loss of tissue turgor. The patient is oliguric with a concentrated urine. Plasma sodium is increased, plasma urea is slightly increased and plasma osmolality is normal or increased. The haematocrit rises only in the later stages of water depletion.

TREATMENT

5% dextrose or, if, as is more usual, sodium has been lost as well, 0.18% saline in dextrose 4% should be administered intravenously. The management of diabetes insipidus is discussed in Chapter 16.

Water intoxication

CAUSES

Water intoxication is *usually iatrogenic* and caused by excessive intravenous administration of hypotonic solutions (e.g. 5% dextrose) in the presence of a reduced ability to excrete water, often caused by *increased levels of antidiuretic hormone* (ADH) in response to stress (e.g. peri-operatively) or in association with an 'inappropriate' secretion of ADH. It may also complicate *absorption of irrigation fluid* during urological surgery.

DIAGNOSIS

Acute severe water intoxication can cause confusion which may progress to convulsions and coma. Plasma sodium is low, often less than 120 mmol/l.

TREATMENT

Mild water intoxication can be treated simply by restriction of intake; in more severe cases 1.8% saline can be administered. If renal function is impaired, the latter may be dangerous and dialysis will be required. In some patients with inappropriate ADH secretion, fluid restriction alone may be insufficient and in such cases drugs that antagonize ADH (e.g. *demeclocycline*) may be used in doses above 600 mg/day to induce nephrogenic diabetes insipidus.

Hyponatraemia

CAUSES

A low plasma sodium (< 135 mmol/l) can be caused not only by *water intoxication*, but also by *depletion of total body sodium*. Some commonly encountered causes in intensive care patients are:

- diuretic therapy;
- renal disease;
- end-stage liver disease;
- fluid losses from the alimentary tract or intra-abdominal drains.

Hyponatraemia is often exacerbated by the use of hypotonic intravenous fluids (e.g. 5% dextrose, 0.18% saline in dextrose 4%) to replace isotonic losses (e.g. from the alimentary tract) or to maintain blood sugar levels in hepatic insufficiency.

In hyperlipidaemia the plasma sodium concentration may be *spuriously low* because the sodium is confined to the aqueous phase, whereas its concentration is expressed in terms of the total plasma volume.

DIAGNOSIS

Significant sodium depletion will cause a fall in intravascular volume and stimulate the release of aldosterone. In true hyponatraemia, therefore, urinary potassium excretion increases while sodium ions are retained. In hyperlipidaemia (or 'pseudo-hyponatraemia') the concentration of other plasma electrolytes (potassium, chloride and bicarbonate) will also be reduced. Failure to recognize pseudohyponatraemia can have dangerous consequences (Editorial, 1980).

TREATMENT

Usually, the situation can be resolved by the administration of 0.9% saline; very rarely, it may be necessary to use hypertonic sodium chloride and frusemide (Arieff, 1993), and in the most severe cases associated with renal impairment, haemofiltration may be required (Larner et al., 1988). Although conventionally too rapid correction of profound hyponatraemia is thought to increase the risk of precipitating *central pontine myelinolysis* (Sterns et al., 1986; Swales, 1987), this contention has recently been questioned (Arieff, 1993). Nevertheless, in cases of symptomatic hyponatraemia the rise in plasma sodium should not be allowed to exceed about 25 mmol/l during the initial 24–48 hours.

Similarly the true nature of a controversial cause of hyponatraemia in the critically ill, the '*sick cell syndrome*' (Flear & Singh, 1973) has been questioned. This was thought to occur only in the most severely ill patients and was said to account for the close association between a low plasma sodium and a poor prognosis. It was postulated that a defect at cellular level, possibly an increase in membrane permeability or a failure of the sodium pump due to an inadequate supply of energy in the form of adenosine triphosphate (ATP) caused sodium ions to enter the cell in exchange for potassium ions, which were then lost in the urine. An alternative explanation is that this abnormality is simply a response to total body potassium depletion that causes intracellular hypotonia and a redistribution of body water.

Hypernatraemia

CAUSES

Hypernatraemia (a plasma sodium > 145 mmol/l) occurs most commonly in situations of predominant *water depletion*. It may also occur in association with *salt retention* in acute renal failure and in this situation can be exacerbated by the administration of excessive sodium ions, often as 8.4% sodium bicarbonate given in an attempt to correct a metabolic acidosis.

TREATMENT

Pure water depletion should be treated with hypotonic intravenous fluids or dialysis, but rapid falls in plasma sodium greater than 2 mmol/h may precipitate cerebral oedema and must be avoided. This has been implicated in the morbidity and mortality of diabetic ketoacidosis.

Hypokalaemia

CAUSES

Potassium depletion is one of the commonest abnormalities of fluid and electrolyte balance encountered in the intensive care unit. Hypokalaemia can be defined as a plasma potassium concentration of less than 3.0 mmol/l and is usually related to *inadequate replacement of excessive urinary or gastrointestinal losses*. For a number of reasons, critically ill patients are particularly prone to the development of hypokalaemia. Elevated levels of *aldosterone* are found in both cardiac and liver failure as well as part of the stress response, while the administration of *steroids* and *diuretics* also increase urinary potassium losses. Enormous quantities of potassium may be lost in the urine during the recovery phases of *acute renal failure*, and severe hypokalaemia may itself lead to tubular dysfunction.

DIAGNOSIS

Hypokalaemia may be detected by recognizing the associated *electrocardiographic (ECG) changes* of ST segment depression, decreased T wave amplitude and U waves (**Fig. 10.2**). Hypokalaemia can also cause supraventricular tachycardias, particularly in the presence of digoxin, as well as more serious ventricular arrhythmias.

There is a reciprocal relationship between the urinary excretion of hydrogen ions and potassium ions; therefore, when hydrogen ions are being reabsorbed by the renal tubules, potassium ions are excreted to maintain ionic equilibrium. Likewise, if total body potassium levels are low, this ion is conserved and hydrogen ions are lost in the urine. This leads to a '*hypokalaemic metabolic alkalosis*' with a paradoxically acid urine.

TREATMENT

Treatment is with potassium chloride by infusion, either alone or combined with dextrose and insulin. Concentrated solutions are extremely irritant and must therefore be administered via a centrally placed catheter. If potassium is given too rapidly, plasma concentrations may reach dangerous levels before equilibration between extra- and intracellular compartments has occurred. Except in exceptional circumstances, intravenous administration of potassium should not exceed 40 mmol/h.

Sometimes plasma potassium levels are within the normal range, but if there is an unexplained metabolic alkalosis with an acid urine, careful administration of potassium chloride, sometimes combined with dextrose and insulin, will often correct the alkalosis.

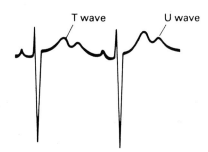

Fig 10.2 Electrocardiographic changes in hypokalaemia—lead V3, showing U waves. These are best seen in the anterior chest leads. Because of T wave flattening and ST depression, the U wave may sometimes be mistaken for a T wave.

Hyperkalaemia

CAUSES

Hyperkalaemia can be defined as a plasma potassium greater than 5 mmol/l. It is frequently *iatrogenic* and caused by excessive potassium administration, often when the onset of acute renal failure has not been immediately recognized. Also administration of suxamethonium to patients with diffuse tissue damage (e.g. muscle trauma, burns, tetanus or paralysis) can release large quantities of potassium into the circulation. There is a risk of this complication from 5 to 15 days after the injury and the danger persists for 2-3 months in those who have sustained burns or trauma, and for perhaps 3-6 months in those with upper motor neurone lesions (Gronert & Theye, 1975). It is of particular importance in patients with renal failure. Other causes of hyperkalaemia include *hypercatabolism*, *'crush syndrome'* and, occasionally, *massive blood transfusion*.

DIAGNOSIS AND TREATMENT

The *ECG changes* associated with hyperkalaemia are peaked T waves and widening of the QRS complexes, followed by bradycardia and asystole (**Fig. 10.3**). Treatment is therefore urgent. Obviously potassium administration should be stopped, and in extreme emergencies *10 ml 10% calcium chloride* injected intravenously will temporarily antagonize the cardiac effects of hyperkalaemia. An intravenous injection of *50 ml 50% dextrose containing 20 units soluble insulin* will drive potassium into the cells. Alkalinization with *sodium bicarbonate* and, if possible, *hyperventilation* will also shift potassium into the intracellular compartment, as well as enhance potassium excretion via the kidneys. The former has by far the greater effect on plasma potassium levels. Sodium bicarbonate should be avoided in patients prone to sodium overload (e.g. those with renal failure). Potassium levels may be further reduced by the slow intravenous administration of a β_2 *adrenoreceptor*

agonist (e.g. salbutamol 500 µg), which will promote cellular uptake of potassium by a cyclic adenosine monophosphate (AMP)-dependent activation of the Na^+/K^+ pump. Nebulized salbutamol (10 mg) can also be used. Rectally administered sodium or calcium *exchange resins*, which physically remove potassium cations, have an onset of action within about 30 minutes that should last for up to six hours. In many cases, however, these measures only defer the dangerous consequences of hyperkalaemia while arrangements are made for definitive treatment with *haemofiltration* or *dialysis*.

Hypomagnesaemia (Zaloga, 1989)

CAUSES

Critically ill patients may develop hypomagnesaemia in association with:

- the excessive use of diuretics;
- the administration of insulin in diabetic ketoacidosis;
- large gastrointestinal fluid losses;
- malabsorption;
- long-term parenteral nutrition with insufficient supplementary magnesium.

DIAGNOSIS AND TREATMENT

Magnesium is important for normal neuromuscular function and the features of deficiency are similar to those of hypocalcaemia, with *tetany, muscle weakness* and *cardiac arrhythmias*. Most patients, however, remain asymptomatic and in general clinical signs and symptoms correlate poorly with plasma magnesium levels, probably because magnesium is a predominantly intracellular ion with less than 1% of the total body content being extracellular. Even red cell or mononuclear cell magnesium concentrations are not a reliable guide to tissue levels.

Treatment is with oral magnesium hydroxide, intramuscular magnesium chloride or the slow intravenous infusion of 10 mmol magnesium sulphate repeated as necessary according to plasma estimations. Recently it has been suggested that magnesium depletion can be diagnosed and treated by administering 30 mmol of magnesium sulphate in 100 ml of 5% dextrose over 8 hours. Magnesium deficiency is diagnosed if the body retains more than 30% of the infused dose (Arnold *et al.*, 1995).

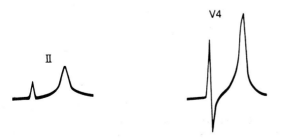

Fig 10.3 Electrocardiographic changes in hyperkalaemia—leads II and V4. Note the tall peaked narrow T waves and broad QRS complexes. There is also atrial standstill.

Hypermagnesaemia

CAUSES

Hypermagnesaemia occurs most commonly as a result of *excessive magnesium administration* and/or *renal failure*.

DIAGNOSIS AND TREATMENT

The main adverse effects of hypermagnesaemia are on *cardiac conduction*, with prolongation of the PR interval and QRS complexes and peaked T waves. At even higher levels, *hyporeflexia, respiratory paralysis* and *coma* may occur, with *cardiac arrest* as the terminal event.

Intravenous *calcium chloride* may be used as emergency treatment for the cardiac conduction defects. *Haemofiltration/dialysis* may be required in the most severe cases.

NUTRITIONAL SUPPORT (Grimble *et al.*, 1992)

In normal individuals short periods of starvation are of little consequence and the same is true for adequately nourished intensive care patients who resume eating within 24–48 hours (e.g. those admitted electively following cardiac surgery). In the majority of critically ill patients, however, nutritional support should be instituted as soon as practicable (usually within 2–3 days of the acute episode) in an attempt to prevent serious reductions in body cell mass as well as to ensure adequate supplies of protein and energy for tissue repair and resisting infection. Many patients are malnourished when admitted and if loss of muscle bulk is allowed to progress, muscle weakness may delay mobilization and compromise the patient's ability to breathe spontaneously (see also Chapters 6 and 7). In addition, malnutrition may be associated with abnormalities of the lung parenchyma, as well as an increased susceptibility to pulmonary infection (Askanazi *et al.*, 1982). It has also been shown that ventilator-dependent patients who respond to nutritional support by increasing protein synthesis are more likely to wean from respiratory support than those who do not (Larca & Greenbaum, 1982).

Objective measures of the patient's nutritional state might help the clinician to assess the need for nutritional support. Unfortunately, although the parameters that can be assessed reasonably easily (e.g. serum albumin and transferrin levels, the triceps skin-fold thickness and cutaneous responses to recall antigens, Forse *et al.*, 1981) can define the nutritional status of a population of patients, they are generally relatively insensitive and lack specificity. Recent studies have confirmed that malnourished patients can be accurately identified on the basis of a subjective clinical assessment of their nutritional status without reference to a rigid scoring system (Detsky, 1991).

Many believe that the efficacy and safety of nutritional support is improved when supervised by a multidisciplinary nutrition team. The exact composition of such teams will vary according to local circumstances, but most will include at least one clinician (physician, surgeon, intensive care specialist), a dietitian, a pharmacist, a clinical biochemist and a nurse specialist.

Enteral nutrition (Dobb, 1992)

In the past many critically ill patients were fed intravenously, but because of the high incidence of complications associated with total parenteral nutrition (TPN, see later in this chapter) the enteral route, which may also be associated with certain specific benefits, is now preferred. There is, for example, increasing evidence that the enterocytes of the small intestine obtain a proportion of their nutrients directly from the gut lumen and that when deprived of this source of nourishment, the mucosa undergoes villous atrophy, impairing its barrier function. It is thought that enteral nutrition, perhaps especially if it includes glutamine (Souba *et al.*, 1990) and fibre, maintains intestinal mucosal integrity, reduces bacterial translocation (Alexander, 1990) (see Chapter 4), enhances autoregulation of blood flow to the gut and maintains gastrointestinal motility. Moreover, when the enteral route is used, nutrients enter the bloodstream via the normal route and are presented directly to the liver for processing. A prospective study has shown that following major abdominal trauma, postoperative enteral nutrition significantly reduced septic complications when compared with TPN (Moore *et al.*, 1989). This finding has been confirmed by a recent meta-analysis of prospective trials comparing enteral and parenteral nutrition (Moore *et al.*, 1992).

ADMINISTRATION

Intragastric tube feeding can be commenced provided that the gastric aspirate is not excessive (e.g. not more than 40 ml/h). Enteral feeding may also be administered via a *gastrostomy* and it has been shown that endoscopically guided *percutaneous gastrostomy* is a simple, safe and well-tolerated procedure. In patients with impaired gastric emptying, it may be advantageous to position a *fine tube in the jejunum* (usually this is most easily achieved endoscopically), or alternatively a *jejunostomy* can be fashioned at the time of surgery e.g. following oesophago-gastrectomy or trauma surgery (Moore & Moore, 1991).

Fine-bore nasogastric and nasojejunal tubes are more comfortable, as well as less likely to cause oesophageal ulceration and stricture than traditional tubes; they are ideal for long-term use. Most fine-bore tubes are supplied with a wire introducer, some can be stiffened by placing them in a refrigerator and others have mercury-weighted tips. Whichever is used it is possible to push these fine-bore tubes past the low-pressure cuff of an endotracheal or tracheostomy tube and into the lungs. Unconscious or debilitated patients and those with bulbar palsy may not react to the presence of such a tube in their major airways, and it is essential to check its position before starting the feed. Although it can be more difficult to aspirate gastric contents through some fine-bore tubes, it is usually possible to inject sufficient air to be heard entering the stomach through a stethoscope placed over the epigastrium. Nevertheless a radiograph should always be taken to verify that the tube is correctly positioned.

The majority of intensive care patients are unable to protect their own airways. Some patients are supine and the presence of a nasogastric tube renders the gastro-oesophageal sphincter incompetent, allowing reflux of gastric contents. The presence of a cuffed endotracheal or tracheostomy tube is not a certain barrier to inhalation since liquids may find their way past a low-pressure cuff. In such patients, therefore, fluid must not be allowed to accumulate in the stomach and the naso-gastric tube must be of a sufficient size to allow aspiration. Some fine-bore tubes are sufficiently rigid and have a large enough lumen to allow aspiration of gastric contents and can therefore be used in those who are tolerating a gastric feed even when they are unable to protect their airways. In the early stages of critical illness, in patients at high risk of aspiration and for short-term use, however, larger bore nasogastric tubes are still usually preferred. It is also easier to be certain of the position of these larger tubes. Patients should be nursed with at least a 30° head-up tilt.

The feed should be administered at a constant rate, preferably using an infusion pump, to reduce the incidence of diarrhoea (Jones et al., 1980). To avoid the risk of regurgitation, the feed can be discontinued every five hours and the stomach aspirated after a one-hour 'rest period'. In addition, feeding can be discontinued during the night to simulate a more normal dietary pattern. There appears to be no advantage in commencing enteral nutrition with $\frac{1}{4}$- or $\frac{1}{2}$-strength feeds, although it is sensible to use reduced volumes initially (e.g. 30–50 ml rather than 100 ml/h) until it is clear that there is no problem with gastric emptying. Volumes of aspirate up to 150 ml can be returned and the feed continued. If larger quantities are obtained, indicating gastric stasis, up to 150 ml can be returned, but the excess should be discarded, the volume of feed administered should be reduced and metoclopramide (5–10 mg intravenously or intramuscularly 8-hourly as required) or cisapride (10 mg nasogastrically 6-hourly) can be given to encourage gastric emptying. Some recommend continuing the enteral feed at a rate of 10 ml/h in all cases in the belief that this may help to preserve gastrointestinal mucosal integrity.

CHOICE OF FEED (Heyland et al., 1994)

In general, one of the proprietary low-residue whole-protein feeds should be used. These provide approximately 75 g of protein and 2000 kcal in 2 litres of feed, with a non-protein calorie:nitrogen ratio that is usually less than 200:1. The majority are lactose-free and contain most of the daily requirements of electrolytes, trace elements and vitamins. Low-sodium feeds may be useful in hypernatraemic patients and feeds containing 2 kcals/ml can be used to limit fluid intake. Although it has been suggested that hyperosmolar feeds may be more likely to produce diarrhoea, this was not the case in one study (Keohane et al., 1984). It is possible that modified enteral formulations containing arginine, ribonucleic acid (RNA) and ω-3 fatty acids may restore or enhance immune function in critically ill and septic patients, but this remains unproven (Cerra et al., 1991).

COMPLICATIONS

Diarrhoea is a common problem in the critically ill and appears to be closely related to concomitant antibiotic therapy (Keohane et al., 1983b, 1984). Occasionally, *Clostridium difficile* infection may be responsible, but lactase deficiency is probably a rare cause of diarrhoea (Keohane et al., 1983b). If diarrhoea does occur, some form of roughage may be added to the feed and agents such as codeine phosphate (30–60 mg orally or nasogastrically 4-hourly) or loperamide (4 mg initially, followed by 2 mg after each loose stool up to a maximum of 16 mg daily orally or nasogastrically) can be used to reduce gastrointestinal motility. Other complications of enteral nutrition include:

- regurgitation and aspiration;
- oesophageal ulceration with bleeding and stricture formation (particularly with large-bore tubes);
- hyperglycaemia;
- deficiencies of potassium, phosphate and zinc;
- mild abnormalities of liver function.

Total parenteral nutrition

INDICATIONS

Parenteral nutrition will be required in those patients in whom enteral feeding is contraindicated (e.g. small bowel anastomoses, intrinsic small bowel disease) or fails due to gastric stasis, ileus, intractable diarrhoea or malabsorption. TPN may also be required when it proves impossible to provide sufficient energy via the enteral route.

Perioperative TPN

It has been recognized for many years that there is an increased risk of complications in surgical patients with pre-existing protein/energy malnutrition (Studley, 1936) and that this is largely related to sepsis, presumably associated with inadequate immune responses (Forse et al., 1981) and impaired tissue repair. While it is undoubtedly possible to provide adequate nutritional support for an indefinite period using home TPN in otherwise healthy patients with severe irreversible malabsorption (e.g. a 'short-bowel' syndrome) there is little evidence that perioperative TPN improves outcome in surgical patients (Detsky, 1991). A meta-analysis of 11 studies concluded that any possible benefit of preoperative TPN in well-nourished patients was small and clinically unimportant, although it was suggested that it might be of greater value in malnourished patients (Detsky et al., 1987). A more recent multicentre study, however, not only confirmed the lack of efficacy of TPN in borderline malnourished patients, who had more infectious complications when given TPN, but also failed to prove unequivocal benefit, despite some encouraging trends, even in severely malnourished patients (Veterans Affairs Total Parenteral Nutrition Cooperative Study Group, 1991). It would seem that in the absence of severe malnutrition most patients are probably best served by prompt surgery.

TPN in the acute phase of critical illness

It has also proved difficult to establish the value of TPN during the acute phase of a non-surgical critical illness, although it is known that patients who lose more than 30% of their initial body weight in the course of an acute illness have only a remote chance of survival (Detsky, 1991). Certainly during the first 48–72 hours of the acute episode, TPN may seriously complicate management and even with aggressive nutritional support it is often impossible to achieve a positive nitrogen balance in critically ill patients. This reflects the use of amino acids as oxidative fuels (Cerra et al., 1987) with reduced protein synthesis and increased protein catabolism, combined with impaired fat and glucose tolerance. In practice, the ability to meet the notional nutritional requirements of critically ill patients may also be limited by the need for fluid restriction, glucose intolerance or impaired renal function. Nevertheless the provision of adequate nutritional support should always be given a high priority; diuretics or haemofiltration should be used to prevent fluid overload, early haemofiltration/dialysis should be instituted to prevent azotaemia and supplemental parenteral nutrition should be given when enteral feeding alone is insufficient.

ADMINISTRATION

Insertion and care of central intravenous catheters for TPN

The *infraclavicular approach to the subclavian vein* is the preferred route for insertion of the intravascular catheter since it allows the patient unrestricted movement of the upper limb, head and neck, and minimizes movement of the catheter at the skin puncture site. Intravenous feeding is never an emergency and catheter placement should be performed as a planned procedure with full aseptic precautions. A *silicone catheter* should be used as these are the least thrombogenic and some authorities recommend the use of a *subcutaneous 'tunnel'*. This may reduce the incidence of catheter-related sepsis (Keohane et al., 1983a), probably because infection originating at the site of exit of the catheter from the skin must travel some distance before gaining access to the bloodstream. Large-bore *Hickman silicone catheters* inserted surgically or percutaneously seem to be associated with a lower risk of obstruction, and are being used increasingly frequently.

The puncture sites should be sprayed with an antiseptic such as povidone-iodine (an alternative is povidone-iodine ointment) and a transparent adhesive dressing applied. This allows frequent inspection of the wound for signs of infection, while avoiding the need to disturb the dressing. Central lines should be removed if signs of infection (unexplained fever, pus or erythema at puncture sites) or thrombophlebitis develop. Alternatively if one lumen of a non-tunnelled triple lumen central venous catheter is used it should be changed every 5–8 days depending on local policies.

Correct positioning of the catheter must be confirmed before intravenous feeding is started. It should be possible to aspirate venous blood freely and a chest radiograph should be performed to confirm that the catheter tip is in the superior vena cava. An infusion pump should be used to ensure that the solution is administered constantly at the required rate throughout the 24-hour period.

Once inserted, the catheter port should be used only for intravenous feeding and never for administering drugs, blood or blood products, or for sampling blood. Except under exceptional circumstances, the use of two- or three-way taps and Y-connectors must be avoided. Recently, double-lumen Hickman catheters have been introduced, which can be used to ensure that one lumen is dedicated solely to the administration of TPN, even in those in whom venous access is restricted.

Peripheral parenteral nutrition

The central venous route for the administration of parenteral nutrition was originally developed in order to avoid the thrombophlebitis that complicated peripheral infusion of hyperosmolar nutrient solutions. More recently it has been recognized that thrombophlebitis associated with peripheral administration of nutritional support is related not only to the osmotic load of the infusion mixture, but also to the irritant effect of the cannula and infection. Admixtures consisting of a 3.5% solution of amino acids, with a lower concentration of glucose (5–10%), the majority of calories provided as fat emulsion and an osmolarity of less than 900 mosm/l minimize the risk of chemical phlebitis and have been shown in clinical studies to be suitable for peripheral administration (Jeejeebhoy & Marliss, 1983). Since most courses of TPN rarely exceed 14 days, preservation of the peripheral vein for around five days allows peripheral parenteral nutrition to be given to most patients with just two or three cannula changes. Peripheral parenteral nutrition therefore has a role for patients in whom adequate nutritional support cannot be provided by the enteral route and when there are difficulties with central venous access. It is also useful when it is anticipated that parenteral nutrition will be required for only a relatively short period (e.g. < 1 week).

Paediatric silicon feeding lines are used in some centres to minimize thrombophlebitic complications (Madan *et al.*, 1992). A number of other techniques have been used in an attempt to reduce the incidence of peripheral venous thrombophlebitis. These have included:

● in-line filters;
● heparin and steroid additives;
● buffering;
● transdermal administration of glyceryl trinitrate.

SELECTION OF THE APPROPRIATE INTRAVENOUS FEEDING REGIMEN

Intravenous feeds must provide the patient with protein, energy (carbohydrate and fats), electrolytes, water, vitamins and trace elements.

Protein is administered in the form of solutions containing a balanced mixture of essential and semi-essential amino acids. The body can only use L-amino acids and approximately 25% of the total nitrogen content should consist of essential amino acids, while a mixture of non-essential amino acids is also required for efficient protein synthesis. High concentrations of a single non-essential amino acid such as glycine should be avoided.

Depending on the degree of catabolism, patients will require in the order of 1.25 g of protein/kg/day (i.e. 0.2 g/kg/day of nitrogen or 1.5 g/kg/24 h of amino acids). In malnourished individuals, restoration of body cell mass is very slow and appears to be directly related to the total energy intake, provided adequate quantities of protein are also given. Increasing the protein intake to more than 1.5–2 g/kg/day will not, however, accelerate weight gain (Shizgal & Forse, 1980). Surprisingly, it is possible to achieve protein sparing in a previously well-nourished patient following moderately severe trauma (e.g. elective surgery) by administering only amino acids via a peripheral vein. In this way, body cell mass may be preserved until full nutritional support is established either enterally or parenterally. In practice, however, this technique is rarely used.

Glucose is the *carbohydrate* of choice, the only disadvantages being the development of hyperglycaemia and, when excessive amounts of glucose are given, fatty liver. Critically ill patients are usually relatively intolerant of glucose because of high circulating levels of insulin antagonists. Furthermore, exogenously administered steroids and other drugs such as thiazide diuretics, are diabetogenic. Extra insulin is therefore usually required, and potassium may be added as well. Administration of this mixture may reduce the catabolic response (Hinton *et al.*, 1971).

Fat solutions are an excellent source of calories and are usually given as the soya bean preparation Intralipid (10 or 20%). They also prevent the development of essential fatty acid deficiency and are a source of cholesterol and phosphate (as phospholipids), although the latter may not be readily available. Fat solutions are non-irritant and can be administered via a peripheral vein (see earlier in this chapter) because they are iso-osmolar, with a neutral pH. Although in the past it was considered sufficient to administer Intralipid peripherally once or twice a week, the present trend is to return to administering fat solutions daily. Some patients, especially those with hepatic disease, acute pancreatitis or extensive sepsis are intolerant of fat. Before obtaining blood samples it is therefore important to check that the plasma is not lipaemic. If fat globules are seen, there is a risk of contaminating autoanalysers. Although there is some evidence that fat emulsions can interfere with immune responses and pulmonary function, in practice these theoretical risks do not seem to be clinically significant (Askanazi *et al.*, 1982; Radermacher *et al.*, 1992).

Energy requirements can be estimated assuming a resting metabolic rate of 30 kcal/kg/day, which may be increased by around 10% in the critically ill and by up to 50% in those with severe burns or major trauma. Current evidence, however, suggests that hypermetabolic and septic critically ill patients should be given energy intakes close to their basal requirements. The optimum combination of carbohydrate and lipid as non-protein energy substrates remains to be clarified. In general it is usual to give 30–40% of the total calorie intake as lipid and to provide 100–200 kcal of non-protein energy for each gram of nitrogen. In the hypercatabolic patient the optimal calorie:nitrogen ratio may fall to less than 140:1, whereas in those who are less catabolic the ratio may be closer to 200:1. While inadequate provision of energy substrates results in depletion of body stores, the administration of excessive quantities of non-protein energy may lead to the development of generalized fat deposition and a 'fatty' liver. Moreover, such over-provision, even when accompanied by large quantities of protein, often fails to reverse the negative nitrogen balance in catabolic patients.

Appropriate solutions should be included in the regimen to provide adequate quantities of sodium, potassium, magnesium, calcium and phosphate. Deficiency of the latter is associated with a reduced red cell 2,3-diphosphoglycerate concentration and an increase in the oxygen affinity of haemoglobin, as well as respiratory muscle weakness (see Chapters 6 and 7). Extra iron may also be required, and in long-term intravenous feeding, replacement of trace elements such as copper, manganese and zinc will become important. Deficiency of the latter may be associated with impaired wound healing. All water- and fat-soluble vitamins must also be provided.

In many centres, the various constituents of the appropriate 24-hour feeding regimen, including fat, are premixed by the pharmacy in a *single bag* (usually containing 1.5–3 litres of solution) using an aseptic technique. The giving set is changed with each new feeding bag or at the end of each 24-hour cycle. If facilities for making up a feeding bag are not available, the various constituents of the regimen should be administered simultaneously using three-way taps or Y-connectors.

COMPLICATIONS (**Table 10.2**)

Probably the most dangerous complication of intravenous feeding is the development of *infection* and *bacteraemia*. Conventional TPN fails to prevent the intestinal mucosal atrophy normally associated with starvation and has been associated with bacterial translocation from the gut lumen (Alverdy *et al.*, 1988) (see

Table 10.2 Complications of parenteral nutrition.

Catheter-related
  Complications related to insertion (see Chapter 3)
  Displacement
  Fracture and embolism
  Occlusion
  Venous thrombosis
  Infection and bacteraemia

Metabolic
  Hyperglycaemia
  Hypoglycaemia (sudden cessation of feeding)
  Hypo/hyperkalaemia
  Hypophosphataemia
  Metabolic acidosis

Fluid overload

Deficiencies of vitamins and trace elements

Hepatobiliary
  Abnormal liver function tests
  Jaundice

Intestinal
  Villous atrophy
  Bacterial translocation/endotoxaemia

Chapter 4). Not only does TPN provide no fibre, but standard preparations lack *glutamine*, which is unstable in solution. Since glutamine is the main source of energy for the gastrointestinal mucosa, formulations of TPN containing glutamine in peptide form have been developed and recently it has been claimed that administration of about 15% of the daily intake of amino acids as glutamine can prevent these atrophic mucosal changes (Van der Hulst *et al.*, 1993). If confirmed, this will clearly have a profound impact on the formulation of intravenous feeds (Powell-Tuck, 1993).

TPN may also be complicated by *displacement of the catheter, mechanical problems, fluid overload, metabolic acidosis, electrolyte imbalance* and *deficiencies of vitamins and trace elements. Metabolic derangements* may occur in up to 5–10% cases (Wolfe *et al.*, 1986). Many of these metabolic problems relate to the components of the infusions. Intravenous fat emulsions have replaced glucose as the main source of energy because they are a more concentrated source of calories and because of the problems caused by overfeeding with glucose such as hyperglycaemia and fatty liver (Driscoll & Blackburn, 1990). Although the newer preparations are safer than their predecessors, reports of various hepatobiliary abnormalities with TPN continue

(Fisher, 1989). Most commonly there is an increase in alkaline phosphatase, but in some cases bilirubin levels are also elevated, sometimes to the extent that the patient becomes jaundiced. Transaminase levels may also rise. These abnormalities of liver function are probably most often due to the provision of energy (either as fat or carbohydrate) in excess of requirements, which leads to *fatty infiltration of the liver*. Another contributory factor may be *intrahepatic cholestasis*, possibly due to changes in the composition of bile. Of course, in critically ill patients, many other factors including shock and sepsis can precipitate liver dysfunction. In adults, changes in liver function induced by TPN are almost always reversible (e.g. by reducing the energy input or by changing to enteral nutrition), but in children, for reasons that are not entirely clear, they can persist and lead to chronic liver disease.

MONITORING PATIENTS RECEIVING TPN

Careful monitoring of patients receiving TPN is therefore required if these complications are to be avoided (**Table 10.3**). It is clearly important to keep an accurate *daily record of fluid balance* and the patient should be *weighed* daily if this is practicable. Urea, creatinine, electrolytes and blood sugar should also be measured daily. In particular, if, as is usual, the patient is receiving an insulin infusion, blood sugar should be determined frequently by the nursing staff at the bedside. Initially, this may be performed hourly, but once a stable regimen is established, the frequency of blood sugar estimations can be progressively reduced to four-hourly. Liver function tests (including estimation of calcium and phosphate), and a full blood count should be performed at least twice weekly. Plasma magnesium should be measured once a week, and blood levels of vitamin B_{12},

Table 10.3 Monitoring parenteral nutrition.	
At least daily	Frequent bedside estimation of blood sugar
	Body weight (if practicable)
	Urea, electrolytes and blood sugar
At least twice weekly	Liver function tests (including Ca^{2+} and PO_4^{2-})
	Full blood count
At least weekly	Mg^{2+}
	Nitrogen balance
Monthly	Vitamin B_{12}
	Folate
	Iron and total iron binding capacity
	Zinc

folate, iron, total iron binding capacity and zinc should be estimated monthly. Normally, all these investigations should also be performed before feeding begins. A 24-hour collection of urine for determination of urea, electrolyte and creatinine concentrations allows calculation of creatinine clearance and nitrogen balance. Estimating total urinary nitrogen excretion from urinary urea excretion is, however, of dubious value, especially in unstable critically ill patients (Konstantinides *et al.*, 1991). A new technique of pyrochemoluminescence, which measures total nitrogen in urine or other body fluids may improve the accuracy of routine clinical determination of nitrogen balance.

GROWTH FACTORS (Ross *et al.*, 1991)

The characteristic hormonal response to critical illness plays an important role in the persistent catabolism and resistance to nutritional support that accompanies trauma, sepsis and major surgery. In the context of nutritional support, changes in the growth hormone insulin-like growth factor axis are of particular interest.

Growth hormone (GH) has direct metabolic effects, which include lipolysis and insulin antagonism, as well as indirect anabolic actions mediated by insulin-like growth factor-1 (IGF–1), a peptide that is structurally similar to insulin. IGF–1 is synthesized predominantly in the liver and released into the circulation where its activity is modified by a variety of binding proteins (IGFBP–1 to 6). In critical illness IGF–1 levels are uniformly low and despite increased basal levels of GH and insulin there is resistance to the anabolic action of these hormones. This may represent an adaptive response away from the indirect metabolic actions of GH towards direct stimulation of lipolysis and insulin antagonism in order to increase the availability of energy substrates in the fasted patient. In long-stay critically ill patients receiving nutritional support, however, administration of supraphysiological doses of GH, either alone or in combination with IGF–1, has the potential to increase protein synthesis and enhance muscle and hepatic uptake of amino acids and glucose. Certainly administration of recombinant human GH can improve nitrogen retention in parenterally and enterally fed patients (Ziegler *et al.*, 1990), although in septic patients GH may exert only a limited effect on nitrogen economy. The influence of growth factor administration on weaning from mechanical ventilation, immune function, length of stay, morbidity and mortality in critically ill patients has yet to be determined.

SEDATION, ANALGESIA AND MUSCLE RELAXATION

Most patients admitted to intensive care will require analgesia and, in the majority, administration of a sedative will be indicated to allay anxiety, help to relieve discomfort and encourage sleep. Sedatives may also be used to manage acute confusional states (see later in this chapter) and during diagnostic or invasive procedures. The combination of an opiate and a sedative or intravenous anaesthetic agent is generally used to facilitate mechanical ventilation and to obtund the physiological response to stress. Morphine and the benzodiazepines are the most common sedative agents used in intensive care and are often administered in combination (Bion & Ledingham, 1987). In selected cases, neuromuscular blockade may be indicated and, in some, heavy sedation or even anaesthesia may be required to control intracranial hypertension or seizures (see Chapter 14).

The properties that should be considered when choosing the most appropriate sedative for an individual patient include:

- sedation potential;
- anxiolysis;
- analgesia;
- amnesia;
- rate of onset and duration of action;
- predictability of effect;
- speed of reversal on cessation;
- degree of respiratory depression;
- cardiovascular depression;
- gastrointestinal effects;
- venous irritation;
- addictive potential;
- cost;
- interaction with other drugs.

As the goals of sedation vary between patients it is unlikely that any one agent will be suitable in all circumstances. For example, in a patient on controlled ventilation, respiratory depression is of little consequence, while a patient with Guillain–Barré syndrome may have little need for analgesia, although the establishment of adequate sleeping patterns and normal gastrointestinal function will be important.

Assessing the levels of sedation

The level of sedation can be assessed as described by Ramsay et al. (1974) for patients sedated with an infusion of the anaesthetic induction agent althesin (alphaxalone-alphadolone). Six levels of sedation were used:

1. anxious and agitated or restless, or both;
2. cooperative, orientated and tranquil;
3. responds to commands only;
4. asleep, but with a brisk response to light glabellar tap or loud auditory stimulus;
5. asleep, sluggish response to light glabellar tap or loud auditory stimulus;

6. asleep, no response.

It is suggested that levels 2–5 can be considered suitable for patients requiring sedation in the intensive care unit. This method of assessment allows sedation to be tailored to individual patients' needs and also facilitates comparative clinical studies between different agents or techniques.

Subsequent refinements to Ramsay's original scheme have included an assessment of compliance with artificial ventilation and tracheal suction, although to trigger coughing or resisting the ventilator intentionally is clearly undesirable in head-injured patients or those with reactive airways.

Physical methods for assessing sedation have also been developed, but are not yet used routinely. For example, the level of cortical electrical activity can be assessed using the *cerebral function monitor* (CFM) or *cerebral function analysing monitor* (CFAM) (see Chapter 14), and *auditory evoked potentials* have been used to assess the depth of sedation or anaesthesia (Thornton et al., 1989). Recently, the measurement of *lower oesophageal contractility* has been used to assess the depth of anaesthesia and sedation. A balloon-tipped catheter is inserted into the lower oesophagus to measure pressure changes related to oesophageal contraction and relaxation. The oesophageal smooth muscle is not affected by muscle relaxants and the frequency of tertiary non-peristaltic spontaneous activity is decreased with sedation and anaesthesia. This technique has been used to aid in the diagnosis of a sedative overdose complicated by concomitant renal failure (Sinclair & Suter, 1988).

Analgesia

OPIATES

Because intramuscular administration of opiates is associated with irregular absorption, fluctuating blood levels and periods of pain between doses, analgesics are best administered to critically ill patients by continuous intravenous infusion (**Table 10.4**). The dose can be adjusted according to the individual's requirements, guided, for example, by the clinical response to nursing or medical interventions. *Patient-controlled analgesia* (PCA, **Table 10.5**) may be preferred for patients who are sufficiently alert and cooperative.

Morphine, papaveretum and pethidine remain the most commonly used opiates. *Fentanyl*, which is a potent lipid-soluble synthetic opioid, is rapidly redistributed to the tissues and has a shorter duration of action, although long-term administration prolongs its elimination half-life. The ultra-short-acting agent *alfentanil* may be useful, especially in patients with renal failure.

Table 10.4 Guidelines for adult doses for some of the opioids commonly administered to mechanically ventilated patients.

Drug	Intravenous bolus dose	Intravenous infusion rate
Morphine	2.5 mg	1–5 mg/h
Pethidine	10 mg	10–20 mg/h
Phenoperidine	1–2 mg	2–4 mg/h
Fentanyl	50–100 μg	100–200 μg/h
Alfentanyl	1–5 mg	1–6 mg/h

Table 10.5 Guidelines for bolus doses and lock out intervals for opioids in patient-controlled analgesia systems.

Opioid	Bolus dose (mg)	Lock out time interval (minutes)
Morphine	0.5–3	5–20
Pethidine	5–30	5–15
Fentanyl	0.02–0.1	3–10

The side-effects of the opioids are dose related and include:

- nausea and vomiting;
- dysphoria;
- decreased gut motility;
- ventilatory depression;
- cardiovascular depression (less with fentanyl).

High doses of pethidine may produce muscle twitching and convulsions due to the accumulation of norpethidine. It is also important to remember that morphine elimination is reduced in renal failure (Ball *et al.*, 1985) and that there may be accumulation of the pharmacologically active metabolite morphine-6-gluronide (Osborne *et al.*, 1986). *Naloxone* (0.1–0.4 mg intravenously) can be used to antagonize opioid side-effects (see Chapter 18).

NON-OPIATE ANALGESICS

Although the opioids are the most commonly used analgesics in critically ill patients, less severe pain, discomfort from bones, joints or muscles following prolonged immobilization and inflammatory disorders (e.g. pleuritic chest pain) may not require, and may respond poorly to, opioid administration. Non-steroidal anti-inflammatory drugs (NSAIDs), which block prostaglan-

din biosynthesis by inhibiting cyclo-oxygenase, may be useful in such cases and there has been increasing interest in the perioperative use of NSAIDs as an alternative or as a supplement to opioid analgesics (Dahl & Kehlet, 1991).

Aspirin is contraindicated in children under 12 years of age because of its links with Reye's syndrome, otherwise a dose of 300–900 mg may be given orally every 4–6 hours to a maximum of 4 g in 24 hours. *Paracetamol*, 500 mg–1 g can be given orally or rectally every 4–6 hours to adults. Since these less-powerful analgesics are also available in many different combinations (e.g. co-codamol contains paracetamol combined with codeine phosphate), it is essential that the precise contents of these commercial preparations are known. *Diclofenac* is available not only as an oral sustained-release preparation and a suppository, but also as a parenteral preparation for intramuscular administration. *Ketorolac* may also be given orally, intramuscularly or intravenously, initially 10 mg four times a day. The dose should be reduced in the elderly and those with renal failure.

The use of NSAIDs in critical illness is, however, significantly limited by *side-effects* related to inhibition of prostaglandin biosynthesis such as:

- platelet aggregation;
- gastrointestinal haemorrhage;
- renal impairment (see Chapter 12);
- bronchospasm.

Sometimes severe muscular pain or chronic pain syndromes similar to sympathetic dystrophy are encountered in patients recovering from critical illness neuropathy. These types of pain may not respond to opioids, but require involvement of a specialist pain team to coordinate the use of membrane-stabilizing agents such as carbamazepine, tricyclic antidepressants or α adrenoreceptor modulation.

REGIONAL BLOCKADE

Regional techniques have been shown to have a number of advantages over intravenous analgesia for the relief of postoperative pain (Allen *et al.*, 1986), particularly when combined with general anaesthesia. This combination can ameliorate the stress response to surgery and may be associated with less sedation, allowing more effective expectoration (Shulman *et al.*, 1984).

Epidural analgesia

Epidural analgesia is associated with measurable improvements in lung function, as well as allowing the patient to cough and deep breathe and facilitating mobilization. It is particularly advantageous after chest or abdominal surgery and in the management of chest injuries (see Chapter 9). Unfortunately in many critically ill patients, placement of an extradural catheter is contraindicated (e.g. because of general or local infection or a coagulopathy). It is controversial whether epidural injections can be undertaken in patients who have received subcutaneous heparin or NSAIDs.

For the control of lower limb, pelvic and abdominal pain, the epidural catheter can be inserted in the lumbar region at L1-2 or L2-3; an initial dose of 10-15 ml of 0.5% bupivacaine can be followed by an infusion of 0.125% bupivacaine at 5-20 ml/h (the use of a continuous infusion rather than repeated bolus doses is less likely to be associated with acute episodes of hypotension). In those with upper abdominal or thoracic pain the epidural catheter is best inserted in the mid-thoracic region between T7 and T10. Here an initial dose of 4-6 ml of 0.5% bupivacaine can be followed by an infusion of 6-10 ml/h of 0.125% bupivacaine.

Epidural administration of opiates may be associated with less hypotension and produces longer lasting, although less dense, analgesia. Opiates act synergistically with local anaesthetic agents and the combination may reduce the potential for side-effects, as well as minimizing the tendency for local anaesthetic agents to exhibit tachyphylaxis (**Table 10.6**).

As well as determining the sensory level of the block, careful observation of cardiorespiratory performance is necessary for all epidural techniques, but particularly when local anaesthetics and opiates are used in combination, when there is a significant risk of delayed insidious opiate-induced respiratory depression as well as the sudden cardiovascular collapse that may follow local anaesthetic-induced sympathetic blockade. Opiate-induced respiratory depression following epidural injection is least likely to occur with the most lipid-soluble agents such as fentanyl and diamorphine. Other side-effects of epidural opiates include nausea and vomiting, urinary retention and pruritus. It may be possible to antagonize these side-effects with naloxone without reducing analgesia. It should not be forgotten that none of the opioids are licensed for use by the epidural or intrathecal route. Other potential complications of epidural analgesia include:

- subarachnoid injection of local anaesthetic leading to coma, bradycardia, hypotension and respiratory arrest;
- intravascular injection;
- high block leading to respiratory muscle paralysis;
- epidural haematoma or abscess.

Interpleural blockade

Local anaesthetic agents can be infused continuously into the interpleural space. Alternatively their administration can be patient-controlled. This technique has been used for the management of multiple rib fractures, as well as following upper abdominal surgery (Murphy, 1993) and thoracic procedures (Ferrante et al., 1991).

Intercostal nerve blocks

Intercostal nerve blocks can provide good analgesia in the relevant dermatomes and may be useful to allow patients with, for example, thoracotomy wounds or rib fractures (not more than three or four) to cough without pain. Unfortunately multiple injections are required and there is a risk of pneumothorax. The action of bupivacaine can be prolonged by the addition of adrenaline.

Sedatives

BENZODIAZEPINES

Benzodiazepines interact with specific receptors in the central nervous system to facilitate the inhibitory effect of γ-aminobutyric acid (GABA) on synaptic transmission, thereby producing sedation and anxiolysis. Other properties of the benzodiazepines include amnesia, some cardiorespiratory depression in larger doses and a minor degree of muscle relaxation. In some cases there may be paradoxical confusion and agitation. Withdrawal symptoms may be seen following long-term use.

Diazepam or *diazepam emulsion* (a soya bean oil/water emulsion, which is less irritant and painful on intravenous injection) remains a popular benzodiazepine for bolus intravenous administration. Although blood levels initially fall rapidly due to redistribution,

Table 10.6 Suggested adult doses of opioid drugs given extradurally.

Opioid	Extradural bolus dose
Diamorphine	2.5–5 mg
Fentanyl	100–200 μg

Bupivicaine	0.125% plus	
Diamorphine	5 mg	
or		diluted in a total volume
Morphine	10 mg	of 50 ml
or		
Fentanyl	100 μg	

Extradural infusion 4–10 ml/hr initially and adjusted according to patient response

the elimination half-life is 20–50 hours and cumulation is a significant problem. Moreover diazepam is metabolized in the liver to produce active metabolites such as nordiazepam and oxazepam. Consequently *midazolam*, which is more potent and rapidly acting, with a shorter elimination half-life and inactive metabolites is increasingly preferred (**Table 10.7**). It is also less irritant than diazepam when given intravenously. In critically ill patients, midazolam is frequently administered as a continuous intravenous infusion. Nevertheless the unpredictable pharmacokinetics of midazolam, especially in hepatic insufficiency and when liver blood flow is reduced, mean that in the long term, cumulative effects may present a significant problem (Shelley *et al.*, 1987; Dirksen *et al.*, 1987).

INTRAVENOUS ANAESTHETIC AGENTS

The barbiturate *thiopentone* is occasionally administered as a continuous intravenous infusion to control raised intracranial pressure or to treat convulsions refractory to more conventional measures (see Chapter 14). Its use may be complicated by cardiovascular and respiratory depression. The effects of thiopentone are cumulative and prolonged recovery must be anticipated.

Propofol is rapidly metabolized, principally in the liver, and its effects are not cumulative. Sedation with this agent is easily controllable and has been associated with more rapid weaning from ventilation than midazolam (Aitkenhead *et al.*, 1989). It causes dose-related falls in blood pressure, largely due to a reduction in systemic vascular resistance. Although originally used in intensive care to provide sedation after cardiac surgery (Grounds *et al.*, 1987) propofol is increasingly being used in general intensive care patients (Harris *et al.*, 1990; Nimmo

et al., 1994). It is not, however, recommended for paediatric practice because there is no licence in the UK for its use in children and a number of adverse effects have been reported. One report from four British intensive care units, for example, described five children with upper respiratory tract infections sedated with propofol (Parke *et al.*, 1992). All the children developed lipaemic serum, metabolic acidosis and myocardial failure; all died. In three of the children, a fatty liver was found at autopsy. There are also concerns about the cost of propofol when used as a continuous infusion in critically ill patients.

INHALATIONAL ANAESTHETIC AGENTS

It has been suggested that inhalational anaesthetic agents and in particular *isoflurane* (Kong *et al.*, 1989; Willatts & Spencer, 1994) may be used as alternatives to intravenous agents. The low blood/gas solubility of isoflurane allows rapid changes in the level of sedation and since less than 0.2% of the absorbed dose is metabolized there is litle potential for organ toxicity or accumulation. The main controversies still relate to the potential adverse cardiovascular effects of isoflurane and practical issues regarding the special equipment required for its administration and scavenging.

MAJOR TRANQUILIZERS

Butyrophenones (e.g. haloperidol, 5–10 mg orally or intramuscularly, as required) can be particularly useful in severe agitation or psychosis (see later in this chapter). They have an antiemetic effect and are not usually associated with cardiovascular depression, even in high doses. They have largely replaced the phenothiazines.

Chlormethiazole (see **Table 10.7**) has been used as a prolonged infusion in the critically ill, as well as for acute alcohol withdrawal, toxic confusional states, pre-eclampsia, status epilepticus and eclampsia.

KETAMINE

Ketamine is a phencyclidine derivative widely used in emergency situations to produce dissociative anaesthesia with cardiovascular stability, maintained muscle tone and profound analgesia. It has also proved useful in mechanically ventilated patients with severe asthma (Park *et al.*, 1987) (see Chapter 6). The initial intravenous dose is 1–4.5 mg/kg followed by an infusion of 10–45 µg/kg/min adjusted according to response. Emergence delirium, vivid dreams and occasionally hallucinations have limited its usefulness during routine

Table 10.7 Guidelines for bolus doses and infusion rates for sedative and anaesthetic agents in mechanically ventilated patients. Age, obesity, simultaneous medication, hepatic and renal dysfunction may change dose requirements.

Sedative or analgesic agent	Bolus dose	Infusion rate
Diazepam	2.5–5 mg	1–4 mg/h
Lorazepam	1–2 mg	Not suitable
Midazolam	2.5–5 mg	0.5–6 mg/h
Propofol	1–2.5 mg/kg	1–4 mg/kg/h
Chlormethiazole	250 mg	According to response
Thiopentone	250–500 mg	100–200 mg/h

anaesthesia, but these can be ameliorated by benzo-diazepine administration.

Muscle relaxation

In the critically ill, muscle relaxants are used to facilitate endotracheal intubation, to reduce the incidence of barotrauma during mechanical ventilation and to decrease metabolic requirements in ventilated patients with reduced cardiorespiratory reserves (see Chapter 7). Muscle relaxants may also be used to control abnormal movements refractory to the administration of sedative or hypnotic agents alone. The use of muscle relaxants in the intensive care unit is more complicated than in the operating theatre because treatment is prolonged, and their activity may be influenced by associated therapies, as well as the severity of the patient's condition. There have also been difficulties because their adminis-tration is usually not monitored using peripheral nerve stimulators.

If precise control of the degree of muscle relaxation is not required, on-demand repeat injections are accept-able, otherwise a continuous intravenous infusion is increasingly preferred (**Table 10.8**). Nevertheless it must be remembered that even with atracurium, the muscle relaxant with the smallest interpatient pharmacodynamic variation, the individual dose require-ments for continuous infusion may vary as much as five fold (Yate *et al.*, 1987).

The *side-effects* of neuromuscular blocking drugs include various histaminic reactions as well as severe or even life-threatening bronchospasm. Although cardio-vascular changes are generally negligible, bolus injection of muscle relaxants may be accompanied by brady- or tachyarrhythmias, and even cardiac arrest. In particular, succinylcholine is contraindicated in a variety of con-ditions in which muscle fasciculations might precipitate hypertonia or systemic hyperkalaemia (see Chapters 7, and 9).

The duration of action of all non-depolarizing muscle relaxants can be prolonged in critically ill patients. This

---

Table 10.8 Suggested adult doses of neuromuscular blocking agents given to critically ill mechanically ventilated patients.

Neuromuscular blocking drug	Bolus dose	Infusion rate
Suxamethonium	0.5–1.5 mg/kg	Not suitable
Pancuronium	0.5–4 mg	Not suitable
Vecuronium	40–100 µg/kg	50–80 µg/kg/h
Atracurium	300–600 µg/kg	300–600 µg/kg/h

---

may be attributable to immobilization, metabolic dis-orders, malnutrition and concomitant steroid or amino-glycoside antibiotic therapy. It may be more likely to follow the uncontrolled administration of the neuro-muscular blocking drug *vecuronium* especially in the presence of renal impairment (Segredo *et al.*, 1990).

Atracurium besilate is the only agent whose action is not dramatically increased in cases of multiple organ failure because of its rapid spontaneous degradation in all clinical situations except deep hypothermia. Perhaps understandably muscle relaxant administration has been implicated as a cause of the neuromuscular weakness sometimes encountered in patients who survive life-threatening illness. It would seem, however, that in many cases the development of acquired neuromuscular disorders in intensive care patients is unrelated to the use of these agents (see Chapters 7 and 14).

PREVENTION OF DEEP VENOUS THROMBOSIS AND PULMONARY THROMBOEMBOLISM (Weinmann & Salzman, 1994)

The pathophysiological processes involved in the causa-tion of deep venous thrombosis (DVT) and pulmonary embolism (PE) were first studied by Rudolf Virchow. He proposed three main predisposing factors:

- damage to the vessel wall;
- diminution of blood flow;
- increased coagulability of the blood.

These three factors (Virchow's triad) are still thought to account for most cases of thromboembolism com-plicating critical illness. Venous thromboembolism is a particularly common complication of major trauma (Geerts *et al.*, 1994), infectious polyneuritis (see Chap-ter 14) and pregnancy (see Chapter 17). In these pa-tients some form of screening practice, such as repeat duplex scanning studies, may be advantageous. This is particularly the case if prophylactic subcutaneous hep-arin has to be discontinued because of heparin-induced thrombocytopenia. In most intensive care patients, pass-ive leg exercises combined with *low-dose heparin* (5000 u subcutaneously 2–3 times daily) and early mo-bilization offers sufficient protection. Low-dose heparin may be contraindicated in neurosurgical and ortho-paedic patients, as well as in some trauma patients (e.g. those with head or ophthalmic injuries) and those with a documented bleeding diathesis. In such cases *inter-mittent pneumatic compression* of the legs may be equally effective. *Elastic stockings* may also be ben-eficial, especially when combined with other measures.

PREVENTION OF STRESS ULCERATION

Acute gastrointestinal haemorrhage associated with peptic ulceration can be a serious and potentially life-threatening complication of critical illness (see also Chapter 15). Those with burns (*Curling's ulcers*), head injuries (*Cushing's ulcers*), multiple trauma, renal failure, respiratory failure, jaundice, hypotension and severe sepsis are among those at greatest risk (Priebe *et al.*, 1980).

Many authors believe that the incidence of gastrointestinal haemorrhage from stress ulceration has decreased in the past ten years, in part due to the widespread use of prophylactic measures, but also as a result of more effective treatment of acute hypoxaemia and shock, as well as improved respiratory care (Tryba, 1994). The use of enteral alimentation has also been associated with a significant decrease in the risk of gastrointestinal haemorrhage (Pingleton & Hadzima, 1983). Nevertheless recent evidence suggests that in the absence of prophylactic measures the frequency of acute upper gastrointestinal mucosal injury approaches 90% within three days of admission to intensive care (Eddleston *et al.*, 1994).

Current evidence suggests that antacids, H_2-receptor blockade and sucralfate are approximately equally effective as prophylaxis against stress ulceration.

Antacid therapy is directed at maintaining the gastric pH consistently higher than 3.5, the value at which the incidence of bleeding diminishes significantly. This regimen has proved effective in many studies, but is inconvenient to administer and can result in diarrhoea and metabolic abnormalities.

H_2-receptor blockers can be administered orally or intravenously, by either bolus or continuous infusion, the intention being to maintain the gastric pH above 3.5. These agents also increase mucosal blood flow as well as stimulate mucus production and prostaglandin synthesis (Friedman *et al.*, 1982; Schuman *et al.*, 1987).

Sucralfate is an aluminium hydroxide salt of sucrose octasulphate that can be administered orally or nasogastrically. It is only a weak antacid, but has antipepsin activity, stimulates prostaglandin synthesis and forms a protective coating over inflamed areas of mucosa (Tryba *et al.*, 1985). It may be associated with a lower incidence of nosocomial infection than agents that cause marked reductions in gastric acidity (Driks *et al.*, 1987).

Prostaglandin E_2 derivatives have been used as stress ulcer prophylaxis in several studies, but at present have not proved to be effective. Misoprostol has been specifically recommended for protection against gastric injury induced by NSAIDs.

It is difficult to provide definitive recommendations for prophylactic therapy (Mackenzie, 1993). Recent research has suggested that prophylaxis against stress ulcers can be safely withheld from critically ill patients unless they have a coagulopathy or require mechanical ventilation (Cook *et al.*, 1994), especially if they were admitted with sepsis or shock (Schuster, 1993). Many also believe that those who are tolerating large-volume enteral alimentation do not require prophylaxis against gastrointestinal haemorrhage. In patients not receiving enteral nutrition, sucralfate 1 g up to six times daily can be administered via the nasogastric tube while ranitidine 50 mg three times daily by intravenous injection can be given to high-risk patients (e.g. those receiving pharmacological doses of steroids) and when sucralfate administration is impossible. It should not be forgotten that although prophylaxis for gastrointestinal bleeding reduces morbidity (Cook *et al.*, 1991) and possibly the duration of intubation and length of intensive care unit stay (Eddleston *et al.*, 1994), it has not been shown to influence mortality.

PSYCHOLOGICAL AND BEHAVIOURAL PROBLEMS

Patients treated in intensive care units can develop various psychiatric disturbances, which may become manifest either in the unit or following discharge (Baxter, 1974). In many cases the psychiatric disorder has an organic cause, whereas in others it is a result of the emotional impact of the critical illness. A number of patients, especially those admitted after accidents or self-harm, have a pre-existing psychiatric disorder.

Delirium

Delirium is the most commonly encountered serious mental disturbance and usually presents as reduced awareness, apathy and drowsiness. Some patients become restless, hyperactive and even violent, with hallucinations and delusions of persecution. Characteristically, the severity of the mental disturbance fluctuates, with lucid intervals during the day and deterioration at night. Metabolic disturbances such as dehydration, hyponatraemia, alkalosis, hyper- and hypoglycaemia, uraemia, hyperchloraemia and hypokalaemia may all predispose to delirium, which is also commoner in the older age groups; children appear to be particularly resistant.

Acute functional psychoses

Patients in intensive care units often experience extreme stress, anxiety and fear of impending death. Critically ill patients are often unable to speak, some are unable to communicate at all and their movement is restricted. In addition, they are severely deprived of sleep, and stages 3 and 4 and REM (rapid eye movement) sleep are severely or completely suppressed (Aurell & Elmqvist, 1985). They also suffer from reduced stimulation, social isolation and physical confinement. Such sensory deprivation is known to induce hallucinations of sound, vision, touch and movement as well as reduced vigilance and an underestimation of time. Patients may also be subjected to repetitive stimulation (e.g. flashing lights on monitors and infusion pumps, the sound of alarms and ventilators) and occasional serious discomfort or pain. Any impairment of cerebral function (e.g. caused by drugs or metabolic derangement) will exaggerate the psychological response of the patient to these environmental stresses and predispose to the development of an acute functional psychosis. These present as thought disorder, delusions or hallucinations in a patient who is fully conscious and orientated with an intact memory (Kiely, 1976). Unlike true delirium, which always has an organic cause, acute functional psychoses resolve when the patient is removed from the intimidating environment that triggered the acute disorientation syndrome (Lloyd, 1993).

Cardiopulmonary bypass has been particularly associated with psychiatric disturbances, although the incidence of serious mental disturbance in this category of patient is now relatively low. This is probably due to a number of factors including shorter bypass times, careful preoperative preparation and attention to environmental factors within the intensive care unit.

Anxiety and depression

Intensive care patients may also exhibit a variety of less severe psychological reactions to their predicament. These range from overwhelming fear, tension and sustained anxiety to severe, often agitated, depression and 'negativism' (Kiely, 1976). Patients may therefore exhibit obsessive compulsive behaviour in which they analyse every aspect of their situation and illness in minute detail; alternatively, they may display repression by rejecting their problem and allowing staff a 'free hand'. Some patients become totally dependent, while others are wholeheartedly involved in their own treatment, denying any feelings of fear or hopelessness.

Pre-existing disorders

Many patients admitted to intensive care units will have pre-existing psychological problems. These will then manifest themselves, sometimes in exaggerated form, as the patient recovers. It has been suggested that certain abnormal personality traits or mental diseases may predispose to particular types of physical illness; cases of self-poisoning, drug addiction and alcohol abuse are the more obvious examples.

The features of *narcotic addiction* include pinpoint pupils and transitory elation, which is followed by marked anxiety and restlessness. Anorexia, constipation and extreme weight loss are common, as is loss of libido. Examination may reveal multiple injection sites, sometimes with bruising, abscesses and septic thrombophlebitis. *Signs and symptoms of withdrawal* include:

- running eyes and nose;
- sneezing;
- perspiration;
- gooseflesh;
- vague aches and pains;
- anxiety, restlessness, aggression;
- dilated pupils.

Nausea, vomiting, abdominal pain, diarrhoea, limb cramps, sleeplessness and agitation may also occur.

Alcohol withdrawal is characterized by nervous system excitation, which varies from mild sleeplessness and irritability to *delirium tremens*. In mild cases there is:

- tremor;
- perspiration;
- nervousness;
- dyspepsia;
- weakness;
- anorexia;
- hyperreflexia;
- insomnia.

Severe cases exhibit:

- hypertension;
- tachycardia;
- fever;
- hallucinations (visual, tactile or auditory);
- disorientation;
- convulsions.

Delirium tremens is characterized by:

- delirium;
- clouding of consciousness;
- convulsions.

In addition, alcohol can exacerbate pre-existing psychiatric disorders such as aggressive psychopathy, manic-depressive psychoses and paranoid schizophrenia.

Prevention

Prevention of these psychological disturbances involves maintaining the patient's contact with reality, together with frequent explanation and reassurance, control of metabolic disturbances and the provision of adequate analgesia and anxiolysis.

For those who are conscious and alert, some form of occupational therapy is required; this may take the form of radio, television or 'talking' books. As normal an environment as possible should be maintained (e.g. darkness and, if possible, uninterrupted sleep at night with natural daylight and wakefulness during the day). Night sedation (e.g. with temazepam 10-20 mg orally) is often useful in this respect. It has been suggested, however, that even when conditions are optimal, critically ill patients are seriously deprived of sleep and that this is due to some fundamental derangement of the sleep–wake regulating mechanism (Aurell & Elmqvist, 1985).

It is also important that intensive care units are provided with windows (see Chapter 1), preferably with a view, and frequent information regarding the time, day of the week and season of the year should be provided. It has been suggested that a digital clock/radio and possibly a calendar would therefore be very useful. The patient should be allowed as much privacy as possible, while monitoring and other equipment should be unobtrusively sited, preferably behind the bed. Finally, all procedures must be fully explained before they are performed and frequent encouragement must be provided about the progress of the illness. It is important to remember that some patients who appear to be unconscious may not be; they will require local anaesthesia or intravenous sedation to avoid awareness before painful therapeutic interventions, procedures to establish invasive monitoring or elective DC cardioversion.

Fortunately, many patients have complete or partial amnesia for their time on the intensive care unit, particularly for the periods when they were most seriously ill. This may be at least partly due to the provision of adequate analgesia and sedation, which is in any case essential for the patient's comfort. These psychological aspects of patient care are particularly dependent on the nurses who spend many hours at the bedside of one individual patient and have the opportunity to establish a close and understanding relationship.

Treatment

Although the patient's inevitable anxiety can usually be safely controlled using benzodiazepines, severe depression is less easily treated. *Tricyclic antidepressants* are often ineffective and may be associated with dangerous cardiovascular side-effects. Acute psychotic reactions may require treatment with either benzodiazepines or butyrophenones to avoid self-harm. *Halo-*

peridol, which has minimal autonomic effects, is probably the agent of choice in the critically ill (Kiely, 1976) and intramuscular injection of this agent in a dose of 5–10 mg, repeated as necessary, is effective in most cases. Alternatively *diazepam* 2.5-5 mg in repeated intravenous doses may be required. A continuous intravenous infusion of 0.8% *chlormethiazole* may prove useful to control patients during withdrawal from alcohol or other drugs, but large volumes (60–90 ml/h) may be required and this can lead to fluid overload. If necessary, symptoms of narcotic withdrawal can be controlled with *methadone*, 10–20 mg, which can be repeated 1–2 hours later and should be effective for about 12 hours.

Relatives

The morale of relatives is also most important and they should receive every possible care and attention. In particular, they should be given frequent detailed explanations about the patient's treatment and progress. As far as possible, free visiting should be allowed since this is beneficial not only to the relatives, but also to the patients, helping them to maintain contact with reality. Visitors should be encouraged to talk to and touch the patient.

Long-term outcome

Until recently little was known about the long-term psychological effects of hospitalization following critical illness on either the patients or their next of kin. It is now well recognized that those who have been in exceptionally threatening or catastrophic accidents are prone to prolonged psychological reactions, particularly *post-traumatic stress disorder* and other phobic anxiety syndromes. Characteristic features of post-traumatic stress disorder include:

- flashback memories of the original accident;
- recurrent nightmares;
- emotional numbing;
- autonomic hyperarousal;
- avoidance behaviour (Perry *et al.*, 1992; Roca *et al.*, 1992).

More long-term studies of patients treated in intensive care are required to determine the prevalence of these disorders and their natural course. General practitioners are best placed to evaluate psychological symptoms once patients have left hospital. They may also arrange treatment with antidepressant drugs or psychotherapy and counselling to the patient and their relatives.

REFERENCES

Aitkenhead AR, Willatts SM, Coates PD *et al.* (1989) Comparison of propofol and midazolam for sedation in critically ill patients. *Lancet* **2**: 704-709.

Alexander JW (1990) Nutrition and translocation. *Journal of Parenteral and Enteral Nutrition* **14** (Suppl): 170-174.

Allen PD, Walman T, Concepcion M *et al.* (1986) Epidural morphine provides post-operative pain relief in peripheral vascular and orthopaedic surgical patients: a dose-response study. *Anesthesia and Analgesia* **65**: 165-170.

Alverdy JC, Aoys E & Moss GS (1988) Total parenteral nutrition promotes bacterial translocation from the gut. *Surgery* **104**: 185-190.

Arieff AI (1993) Management of hyponatraemia. *British Medical Journal* **307**: 305-308.

Arnold A, Tovey J, Mangat P, Penny W & Jacobs S (1995) Magnesium deficiency in critically ill patients. *Anaesthesia* **50**: 203-205.

Askanazi J, Weissman C, Rosenbaum SH *et al.* (1982) Nutrition and the respiratory system. *Critical Care Medicine* **10**: 163-172.

Aurell J & Elmqvist D (1985) Sleep in the surgical intensive care unit: continuous polygraphic recording of sleep in nine patients receiving postoperative care. *British Medical Journal* **290**: 1029-1032.

Ball M, Moore RA, Fisher A, McQuay HJ, Allen MC & Sear J (1985) Renal failure and the use of morphine in intensive care. *Lancet* **1**: 784-786.

Baxter S (1974) Psychological problems of intensive care. *British Journal of Hospital Medicine* **11**: 875-885.

Bion JF & Ledingham IMCA (1987) Sedation in intensive care—a postal survey. *Intensive Care Medicine* **13**: 215-216.

Cahill GF Jr (1970) Starvation in man. *New England Journal of Medicine* **282**: 668-675.

Cerra F, Blackburn G, Hirsch J, Mullen K & Luther W (1987) The effect of stress level, amino acid formula, and nitrogen dose on nitrogen retention in traumatic and septic stress. *Annals of Surgery* **205**: 282-287.

Cerra FB, Lehmann S, Konstantinides FN *et al.* (1991) Improvement in immune function in ICU patients with enteral nutrition supplemented with arginine, RNA and menhaden oil is independent of nitrogen balance. *Nutrition* **7**: 193-199.

Cook DJ, Witt LG, Cook RJ & Guyatt GH (1991) Stress ulcer prophylaxis in the critically ill: a meta-analysis. *American Journal of Medicine* **91**: 519-527.

Cook DJ, Fuller HD, Guyatt GH *et al.* (1994) Risk factors for gastrointestinal bleeding in critically ill patients. *New England Journal of Medicine* **330**: 377-381.

Dahl JB & Kehlet H (1991) Non-steroidal anti-inflammatory drugs: rationale for use in severe postoperative pain. *British Journal of Anaesthesia* **66**: 703-712.

Detsky AS (1991) Parenteral nutrition—is it helpful? *New England Journal of Medicine* **325**: 573-575.

Detsky AS, Baker JP, O'Rourke K & Goel V (1987) Perioperative parenteral nutrition: a meta-analysis. *Annals of Internal Medicine* **107**: 195-203.

Dirksen MSC, Vree TB & Driessen JJ (1987) Clinical pharmacokinetics of long term infusion of midazolam in critically ill patients. *Anaesthetics and Intensive Care* **15**: 440-444.

Dobb G (1992) Enteral nutrition for the critically ill. In: JL Vincent (ed), *Yearbook of Intensive Care and Emergency Medicine*. Springer Verlag, Berlin, pp. 609-619.

Driks MR, Craven DE, Celli BR, *et al.* (1987) Nosocomial pneumonia in intubated patients given sucralfate as compared with antacids or histamine type 2 blockers. The role of gastric colonization. *New England Journal of Medicine* **317**: 1376-1382.

Driscoll DF & Blackburn GL (1990) Total parenteral nutrition 1990. A review of its current status in hospitalised patients and the need for patient-specific feeding. *Drugs* **40**: 346-363.

Eddleston JM, Pearson RC, Holland J, Tooth JA, Vohra A & Doran BH (1994) Prospective endoscopic study of stress erosions and ulcers in critically ill adult patients treated with either sucralfate or placebo. *Critical Care Medicine* **22**: 1949-1954.

Editorial (1980) Dangerous pseudohyponatraemia. *Lancet* **ii**: 1121.

Ferrante FM, Chan VW, Arthur GR & Rocco AG (1991) Interpleural analgesia after thoracotomy. *Anaesthesia and Analgesia* **72**: 105-109.

Fisher RL (1989) Hepatobiliary abnormalities associated with total parenteral nutrition. *Gastroenterology Clinics of North America* **18**: 645-666.

Flear CTG & Singh CM (1973) Hyponatraemia and sick cells. *British Journal of Anaesthesia* **45**: 976-994.

Forse RA, Christou N, Meakins JL, MacLean JD & Shizgal HM (1981) Reliability of skin testing as a measure of nutritional state. *Archives of Surgery* **116**: 1284-1288.

Friedman CJ, Oblinger MJ, Suratt PM *et al.* (1982) Prophylaxis of upper gastrointestinal hemorrhage in patients requiring mechanical ventilation. *Critical Care Medicine* **10**: 316-319.

Geerts WH, Code KI, Jay RM, Chen E & Szalai JP (1994) A prospective study of venous thromboembolism after major trauma. *New England Journal of Medicine* **33**: 1601-1606.

Grimble GK, Payne-James JJ & Silk DBA (1992) Advances in nutrition in the critically ill. *Baillière's Clinical Anaesthesiology* **6**: 213-252.

Gronert GA & Theye RA (1975) Pathophysiology of hyperkalemia induced by succinylcholine. *Anesthesiology* **43**: 89-99.

Grounds RM, Lalor JM, Lumley J, Royston D & Morgan M (1987) Propofol infusion for sedation in the intensive care unit: preliminary report. *British Medical Journal* **294**: 397-400.

Harris CE, Grounds RM, Murray AM, Lumley J, Royston D & Morgan M (1990) Propofol for long-term sedation in the intensive care unit. A comparison with papaveretum and midazolam. *Anaesthesia* **45**: 366-372.

Heyland DK, Cook DJ & Guyatt GH (1994) Does the formulation of enteral feeding products influence infectious morbidity and mortality rates in the critically ill patients? A critical review of the evidence. *Critical Care Medicine* **22**: 1192-1202.

Hinton P, Allison SP, Littlejohn S & Lloyd J (1971) Insulin and glucose to reduce catabolic response to injury in burned patients. *Lancet* **i**: 767-769.

Jeejeebhoy KN & Marliss EB (1983) Energy supply in total parenteral nutrition. In: Fischer JE (ed), *Surgical Nutrition*. Boston, Little, Brown, pp. 645-662.

Jones BJM, Payne S & Silk DBA (1980) Indications for pump assisted enteral feeding. *Lancet* **i**: 1057-1058.

Keohane PP, Jones BJM, Attrill H *et al.* (1983a) Effect of catheter tunnelling and a nutrition nurse on catheter sepsis during parenteral nutrition. A controlled trial. *Lancet* **ii**: 1388-1390.

Keohane PP, Attrill H, Jones BJM *et al.* (1983b) The roles of lactose and *Clostridium difficile* in the pathogenesis of enteral feeding associated diarrhoea. *Clinical Nutrition* **1**: 259-264.

Keohane PP, Attrill H, Love M, Frost P & Silk DBA (1984) Relation between osmolality of diet and gastrointestinal side effects in enteral nutrition. *British Medical Journal* **288**: 678-680.

Kiely WF (1976) Psychiatric syndromes in critically ill patients. *Journal of the American Medical Association* **235**: 2759-2761.

Kong KL, Willatts SM & Prys-Roberts C (1989) Isoflurane compared with midazolam for sedation in the intensive care unit. *British Medical Journal* **298**: 1277-1280.

Konstantinides FN, Konstantinides NN, Li JC, Myayr ME & Cerra FB (1991) Urinary urea nitrogen: too insensitive for calculating nitrogen balance studies in surgical clinical nutrition. *Journal of Parenteral and Enteral Nutrition* **15**: 189-193.

Larca L & Greenbaum DM (1982) Effectiveness of intensive nutritional regimes in patients who fail to wean from mechanical ventilation. *Critical Care Medicine* **10**: 297-300.

Larner AJ, Vickers CR, Abu D, Buckels JAC, Elias E & Neuberger J (1988) Correction of severe hyponatraemia by continuous arteriovenous haemofiltration before liver transplantation. *British Medical Journal* **297**: 1514-1515.

Lloyd GG (1993) Psychological problems and the intensive care unit. *British Medical Journal* **307**: 458-459.

Mackenzie SJ (1993) Stress ulcer prophylaxis: routine or targeted? Pathogenesis, significance and prophylactic measures. *British Journal of Intensive Care* **3**: 339-344.

Madan M, Alexander DJ & McMahon MJ (1992) Influence of catheter type on occurrence of thrombophlebitis during peripheral intravenous nutrition. *Lancet* **339**: 101-103.

Moore EE & Moore FA (1991) Immediate enteral nutrition following multisystem trauma: a decade perspective. *Journal of the American College of Nutrition* **10**: 633-648.

Moore FA, Moore EE, Jones TN, McCroskey BL & Peterson VM (1989) TEN versus TPN following major abdominal trauma-reduced septic morbidity. *Journal of Trauma* **29**: 916-923.

Moore FA, Feliciano DV, Andrassy RJ, *et al.* (1992) Early enteral feeding compared with parenteral reduces post-operative septic complications. The results of a meta-analysis. *Surgery* **216**: 172-183.

Murphy DF (1993) Interpleural analgesia. *British Journal of Anaesthesia* **71**: 426-434.

Nimmo GR, Mackenzie SJ & Grant IS (1994) Haemodynamic and oxygen transport effects of propofol infusion in critically ill adults. *Anaesthesia* **49**: 485-489.

Osborne RJ, Joel SP & Slevin ML (1986) Morphine intoxication in renal failure: the role of morphine-6-glucuronide. *British Medical Journal* **292**: 1548-1549.

Park GR, Manara AR, Mendel L & Bateman PE (1987) Ketamine infusion. *Anaesthesia* **42**: 980-983.

Parke TJ, Stevens JE, Rice ASC *et al.* (1992) Metabolic acidosis and fatal myocardial failure after propofol infusion in children: five case reports. *British Medical Journal* **305**: 613-616.

Perry S, Difede J, Musngi G, Francis AJ & Jacobsberg (1992) Predictors of posttraumatic stress disorder after burn injury. *American Journal of Psychiatry* **149**: 931-935.

Pingleton SK & Hadzima S (1983) Internal alimentation and gastrointestinal bleeding in mechanically ventilated patients. *Critical Care Medicine* **11**: 13-16.

Powell-Tuck J (1993) Glutamine, parenteral feeding and intestinal nutrition. *Lancet* **342**: 451-452.

Priebe JH, Skillman JJ, Bushnell LS, Long PC & Silen W (1980) Antacid versus cimetidine in preventing acute gastrointestinal bleeding. *New England Journal of Medicine* **302**: 426-430.

Radermacher P, Santak B, Strobach H, Schror K & Tarnow J (1992) Fat emulsions containing medium chain triglycerides in patients with sepsis syndrome: effects on pulmonary hemodynamics and gas exchange. *Intensive Care Medicine* **18**: 231-234.

Ramsay MAE, Savege TM, Simpson BRJ & Goodwin R (1974) Controlled sedation with alphaxalone alphadolone. *British Medical Journal* **ii**: 656-659.

Roca RP, Spence RJ & Munster AM (1992) Post-traumatic adaptation and distress among adult burn survivors. *American Journal of Psychiatry* **149**: 1234-1238.

Ross RJM, Miell JP & Buchanan CR (1991) Avoiding autocannibalism: consider growth hormone and insulin-like growth factor I. *British Medical Journal* **1**: 1147-1148.

Schuster DP (1993) Stress ulcer prophylaxis: in whom? with what? *Critical Care Medicine* **21**: 4-6.

Segredo V, Matthay MA, Sharma ML *et al.* (1990) Prolonged neuromuscular blockade after long-term administration of vecuronium in two critically ill patients. *Anesthesiology* **72**: 566-570.

Shelley MP, Mendel L & Park GR (1987) Failure of critically ill patients to metabolise midazolam. *Anaesthesia* **42**: 619-626.

Shizgal HM & Forse RA (1980) Protein and calorie requirements with total parenteral nutrition. *Annals of Surgery* **192**: 562-569.

Shulman M, Sandler AN, Bradley JW, Young PS & Brebner J (1984) Post thoracotomy pain and pulmonary function following epidural and systemic morphine. *Anesthesiology* **61**: 569-575.

Shuman RB, Schuster DP & Zuckerman GR (1987) Prophylactic therapy for stress ulcer bleeding: a reappraisal. *Annals of Internal Medicine* **106**: 562-567.

Sinclair ME & Suter PM (1988) Detection of overdosage of sedation in a patient with renal failure by absence of lower oesophageal motility. *Intensive Care Medicine* **14**: 69-71.

Souba WW, Herskowitz K, Salloum RM, Chen MK & Austgen TR (1990) Gut glutamine metabolism. *Journal of Parenteral and Enteral Nutrition* **14** (Suppl): 45-50S.

Sterns RH, Riggs JE & Schochet SS Jr (1986) Osmotic demyelination syndrome following correction of hyponatremia. *New England Journal of Medicine* **314**: 1535-1542.

Studley HO (1936) Percentage of weight loss: a basic indicator of surgical risk in patients with chronic peptic ulcer. *Journal of the American Medical Association* **106**: 458-460.

Swales JD (1987) Dangers in treating hyponatraemia. *British Medical Journal* **294**: 837.

Thornton C, Barrowcliffe MP, Konieczko KM, *et al.* (1989) The auditory evoked response as an indicator of awareness. *British Journal of Anaesthesia* **63**: 113-115.

Tryba M (1994) Stress ulcer prophylaxis. *Intensive Care Medicine* **20**: 311-313.

Tryba M, Zervouner F, Torok M & Zenz M (1985) Prevention of acute stress bleeding with sucralfate, antacids or cimetidine. *American Journal of Medicine* **79**: 55-61.

Van der Hulst RR, Van Kreel BK, Von Meyenfeldt M F, *et al.* (1993) Glutamine and the preservation of gut integrity. *Lancet* **341**: 1363-1365.

Veterans Affairs Total Parenteral Nutrition Cooperative Study Group (1991) Perioperative total parenteral nutrition in surgical patients. *New England Journal of Medicine* **325**: 525-532.

Weinmann TE & Salzman EW (1994) Deep vein thrombosis. *New England Journal of Medicine* **331**: 1630-1640.

Willatts SM & Spencer EM (1994) Sedation for ventilation in the critically ill: a role for isoflurane? *Anaesthesia* **49**: 422-428.

Wolfe BM, Ryder MA, Nishikawa RA, Halsted CH & Schmidt BF (1986) Complications of parenteral nutrition. *American Journal of Surgery* **152**: 93-99.

Yate PM, Flynn PJ, Arnold RN, Weatherly BC, Simmons RJ & Dopson T (1987) Clinical experience and plasma concentrations during the infusion of atracurium in the intensive therapy unit. *British Journal of Anaesthesia* **59**: 211-217.

Zaloga GP (1989) Interpretation of the serum magnesium level. *Chest* **95**: 257-258.

Ziegler TR, Young LS, Ferrari-Baliviera E, Demling RH & Wilmore DW (1990) Use of human growth hormone combined with nutritional support in the critical care unit. *Journal of Parenteral and Enteral Nutrition* **14**: 574-581.

11 Infection in the Critically Ill

The incidence of hospital-acquired (nosocomial) infection has increased dramatically over the last half century. Currently approximately 5–10% of hospitalized patients develop a nosocomial infection, a significant proportion require admission to an intensive care unit (ICU) and overall around 3% die as a result of their infection. In intensive care units the prevalence of nosocomial infections has been estimated to be 18–36%.

The organisms predominantly responsible for hospital-acquired infections have altered since antibiotics were introduced into clinical practice. In the 1940s, the majority of fatal infections were caused by streptococci (*Streptococcus pyogenes* and *S. pneumoniae*) or staphylococci. Later, the emergence of resistant strains of *Staphylococcus aureus* caused concern, but during the late 1950s and the 1960s there was a progressive increase in the number of cases of sepsis and the streptococci and staphylococci were largely superseded as a cause of life-threatening infection in hospitalized patients by the aerobic Gram-negative bacilli (Altemeier *et al.*, 1967). Initially, the dominant organism was *Escherichia coli*, but subsequently other Gram-negative bacteria, such as *Klebsiella* spp., *Proteus* spp., *Pseudomonas* spp., *Enterobacter* and *Citrobacter* spp. assumed greater importance. An increasing number of these organisms have since developed antibiotic resistance, probably encouraged by the widespread use of broad-spectrum antimicrobial agents, many of which were intrinsically more active against Gram-positive bacteria. This problem is partly a result of 'natural selection' and spontaneous mutation, but has been compounded by the ability of Gram-negative organisms to transfer resistance from one strain to another, for example within the bowel lumen, as 'R' factors or 'plasmids'. More recently Gram-positive infections have again assumed greater prominence and during the 1980s Gram-positive cocci resistant to multiple antibiotics have emerged as important pathogens. Unusual pathogens are encountered increasingly frequently in immunocompromised hosts, and fungal infection is always a danger in such patients, especially when they have received broad-spectrum antibiotics.

FACTORS PREDISPOSING TO INFECTION IN HOSPITALIZED PATIENTS

The changing pattern of infection, and the increasing incidence of nosocomial infections is not, of course, solely attributable to the effects of antibiotic therapy; alterations in both the susceptibility of the hospital population and the procedures to which they are subjected have also contributed to this phenomenon.

An increasing number of hospitalized patients survive with impaired immune responses. These may result from their disease, for example:

- renal failure;
- diabetes mellitus;
- malignancy;
- human immunodeficiency virus (HIV) infection;
- severe trauma;
- burns.

Alternatively impaired immune responses may be due to therapy with:

- immunosuppressants;
- cytotoxics;
- steroids;
- radiotherapy.

Furthermore, the risk of infection increases:

- at the extremes of age;
- in the presence of malnutrition;
- with the severity of the underlying disease.

Critical illness is associated with impaired immunity, the aetiology of which is complex and probably multifactorial. There are widespread abnormalities of macrophage, T and B cell function, neutrophil chemotaxis and intracellular killing.

Cell-mediated immunity (CMI), as measured by the delayed-type hypersensitivity skin reaction to recall antigens, has been shown to be impaired in the critically ill and persistent anergy is associated with a poor prognosis (Bradley *et al.*, 1984). In addition, the lymphocyte response to mitogens may be impaired by a number of factors, including surgery, trauma, burns, infection, malignancy and malnutrition. Various causes have been suggested including the effects of anaesthesia, blood transfusion and a negative nitrogen balance. Circulating depressant factors, increased suppressor cell, mainly T-cell, activity and defective T-helper cell function may also be involved (Wolfe *et al.*, 1981). This CMI is of most importance in combating infections with poorly encapsulated organisms such as *Pseudomonas* spp.

Neutrophil chemotaxis and *intracellular killing* may also be impaired. Chemotaxis may be impaired by an intrinsic intracellular defect, or defective production of chemotactic factors, but inhibition is most likely to be mediated by circulating depressant factors. Neutrophil function may also be depressed by phosphate deficiency and the administration of volatile anaesthetic agents. Some of the most seriously ill patients also become *leucopenic* and this is recognized as a bad prognostic sign in the presence of infection.

Depletion of *complement*, reduced *fibronectin* levels (O'Connell *et al.*, 1984) and *defective phagocytosis* due to reduced opsonic activity may also predispose to infective complications. Not uncommonly, immunoglobulin levels are also reduced as a result of extravascular leakage, reduced synthesis and increased consumption. Moreover B cell numbers are decreased, and the percentage of resting B cells available to be activated to produce antibodies is reduced so that inadequate levels of secretory antibodies are available at mucosal sites (Abraham & Chang, 1990). Presumably this contributes to the increased incidence of bacterial colonization at these surfaces and the increased susceptibility to bloodstream invasion.

These highly susceptible patients are now more frequently subjected to:

- extensive surgery;
- invasive procedures—intravascular and urethral catheterization, insertion of intercostal drains, tracheal intubation or tracheostomy;
- parenteral nutrition.

It is not surprising, therefore, that persistent or recurrent sepsis is such an intractable problem in the critically ill.

SOURCES AND PREVENTION OF INFECTION

Endogenous (autogenous) infection

Very often, the source of infection is the patient's own skin or, most importantly, oropharyngeal cavity and gastrointestinal tract. Potentially pathogenic microorganisms (PPM) involved in infection in the ICU can be divided conveniently into those present in otherwise healthy people (the so-called 'community PPM') and those commonly present in the hospital environment (i.e. in individuals with underlying disease; the so-called

'hospital PPM') (**Table 11.1**). This classification also implies that individuals with a chronic illness, but resident in the community may carry hospital PPM. There are three basic patterns of infection in the ICU:

- primary endogenous;
- secondary endogenous;
- exogenous.

In *exogenous infection*, there is no preceding microbial carriage in the throat and/or gut. In *endogenous (autogenous)* infection, oropharyngeal and/or intestinal carriage precedes infection. A *primary endogenous infection* is caused by a PPM carried by the patient on admission to the ICU, whereas a *secondary endogenous infection* is caused by PPMs acquired in the ICU. Endemic infection in the ICU is more often primary endogenous (Van Saene *et al.*, 1994).

In health *colonization of the alimentary tract* by aerobic bacteria is resisted by:

- the integrity of the mucosal lining;
- normal gastrointestinal motility, including swallowing and peristalsis;
- the desquamation of mucosal cells;
- mucus production;
- secretory IgA.

Normal flora, mainly the resident anaerobes, also inhibit the proliferation of aerobic organisms. These protective mechanisms are frequently impaired in the critically ill, leading to colonization of the oropharynx and gastrointestinal tract by large numbers of aerobic Gram-negative bacteria such as *E. coli*, *Klebsiella* spp., *Proteus* spp. and *Pseudomonas aeruginosa*, as well as by *S. aureus* and yeasts, especially *Candida* spp.

Table 11.1 Potentially pathogenic microorganisms (PPM) causing infections in intensive care unit patients.

Previously healthy ('community' PPM)

Streptococcus pneumoniae
Haemophilus influenzae
Moraxella catarrhalis
Escherichia coli
Staphylococcus aureus
Candida albicans

With underlying disease ('hospital' PPM)

Klebsiella spp.
Proteus spp.
Morganells spp.
Enterobacter spp.
Citrobacter spp.
Serratia spp.
Acinetobacter spp.
Pseudomonas spp.

An important factor promoting colonization and subsequent overgrowth of abnormal flora in the critically ill appears to be increased adherence of bacteria to the mucosa due to alteration of the epithelial surface. *Oropharyngeal colonization* is more likely in those with a tracheal or nasogastric tube in place, pre-existing pulmonary disease, or uraemia, and in patients receiving antibiotics. It becomes increasingly likely the longer patients stay in hospital and the more severely ill they are, and in older age groups.

Colonization of the stomach with Gram-negative organisms is also common in critically ill patients, particularly when gastric pH is elevated by antacid prophylaxis (see Chapter 10), and in those with gastroduodenal reflux (Inglis *et al.*, 1992). It has been suggested that under these circumstances regurgitation and aspiration of gastric contents may contribute to colonization or infection of the oropharynx and respiratory tract (Du Moulin *et al.*, 1982). In a more recent study, however, the frequency of gastric colonization was confirmed, but there was no evidence that microorganisms migrated to the nasopharynx or that there was a relationship between such colonization and clinically important infection. Neither was there any relationship between gastric pH and colonization (Cade *et al.*, 1992).

The vector in many cases of autogenous infection is the patient's own hands, or those of his attendants. The patient must therefore be prevented from handling infected areas and transferring organisms to vulnerable sites elsewhere (e.g. a tracheostomy stoma). Meticulous hygiene is essential to protect the patient from endogenous infection, necessitating frequent changes of bed linen, cleaning of contaminated areas and hand washing.

SELECTIVE DECONTAMINATION OF THE DIGESTIVE TRACT

Decontamination of the digestive tract is designed to prevent autogenous or endogenous infection by reducing the numbers of PPM in the oropharynx and gastrointestinal tract (Stoutenbeek *et al.*, 1994). The technique was originally introduced to reduce infective complications in neutropenic oncology patients; at first unselective decontamination was often used, but this was associated with a risk of overgrowth of Gram-negative bacteria acquired from the hospital environment, probably because of a decrease in the numbers of anaerobic bacilli. Selective decontamination of the digestive tract (SDD) aims to avoid this problem by eliminating carriage of aerobic bacilli and yeasts while preserving the normal anaerobic flora and thereby maintaining *colonization resistance*. As well as minimizing the risk of nosocomial infection, SDD can potentially reduce the incidence of multiple organ failure by decreasing the load of bacteria and endotoxin within the gut lumen and limiting the

extent of translocation of PPM and absorption of faecal endotoxin (see Chapter 4). Successful decontamination of individual patients might also reduce the general level of contamination within the intensive care unit, thereby contributing to an overall reduction in infection rates.

Various regimens have been used to achieve SDD. Most use a combination of non-absorbable antibacterial and antifungal agents instilled via the nasogastric tube, together with a topical preparation applied to the oropharynx; many have also included a variable period of intravenous antimicrobial prophylaxis. It is suggested that with this combined approach the parenteral antibiotic component might prevent primary endogenous infection (caused by PPM carried on admission) and, together with the topical antimicrobials, might lower the incidence of secondary endogenous infection (caused by newly acquired microorganisms colonizing the digestive tract).

The use of SDD in critically ill patients was first described by Stoutenbeek *et al.* in 1984. They administered tobramycin, polymyxin (which binds endotoxin) and amphotericin B via the nasogastric tube, combined with systemic cefotaxime for at least four days, to a group of multiple trauma patients; they also emphasized the importance of decontaminating the oropharyngeal cavity using a sticky paste containing 2% tobramycin, polymyxin and amphotericin B. The infection rate fell from 81% in historical controls to 16% in treated patients, although the effect on mortality was not reported. A subsequent prospective study with consecutive controls confirmed the reduction in colonization rates and the incidence of acquired infection, and also demonstrated a significant reduction in mortality in the trauma subgroup. There was also a tendency for improved outcome in longer-stay patients (i.e. in hospital for more than seven days) and in those with mid-range acute physiology, and chronic health evaluation (APACHE) scores (Ledingham *et al.*, 1988). In a later randomized study in a heterogeneous group of intensive care patients (Ulrich *et al.*, 1989), a regimen consisting of gastrointestinal and nasopharyngeal decontamination with polymyxin E, norfloxacin, amphotericin B and systemic trimethoprim significantly reduced the incidence of Gram-negative respiratory, urinary tract and line-related infections. Mortality was also significantly reduced. More recently a prospective double-blind randomized placebo-controlled study in mechanically ventilated ICU patients confirmed that SDD can dramatically reduce the incidence of nosocomial infections, but failed to demonstrate any improvement in survival, or any reduction in the incidence of multiple organ failure. There was also a substantial increase in the cost of antimicrobial drugs (Gastinine *et al.*, 1992). Another prospective, randomized, double-blind study reached a similar conclusion (Hammond *et al.*, 1992).

A number of meta-analyses have since been performed in an attempt to resolve some of the controversy surrounding the use of SDD in the critically ill. The first, which included only 491 patients in six controlled and six randomized studies (Vandenbroucke-Grauls & Vandenbroucke, 1991) concluded that at best SDD had only a very limited effect on survival of ICU patients, despite a clear reduction in the incidence of respiratory tract infections. The second, larger meta-analysis included 4142 patients in 22 studies. The findings were in agreement with the previous review in that the incidence of respiratory tract infections was significantly reduced (by about 60%), but the authors concluded that in long-stay (> five days) and mechanically ventilated (> 48 hours) general intensive care patients, the effect on mortality remained uncertain, being at best only a moderate improvement in survival. Moreover, there appeared to be only a weak association between the reduction in infection rates and improved survival. A beneficial effect on mortality seemed most likely when combined topical and systemic treatment was used since in these cases there was a significant 20% reduction in the odds of death. The authors also pointed out that in no trial has there been any suggestion that SDD worsens outcome (Selective Decontamination of the Digestive Tract Trialists Collaborative Group, 1993). Since then two further meta-analyses of 2270 patients in 16 studies (Kollef, 1994) and of 3395 patients in 25 randomized studies (Heyland et al., 1994) have been performed. Although both analyses concluded that SDD reduces the incidence of acquired pneumonia, they indicated that its effect on mortality was small or non-existent (Heyland et al., 1994; Kollef, 1994). There was, however, a suggestion that when topical antibiotics were combined with a short course of intravenous antibiotics the reduction in mortality was significant.

The obvious discrepancy between the dramatic reduction in nosocomial infection produced by SDD and at best only moderate improvement in survival suggests that many of those who die in ICUs, especially medical patients, do so with, but not because of, infection. Nevertheless there is some evidence that SDD can improve survival in burns patients, perhaps by reducing colonization of wounds, urine and gastric aspirate, and the incidence of respiratory infections (Mackie et al., 1992) and may be beneficial in patients with fulminant hepatic failure (Rolando et al., 1993). Finally it has been suggested that SDD is most likely to be effective in longer-stay patients with a curable underlying condition (e.g. trauma) and a moderately severe acute illness (mid-range APACHE scores).

There has been considerable concern that SDD, which contradicts traditional microbiological advice to use narrow-spectrum antibiotics only to treat clearly established infection and not colonization, might select out resistant microorganisms. In general these fears do not seem to have been justified, but some remain concerned that the widespread use of these regimens could lead to the emergence of antibiotic-resistant bacilli. It also remains unclear whether combined systemic and topical regimens are superior to the use of topical antimicrobials alone.

A number of factors have complicated interpretation of the large number of published trials of SDD. These include the variety of antimicrobial regimens used (e.g. some have omitted the systemic component), the different patient groups studied, the variable quality of microbiological surveillance (it is important to confirm decontamination microbiologically), and the different criteria used for the diagnosis of pneumonia. Moreover, not all studies have been prospective, randomized and double-blind, and the use of concurrent controls may influence the results by acting as a source of acquired infection for the treatment group.

Some are convinced that SDD does have a role in intensive care since it undoubtedly reduces colonization rates and the incidence of infection, and because there is evidence to suggest that in certain subgroups (e.g. trauma, elective surgery, long-term mechanical ventilation, mid-range APACHE scores) mortality may also be reduced (Reidy & Ramsey, 1990). The validity of using mortality as the end point for the efficacy of a regimen designed to prevent nosocomial infections has also been questioned. Others remain unconvinced and believe that greater attention to accepted standards of microbiological practice is likely to be more effective (Atkinson & Bihari, 1993). Most, however, would agree that the important question as to whether SDD has a clinically significant effect on survival in selected subgroups of patients remains to be answered. It has been recommended that further large (1500–16,200 patients) clinical trials should be performed to answer this question (Selective Decontamination of the Digestive Tract Trialists Collaborative Group, 1993; Heyland et al., 1994).

Exogenous infection

Exogenous infection is unusual, but hospitals, patients, staff and contaminated equipment act as a reservoir of PPM. Critically ill patients are therefore at risk of acquiring an exogenous infection from:

- the environment, such as ventilation equipment;
- their attendants;
- their fellow patients.

The precautions taken to prevent exogenous infection vary from one unit to another, reflecting the lack of evidence as to the efficacy of many of the measures that can be adopted. For example, in some, clean gowns and overshoes are worn by all staff and visitors who enter the unit. Although this has not been shown to reduce the incidence of infection conclusively, it has the advantage of limiting the number of casual visitors and emphasizing the need for personal cleanliness.

The greatest risk to the patient, however, is from PPM transmitted from other patients or from contaminated areas of the unit such as the sinks, usually on the hands of the staff. The most important preventive measure is therefore *thorough handwashing* between patients (Daschner, 1985); the use of an antimicrobial agent (chlorhexidine) is probably more effective than soap and alcohol (Doelbing *et al.*, 1992). *Fomites*, such as stethoscopes, may also be responsible for transmitting organisms between patients. In some units, disposable aprons, and even gloves, are worn at all times and are changed when moving from one patient to another. In others, such precautions are only employed when a patient is known to harbour resistant organisms. Caps and masks are generally considered to be unnecessary, except when performing aseptic procedures, while environmental monitoring is expensive, tedious and probably of little value (Daschner, 1985).

Unit design (see Chapter 1) is an important element in minimizing transmission of PPM. There must be adequate space around each bed and some single cubicles should be available for barrier or reverse barrier nursing. These cubicles can be equipped with unidirectional plenum ventilation. Adequate handwashing facilities are essential and a basin should be provided adjacent to each bed area.

Staff must be trained in the correct procedures for reducing transmission, and must be motivated to perform them to a high standard at all times. If staffing levels are inadequate, these procedures may be overlooked and movement between patients will increase, particularly in times of stress; as a consequence, the incidence of transmission and subsequent secondary endogenous and/or exogenous infection may rise.

Infection control teams

Preventive measures are most likely to be successful when supervised by an infection control team. This group can assume responsibility for monitoring rates of infection, antibiotic usage and sensitivity patterns and reporting these to clinicians. They can also establish procedures for sterilization and disinfection, develop and enforce policies to contain infection, including isolation procedures, and promote effective preventive measures, such as handwashing. The team should also be concerned with staff health and safety and should, for example, develop procedures for the management of needlestick injuries and supervise vaccinations.

Enhancing host defences

Measures that may improve host defences include:

- nutritional support;
- active and passive immunization;
- granulocyte transfusions;
- immune stimulation (e.g. BCG and levamisole);
- fibronectin, fresh frozen plasma (FFP), cryoprecipitate, γ-globulin.

In the future it may be possible to restore macrophage and T cell function by administering cytokines such as interferon-γ (Ertel *et al.*, 1992) and interleukin-10 (IL-10).

NOSOCOMIAL INFECTIONS IN THE CRITICALLY ILL

The majority of hospital-acquired infections involve the urinary tract (42%), surgical wounds (20%), the respiratory tract (14%) or the bloodstream (8%).

Nosocomial pneumonia

Nosocomial pneumonia represents 10–30% of all nosocomial infections in the critically ill and is associated with a high mortality of 20–50%. Most (around 60%) are caused by Gram-negative bacteria, but more recently there has been an increase in pneumonia due to Gram-positive organisms, including methicillin-resistant *S. aureus* (MRSA).

PREDISPOSING FACTORS (**Table 11.2**)

Critically ill patients with tracheal tubes or tracheostomies in place are particularly liable to develop secondary pulmonary infection. Many of the normal barriers to the introduction of microorganisms have been bypassed, while colonization of tracheostomy wounds, the oropharynx, upper airways and the stomach is common (see above). Moreover, mucociliary transport can be impaired by opiates, high inspired oxygen concentrations, inadequate humidification and trauma from tracheal suctioning. Laryngeal dysfunction predisposes to aspiration and may be related to neurological abnormalities, drug administration or the presence of a tracheal and/or nasogastric tube. Macrophage function may be defective, while retention of secretions, pulmonary oedema and destruction of the normal bacterial flora by antibiotics all increase the risk of infection. Bacteria may also be introduced during endotracheal suction. The risk of pneumonia is increased in:

- the elderly;
- the immunosuppressed;
- those with chronic lung disease;
- following surgery (particularly thoraco-abdominal);
- after large volume aspiration;
- when consciousness is depressed.

DIAGNOSIS

Diagnosis can be difficult, especially in those with pre-existing lung pathology such as adult respiratory distress syndrome (ARDS). The diagnosis should be suspected when:

- the patient develops a fever;
- there are new infiltrates on the chest radiograph;
- there is a change in the quantity or appearance of the sputum;
- lung function deteriorates;
- there is an otherwise unexplained deterioration in the patient's general condition.

Unfortunately in most critically ill patients there are several potential sources of fever, the significance of

Table 11.2 Factors predisposing to nosocomial pneumonia.

Tracheal intubation/tracheostomy	Bypass normal defences
Colonization	Oropharynx Upper airways Stomach Tracheostomy wound
Impaired mucociliary transport	Opiates High inspired oxygen concentrations Inadequate humidification Tracheal suctioning
Laryngeal dysfunction	Neurological abnormalities Drug administration Endotracheal tube Nasogastric tube
Impaired macrophage function	
Retention of secretions	
Pulmonary oedema	
Destruction of normal bacterial flora by antibiotics	

purulent sputum is often uncertain, and the appearance of new infiltrates on the chest radiograph may represent not only infection, but also ARDS, pulmonary oedema, infection or atelectasis. Not surprisingly, therefore, the clinical diagnosis of nosocomial pneumonia has been shown to be incorrect in about one-third of cases when compared to histological findings (Andrews *et al.*, 1981).

INVESTIGATIONS (Tobin & Grenvik, 1984; MacFarlane, 1985)

Sputum, either expectorated or obtained by endotracheal suction, should be sent for culture and determination of antibiotic sensitivities. It is important that the specimen is immediately stained and examined microbiologically. In some cases it may not be possible to obtain an adequate quantity of sputum from the lower airways and expectorated samples are often contaminated with bacteria or fungi during their passage through the upper airways. Although aspirates obtained via an endotracheal or tracheostomy tube are less likely to be contaminated than expectorated sputum, they can still produce false-positive cultures. *Blood cultures* are rarely positive (10–20% of cases), but when an organism is isolated it is very likely to be the cause of the pneumonia.

Because clinical criteria for the diagnosis of nosocomial pneumonia are unreliable, and the results obtained from standard microbiological studies of central tracheobronchial secretions are frequently misleading (Berger & Arango, 1985), some recommend that both the diagnosis and the causative organism should be pursued more aggressively using *invasive techniques*. It is often particularly difficult to identify the causative organism in immunocompromised patients with an opportunistic infection and some of these more invasive procedures are especially useful in such cases (see later).

Transtracheal needle aspiration (TTA)

In unintubated patients oropharyngeal contamination can be avoided by sampling via the cricothyroid membrane. The risk of complications with this technique is low, haemorrhage being the main concern, and the diagnostic yield is excellent in bacterial pneumonia, provided antibiotics have not already been given. There is, however, a significant incidence of false-positive results.

Fibre-optic bronchoscopy

Diagnostic material can be obtained during fibre-optic bronchoscopy by:

- aspiration;
- bronchial brushings;
- bronchoalveolar lavage;
- transbronchial lung biopsy.

Complications include:

- hypoxaemia;
- bronchospasm;
- cardiac arrhythmias;
- pneumothorax;
- haemorrhage;
- infection.

Because directly aspirated material and samples obtained by conventional bronchial brushings are likely to be contaminated by organisms colonizing the large airways *protected specimen brushing* (PSB) has been advocated for the diagnosis of bacterial pneumonia. This technique involves passing a double lumen catheter with a protected brush through the fibre-optic bronchoscope to collect uncontaminated specimens from suspected areas of infection. The sample can then be cultured quantitatively; growth of more than 10^3 colony forming units/ml is generally considered significant. The overall sensitivity of PSB may be as high as 93% and the incidence of false-positives is low. The number of false-negative results can be minimized by sampling from several areas of lung. PSB is most useful when secondary bacterial infection occurs in a patient who is already receiving antibiotics to which the new infecting organism is resistant. It is probably of little value in patients with recent clinical evidence of a chest infection who have been given new antibiotics. PSB specimens should, therefore, always be obtained before starting a new course of antibiotics. Bronchial brushings can also be useful for the detection of *Pneumocystis carinii* and fungi. Complications of brush biopsy include pneumothorax, haemorrhage and infection.

Bronchoalveolar lavage (BAL) (Morrison & Stockley, 1988) has also been advocated for the diagnosis of nosocomial bacterial pneumonia, although contamination with upper airway organisms is again a problem and some therefore consider this technique to be most suitable for demonstrating parasites and fungi. Immediate microscopic analysis of BAL fluid may allow rapid identification of the causative organism in patients with pneumonia. In one experimental study quantitative cultures of PSB specimens correlated well with the bacterial content of lung tissue, but the results obtained with BAL were superior (Johanson *et al.*, 1988). In general BAL is rather more sensitive than PSB since a wider area of the lung is sampled, but the most accurate diagnostic information in bacterial pneumonia is probably obtained when BAL is combined with PSB. BAL has also been used successfully to diagnose opportunistic pulmonary infections in immunocompromised hosts. Compli-

cations of BAL include worsening hypoxaemia and infection.

It is almost always possible to obtain lung tissue using *transbronchial biopsy* and an aetiological diagnosis is made in 40–80% of cases. However, the incidence of complications, particularly pneumothorax is highest with this technique, especially in those undergoing mechanical ventilation, and its use is therefore normally restricted to establishing the cause of pulmonary infiltrates in spontaneously breathing patients, especially those who are immunocompromised. In patients with malignant disease, sampling errors and false-negatives may occur: in particular the biopsy may show only 'non-specific interstitial pneumonitis' in nearly half the cases, many of whom may in fact have active infection. The incidence of haemorrhage is low provided thrombocytopenic patients receive a platelet transfusion before the procedure. Uraemic patients are more likely to bleed. Supplemental oxygen must be given during the procedure.

Percutaneous transthoracic needle biopsy

Percutaneous transthoracic needle biopsy produces a reasonable diagnostic yield, but the incidence of pneumothorax is around 25%, although significant haemoptysis is unusual. Its use is confined to spontaneously breathing patients who are sufficiently alert and cooperative to be able to stop breathing for 5-second periods while the needle is advanced.

Open lung biopsy

A small segment of lung can be excised through a minithoracotomy; this usually allows a histological and microbiological diagnosis to be made. Pneumothorax, haemothorax and infection may all occur, but in experienced hands the morbidity and mortality of this procedure is acceptably low. Open lung biopsy is indicated when transbronchial techniques fail to establish the diagnosis and when a definitive diagnosis must be established with the first procedure. It is probably safer than transbronchial biopsy in mechanically ventilated patients and those with uncorrectable hypoxaemia or a bleeding disorder. In immunosuppressed patients with pulmonary infiltrates a specific diagnosis can be established in about 70% of cases, while a non-specific interstitial pneumonitis is found in the remainder.

Choosing the most suitable investigation

The choice of the most suitable technique in an individual patient depends on a number of factors including:

- the presumed diagnosis (bacterial, fungal, viral or protozoan);
- the presence of coagulation disorders;
- the severity of respiratory failure;
- the experience of available personnel.

PREVENTION OF NOSOCOMIAL PNEUMONIA

The *ventilator tubing* frequently becomes contaminated, usually with organisms from the patient's own airways, and should therefore be changed every 48 hours to avoid proliferation of these bacteria, reinfection of the patient and contamination of the ventilator. *Humidifier water* can also become contaminated and should be changed regularly, although heating to 60°C should effectively prevent contamination.

The *ventilators* themselves are a potential source of infection and autoclavable patient circuits are now standard. Disposable heat and moisture exchanging *filters* can be positioned in the inspiratory and expiratory limbs of the circuit (see Chapter 7), while heated filters are incorporated in some ventilators. An aseptic technique should be used for tracheal suction.

Urinary tract infections

Urinary tract infections account for about 40% of all nosocomial infections, but mortality rates are generally low. Most are related to the presence of a urinary catheter, which provides a route for infection with faecal organisms colonizing the perineal region. Bacteria gain access to the bladder by intra- or extraluminal migration. It is therefore important to catheterize the bladder only when clearly indicated, not simply for convenience. Urethral catheterization must be performed aseptically. The catheter must be carefully secured and connected to a closed drainage system, and continuous, unobstructed drainage must be ensured.

Infection related to intravascular devices

Approximately 11–16% of central venous and pulmonary artery catheters may become contaminated with PPMs and the incidence of catheter-related blood infections is around 2–5% (Pinilla *et al.*, 1983; Cobb *et al.*, 1992). Intra-arterial cannulae are less likely to become contaminated (approximately 4–5%) and are rarely, if ever, responsible for blood infections (Pinilla *et al.*, 1983) (see also Chapter 3).

Infection related to intravascular devices may be due to poor aseptic technique during cannulation or inadequate care of the cannula, the infusion lines or the skin puncture site. Sometimes thrombus, which acts as a culture medium, forms on the catheter and becomes secondarily contaminated during a bacteraemic episode or via a contaminated infusion set. This is particularly likely to occur in patients receiving parenteral nutrition. Infection related to intravascular devices may be complicated by bacteraemia, suppurative phlebitis and infective endocarditis. The organisms most often implicated are coagulase-negative staphylococci, which accounted for 80% of infections related to catheters in one series (Pinilla *et al.*, 1983) and *S. aureus*, although occasionally aerobic Gram-negative bacilli, JK diphtheroids or *Candida* spp. may be responsible.

PREVENTION

All intravascular catheters must be inserted with full aseptic precautions after adequate skin disinfection. Intravenous infusion sets should be changed regularly (e.g. every 48 hours), although the use of in-line bacterial filters may allow less frequent replacement. Central venous cannulae should probably be replaced routinely every 5–8 days, although in one study scheduled replacement every three days was not associated with a lower incidence of bloodstream infection than when cannulae were changed only when clinically indicated (Cobb *et al.*, 1992). It is important to fix intravascular cannulae firmly, to use closed systems, and to avoid contamination of three-way taps. The puncture site should be covered with a transparent dressing and inspected at least daily. Parenteral nutrition must be administered via a dedicated cannula (see also Chapter 10). The use of occlusive antimicrobial dressings, in-line filters, regular flushing, antiseptic cream or spray applied to the puncture site, and subcutaneous tunnelling of feeding lines have not been conclusively shown to reduce the incidence of infection. Rates of infection may be higher with triple lumen than with single lumen catheters (Hilton *et al.*, 1988).

DIAGNOSIS

Catheter-related infection should be suspected if the patient develops signs of sepsis in the absence of an obvious source or if they persist after apparent eradication of a septic focus. The diagnosis is more likely if there are signs of infection at the puncture site (e.g. purulent discharge or lymphangitis) and is supported if blood cultures obtained through the cannula are positive while blood sampled from a separate puncture of a peripheral vein is sterile. Quantitative blood cultures of simultaneous catheter and peripheral samples are thought to be useful in distinguishing between catheter-related and other sources of bacteraemia. Catheter infection is confirmed by a positive culture from its tip or the subdermal segment, while catheter-related bacter-aemia is diagnosed when the same organism is isolated from the blood.

TREATMENT

Intravascular catheters should be removed and their tips sent for culture. Some recommend that the subdermal segment of the catheter should also be cultured. If the fever subsides it can be assumed that one or other of the cannulae was responsible and occasionally the use of antibiotics can be avoided. Ideally replacement of central venous cannulae should be delayed to allow elimination of residual organisms and in some cases it may subsequently be possible to use only peripheral venous access.

Because Hickman catheters are more difficult to insert and remove it may be reasonable to attempt to clear the infection by injecting antibiotics through the catheter. When venous access is limited it may be necessary to change the catheter over a guide wire, although this can be associated with an increased risk of bloodstream infection in the following three days. Replacement at a new site, on the other hand, increases the risk of mechanical complications (Cobb *et al.*, 1992).

Wound infections

Wound infections account for 20–25% of all nosocomial infections and are usually caused by autogenous infection at the time of surgery. A wound infection is diagnosed when there is a purulent discharge and a PPM is isolated in high concentrations. Commonly implicated organisms include *E. coli*, enterococci, *P. aeruginosa*, *Enterobacter* spp. and *Citrobacter* spp.

Wound infections are more common in the elderly, the poorly nourished, in those with renal failure or diabetes mellitus and in patients receiving steroids. The risks are greater following prolonged surgery and contaminated or dirty procedures.

THE RATIONAL USE OF ANTIBIOTICS

Critically ill patients often receive prolonged courses of the most expensive broad-spectrum antibiotics and although the use of such agents may be life-saving, there is considerable potential for their abuse. In order to limit the emergence and spread of resistant organisms, antibiotics must be used rationally and sparingly.

- They should be prescribed only when clearly indicated.

- Narrow-spectrum agents should be used whenever possible.
- They should usually be given for only a short period (e.g. five days).
- Prophylactic administration should be carefully controlled.
- Unnecessary treatment of colonization must be avoided (but see SDD above).

Unfortunately, it is often extremely difficult to distinguish colonization from infection, particularly in the respiratory tract (see above). Usually, the distinction can only be made on clinical grounds and is based on the presence of the usual signs of infection (pyrexia, leucocytosis, visibly purulent sputum, haemodynamic changes), combined with the recognition of a source of sepsis and a pure, or heavy, growth of a pathogen from the suspected site. If blood cultures are positive and grow the same organism as that isolated from the presumed source of infection, it is probable that this is the pathogen.

Very often, antimicrobial agents have to be given before the organism has been identified. Under these circumstances, material from all possible sites of infection and blood should be obtained and sent for culture and antimicrobial sensitivities before the first dose of antibiotic is administered. Sometimes, an immediate Gram stain will provide a valuable clue as to the probable pathogen. Otherwise, a rational choice of antibiotic should be made on the basis of the organisms most likely to arise from the presumed site of sepsis and the known local patterns of infection. Many hospitals produce policies that guide the choice of antibiotic regimen in particular clinical situations (**Table 11.3**) and these help to rationalize the use of antimicrobial agents within the hospital environment. Close cooperation with the microbiology department is essential at all times, particularly in view of the increasing prevalence of antibiotic resistant pathogens; infection with such an organism is more likely to prolong hospitalization, to increase the risk of death, and to require treatment with more toxic or more expensive antibiotics (Holmberg *et al.*, 1987).

In some units, sputum, urine, and other available material are regularly cultured, (e.g. twice a week). The results may then guide the initial choice of antibiotic. Similarly, intravascular cannulae should always be sent for culture on removal. Surveillance cultures including nose, throat and rectal swabs, as well as sputum and urine can be obtained routinely on admission, and afterwards twice weekly.

In general, if the pathogen has been identified and its drug sensitivities are known, administration of a single antibiotic, if possible with a narrow spectrum of activity, is preferable to the use of combinations. The latter may, however, be required for empirical therapy to prevent the emergence of resistant strains (e.g. in the

Table 11.3 Suggested antibiotic regimens.

Nature of infection	Possible causative organisms	Recommended antibiotic regimen
Pneumonia Acquired in the community	*Streptococcus pneumoniae* *Haemophilus influenzae* *Mycoplasma pneumoniae* *Legionella pneumophila*	Amoxycillin and erythromycin (can substitute cefuroxime for amoxycillin in those allergic to penicillin)
	Staphylococcal pneumonia possible	Add flucloxacillin
	Staphylococcal pneumonia confirmed, not responding to flucloxacillin	Add sodium fucidate to flucloxacillin
	Documented pneumococcal pneumonia	Penicillin
Acquired in hospital	As above plus aerobic Gram-negative bacilli.	Cefuroxime, cefotaxime or ceftazidime
	If *Mycoplasma* or Legionnaire's disease is a possibility	Add erythromycin
	Pseudomonas pneumonia and/or bacteraemia a possibility	Aminoglycoside and piperacillin (ceftazidime is an alternative)
Aspiration pneumonia		Cefuroxime and metronidazole
Exacerbation chronic obstructive pulmonary disease	*Haemophilus influenzae* *Streptococcus pneumoniae* *Moraxella catarrhalis* (*Pseudomonas aeruginosa*)	Amoxycillin and erythromycin Co-amoxiclav Cefuroxime or cefotaxime Ciprofloxacin
Intra-abdominal infection	Gram-negative bacilli, staphylococci and anaerobes (e.g. *Bacteroides fragilis*)	Aminoglycoside (gentamicin, tobramycin or netilmicin) or a second- or third-generation cephalosporin combined with metronidazole
	For enterococci	Add ampicillin (particularly effective for biliary tract infections)
	Pseudomonas aeruginosa possibility	Add ticarcillin or piperacillin (will also cover *Streptococcus faecalis*)
Pelvic infections	Anaerobes Gram-negative bacilli	Metronidazole plus ampicillin or an aminoglycoside
	If clostridial or group A streptococcal infection suspected	Add penicillin to above
	If staphylococcal infection suspected	Add flucloxacillin to above
Urinary tract infections	*Escherichia coli; Proteus* spp. *Klebsiella* spp.	Ampicillin or amoxycillin Co-trimoxazole is an alternative Aminoglycoside if organism resistant to above and there is no renal failure
Intravascular catheter infection	Coagulase negative staphycococci, *Staphylococcus aureus, Enterococcus* or *Streptococcus* spp., coliforms, *Pseudomonas aeruginosa, Corynebacterium* spp.	Flucoxacillin and gentamicin or vancomycin and ciprofloxacin if methicillin resistant *S. aureus* (MRSA) possible
Necrotizing fasciitis	Mixed aerobic and anaerobic organisms Group A streptococcus	Third generation cephalosporin, aminoglycoside and metronidazole for synergistic infection. Penicillin for streptococcal infection

Table 11.3 Continued

Nature of infection	Possible causative organisms	Recommended antibiotic regimen
Neurological infections Meningitis	Neisseria meningitidis Streptococcus pneumoniae Haemophilus influenzae (In neonates group B streptococci and Escherichia coli predominate)	Cefotaxime in high doses
Brain abscess		Chloramphenicol often used
Wound infections	Coagulase-negative staphylococci, coliforms, Staphylococcus aureus, Enterococcus or Streptococcus spp.	Flucloxacillin and gentamicin Add metronidazole for traumatic wounds or when mucosal surface has been breached Vancomycin and ciprofloxacin if MRSA possible
Unusual pathogens	Pneumocystis carinii	High-dose co-trimoxazole
	Mycoplasma pneumoniae, Legionella pneumophila	Erythromycin
	Chlamydia psittaci, Coxiella burnetti	Tetracycline
	Fungi	Amphotericin (can be combined with 5-fluorocytosine)

treatment of tuberculosis) and for the treatment of mixed infections. Furthermore, certain antibiotic combinations are synergistic (e.g. penicillin and gentamicin against *S. faecalis*) and may therefore be particularly useful for the treatment of life-threatening infections. On the other hand, the combination of some bacteriostatic and bactericidal agents might be antagonistic, although this is no longer generally considered to be clinically important. Bactericidal antibiotics are probably superior in the treatment of endocarditis, and for neutropenic patients, but there is no evidence that they offer any advantages in other situations.

In a proportion of patients, failure of organism-sensitive antibiotic to prevent death from sepsis may be related to antibiotic-mediated endotoxin liberation (Editorial, 1985). It might be possible to prevent some of these deaths by developing treatments to neutralize endotoxin and its mediators (see Chapter 4) or by developing antibiotics with a reduced propensity to liberate endotoxin.

Pneumonia

The appropriate initial regimen for a patient with pneumonia depends largely on whether the infection was acquired in hospital or in the community.

Pneumonias contracted outside the hospital environment can be treated initially with a combination of amoxycillin and erythromycin. The former will cover the common respiratory pathogens, such as *Haemophilus influenzae* and pneumococcus, while the latter may be effective against *Mycoplasma pneumoniae* and *Legionella pneumophila*. A second-generation cephalosporin, such as cefuroxime, may be substituted for amoxycillin in those allergic to penicillin (although there is some cross-sensitivity) and to broaden the spectrum of activity for pneumonias acquired in hospital. Because an increasing number of community-acquired *H. influenzae* are resistant to amoxycillin, some recommend using cefuroxime or cefotaxime in all cases.

If *Staphylococcal pneumonia* is a possibility (e.g. during an influenza epidemic), flucloxacillin or, possibly, cefotaxime should be used. If this diagnosis is subsequently confirmed and the patient is not responding, the addition of sodium fucidate may prove to be more effective. Penicillin remains the drug of first choice in patients with documented *Pneumococcal pneumonia*.

If *Pseudomonas pneumonia* (or bacteraemia) is a possibility it is usually preferable to administer an antipseudomonal penicillin such as ticarcillin or piperacillin, usually in combination with an aminoglycoside. Alternatively, ceftazidime, which has good antipseudomonal activity, can be used.

Aspiration pneumonia can be treated with cefuroxime and metronidazole.

In general, aminoglycosides penetrate poorly into lungs and sputum and are therefore rarely used for pulmonary infections, except when bloodstream invasion is suspected.

Exacerbations of chronic obstructive pulmonary disease (Hosker et al., 1994)

Ampicillin or amoxycillin is usually given first and is nearly always effective in those cases due to pneumococcus. Because 10-14% of sputum isolates of *H. influenzae* are resistant to ampicillin, co-amoxiclav (amoxycillin and clavulanic acid) may be used as an alternative. Ciprofloxacin may also be more effective than ampicillin. A second-generation oral cephalosporin such as cefaclor may be effective, and intravenous cefuroxime or cefotaxime can be useful in more seriously ill hospitalized patients. Chloramphenicol and tetracycline remain useful second-line agents.

Intra-abdominal infection

Infections arising from sites within the abdomen usually require combination therapy to provide an adequate spectrum of activity, at least until the results of cultures and drug sensitivities are available. In this situation, an aminoglycoside is usually administered in combination with metronidazole. There is little to choose between gentamicin and tobramycin, both of which are active against the majority of aerobic Gram-negative bacilli, as well as staphylococci. In order to achieve effective therapy, without the risk of oto- or nephrotoxicity, it is important to monitor the blood levels of both these agents. (There is some evidence that netilmicin is a less-toxic alternative to the older aminoglycosides.) Amikacin should be reserved for the treatment of documented infection with gentamicin-resistant organisms. Second- or third-generation cephalosporins can be used as alternatives, or in addition to an aminoglycoside.

Metronidazole is given to control infection caused by anaerobic organisms such as *Bacteroides fragilis*, and has superseded clindamycin and lincomycin, both of which were particularly implicated in the causation of pseudomembranous colitis. This combination will not cover *S. faecalis* and may be ineffective against some strains of *P. aeruginosa*. The addition of ampicillin will provide activity against *S. faecalis*, while the use of an antipseudomonal penicillin will cover both these organisms. Furthermore, since ampicillin is concentrated in the bile it is particularly effective in the treatment of biliary tract infections.

Pelvic infections

Pelvic sepsis arising from the female genital tract is frequently associated with anaerobic infection and will always require treatment with metronidazole, initially in combination with ampicillin or amoxycillin. An amino-glycoside can be substituted for the ampicillin in the most seriously ill or in those who fail to respond.

If clostridial infection is suspected (e.g. following a criminal abortion), penicillin should be used, while if staphylococcal infection is a possibility (e.g. in tampon-associated toxic shock syndrome), vancomycin (or possibly flucloxacillin) must be administered.

Urinary tract infections

Urinary tract infections often respond well to ampicillin or amoxycillin since both are active against most strains of *E. coli*, *Proteus* and *Klebsiella* and have the advantage of excellent diffusion into the urinary tract. Co-trimoxazole also has good tissue penetration and can be used as an alternative to ampicillin. Provided there is no renal impairment, an aminoglycoside can be effective if culture and sensitivities indicate that it is appropriate.

Wound infections

In the absence of a systemic response, localized infection is treated by the topical application of disinfecting agents such as taurolin 2% at least twice a day. Local collections of pus and abscesses must be drained. Systemic antibiotics are only indicated when there are signs of generalized inflammation. Organisms commonly implicated include coliforms, *S. aureus*, enterococci or *Streptococcus* spp. Coagulase-negative staphylococci may be contaminants. Empirical therapy can be with flucloxacillin and gentamicin, combined with metronidazole if the wound is traumatic or a mucosal surface has been breached. When MRSA is prevalent, vancomycin and ciprofloxacin is a suitable combination.

Intravascular device infection

Localized entry site infections can be treated with a topical application of a disinfecting agent such as taurolin 2%, sometimes combined with a systemic antibiotic. Empirical therapy, when indicated, must cover *S. aureus* and Gram-negatives, and the combination of flucloxacillin and gentamicin is suitable (vancomycin and ciprofloxacin can be used if MRSA is prevalent).

Neurological infections

The three most common pathogens in acute bacterial meningitis are *Neisseria meningitidis*, *S. pneumoniae* and *H. influenzae*, although in neonates group B streptococci and *E. coli* predominate. Cefotaxime is now the antibiotic of choice. In those with an abscess, chloramphenicol, which has excellent penetration, is still often used.

Necrotizing fasciitis (Burge and Watson, 1994)

Necrotizing fasciitis is a serious, but uncommon, soft tissue infection that spreads rapidly along fascial planes, causing necrosis of subcutaneous fat and, in some cases, the epidermis. Gas production is frequently prominent and the overlying skin may become gangrenous. Necrosis is usually limited in depth to the plane of the muscle fascia. Necrotizing fasciitis may be caused by a 'synergistic' infection with a mixture of enteric Gram-negative rods and anaerobes (e.g. *Bacteroides* spp., *Clostridium* spp. and anaerobic streptococci) or by infection with invasive group A streptococci alone (Chelsom *et al.*, 1994). Organisms often gain access to the subcutaneous tissues through a trivial skin wound. The condition is more common in diabetics.

CLINICAL PRESENTATION AND DIAGNOSIS

The patient is usually extremely toxic, often with disproportionate pain and, in the early stages, only minor skin changes. When the male genitals (usually the scrotum) are involved the condition is called *Fournier's gangrene*; in these cases infection may spread rapidly to the perineum, pelvis and abdominal wall. Microscopy of aspirate from the subcutaneous tissues may reveal the organisms. Characteristic findings at surgery include grey, oedematous fat, which strips off the underlying fascia with a sweep of the finger.

TREATMENT

Radical surgical excision until normal tissue is exposed improves survival, albeit at the cost of greater deformity. The aim is to perform definitive surgery, no matter how radical, at the first operation. Extensive cleansing with taurolin 2% is generally recommended. *Systemic antibiotics* should include a second- or third-generation cephalosporin and an aminoglycoside combined with metronidazole. In those with suspected invasive streptococcal disease benzylpenicillin should be administered intravenously. If readily available *hyperbaric oxygen* treatment should be considered.

PROGNOSIS

When aggressive surgery is performed early at an experienced centre mortality rates as low as 10% or less can be achieved. Otherwise up to 60% of patients may die.

Many of those who do survive are left with considerable scarring and deformity.

Prophylactic antibiotics

The use of prophylactic antibiotics is controversial, but in general this practice encourages the emergence of resistant strains with which the patient, whose normal bacterial flora is destroyed, then becomes colonized. Situations in which the use of prophylactic antibiotics is generally accepted include:

- cardiac surgery (gentamicin and flucloxacillin);
- skull fracture with leakage of cerebrospinal fluid (ampicillin and flucloxacillin or cefotaxime);
- insertion of prosthetic vascular grafts (flucloxacillin);
- the prevention of gas gangrene following major trauma or amputation of an ischaemic limb (penicillin).

ANTIBIOTIC-ASSOCIATED DIARRHOEA

Antibiotic-associated diarrhoea is a common complication of antibiotic therapy and can significantly complicate the management of critically ill patients. Mild forms may simply be a consequence of alterations in the bacterial flora, but in some instances there may be a low-grade *Clostridium difficile* infection. Particularly severe diarrhoea occurs in the small proportion of patients who develop *pseudomembranous colitis*, which is caused by the toxin produced by *C. difficile* (George *et al.*, 1978). This condition is usually encountered in patients receiving broad-spectrum antibiotics and was originally described in association with the administration of lincomycin and clindamycin. Since then most other antibiotics have also been incriminated.

There is evidence that *C. difficile* is frequently transmitted between hospitalized patients and that the organism is often present on the hands of hospital personnel (McFarland *et al.*, 1989). A significant proportion of those who acquire the organism during their hospitalization remain asymptomatic and a few patients are already carrying *C. difficile* when they are admitted. The diagnosis of *C. difficile* colitis is made by growing the organism from the stools and by identifying the toxin.

C. difficile is always sensitive to vancomycin, which should be administered orally, but metronidazole may also be effective. Sometimes patients relapse or develop a persistent carrier state.

UNUSUAL PATHOGENS—DIAGNOSIS AND TREATMENT

Clearly, not all the infections seen on the ICU are caused by common PPM. This applies particularly to pulmonary infections, which are sometimes caused by unusual pathogens such as:

- *Mycobacterium tuberculosis*;
- viruses;
- *M. pneumoniae*;
- *Chlamydia psittaci* (psittacosis);
- *L. pneumophila* (Legionnaires' disease);
- *Coxiella burnetti* (Q fever);
- protozoans (e.g. *P. carinii*);
- fungi.

Mycoplasma pneumoniae

M. pneumoniae is a relatively common cause of pneumonia and is often seen in teenagers or young adults. It presents as an atypical pneumonia with 'flu' like symptoms, sometimes associated with extrapulmonary complications such as:

- myocarditis and pericarditis;
- rashes and erythema multiforme;
- haemolytic anaemia and thrombocytopenia;
- myalgia and arthralgia;
- meningo-encephalitis and other neurological abnormalities;
- gastrointestinal symptoms (e.g. vomiting, diarrhoea).

The chest radiograph usually shows involvement of only one lower lobe, although sometimes there is dramatic shadowing in both lower lobes.

The white blood count is not raised, cold agglutinins occur in half the cases, and the diagnosis is confirmed by a rising antibody titre.

Treatment is with erythromycin although tetracycline is also effective.

Chlamydia psittaci

Characteristically psittacosis presents as a low-grade illness developing over several months in a patient who has been in contact with infected birds, especially parrots. Symptoms include malaise, high fever, cough and muscular pains. The liver and spleen are sometimes enlarged and scanty 'rose spots' may be seen on the abdomen. Sometimes there is no history of contact with infected birds and occasionally the patient presents with a high swinging fever and dramatic prostration with photophobia and neck stiffness that can be confused with meningitis.

The chest radiograph shows a diffuse or segmental pneumonia and the diagnosis is confirmed by a rising titre of complement-fixing antibody. It may be possible to isolate the causative organism in psittacosis, but this is dangerous and only performed in specialist centres.

Treatment is with tetracycline or, alternatively, rifampicin.

Coxiella burnetti

Q fever presents as a primary atypical pneumonia, which sometimes runs a chronic course and is occasionally associated with endocarditis.

The chest radiograph often shows multiple lesions. The diagnosis is confirmed by a rising titre of complement-fixing antibody.

Treatment is with erythromycin or tetracycline.

Legionella pneumophila

Infection with *L. pneumophila* may occur as outbreaks in previously fit individuals when institutional shower facilities or cooling systems have been contaminated, as well as in immunocompromised patients or older male smokers. Sporadic cases, where the source is unknown may also be seen. Characteristically the patient presents with malaise, headache, myalgia and a fever of up to 40°C with rigors. Gastrointestinal symptoms such as nausea, vomiting, diarrhoea and abdominal pain are common. Some patients have mental confusion and other neurological signs, and some have haematuria and occasionally renal failure develops. The diagnosis of legionnaires' disease is extremely likely if the patient has three of the four following features.

- a prodromal 'flu' like illness;
- a dry cough, confusion or diarrhoea;
- lymphopenia without marked leukocytosis;
- hyponatraemia.

The chest radiograph usually shows unilateral lobar and then multilobar shadowing, sometimes with a small pleural effusion. Cavitation is rare.

It is possible to visualize *L. pneumophila* using direct immunofluorescent staining of pleural fluid, sputum or bronchial washings. The diagnosis is confirmed by rising antibody titres and the organism can be cultured, although this takes up to three weeks.

Erythromycin is the antibiotic of choice, but rifampicin can also be used.

Pneumocystis carinii

Clinical features of *P. carinii* pneumonia (PCP) include a high fever, breathlessness and a dry cough. Marked hypoxaemia is characteristic. In patients with acquired immunodeficiency syndrome (AIDS) the onset may be more insidious, and is sometimes associated with diarrhoea and weight loss.

Chest radiography typically reveals diffuse bilateral alveolar and interstitial shadowing spreading out from the perihilar region in a butterfly pattern.

The diagnosis of PCP can usually be established by BAL, although in some cases transbronchial biopsy is required, followed by Giemsa staining.

Treatment is with high-dose co-trimoxazole (120 mg/kg daily in divided doses) given intravenously for two weeks and continued for a further week orally. Side-effects occur in up to 80% of patients and include nausea, skin rashes, megabloblastic bone marrow change and agranulocytosis. Nebulized pentamidine (600 mg once a day for 21 days) rarely produces unwanted effects and has been shown to be effective in milder cases. In patients with AIDS the incidence of recurrent PCP can be reduced by once monthly nebulized pentamidine or low-dose cotrimoxazole 960 mg once daily.

Cytomegalovirus

Infection with cytomegalovirus (CMV) is most commonly encountered in the immunocompromised (Editorial, 1981), particularly those with AIDS and recipients of bone marrow or solid organ transplants. The virus may be transmitted by transfusion with infected blood. Whereas in healthy adults CMV causes an illness similar to infectious mononucleosis, in immunocompromised patients infection may be disseminated, with encephalitis, retinitis, diffuse involvement of the gastrointestinal tract and pneumonitis.

Serological tests can be used to detect past (IgG) or current (IgM) infection and the virus can be identified in tissue culture. Transbronchial biopsy can be useful to establish the diagnosis of CMV pneumonitis.

In immunosuppressed patients treatment with ganciclovir (5 mg/kg 12-hourly for 14–21 days) reduces retinitis and gastrointestinal damage and can eliminate CMV from blood, urine and respiratory secretions. It is less effective against pneumonitis and encephalitis. Drug resistance has been reported.

Fungal infections

Fungal infections usually occur in patients who have received prolonged treatment with broad-spectrum antibiotics, particularly if they are also immunosuppressed. Colonization of the throat, tracheostomy wounds, stomach and gut is relatively common and rarely requires treatment. When fungi are obtained in significant quantities from diagnostic samples such as sputum or urine, however, it can be difficult to make the important distinction between colonization and invasive infection.

Because yeast cells adhere firmly to plastic, oropharyngeal and rectal carriage of yeasts frequently leads to contamination of tubes and catheters. Treatment of colonization should therefore include changing of endotracheal tubes, nasogastric tubes and urinary catheters, for example, and the application of topical antifungals. This will usually lead to clearance of yeasts from the lower airways and bladder.

Fungaemia carries an extremely high mortality and requires prolonged systemic administration of potentially toxic drugs such as amphotericin. Positive blood cultures may indicate significant infection, while a rising *Candida* antibody titre also suggests invasive disease. Attempts to detect *Candida* antigen in blood are still being evaluated. Endophthalmitis (hard, greyish-white exudates seen on retinoscopy) is occasionally present and confirms invasive fungal disease. Candida pneumonia following aspiration of contaminated oropharyngeal secretions is extremely unusual, except in immunocompromised patients in whom fungaemia may also be due to translocation from the gut. Nevertheless if a heavy growth of fungus with pus cells is obtained repeatedly from the sputum of a ventilated patient in the presence of chest radiographic signs of consolidation, treatment for systemic fungal infection may be indicated, although more invasive techniques will normally be required to establish the diagnosis with certainty.

Pulmonary aspergillosis may produce a mycetoma with a characteristic, mobile crescentic translucency seen on the chest radiograph. The serum from such patients may contain *Aspergillus* precipitins.

As well as administering specific antifungal agents, successful treatment depends on removing all possible sources of continuing infection such as intravascular catheters and prosthetic heart valves. *Amphotericin* probably remains the most effective, and is certainly the longest established, antifungal agent, sometimes effecting a cure in disseminated candidiasis and producing a beneficial effect in some cases of aspergillosis. Some degree of renal impairment usually develops soon after commencing amphotericin, but if treatment is continued the glomerular filtration rate usually stabilizes at 20–60% of normal. Renal function almost always improves rapidly once treatment is discontinued. Other adverse effects include anaemia, hypokalaemia, thrombocytopenia and hepatic dysfunction. Liposomal and colloidal forms of amphotericin are less toxic, but more expensive. There is also some evidence that the combination of amphotericin with the less toxic *5-fluorocytosine* is synergistic and in this way the dose, and adverse effects, of amphotericin may be reduced. *Fluconazole* may be a useful agent for the treatment of *C.*

albicans and cryptococcal infections in immunocompromised patients. If therapy is effective, improvement occurs within a few days, but treatment usually has to continue for several weeks, or even months.

THE IMMUNOCOMPROMISED PATIENT

Acquired immunodeficiency syndrome

Acquired immunodeficiency syndrome (AIDS) is a consequence of infection with human immunodeficiency virus (HIV), which infects and destroys CD4 lymphocytes and impairs the function of those that remain, leading to a progressive impairment of CMI. Antibody-mediated immune responses are also defective and some patients, especially children, are particularly prone to recurrent bacterial infection. HIV-1 and the related HIV-2 are both retroviruses, which can be further classified as lentiviruses ('slow' viruses) because of their slowly progressive clinical effects.

Individuals who have an increased risk for infection with HIV are:

- those who have multiple sexual partners (it is particularly common among homosexuals or bisexuals in North America, Western Europe and Australasia, while in much of Sub-Saharan Africa, Asia and Latin America, heterosexuals and prostitutes are at considerable risk, and heterosexual spread is increasingly common in Europe);
- intravenous drug users who share needles;
- children born to infected women;
- recipients of blood and blood products (e.g. haemophiliacs and transfusion recipients, especially in countries where blood donation is not screened).

CLINICAL FEATURES

Some weeks after infection with the virus there may be an *acute febrile illness*, which is easily mistaken for influenza or infectious mononucleosis. Occasionally this initial illness may lead to transient severe immunosuppression sufficient to cause oesophageal candidiasis, or rarely, *Pneumocystis* pneumonia. There is then a *symptom-free period*, which may last for months or several years. Some symptomless individuals show *persistent generalized lymphadenopathy (PGL)*, but this does not signify increased risk of progression. Early symptomatic HIV disease (*AIDS-related complex (ARC)*) includes:

- progressive weight loss;
- fatigue;
- mild chronic diarrhoea;

- 'minor' opportunistic infections (e.g. oral candidiasis, herpes zoster, viral (hairy) leucoplakia.

Neurological manifestations (e.g. dementia, subacute encephalitis, peripheral neuropathy, atypical aseptic meningitis) rarely occur in isolation, but are usually associated with ARC or AIDS.

A high proportion of individuals infected with HIV will eventually develop AIDS; the proportion increases with time, about 50% develop symptomatic disease within 10 years and about 65% at 14 years. Some, however, remain well for many years. AIDS is characterized by major opportunistic infections and tumours, which include the following.

- Bacterial infections, which are often disseminated—*Listeria monocytogenes*, *Salmonella* (non-typhi), *Mycobacterium avium-intracellulare*, *M. kansasii*, *M. tuberculosis*.
- Viral infections—herpes simplex (ulcerating), cytomegalovirus (retinitis, colitis, oesophageal ulcers, pneumonitis, encephalitis), herpes zoster, JC virus (progressive multifocal leukoencephalopathy).
- Fungal infections—*Candida* oesophagitis; *cryptococcus neoformans* (meningitis or disseminated), *Histoplasma* spp.
- Protozoal infections—*P. carinii* pneumonia (PCP); *Cryptosporidium* spp., *Isospora belli*, *Strongyloides stercoralis* (hyperinfection), *Toxoplasma gondii*.
- Malignancies—Kaposi's sarcoma, primary brain lymphomas, Burkitt's or other B cell lymphomas and squamous cell carcinoma of anus.

DIAGNOSIS

The diagnosis should be suspected in individuals presenting with any of the clinical features outlined above in the absence of other causes for immunodeficiency, especially if they have indulged in high-risk behaviour. PCP remains the index diagnosis in approximately half the cases of AIDS, while the incidence of Kaposi's sarcoma in homosexual men is falling (Peters *et al.*, 1991).

Acute clinical management is concerned primarily with the opportunistic diseases and attention must be focused on prompt identification and treatment of these.

Before confirming a suspected diagnosis of HIV infection by testing for the presence of antibody to HIV, the patient must be carefully counselled, preferably by someone experienced in the implications of a positive test. In some acutely ill patients of unknown HIV status, it may be wise to defer consideration of HIV testing until the wider issues can be discussed and the patient more adequately informed and counselled.

Because the enzyme-linked immunosorbent assay (ELISA) used to test for antibody to HIV may produce both false-positive and false-negative results, confirmatory tests are required and expert advice should be sought if there are unexpected findings. False positives with some methods may occur in patients with autoimmune disease, chronic liver disease or myeloma, while the test may be falsely negative in those who have not yet seroconverted (this is common during the first two months after infection) or in patients with defects of antibody production.

Multiple immunological abnormalities may be detected in patients with AIDS including:

- lymphopenia, especially of CD4 (T helper) cells;
- defects in the function of CD4 cells;
- B cell abnormalities with polyclonal activation of B cells and hypergammaglobulinaemia;
- macrophage defects.

MANAGEMENT ON INTENSIVE CARE

Intensive care is only occasionally indicated for severe complications of AIDS; approximately two-thirds of such patients are admitted with respiratory failure, usually due to PCP. Other complications which may require intensive care include:

- hypotension (sepsis, dehydration due to diarrhoea and vomiting, adrenal insufficiency);
- severe central nervous system disease (cryptococcal meningitis, toxoplasmosis, listeriosis);
- seizures;
- cardiac tamponade (usually due to tuberculosis);
- gastrointestinal haemorrhage;
- drug toxicity (e.g. Stevens–Johnson syndrome);
- complications of a diagnostic procedure (e.g. pneumothorax following transbronchial biopsy or respiratory decompensation following bronchoalveolar lavage).

The small number of patients who are admitted for reasons unrelated to their immune deficiency (e.g. following surgery) have a much better prognosis than those with life-threatening complications of AIDS.

Pulmonary disease associated with AIDS (Stover et al., 1985)

Most commonly pulmonary disease associated with AIDS is due to infection, usually with *P. carinii*, although mycobacteria (especially tuberculosis), pyogenic bacteria, fungi or CMV may also be responsible. In some cases respiratory failure is due to lymphocytic pneumonitis or pulmonary infiltration with Kaposi's sarcoma (often complicating bacterial infection).

Pathophysiology of PCP. In PCP the alveoli are filled with microorganisms and there is alveolar epithelial damage with increased pulmonary microvascular permeability. The alveoli are flooded with proteinaceous fluid and depleted of surfactant.

Presentation and diagnosis. Typically patients present with a history of several weeks of fever and malaise with dry cough and tachypnoea. On auscultation there may be no abnormal findings, but diffuse crackles throughout both lung fields can be heard in severe cases.

Except in those with bacterial pneumonia, the chest radiograph usually shows diffuse shadowing, which in PCP is of a mixed interstitial and alveolar pattern. Mediastinal adenopathy is uncommon and when present suggests mycobacterial infection or lymphoma. Pleural effusions may be seen in association with pulmonary Kaposi's sarcoma (when they are usually haemorrhagic), and should also raise the possibility of tuberculosis.

Diagnostic methods have been discussed elsewhere in this chapter.

Treatment. Patients with severe respiratory failure may benefit from continuous positive airways pressure (CPAP) or intermittent positive pressure ventilation (IPPV) with positive end-expiratory pressure (PEEP) (see Chapter 7), although in those with PCP any increase in P_aO_2 is often relatively modest. Because the lungs are often very stiff high inflation pressures are required and the risk of pneumothorax or barotrauma is high (see Chapter 7).

The treatment of specific infections have been considered earlier in this chapter, but of particular importance in patients with severe AIDS-related PCP is the observation that the early addition of short intensive courses of corticosteroids (e.g. 40 mg methylprednisolone 8-hourly for 3–6 days) to standard therapy improves survival and reduces the incidence of respiratory failure (Bozzette *et al., 1990; Gagnon et al.,* 1990). Steroids may also improve outcome in those who require ventilatory support (Montaner *et al.,* 1989).

PROGNOSIS

The median survival time for patients presenting with AIDS doubled from 10 to 20 months during the late 1980s and this was accompanied by an improvement in their quality of life (Peters *et al.,* 1991). This reduction in mortality may be related to:

- treatment with zidovudine (reduced frequency and severity of opportunistic infections);
- earlier presentation, diagnosis and treatment;
- more effective therapy for opportunistic infections;
- prophylaxis against PCP (usually secondary prophy-

laxis with, for example, nebulized pentamidine; primary prophylaxis is rarely used);

● the use of corticosteroids in severe PCP.

As a result a larger proportion of deaths are now attributable to Kaposi's sarcoma or cerebral lymphoma, and there is an increasing incidence of other disorders, which are often refractory to treatment such as:

● cryptosporidiosis;
● progressive multifocal leucoencephalopathy;
● *M. avium-intracellulare*;
● late relapses of cryptococcal meningitis with secondary hydrocephalus.

The mortality of patients who require mechanical ventilation for PCP complicating AIDS has generally been reported to be as high as 80–100%, but lower in-hospital mortality rates of around 60% have been achieved (El-Sadr & Simberkoff, 1988), probably reflecting differing criteria for intervention. Survival is more likely in those with a shorter duration of symptoms before admission, as well as in patients with less severe hypoxia and when gas exchange improves rapidly following the institution of respiratory support. The prognosis is also more favourable when deterioration is precipitated by bronchoscopy (El-Sadr & Simberkoff, 1988). The mean survival time for those who recover from PCP following a period of mechanical ventilation is probably the same as that of patients with PCP who do not require respiratory support (El-Sadr & Simberkoff, 1988). In another series the in-unit mortality of AIDS patients with respiratory failure requiring ventilatory support was 66%, although after three months survival had fallen to 15%. The overall three-month survival for all those with AIDS admitted to intensive care for life-sustaining support was 26% (Rogers *et al.*, 1989).

There can therefore be no doubt that a minority of patients with AIDS can benefit from intensive care and arbitrary policies denying intensive care to such patients when it is medically indicated are not warranted (Wachter *et al.*, 1989). ICU staff may have a variety of concerns about the provision of intensive care for these patients including their relative youth, the generally poor long-term prognosis and the risks of occupational infection. Many of these anxieties can be ameliorated by allowing informed patients to participate in treatment decisions and by educating staff in basic infection control procedures and the nature of the disease.

MEASURES TO MINIMIZE THE RISK OF CROSS-INFECTION

Although the risk of acquiring HIV infection during occupational exposure to AIDS patients in the ICU is low (Rogers *et al.*, 1989), the importance of minimizing

sharp injuries and accidental exposure to potentially infected body fluids and of adhering to universal precautions (see Chapter 13) cannot be overemphasized. Appropriate measures should be taken for isolating patients with suspected tuberculosis, which is especially common in African patients.

There is no evidence that reverse isolation can reduce the incidence of nosocomial infection in patients with AIDS, as most are already present and are not acquired acutely from the environment (see earlier in this chapter).

Intensive care for patients with malignant disease

The management of malignant disease during the latter half of this century has progressed enormously. Although there have been important developments in the management of some solid tumours, the most dramatic improvements in long-term prognosis have been seen in patients with haematological and lymphoreticular malignancies, a significant proportion of whom can now be cured.

Patients with malignant disease are prone to a wide variety of acute life-threatening disturbances related either to the effects of the tumour itself or to complications of its treatment. The majority of these disorders are potentially reversible and in view of the improved long-term prognosis it is appropriate to admit selected cases to the ICU, provided the prospects for cure or worthwhile palliation of the underlying malignancy are considered to be reasonable.

Dangerous complications directly or indirectly caused by the tumour include:

● pleural or pericardial effusions;
● renal failure induced by ureteric compression;
● pancytopenia due to marrow invasion;
● airway obstruction;
● metabolic disturbances (uraemia, ectopic hormone production):
● hypercalcaemia;
● hyperosmolar coma;
● neurological syndromes;
● massive haemorrhage from an ulcerated lesion;
● superior vena cava obstruction;
● cardiac tamponade;
● gastrointestinal disorders (obstruction, perforation, haemorrhage);
● renal failure (many causes):
● constrictive pericarditis;
● hyperviscosity syndrome (e.g. myeloma).

Life-threatening complications of treatment are most often the result of immunosuppression caused by chemotherapy, radiotherapy or steroids. Such patients are very susceptible to overwhelming infection, particularly during the profound leucopenia induced by aggressive chemotherapy. In the majority of those with haematological malignancy, admission to ICU is precipitated by *pneumonia* and/or *septic shock*, often complicated by *acute respiratory failure* (Lloyd-Thomas *et al.*, 1988).

Sometimes *bleeding*, which is usually a result of marrow suppression with thrombocytopenia or less often DIC, liver failure or the effects of drugs, is of sufficient severity to warrant admission. Other dangerous, less frequent, complications of anti-cancer treatment include:

- cardiac arrhythmias;
- cardiomyopathy induced by irradiation or cytotoxic agents;
- pulmonary fibrosis related to chemotherapy or radiotherapy;
- graft versus host disease (GVHD);
- tumour lysis syndrome;
- gastrointestinal disorders (neutropenic enterocolitis, perforation, haemorrhage, diarrhoea, paralytic ileus).

Patients with malignant disease may also benefit from *elective admission* to the ICU following extensive surgical procedures, particularly if they have co-existent medical disorders. Intensive care may also be required for *postoperative complications*.

INFECTIOUS COMPLICATIONS OF MALIGNANT DISEASE

Infection is a frequent complication of malignant disease and an important cause of death in patients with cancer, particularly those with haematological malignancy in whom it is the commonest factor precipitating admission to the ICU (Lloyd-Thomas *et al.*, 1988).

Impaired resistance to infection in patients with malignant disease (**Table 11.4**)

The increased susceptibility of patients with malignancy to infection may be related to:

- reduced or abnormal granulocytes;
- decreased antibody production;
- impaired cellular immunity (CMI);
- disruption of mucocutaneous barriers;
- obstruction of drainage tracts;
- invasive procedures.

In general immune competence is relatively intact before treatment and the majority of those with impaired cellular and humoral immunity are receiving chemotherapy, radiotherapy or steroids. Neutropenia is by far the most important cause of the increased suscep-

Table 11.4 Immune defects in patients with malignant disease.

Carcinomas and sarcomas	Cell-mediated immunity more compromised than humoral response (degree depends on extent of metastatic spread)
	Effects of chemotherapy
Acute leukaemia	Abnormal neutrophil function
	Deficiency in the maturation of macrophages
	Defects in humoral immunity
	Neutropenia (most profound in those receiving intensive remission induction chemotherapy)
Bone marrow transplantation	Profound marrow aplasia until transplanted marrow starts to function
	Prolonged cellular immune dysfunction
	Prolonged impaired humoral immunity
Chronic leukaemia	Defective cellular and humoral immunity
	Neutropenia
Lymphoproliferative disorders	Markedly impaired cell-mediated immunity
	Impaired humoral immunity in some cases

tibility to infection and there is an inverse correlation between the granulocyte count and both the incidence and the severity of infection. The most pronounced immune suppression is seen in patients in relapse, probably largely as a result of previous courses of chemotherapy.

Organisms causing infection

Bacteria still account for the majority of infections. Most often aerobic Gram-negative bacilli (such as *E. coli*, *Klebsiella* spp., *Pseudomonas* spp., *Proteus* spp. or *Enterobacter* spp.) are implicated, although there has been a recent resurgence in infections due to Gram-positive cocci including coagulase-negative staphylococci. Multiple infections are relatively common. In general anaerobic infections are unusual in leukaemic patients, but are common in those with gastrointestinal and genitourinary malignancies. Less frequently, especially in those with impaired cellular immunity, infection may be due to unusual bacteria such as *L. pneumophila* and *Nocardia asteroides*. Humoral immune dysfunction renders the patient susceptible to infection with encapsulated bacteria (*S. pneumoniae, H. influenzae* and *N. meningitidis*), as well as aerobic Gram-negative bacilli and *Pseudomonas* spp.

The incidence of *fungal* infections in patients with leukaemia has increased and is usually related to a prolonged period of neutropenia combined with suppression of the normal bacterial flora by broad-spectrum antibiotics. Fungi are also an important cause of infection in bone marrow transplant recipients. The majority of fungal infections in cancer patients are caused by organisms such as *Candida* and *Aspergillus* spp., which seldom cause infection unless host defence mechanisms are compromised. When cellular immunity is impaired the risk of infection with fungi such as *C. neoformans* and *Histoplasma capsulatum* is increased.

Infection with *viruses* such as CMV, herpes simplex and varicella zoster is particularly seen in those with impaired cellular immunity as is infection by *protozoa* (*P. carinii* and *Toxoplasma gondii*) and the helminth *Strongyloides stercoralis*.

Sites of infection

Common sites of infection include:

- the lung (commonest);
- mucosal surfaces (oral and perirectal);
- disseminated;
- central nervous system (unusual except cryptococcal meningitis in those with impaired CMI and secondary to bacteraemia or fungaemia);
- genitourinary (unusual except in the elderly and those with urinary catheters or pelvic tumours).

Prevention of infection

Once the patient has been admitted to the ICU measures to prevent infection that have been instituted on the ward (e.g. selective decontamination of the digestive tract) should in general be continued. Careful attention to handwashing and other routine infection control measures (see earlier in this chapter) is essential. Invasive procedures should only be used when clearly indicated; strict attention to an aseptic technique and meticulous care of all intravascular cannulae, skin puncture sites and infusion lines is essential.

Diagnosis of infection

In neutropenic patients the usual signs and symptoms of infection (except fever) are often absent because the patient is unable to mount an adequate inflammatory response. Sputum may not be purulent, cough may be minimal or absent, the appearance of physical signs is delayed and the chest radiograph often appears normal initially. Similarly urinary tract infection may not be accompanied by pyuria, and meningitis may be clinically silent. Finally it is important to appreciate that in these patients an apparently minor infection such as mild perianal cellulitis may cause bacteraemia with fever and chills. The diagnosis of infection in such patients is therefore often based solely on the presence of fever.

Immediately infection is suspected a thorough clinical examination should be performed in an attempt to identify the source. Besides surveillance samples of throat and rectum, diagnostic investigations should include:

- three blood cultures (three sets in each case);
- culture of sputum (obtained if necessary by transtracheal aspiration in those with chest radiographic evidence of pneumonia);
- bronchoscopy and BAL (in selected cases);
- aspiration or biopsy specimens from suspicious mucosal or skin lesions;
- culture of urine;
- lumbar puncture (when indicated);
- removal and culture of indwelling cannulae (except sometimes Hickman cannulae, but should obtain blood cultures through the line);
- blood gas analysis (in those who are tachypnoeic);
- special investigations to establish the identity of the infecting organism (unusual bacteria, fungi, viruses, protozoa).

The appearance of *new pulmonary infiltrates* on the chest radiograph of a patient with malignant disease is not necessarily indicative of infection since there are also a large number of non-infectious causes (**Table 11.5**). Standard diagnostic procedures, including transtracheal aspirate (TTA), often fail to establish the aetiology of lung disease in these immunosuppressed patients, particularly when there is diffuse, bilateral involvement. Invasive procedures (see earlier in this chapter) are therefore often required to establish the diagnosis, although the risks of these techniques are increased in many patients with malignant disease because of associated problems such as thrombocytopenia, coagulopathy, respiratory failure and impaired tissue healing.

Table 11.5 Causes of new pulmonary infiltrates in patients with malignant disease.

Infectious	Bacterial pneumonia
	Fungal pneumonia
	Pneumocystis carinii pneumonia
	Viral pneumonia
Non-infectious	Radiation pneumonitis
	Cytotoxic drug-induced lung disease (e.g. bleomycin, methotrexate, busulphan and procarbazine)
	Malignant infiltration
	Pulmonary leukostasis (in uncontrolled leukaemia with very high blood counts)
	Pulmonary haemorrhage
	Pulmonary oedema
	Non-specific interstitial pneumonitis

Principles of treatment

Unless there is an obvious non-infectious cause, empirical antibiotic therapy must be instituted promptly whenever a neutropenic patient develops a fever. This approach dramatically reduces morbidity and mortality. A combination of two or three agents is usually required to cover the range of potential pathogens, the choice depending on the organisms known to be prevalent at a particular institution and their sensitivity patterns. Most often an aminoglycoside is combined with a cephalosporin or an antipseudomonal penicillin. The chosen combination should be administered intravenously.

Subsequently it may be possible to modify the antibiotic regimen according to the results of cultures and sensitivities to a more specific, less toxic and less expensive combination. Many clinicians, however, would be reluctant to alter a combination that has produced resolution of fever and clinical improvement, regardless of the culture results.

If the patient remains pyrexial and unwell, and there is no microbiological confirmation of the responsible organism, the antibiotic regimen may be changed empirically. In some cases antifungal therapy or treatment for *P. carinii* may also be instituted empirically.

Septic shock

Septic shock is a common cause of admission to the ICU, especially in those with haematological malignancy in whom it often occurs in association with respiratory failure (Lloyd-Thomas *et al.*, 1988). The commonest source of infection in these patients is the lungs.

The principles governing the management of septic shock complicating malignant disease are the same as those for patients without cancer and appropriate treatment is similarly dependent on the percutaneous insertion of intravascular cannulae (see Chapter 4). The risks of these invasive techniques, particularly infection and haemorrhage, are especially high in patients with malignancy. The danger of serious haemorrhage can be minimized by previous administration of FFP and/or platelet concentrates as indicated and by puncturing the smaller peripheral arteries and veins where bleeding is more easily controlled. It may be possible to insert central venous and pulmonary artery catheters via a vein in the antecubital fossa. Failing this the internal jugular vein should be used for central venous access since direct pressure can be applied to control venous bleeding or if the carotid artery is accidentally punctured. The subclavian approach should be avoided. Although cannulation of femoral vessels is thought by some to be associated with an increased risk of infection, this route can be used when others have failed. In practice serious complications related to vascular cannulation are rare.

Prognosis

Mortality rates are high when patients with malignant disease develop an acute illness severe enough to warrant admission to the ICU, particularly in those with respiratory failure (Lloyd-Thomas *et al.*, 1988). An overall hospital mortality rate of around 70–80% can be expected in patients admitted to the ICU with acute complications of haematological malignancies or bone marrow transplantation, rising to 80–90% or higher if respiratory failure develops. The prognosis is even worse for patients requiring prolonged mechanical ventilation, those with septic shock (particularly when combined with pneumonia) and those with residual or relapsed malignancy. Mortality is related to the number of organ failures and the severity of the acute illness. Survival in neutropenic patients depends on rapid recovery of marrow function. Mortality rates are lower when patients with all types of malignancy, including solid tumours, as well as surgical patients and those with metabolic disturbances are considered. The long-term prognosis for those who do survive is also often poor and depends largely on the nature and progress of the underlying malignancy. Nevertheless, for some patients, intensive care is life-saving, the prospects for long-term survival can be good and the quality of life for those with haematological malignancy who do survive long-term has been shown to be excellent (Yau *et al.*, 1991).

Despite these high mortality rates, the authors believe that intensive care is justified for patients with acute life threatening complications of malignancy unless or until it is clear that there is no prospect of recovery from the acute illness or that the underlying malignancy cannot be controlled. To ensure a humane approach to the management of malignant disease and appropriate use of limited resources, it is important that when the prognosis is clearly hopeless, clinicians in consultation with other members of staff and the patient or their relatives, consider withholding or withdrawing aggressive supportive treatment (see Chapter 1).

REFERENCES

Abraham E & Chang YH (1990) Hemorrhage in mice produces alterations in intestinal B cell repertoires. *Cellular Immunology* **128**: 165-174.

Altemeier WA, Todd JC & Inge WW (1967) Gram-negative septicemia: a growing threat. *Annals of Surgery* **166**: 530-542.

Andrews CP, Coalson JJ, Smith JD & Johanson WG Jr (1981) Diagnosis of nosocomial bacterial pneumonia in acute, diffuse lung injury. *Chest* **80**: 254-258.

Atkinson SW & Bihari DJ (1993) Selective decontamination of the gut. *British Medical Journal* **306**: 286-287 (Editorial).

Berger R & Arango L (1985) Etiologic diagnosis of bacterial nosocomial pneumonia in seriously ill patients. *Critical Care Medicine* **13**: 833-836.

Bozette SA, Sattler FR, Chiu J et al. (1990) A controlled trial of early adjunctive treatment with corticosteroids for *Pneumocystis carinii* pneumonia in the acquired immunodeficiency syndrome. California, Collaborative Treatment Group. *New England Journal of Medicine* **323**: 1451-1457.

Bradley JA, Hamilton DNH, Brown MW et al. (1984) Cellular defense in critically ill surgical patients. *Critical Care Medicine* **12**: 565-570.

Burge TS & Watson JD (1994) Necrotising fasciitis. *British Medical Journal* **308**: 1453-1454 (Editorial).

Cade JF, McOwat E, Siganporia R, Keighley C, Presneill J & Sinickas V (1992) Uncertain relevance of gastric colonization in the seriously ill. *Intensive Care Medicine* **18**: 210-217.

Chelsom J, Halstensen A, Haga T & Hoiby EA (1994) Necrotizing fasciitis due to group A streptococci in western Norway: incidence and clinical features. *Lancet* **344**: 1111-1115.

Cobb DK, High KP, Sawyer RG, et al. (1992) A controlled trial of scheduled replacement of central venous and pulmonary-artery catheters. *New England Journal of Medicine* **327**: 1062-1068.

Daschner FD (1985) Useful and useless hygienic techniques in intensive care units. *Intensive Care Medicine* **11**: 280-283.

Doelbling BN, Stanley GL, Sheetz CT et al. (1992) Comparative efficacy of alternative hand-washing agents in reducing nosocomial infections in intensive care units. *New England Journal of Medicine* **327**: 88-93.

Du Moulin GC, Paterson DG, Hedley-Whyte J & Lisbon A (1982) Aspiration of gastric bacteria in antacid-treated patients: a frequent cause of postoperative colonisation of the airway. *Lancet* **ii**: 242-245.

Editorial (1981) Pulmonary problems of the immunocompromised patient. *British Medical Journal* **282**: 2077.

Editorial (1985) A nasty shock from antibiotics? *Lancet* **ii**: 594.

El-Sadr W & Simberkoff MS (1988) Survival and prognostic factors in severe *Pneumocystis carinii* pneumonia requiring mechanical ventilation. *American Review of Respiratory Diseases* **137**: 1264-1267.

Ertel W, Morrison MH, Ayella A, Dean RE & Chaudry IH (1992) Interferon-gamma attenuates hemorrhage-induced suppression of macrophage and splenocyte functions and decreases susceptibility to sepsis. *Surgery* **111**: 177-187.

Gagnon S, Boota AM, Fischl MA, Baier H, Kirksey OW & La Voie L (1990) Corticosteroids as adjunctive therapy for severe *Pneumocystis carinii* pneumonia in the acquired immunodeficiency syndrome. A double-blind placebo-controlled trial. *New England Journal of Medicine* **323**: 1444-1450.

Gastinne H, Wolff M, Delatour F, Faurisson F & Chevret S (1992) A controlled trial in intensive care units of selective decontamination of the digestive tract with nonabsorbable antibiotics. The French Study Group on Selective Decontamination of the Digestive Tract. *New England Journal of Medicine* **326**: 594-599.

George RH, Symonds JM, Dimock F et al. (1978) Identification of *Clostridium difficile* as a cause of pseudomembranous colitis. *British Medical Journal* **i**: 695.

Hammond JM, Potgieter PD, Saunders GL & Forder AA (1992) Double-blind study of selective decontamination of the digestive tract in intensive care. *Lancet* **340**: 5-9.

Heyland DK, Cook DJ, Jaeschke R, Griffith L, Lee HN & Guyatt GH (1994) Selective decontamination of the digestive tract. An overview. *Chest* **105**: 1221-1229.

Hilton E, Haslett TM, Borenstein MT, Tucci V, Isenberg HD & Singer C (1988) Central catheter infections: single versus triple-lumen catheters. Influence of guide wires on infection rates when used for replacement of catheters. *American Journal of Medicine* **84**: 667-671.

Holmberg SD, Solomon SL & Blake PA (1987) Health and economic impacts of antimicrobial resistance. *Review of Infectious Diseases* **9**: 1065-1078.

Hosker H, Cooke NJ & Hawkey P (1994) Antibiotics in chronic obstructive pulmonary disease. *British Medical Journal* **308**: 871-872 (Editorial).

Inglis TJJ, Sproat LJ, Sheratt MJ, Hawkey PM, Gibson JS & Shah MV (1992) Gastroduodenal dysfunction as a cause of gastric bacterial overgrowth in patients undergoing mechanical ventilation of the lungs. *British Journal of Anaesthesia* **68**: 499-502.

Johanson WG Jr, Seidenfeld JJ, Gomez P, De los Santos R & Coalsen JJ (1988) Bacteriologic diagnosis of nosocomial pneumonia following prolonged mechanical ventilation. *American Review of Respiratory Diseases* **137**: 259-264.

Kollef MH (1994) The role of selective digestive tract decontamination on mortality and respiratory tract infections. A meta-analysis. *Chest* **105**: 1101-1108.

Ledingham IMcA, Alcock SR, Eastaway AT, McDonald JC, McKay IC & Ramsay G (1988) Triple regimen of selective decontamination of the digestive tract, systemic cefotaxime, and microbiological surveillance for prevention of acquired infection in intensive care. *Lancet* **i**: 785-790.

Lloyd-Thomas AR, Wright I, Lister TA & Hinds CJ (1988) Prognosis of patients receiving intensive care for life-threatening medical complications of haematological malignancy. *British Medical Journal* **296**: 1025-1029.

McFarland LV, Mulligan ME, Kwok RYY & Stamm WE (1989) Nosocomial acquisition of *Clostridium difficile* infection. *New England Journal of Medicine* **320**: 204-210.

MacFarlane J (1985) Lung biopsy (editorial). *British Medical Journal* **290**: 97-98.

Mackie DP, Van Hertum WAJ, Schumburg T, Kijper EC & Knape P (1992) Prevention of infection in burns: preliminary experience with selective decontamination of the digestive tract in patients with extensive injuries. *The Journal of Trauma* **32**: 570-575.

Montaner JSG, Russell JA, Lawson L & Ruedy J (1989) Acute respiratory failure secondary to *Pneumocystis carinii* pneumonia in the acquired immunodeficiency syndrome. A potential role for systemic corticosteroids. *Chest* **95**: 881-884.

Morrison HM & Stockley RA (1988) The many uses of bronchoalveolar lavage. *British Medical Journal* **296**: 1758.

O'Connell MT, Becker DM, Steele BW, Peterson GS & Hellman RL (1984) Plasma fibronectin in medical ICU patients. *Critical Care Medicine* **12**: 479-482.

Peters BS, Beck EJ, Coleman DG, *et al.* (1991) Changing disease patterns in patients with AIDS in a referral centre in the United Kingdom: the changing face of AIDS. *British Medical Journal* **302**: 203-207.

Pinilla JC, Ross DF, Martin T & Crump H (1983) Study of the incidence of intravascular catheter infection and associated septicaemia in critically ill patients. *Critical Care Medicine* **11**: 21-25.

Reidy JJ & Ramsay G (1990) Clinical trials of selective decontamination of the digestive tract: Review. *Critical Care Medicine* **18**: 1449-1456.

Rogers PL, Lane HC, Henderson DK, Parrillo J & Masur H (1989) Admission of AIDS patients to a medical intensive care unit: causes and outcome. *Critical Care Medicine* **17**: 113-117.

Rolando N, Gimson A, Wade J, Philpott-Howard J, Casewell M & Williams R (1993) Prospective controlled trial of selective parenteral and enteral antimicrobial regimen in fulminant liver failure. *Hepatology* **17**: 196-201.

Selective Decontamination of the Digestive Tract Triallists' Collaborative Group (1993) Meta-analysis of randomised controlled trials of selective decontamination of the digestive tract. *British Medical Journal* **307**: 525-532.

Stoutenbeek CP, Van Saene HKF, Miranda DR & Zandstra DF (1984) The effect of selective decontamination of the digestive tract on colonisation and infection rate in multiple trauma patients. *Intensive Care Medicine* **10**: 185-192

Stoutenbeek CP, van Saene HKF & Liberati A (1994) Prevention of respiratory tract infections in intensive care by selective decontamination of the digestive tract. In: Niederman MS, Sarosi GA, Glassroth J (eds) *Respiratory Infections: a scientific basis for Management*. 1st edn. Philadelphia, WB Saunders Co, pp. 579-594.

Stover DE, White DA, Romano PA, Gellene RA & Robeson WA (1985) Spectrum of pulmonary diseases associated with the acquired immune deficiency syndrome. *American Journal of Medicine* **78**: 429-437.

Tobin MJ & Grenvik A (1984) Nosocomial lung infection and its diagnosis. *Critical Care Medicine* **12**: 191-199.

Ulrich C, Harnick de Weerd JE, Bakker NC, Jacz K, Doornbos L & De Ridder VA (1989) Selective decontamination of the digestive tract with norfloxacin in the prevention of ICU-acquired infections: a prospective randomized study. *Intensive Care Medicine* **15**: 424-431.

Vandenbroucke-Grauls CM & Vandenbroucke JP (1991) Effect of selective decontamination of the digestive tract on respiratory tract infections and mortality in the intensive care unit. *Lancet* **338**: 859-862.

Van Saene HKF, Nunn AJ & Petros AJ (1994) Viewpoint: survival benefit by selective decontamination of the digestive tract (SDD). *Infection Control and Hospital Epidemiology* **15**: 443-446.

Wachter RM, Luce JM, Lo B & Raffin TA (1989) Life-sustaining treatment for patients with AIDS. *Chest* **95**: 647-652.

Wolfe JHN, Saporoschetz I, Young AE, O'Connor NE & Mannick JA (1981) Suppressive serum, suppressor lymphocytes, and death from burns. *Annals of Surgery* **193**: 513-520.

Yau E, Rohatiner AZS, Lister TA & Hinds CJ (1991) Long term prognosis and quality of life following intensive care for life-threatening complications of haematological malignancy. *British Journal of Cancer* **64**: 938-942.

12 Acute Renal Failure

Because of its enormous metabolic activity, the kidney is particularly susceptible to the effects of underperfusion and hypoxaemia. Although acute renal failure (ARF) may occasionally result from a single identifiable event such as hypotension or drug toxicity, it occurs most frequently in the context of multiple organ failure and sepsis. The outcome in this latter category of patient is often poor, particularly in those with respiratory failure.

Prevention of ARF is therefore a fundamental aspect of intensive care practice. This entails:

- early identification of those at risk;
- meticulous cardiovascular support, including rapid expansion of the circulating volume when indicated (Chapter 4);
- the judicious use of inotropes when indicated (Chapter 4);
- careful maintenance of crystalloid balance (Chapter 10);
- aggressive treatment of sepsis (Chapter 4);
- the avoidance of nephrotoxic drugs.

Constant vigilance for the early signs of impaired renal function, followed by immediate corrective measures when required, is also essential. In some circumstances, the use of specific preventive therapy is warranted (see later in this chapter).

DEFINITION AND CAUSES (Table 12.1)

ARF can be defined as a sudden (and usually reversible) failure of the kidneys to excrete the waste products of metabolism, and may be broadly categorized as prerenal, postrenal or intrarenal.

Prerenal failure, in which function is impaired, but there is no parenchymal damage, is due to reduced renal perfusion, usually related to an episode of shock, hypovolaemia or dehydration. Prerenal uraemia can also result from excessive production of waste products, which may then accumulate in those with pre-existing mild renal impairment.

Postrenal failure is caused by an obstruction to urine flow. This may be due to a lesion at the bladder outlet, bilateral upper urinary tract obstruction or unilateral obstruction of a solitary kidney.

The terms *ARF* and *acute tubular necrosis* (ATN) have become virtually synonymous. The latter strictly

Table 12.1 Causes of acute renal failure.

Acute tubular necrosis (ATN)
Bilateral cortical necrosis
Acute glomerulonephritis
   Rapidly progressive crescentic nephritis
   Systemic lupus erythematosus (SLE)
   Necrotizing vasculitis (e.g. polyarteritis nodosa,
     Goodpasture's syndrome)
Malignant hypertension
Acute interstitial nephritis
Severe pyelonephritis (papillary necrosis)
Occlusive renovascular disease
Acute exacerbations of chronic renal impairment
Acute obstructive uropathy

refers to necrosis of kidney tubules, but is now used to describe the clinical syndrome of reversible acute intrinsic renal failure that can follow an episode of renal ischaemia (vasomotor nephropathy) or exposure to a nephrotoxin. It accounts for the majority of cases of ARF encountered in intensive care units.

Nephrotoxins that can precipitate ATN include:

- organic solvents (e.g. carbon tetrachloride);
- antibiotics (e.g. gentamicin);
- heavy metals (e.g. mercuric chloride);
- radiological contrast media;
- myoglobin released from damaged muscle in patients with severe crush injuries compartment syndrome (see Chapter 9) or non-traumatic rhabdomyolysis (e.g. alcohol withdrawal, barbiturate poisoning or uncontrolled seizure activity).

Haemoglobinuria from mismatched blood transfusions or severe haemolytic anaemia may also lead to renal impairment. Extensive *burns* can be complicated by hypovolaemia, infection, rhabdomyolysis, ventricular dysfunction or disseminated intravascular coagulation (DIC) and are therefore frequently associated with ARF. Other situations in which ARF is commonly encountered include *severe sepsis, major gastrointestinal or postpartum haemorrhage, septic abortion, acute pancreatitis, biliary tract infection* and *postoperatively*, especially after *aortic aneurysm repair* and in the elderly or *jaundiced. Raised intra-abdominal pressure* to above about 30 cm H_2O also causes renal dysfunction, perhaps due to direct pressure effects on the kidney or renal vein compression, which can be relieved by decompressing the abdomen. Intra-abdominal pressure can be measured using a water manometer or transducer attached to a urinary catheter filled with sterile water and an increase to above 25 mm Hg has been suggested as a criterion for abdominal re-exploration (Kron *et al.*, 1984). Severe, acute *hyperuricaemia* is a relatively uncommon cause of ARF, the basis of which is uric acid deposition in the distal tubules and collecting ducts. Hyperuricaemic ARF is now seen most frequently as a complication of chemotherapy for lymphomas or leukaemias. Finally, ARF is a common complication of *liver disease*, including fulminant hepatic failure, decompensated cirrhosis and obstructive jaundice, but the term 'hepatorenal syndrome' is non-specific and should probably be avoided (see Chapter 13).

ARF may also, but less commonly, be due to a variety of *glomerular lesions* (e.g. a rapidly progressive crescentic nephritis or a glomerulonephritis related to a systemic illness such as systemic lupus erythematosus (SLE), polyarteritis nodosa (PAN) or Goodpasture's syndrome.

Acute interstitial nephritis is now recognized as an unusual, but important, cause of ARF and is usually a result of an acute or subacute 'allergic' reaction to drugs. While classically described in association with methicillin or other penicillins, diuretics may also be implicated and numerically the non-steroidal anti-inflammatory drugs (NSAIDs) are becoming an increasingly important cause of this condition.

Renal failure due to *vascular lesions* may be embolic (e.g. from a mural thrombus) or thrombotic (e.g. following trauma or vascular surgery) or may occur in association with atheroma or polyarteritis nodosa.

PATHOPHYSIOLOGY OF ACUTE INTRINSIC RENAL FAILURE (Table 12.2)

The production of urine by ultrafiltration of plasma is largely dependent on the glomerular capillary hydrostatic pressure, which in turn is determined by the cardiac output, aorto-renal blood flow and the balance between afferent and efferent renal arteriolar tone.

Table 12.2 Pathogenesis of acute renal failure.
Renal ischaemia
Decreased glomerular ultrafiltration coefficient
Tubular backleak of filtrate
Tubular obstruction

Afferent arterioles constrict in response to $\alpha 1$ agonists, vasoconstrictor prostaglandins such as thromboxane, endothelin and inhibition of nitric oxide (NO) synthase (MacAllister & Vallance, 1994): they are dilated by β_2 and dopaminergic stimulation, as well as vasodilator prostaglandins such as prostacyclin, PGE_1 and PGE_2. Efferent vasoconstriction is mediated principally by angiotensin II, while larger doses of NO synthase inhibitors constrict both the afferent and efferent arteriole and reduce both renal blood flow and glomerular filtration rate (GFR) (MacAllister & Vallance, 1994). Total blood flow to the kidneys is extremely high, nearly one-quarter of the cardiac output, the majority being directed to the renal cortex where the cortical tubules therefore consume only a small proportion of their profuse supply of oxygen. By contrast medullary blood flow is limited to avoid disrupting the gradient of osmolality generated by the countercurrent mechanism within the vasa recta. Moreover the thick ascending limb of Henle's' loop avidly consumes oxygen for sodium transport and oxygen diffuses directly from the descending (arterial) to the ascending (venous) branches of the vasa recta; in this region the balance between oxygen supply and demand is therefore much more precarious.

The medulla is, however, protected from hypoxic injury by various mechanisms. These include the release of adenosine from the breakdown of cellular adenosine triphosphate (ATP), which enhances medullary blood flow while decreasing tubular transport and GFR, and PGE_2 (Brezis *et al.*, 1986), which is a medullary vasodilator and an inhibitor of active transport by medullary thick limbs. The reduction in cortical flow that occurs in response to hypotension may also be considered as a protective mechanism since GFR falls and blood is redistributed to the medulla, thereby helping to restore the balance between tubular oxygen supply and demand. Conversely injury to the susceptible thick ascending limb, which bears the brunt of the damage in ATN, is most likely when renal ischaemia is combined with continuing tubular reabsorptive work due to a preserved or enhanced GFR. Typically such a situation is caused by angiotensin II, which constricts postglomerular vessels and increases filtration fraction.

Except for those cases caused by nephrotoxins, the onset of ATN is almost always related to an episode of reduced renal blood flow and is precipitated by the vasomotor response to hypovolaemia, hypotension, a reduced cardiac output or sepsis. In some cases localized renal arterial pathology or an increased vascular resistance associated with hypertension or toxaemia of pregnancy may be a contributory factor. The reduction in renal blood flow is associated with marked selective cortical ischaemia, probably related to preglomerular vasoconstriction (Reubi *et al.*, 1973). Although it has been suggested that systemic activation of the renin–angiotensin system is an important mediator of these alterations in renal blood flow, it seems more likely that intrarenal renin release with local angiotensin-induced afferent arteriolar constriction is largely responsible (Myers & Moran, 1986). This may be combined with a deficiency of vasodilator prostaglandins (e.g. PGE_2) and an excess of vasoconstrictor prostaglandins (e.g. thromboxane) and leucotrienes (Badr *et al.*, 1986), as well as increased sympathetic activity.

Renal blood flow usually remains low throughout the oliguric phase, even when volume deficits have been replaced and blood pressure restored, but then returns to normal during recovery of renal function. Some therefore attribute the continued reduction in GFR to persistent afferent arteriolar constriction, possibly combined with efferent arteriolar dilatation or to occlusion of small blood vessels by ischaemic cell swelling (Flores *et al.*, 1972). Renal cortical ischaemia does not always persist, however, and, using an ischaemic model of ARF, it has been shown that the tubules remained collapsed despite restoration of renal blood flow to supranormal values, suggesting a defect in glomerular filtration (Cox *et al.*, 1974). This may be explained in part by a loss of glomerular permeability, although tubular injury, involving predominantly the proximal tubules, may be of central importance in the development of oliguria (Myers & Moran, 1986). Tubular obstruction by endothelial cell swelling and/or casts and cellular debris, as well as leakage of tubular fluid across necrotic epithelium into the interstitium may increase tubular hydrostatic pressure with back diffusion and reabsorption of filtrate, thereby contributing to persistent oliguria. Nephrotoxins also cause necrosis of the tubular epithelium but, in contrast to ischaemic injury, the basement membrane remains intact and epithelial regeneration can occur after only a few days.

Simultaneous renal ischaemia and toxic insults act synergistically to increase the probability of ARF, which in most cases seems to be the result of a combination of risk factors (Shusterman *et al.*, 1987). For example, NSAIDS interfere with renal protective mechanisms by blocking prostaglandin synthesis and underperfused kidneys produce more concentrated urine containing increased levels of toxins, nephrotoxic agents such as cyclosporin and radiocontrast media. Similarly increased concentrations of myoglobin (which avidly binds NO) will exacerbate renal vasoconstriction. Common associations include:

- hypoperfusion and pre-existing renal disease, diabetes mellitus or hypertension;
- hypovolaemia and rhabdomyolysis;
- the administration of cyclosporin or amphotericin in the presence of salt depletion;
- the use of NSAIDS or captopril (which reduces capillary hydrostatic pressure by decreasing angiotensin II

production) during an episode of renal underperfusion.

In *critically ill patients*, ARF commonly occurs in association with the systemic inflammatory response syndrome (SIRS), multiple organ dysfunction syndome (MODS), severe sepsis and septic shock (see Chapter 4). This may be partly related to the direct or indirect effects of endotoxin, which impairs renal blood flow in experimental animals even in the absence of hypotension (Hinshaw *et al.*, 1959), and can initiate intravascular coagulation as well as the release of inflammatory mediators including toxic oxygen radicals (see Chapter 4).

Obstructive jaundice may be incriminated in the development of ARF when there is no other obvious cause, but the precise mechanism is unclear. Although the toxic effects of circulating endotoxin or bile have been held responsible for the renal haemodynamic disturbances observed in these patients, others have suggested that jaundice renders the kidneys more sensitive to ischaemia (Dawson, 1964).

ARF is also common in *hepatic failure*; in one study, approximately 80% of patients in grade III or IV coma had some impairment of renal function (Wilkinson *et al.*, 1974). Although most cases are due to identifiable prerenal factors or to vasomotor nephropathy associated with hypotension, gastrointestinal haemorrhage or sepsis, in a few the mechanism is unclear. In decompensated cirrhosis, ARF is probably caused by a redistribution of renal blood flow, with a reduction in total flow and GFR occurring only as late events. This redistribution of flow may largely account for the intense sodium retention that occurs in cirrhosis, with hyperaldosteronism playing a less important role. The ability to handle a water load, concentrate urine and excrete hydrogen ions is also impaired in cirrhotics. ARF may then be precipitated by an episode of gastrointestinal bleeding, a sudden increase in ascites or overvigorous diuretic administration.

In summary, therefore, although it has been suggested that renal cortical ischaemia is the main pathogenic event in ARF, it seems likely that in most cases more than one mechanism is involved and the factors that initiate the damage are not necessarily the same as those that perpetuate renal dysfunction.

DIAGNOSIS AND INVESTIGATIONS
(Table 12.3)

In intensive care patients, *oliguria* (urine output < 0.5 ml/kg/h) is usually the first indication that renal function is impaired. The diagnosis is then confirmed by:

- a progressive rise in blood urea and creatinine levels;

- a metabolic acidosis;
- hyperkalaemia;
- salt and water retention.

Occasionally, an unexpected increase in plasma pot-assium concentration is the earliest sign of impaired renal function, particularly in the presence of extensive tissue injury.

Oliguria is not, however, an essential prerequisite for the diagnosis of ARF, since when renal concentrating ability is reduced, even a urine production of 2–3 l/day may not reflect a sufficiently high GFR to excrete the nitrogenous metabolic waste products, particularly if the patient is hypercatabolic. It is also important to appreciate that in critically ill patients, alterations in cir-culating levels of antidiuretic hormone (ADH), aldos-terone and atrial natriuretic factor (ANF) play an important role in the development of oliguria as do the effects of positive pressure ventilation, positive end-expiratory pressure (PEEP), fluid restriction, and diuretics in those with respiratory failure (see Chapters 6 and 7).

In all cases, and particularly if the patient is anuric or has intermittent complete anuria, *bladder outflow obstruction* must be excluded. This possibility should be suspected in patients with previous symptoms of prostatic enlargement and in those who have suffered recent trauma or surgery to the pelvic area. Examination may reveal an enlarged bladder. If there is any doubt, aseptic bladder catheterization should be performed or, if a urinary catheter is already in place, it should be examined for obstruction. It is usually advisable to obtain the assistance of a urologist if possible and many would recommend that an ultrasound scan should be performed before catheterizing the bladder. Rectal and vaginal examinations should be performed and the external genitalia must be inspected.

Anuria is an ominous sign in patients who have

recently undergone surgery to the aorta in close proxim-ity to the renal arteries. If loss of vascular supply to the kidneys is a serious possibility, then the implications for management are profound. Early *renography*, followed by direct *renal arteriography* if no perfusion is shown, is indicated.

Once bladder outflow obstruction has been excluded, it is important to determine whether the patient has pre-renal, intrarenal or postrenal failure.

The *history* can provide a clue to the aetiology and may establish whether there was any pre-existing renal impairment. Many critically ill patients will be unable to communicate, but relatives or close friends can be interviewed and documented case histories will often be available from the admitting team or referring hos-pital. It is important to establish whether there is any evidence of previous renal disorders (childhood neph-rotic syndrome, haematuria, nocturia, renal colic, hyper-tension, failed medical examinations for insurance pur-poses or for entry into the armed forces) as well as to ask about recognized aetiological factors such as anal-gesic abuse (particularly in patients with arthritis or migraine), 'mainlining' of drugs, ingestion of NSAIDs, and diabetes mellitus, and recent infections, surgery or trauma. The family history may suggest the possibility of polycystic disease. Finally, it is important to enquire about any recent exposure to unusual chemicals or sol-vents at work or in the home.

Old case-notes should be scrutinized for the results of previous urine testing (proteinuria, haematuria), urea and creatinine determinations, and blood pressure recordings. Plain abdominal films, intravenous urograms or ultrasound examinations may also be available and can give an indication of previous kidney size and the presence of stones.

Recent notes may reveal an episode of hypotension (e.g. on the anaesthetic chart) or sepsis, as well as pro-vide a record of drugs administered (look particularly for gentamicin, NSAIDs and contrast media).

Prerenal failure

In prerenal failure the excretory function of the kidneys is impaired by shock, hypovolaemia or dehydration; this causes oliguria and a reduction in GFR, with maximal tubular reabsorption of salt and water. Usually pro-teinuria is absent and the urinary sediment unremark-able. In general, blood urea rises more than creatinine and the urine is concentrated (osmolality > 500 mmol/l) with a high urea and low sodium content (< 20 mmol/l). In some cases, however, there may be a renal 'leak' of sodium in which case urinary sodium content may be higher than 30 mmol/l and oliguria is less marked or absent. Classically, the urine : plasma ratios of osmolality, urea and creatinine are greater than

Table 12.3 Investigations in acute renal failure.
Urea, creatinine Sodium, potassium Blood gases/acid–base
Plasma and urine osmolality Urine sodium and protein content Urine microscopy
Ultrasound scan of kidney Renography Renal arteriography High-dose intravenous urography Ureterography
Renal biopsy

2, 30 and 15 respectively. Unfortunately, in many intensive care patients, values for these urine : plasma ratios are borderline or misleading, especially in non-oliguric renal failure when diuretics have been administered, and in those with pre-existing renal or hepatic disease, cardiac failure or electrolyte disturbances (particularly hypokalaemia). Consequently, they are rarely of value and the distinction can only be made on the basis of a clinical assessment of the state of hydration (oedema, neck veins, blood pressure, postural hypotension) and the response to a volume challenge, guided as necessary by measurements of central venous pressure (CVP) and/or pulmonary artery occlusion pressure (PAOP).

Urinary tract obstruction

Once prerenal failure has been excluded, the most immediate problem is the exclusion or identification of urinary tract obstruction. In most patients, *ultrasound scanning* can reliably identify obstruction as well as provide a reasonable estimate of kidney size, and is the most practical and useful imaging technique in intensive care patients. If ultrasound is inconclusive, *high-dose intravenous urography* provides the same information and very occasionally may define the site of the obstruction. Usually, however, when obstruction is detected, *antegrade or retrograde ureterography* is necessary to define the site. Obstruction requires skilled urological assessment with a view to urgently establishing free drainage of urine.

Acute renal failure

The diagnosis of *intrinsic ARF* is suggested by demonstrating that urine and plasma are iso-osmolar, that the urinary sodium concentration is high (> 30–50 mmol/l) and that the urinary potassium concentration is low (< 10 mmol/l). Proteinuria is present. The differential diagnosis then includes:

- ATN;
- glomerular lesions (acute glomerulonephritis, vasculitis);
- cortical necrosis;
- acute interstitial nephritis;
- renal vascular lesions;
- an acute exacerbation of chronic renal disease.

Renal size must be determined since small kidneys are indicative of underlying chronic renal disease. An ultrasound scan may reveal the size of the kidneys or even suggest polycystic disease. The diagnosis of *rhabdomyolysis* is supported by an elevated serum creatine phosphokinase level and by detecting myoglobin in the urine. The serum potassium is usually markedly elevated

and there may be hypocalcaemia due to a shift of calcium into injured muscle.

GLOMERULAR DISEASE

The possibility that ARF is due to a glomerular lesion should be considered, particularly when there are extrarenal signs such as:

- skin lesions (especially purpura);
- arthritis;
- neurological manifestations (e.g. mononeuritis);
- pulmonary involvement.

Hypertension is usual in these cases. Serum complement levels may be reduced and in some, circulating immune complexes are identified. Examination of the urine may reveal red cell casts and proteinuria, whereas in vasomotor nephropathy the urinary sediment will contain only tubular cells with a few granular casts. If the presentation suggests the possibility of a treatable lesion, *renal biopsy* may be indicated. There is, however, a significant risk of complications with this procedure, particularly haemorrhage, and these should be weighed against the likely benefits.

When glomerular disease presents as ARF, it is usually due to an acute process such as a rapidly progressive crescentic nephritis or a systemic disease such as PAN, SLE or Goodpasture's syndrome. The latter should be suspected when there is pulmonary involvement with haemorrhage and the diagnosis can be confirmed by demonstrating linear deposits of IgG along the glomerular basement membrane and by identifying circulating antiglomerular basement membrane antibody.

RENAL CORTICAL NECROSIS

Renal cortical necrosis usually presents as ARF and cannot normally be distinguished from vasomotor nephropathy in the acute stage. The aetiological factors are often the same and include:

- severe shock;
- major surgery;
- transfusion reactions;
- infections;
- burns.

Cortical necrosis occurs particularly in association with *obstetric disasters*, especially later in pregnancy (Kleinknecht et al., 1973). It has been suggested, therefore, that cortical necrosis occurs especially in those with a hypercoagulable state in whom development of DIC may cause particularly severe renal ischaemia. Cortical necrosis may simply be a more severe form of ATN with less chance of recovery, and should be suspected if oliguria is prolonged. The diagnosis is likely if the kidney size is found to be decreasing and cortical calcification, which appears in approximately half the patients after about six weeks, is virtually diagnostic. In such cases, a renal biopsy may be performed to confirm the diagnosis.

ACUTE INTERSTITIAL NEPHRITIS

Acute interstitial nephritis is suggested by:

- a rash;
- fever;
- joint involvement;
- marked eosinophilia;
- raised serum IgE levels.

Large numbers of eosinophils may be identified in the urine. Renal biopsy confirms the diagnosis.

RENAL VASCULAR LESIONS

Renal vascular lesions present as *sudden oliguria*, or often *complete anuria*, accompanied by hypertension and *loin pain*. Vascular obstruction may be due to embolism (e.g. from a mural thrombus) or thrombosis (e.g. following trauma, due to vascular surgery, or related to PAN or atheroma). The diagnosis can be confirmed by *radio-isotope scan* or *direct renal arteriography*. The latter will be required to define the site of the lesion.

MANAGEMENT AND CLINICAL COURSE (Table 12.4)

Prerenal failure

Prerenal failure should be treated by optimizing the circulating volume, replacing fluid and electrolyte deficits, and restoring the blood pressure. If cardiac output and blood pressure remain low despite volume expansion, inotropes and vasopressors should be administered, the objective being to avoid afferent arteriolar constriction and efferent vasodilation while maintaining an adequate renal perfusion pressure (this will be higher in those with pre-existing hypertension) (see Chapter 4). Hypoxaemia, hypercarbia and, in some cases, metabolic acidosis, should also be corrected. Diuretics should generally be avoided in patients with prerenal oliguria; in this respect it is important to appreciate that there may be a delay of several hours between restoration of the circulating volume and institution of these other measures and restoration of the urine output.

Table 12.4 Management of acute renal failure.
Prerenal oliguria
Optimize the circulating volume
Correct fluid and electrolyte deficits
Restore blood pressure and cardiac output
Incipient renal failure
Mannitol
Frusemide
Dopamine
(Calcium entry blockers)
Early oliguric phase
Fluid restrict
Modify drug doses
Control hyperkalaemia (calcium exchange resins, dextrose and insulin, sodium bicarbonate)
Consider correcting acidosis (rarely indicated)
Consider controlling hypertension
Established acute renal failure
Blood purification—peritoneal dialysis, haemodialysis, haemofiltration (intermittent, continuous—CAVH/CAVHD, CVVH/CVVHD)
Nutritional support
Antacid prophylaxis
Prevent infection
Adjust drug doses
Careful fluid balance
Treat underlying cause
Diuretic phase
Extreme care with fluid and electrolyte balance

Incipient renal failure

Although the treatment of ARF is largely supportive, a number of active measures are usually employed based on the premise that there may be an incipient phase of ATN that can be reversed by prompt intervention. While this is a popular concept, the evidence that such a phase exists is largely anecdotal and the efficacy of measures designed to abort or limit the severity of subsequent established ARF is still debated. Nevertheless, one or more of the following measures are usually employed in most units.

MANNITOL

It has been suggested that this osmotic diuretic, which is also a free radical scavenger and stimulates prostaglandin production, may have a protective effect when used prophylactically in those with obstructive jaundice (Dawson, 1964), during surgery on the abdominal aorta (Barry et al., 1961), and during renal transplantation. It is, however, unclear whether this agent can influence the course of ARF when given after the initiating event. There is some experimental evidence that mannitol can produce potentially beneficial effects in ARF including prevention of cellular swelling (Flores et al., 1972), improved renal haemodynamics (Johnston et al., 1979), and attenuation or prevention of tubular obstruction by increasing proximal intratubular pressures and urine flow rates (Cronin et al., 1978). Although there is some uncontrolled clinical evidence that early administration of mannitol can abort or at least limit the severity of ARF (Luke et al., 1965), this has yet to be substantiated. Furthermore, its use may be complicated by circulatory overload and pulmonary oedema, particularly if a diuresis does not follow its administration, as well as cellular dehydration. Nevertheless, some authorities recommend administering intravenous mannitol (e.g. 20 g of a 20% solution) within up to 48 hours after the renal insult.

FRUSEMIDE

This loop diuretic and vasodilator can increase renal cortical blood flow (Birtch et al., 1967), stimulates production of vasodilator prostaglandins, thereby increasing afferent arteriolar flow (Gerber, 1983), and may specifically improve glomerular filtration rate, (De Torrente et al., 1978). It has also been suggested that frusemide may protect the kidneys from hypoxic/ischaemic insults by decreasing reabsorptive activity, thereby limiting metabolic requirements in the vulnerable thick ascending limb of the tubules (Brezis et al., 1984).

Nevertheless, the clinical value of frusemide in ARF remains uncertain. Minuth et al. (1976) performed a retrospective non-randomized study and claimed that a response to frusemide decreased the need for dialysis, although it did not appear to affect mortality. Some authorities therefore feel that frusemide may be valuable because it converts oliguric renal failure to non-oliguric renal failure, thereby minimizing the risks of hyperkalaemia and fluid overload, facilitating nutritional support and decreasing dialysis requirements. Others believe that frusemide only produces a diuresis in those in whom ARF would in any case have been rapidly reversible. Indeed, a number of controlled studies have shown frusemide to be ineffective (Kleinknecht et al., 1976), while Lucas et al. (1977) showed that administration of

frusemide produced a marked diuresis, but did not improve renal blood flow or the GFR, nor did it prevent the subsequent development of established ARF. There are also theoretical objections to the use of this agent since it may increase the nephrotoxicity of some antibiotics and could actually precipitate ARF when used in the presence of hypovolaemia.

Nevertheless, particularly in view of its potential tubular protective effect, frusemide is still recommended by most clinicians, traditionally in repeated high doses (e.g. 250-500 mg in 100 ml 5% dextrose infused over 20 minutes) or, increasingly often as a continuous intravenous infusion (2-10 mg/h). Some suggest that plasma levels should be measured to reduce the risk of ototoxicity, especially if the patient is also receiving aminoglycosides, but this is not usually possible. If there is no response within 4-8 hours, frusemide is usually discontinued.

DOPAMINE (see also Chapter 4).

Dopamine has been shown to increase renal plasma flow, GFR and sodium excretion (McDonald et al., 1964) and in low doses (1-3 μg/kg/min) may avoid or reverse afferent vasoconstriction. It might therefore be a useful agent for the prevention of ARF in at-risk patients or to abort incipient renal failure, although higher doses, which can cause α1-mediated vasoconstriction, should be avoided. Although theoretically dopamine antagonists such as butyrophenones, phenothiazines and metoclopramide might counteract the effects of low-dose dopamine, it has been shown that in critically ill patients normal doses of metoclopramide do not antagonize the renal effects of a low-dose dopamine infusion (Munn et al., 1993).

In an uncontrolled study, Henderson et al. (1980) administered low-dose dopamine (1 μg/kg/min) to patients in early oliguric ARF, with urine : plasma osmolality ratios of <1.1 : 1.0, who had failed to respond to a large dose of frusemide. They demonstrated a significant increase in urine output, which was subsequently maintained in 7 of the 11 patients after the dopamine was discontinued. Their impression was that by producing a diuresis, dopamine decreased dialysis requirements, simplified management and may have improved outcome. In another study (Parker et al., 1981), administration of dopamine 1.5-2.5 μg/kg/min to oliguric critically ill patients with a falling creatinine clearance increased urine output, creatinine clearance, osmolar clearance and the excreted fraction of filtered sodium without affecting haemodynamics or free water clearance. Again, dialysis requirements were reduced. There is some experimental evidence that the *combination of frusemide and dopamine* may act synergistically in this situation (Lindner, 1983), possibly because the vascular effects of dopamine facilitate penetration of frusemide to its site of action in the macula densa. Finally, it has been suggested that prophylactic administration of low-dose dopamine in high-risk situations (e.g. liver transplantation) can reduce the incidence of renal dysfunction (Polson *et al.*, 1987), although low-dose dopamine appears to be of no value when given to patients undergoing elective major vascular surgery (Baldwin *et al.*, 1994).

Many therefore consider the administration of low-dose dopamine to be justified for prophylaxis in high-risk cases and when oliguria persists despite exclusion and correction of prerenal causes. If a diuresis ensues the infusion is usually continued to simplify management. It has yet to be established, however, whether low-dose dopamine can abort incipient ARF, and in view of its potential adverse effects, in particular precipitation of gut mucosal ischaemia (see Chapter 4) and possibly an increase in tubular work, others believe that until the efficacy and safety of this agent have been clearly demonstrated in prospective controlled trials its use for this indication cannot be recommended (Thompson & Cockrill, 1994). Certainly there is no evidence that low-dose dopamine is beneficial in established intrinsic renal failure.

CALCIUM ENTRY BLOCKERS

Calcium entry blockers may protect the kidneys from an ischaemic insult (Wooley *et al.*, 1988), perhaps by reversing vasospasm as well as protecting the kidney from raised intracellular and mitrochondrial levels of calcium.

Early oliguric phase

In the early oliguric phase, most patients are fluid overloaded due to delayed recognition of the onset of ARF, often exacerbated by 'volume challenges' administered in an attempt to restore urine output. Although the plasma sodium concentration may be low, total body sodium is usually normal or increased. In extreme cases, the combination of *salt and water overload* can produce peripheral and pulmonary oedema, sometimes with hypertension, and these constitute an indication for early dialysis. It is therefore important to *fluid restrict* patients as soon as the diagnosis of intrinsic ARF is certain. Intravenous fluids should be limited to the volume required to replace insensible losses. In general, administration of sodium and potassium should be avoided except to replace specific identified losses exactly. *Drug doses* must be modified appropriately at this time.

Although the rising blood urea and creatinine levels seldom create a problem at this stage, dangerous *hyper-kalaemia* can occur early, particularly if potassium supplements continue to be administered after the onset of renal impairment. A combination of factors contribute to hyperkalaemia including reduced renal excretion and increased cellular release of potassium. The latter may be attributable to direct tissue trauma, haemolysis, protein catabolism, infection, steroids and the effects of acidosis. The rate of increase in plasma potassium, as well as the rise in urea and creatinine levels, therefore depends largely on the degree of catabolism and the extent of any tissue damage, so it is particularly rapid in those with severe trauma, sepsis or rhabdomyolysis.

Hyperkalaemia produces characteristic ECG abnormalities (elevated and pointed T waves, flattened or absent P waves followed by widened QRS complexes) and if unchecked can culminate in cardiac arrest in diastole. Although the rise in potassium levels may be attenuated by the use of *calcium exchange resins* (15–30 g orally or rectally and repeated as necessary), dangerous hyperkalaemia should be treated with *dextrose and insulin* (e.g. 50 ml 50% dextrose with 20 units soluble insulin) and/or correction of the acidosis with 8.4% *sodium bicarbonate* (to encourage cellular uptake of potassium). In more urgent cases, 10–20 ml 10% *calcium chloride* can be used to counteract the effects of hyperkalaemia on the myocardium. These measures will only alleviate the situation temporarily and preparations for dialysis should begin immediately. In extreme cases with marked bradycardia or asystole, isoprenaline or cardiac massage may sustain the patient until hyperkalaemia can be corrected by dialysis.

Because metabolic acidosis develops relatively slowly, and is compensated by hypocarbia, it is not usually a problem at this stage unless it is a significant component of the precipitating illness (e.g. septic shock, low cardiac output or diabetic ketoacidosis). Administration of bicarbonate, (which will exacerbate salt and water overload, may precipitate hypocalcaemia and causes a left shift of the oxyhaemoglobin dissociation curve) is therefore rarely indicated, except to counteract hyperkalaemia and when acidosis is extreme.

Occasionally, severe malignant *hypertension* complicates the early oliguric phase of ARF and this should be controlled (e.g. by administering hydralazine or an infusion of sodium nitroprusside).

Established ARF

In the phase of established ARF, the measures outlined above must be combined with the *removal of uraemic toxins* and with *nutritional support*.

Derangement of other functions of the kidney such as erythropoietin production, the formation of 1,25-dihydroxycholecalciferol and the catabolism of parathyroid hormone, are of limited clinical relevance in established ARF. It is not necessary to administer allo-purinol since the risks of uric acid-induced interstitial nephritis are negligible. Similarly, the administration of aluminium hydroxide or other phosphate-binders to reduce serum phosphate levels is unnecessary because metastatic calcification is extremely unlikely.

COMPLICATIONS OF ESTABLISHED ARF AND URAEMIA (Kleinknecht et al., 1972)

Many of the systemic manifestations of uraemia may be due to 'middle molecules'; blood urea and creatinine levels are only an approximate guide to blood levels of these and other toxic substances. *Gastrointestinal disturbances* are prominent and include stomatitis, anorexia, nausea, vomiting, hiccups and diarrhoea or constipation. The introduction of routine antacid prophylaxis, better nutrition and more aggressive dialysis may all have contributed to the virtual disappearance of gastrointestinal haemorrhage as an immediate cause of death (Cameron, 1986).

Central nervous system (CNS) effects may progress from mild confusion, with decreased responsiveness, to agitation, disorientation, hyperreflexia, twitching, irritability and, occasionally, frank convulsions. The EEG changes usually indicate a non-specific metabolic disturbance. These CNS manifestations tend to occur only in severe uraemia and may resolve slowly, even when uraemia has been controlled with dialysis.

Acute uraemic fibrinous pericarditis, which can cause cardiac tamponade, is now rarely encountered because of the ready availability of dialysis techniques.

Haemopoietic disturbances are common. Erythropoiesis is depressed, presumably by uraemic toxins, and this, sometimes exacerbated by haemolysis and blood loss, is responsible for the inevitable normocytic, normochromic anaemia in which the haemoglobin concentration falls inexorably to around 7 g/100 ml. Decreased erythropoietin production may also contribute to the development of anaemia in ARF. This anaemia is not, in itself, an indication for blood transfusion. *Coagulopathies*, manifested as a purpuric rash or frank haemorrhage, are also common and are usually caused by a defect in platelet function, although they may occasionally be related to DIC (see Chapter 4). The platelet defect is probably due to retained toxins since the abnormality can be corrected by dialysis (Lindsay et al., 1975). These haematological abnormalities resolve during the diuretic phase, when the patient may require supplements of iron, folic acid or, rarely, vitamin B_{12}.

Uraemic patients are very susceptible to *infection* as a result of impaired leucocyte function, antibody formation and cellular immune responses. In one study, 74% of patients with ATN developed an infection and this caused 54% of the deaths (McMurray et al., 1978). The

infection may have been present initially (e.g. related to trauma or surgery) or may arise during the period of ARF (e.g. peritonitis). Pulmonary infections are also common, particularly in those requiring mechanical ventilation.

A number of events may precipitate *respiratory failure* in patients with ARF including:

- pulmonary oedema;
- pneumonia;
- a variety of cerebral disorders (e.g. hypertensive encephalopathy and cerebral oedema, the effects of marked uraemia or the accumulation of sedative drugs).

The combination of acute respiratory failure and acute renal failure is difficult to manage and is associated with a poor prognosis.

BLOOD PURIFICATION

In general, one of the blood purification techniques discussed below should be started early and performed frequently or continuously since this not only controls hyperkalaemia and uraemia, but also facilitates adequate nutritional support and simplifies drug and fluid therapy. In this way the incidence of complications may be reduced (Kleinknecht et al., 1972).

Active intervention is required when there are uraemic symptoms, salt and water overload, or dangerous hyperkalaemia. Other biochemical indices include urea > 30-50 mmol/l, creatinine > 0.7-1.5 mmol/l and bicarbonate < 12 mmol/l. Elective removal of water and electrolytes may be required to accommodate the fluid load of total parenteral nutrition or blood transfusion. In non-catabolic ARF, these limits may not be exceeded for up to six days after the onset of oliguria, whereas early intervention is usually required (within 24-48 hours) in hypercatabolic patients.

Techniques using diffusion (dialysis) (**Fig. 12.1**)

The choice between peritoneal and haemodialysis depends on a number of factors including the available facilities, the expertise of the staff and the type of patient requiring treatment.

Peritoneal dialysis (PD)
Indications and contraindications. PD is relatively simple, efficient and requires the minimum of expertise and equipment. It can be used when haemodialysis is contraindicated or the facilities for its use are not available, when vascular access is difficult and when there is a risk of bleeding or circulatory instability. It is also indicated in the management of some cases of pancreatitis. It

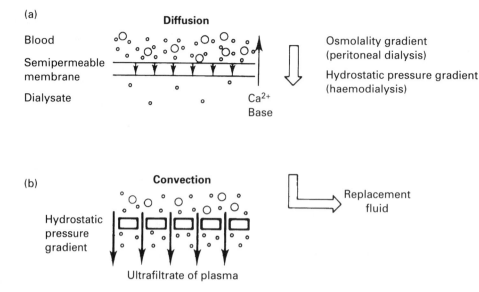

Fig. 12.1 Principles of blood purification. (a) Diffusion—solutes are removed by diffusion across a semipermeable membrane (synthetic in haemodialysis, peritoneum in peritoneal dialysis) according to their concentration gradient. Fluid is removed by hydrostatic pressure (haemodialysis) or osmosis (peritoneal dialysis). (b) Convection—the ultrafiltrate is replaced by a sterile electrolyte solution that has a similar composition to the dialysate used in haemodialysis.

should generally be avoided in those with respiratory difficulty (since it impedes diaphragmatic movement) and in the presence of faecal fistulae, abdominal wall infection, colostomy or tense ascites, as well as following aortic surgery. In patients with intra-abdominal adhesions from previous surgery or distended bowel, there is a significant risk of perforating the bowel during insertion of the catheter. PD may not control uraemia in the hypercatabolic patient.

Technique.

- Before inserting the PD catheter the bladder must be emptied.
- Using an aseptic technique and local anaesthesia, a trocar and semi-rigid teflon catheter is usually inserted in the midline 2-10 cm below the umbilicus, although positions more laterally near the iliac fossae may also be used.
- Once the parietal peritoneum has been penetrated, the catheter is directed downwards into the pelvis. The catheter can be sited more easily, and the risk of bowel perforation reduced by filling the peritoneal cavity with 1-2 litres of dialysis fluid before manoeuvring the catheter.
- Movement of the catheter in relation to the anterior abdominal wall must be restricted by firmly enclosing the exposed portion of the catheter with a foam-rubber pad and an adhesive dressing.

For long-term PD, a soft silastic Tenckhoff catheter is placed surgically.

In adults, a continuous flow system, with minimal dwell time, should be used to reduce the risk of catheter blockage. The aim is to achieve a total exchange of approximately 40 l/day using cycles of 1-2 l. For example, 1-2 l of dialysate is run in as rapidly as possible, is left in the peritoneal cavity for about 30 minutes and then allowed to drain by gravity over about 20 minutes. Each cycle therefore lasts approximately 60 minutes. During early cycles the entire volume instilled may not be removed because a pelvic reservoir of 1-2 l of fluid may be required.

Water is removed in proportion to the osmotic pressure gradient created by the glucose content of the dialysate. A glucose concentration of about 1.5% is approximately isotonic, while solutions containing up to about 4% glucose can be substituted in patients with fluid overload. Dialysate is usually supplied without potassium, but this may be added in the appropriate concentration should there be a tendency to hypokalaemia. During early cycles 500-1000 u heparin can be added to each dialysate exchange to prevent occlusion of the catheter by fibrin clots.

Monitoring. Cycle times as well as the volumes of fluid instilled and removed must be closely monitored. The circulating volume should be regularly assessed and plasma electrolytes, urea and creatinine should be determined at least daily. The most reliable means of assessing fluid balance is, however, body weight. The blood glucose level should be checked frequently, especially when hypertonic solutions, which may precipitate hyperglycaemia, are used. The returned dialysate should be inspected for turbidity and cultured daily.

Complications

- *Inadequate drainage of dialysate* is usually due to malposition of the catheter or obstruction by a fibrin clot. The catheter should be flushed with saline and repositioned or replaced.
- *Leakage of dialysate* around the catheter can usually be controlled with a purse string suture, but when pleural effusions develop, PD should be discontinued.
- *Pain* is usually felt deep in the pelvis and requires repositioning of the catheter, but may also occur at the end of inflow due to overdistension. Persistent pain and tenderness may be indicative of *peritonitis* in which case a sample of the dialysate return should be sent for Gram stain, culture and sensitivities, while broad-spectrum antibiotics are instilled into the peritoneal cavity and dialysis is continued. In those with severe infection, antibiotics should also be administered systemically. Peritonitis can be due to *bowel perforation*, which may be associated with sudden watery diarrhoea and faeculent dialysate return. A conservative approach with antibiotic administration and continued PD via a different catheter is usually adequate, but surgical exploration is indicated in those who fail to respond.
- *Significant bleeding* is an unusual complication of PD.
- *Cardiorespiratory disturbances* may be precipitated by PD and include hypovolaemia, arrhythmias (due to hypokalaemia and increased vagal tone due to abdominal distension), basal atelectasis and chest infections.
- *Metabolic disturbances* associated with PD include hyperglycaemia, hypokalaemia and hypernatraemia.

Haemodialysis (**Fig. 12.2**)

Practical considerations. Haemodialysis removes solutes primarily by passive diffusion across a synthetic semipermeable membrane, the rate of removal depending on solute size and its concentration gradient between plasma and dialysate. Clearance of small molecules such as electrolytes, urea and creatinine is proportional to the permeability of the dialysing membrane, the duration of dialysis and blood and dialysate flow rates. Clearance of larger molecules such as the 'middle molecules' is primarily related to membrane porosity and dialysis duration, and is fairly independent of flow rates. Solute removal can therefore be controlled by adjusting the membrane surface area and the duration of dialysis. Membrane permeability depends on the type of machine used, dialysate flow is not normally a limiting factor for solute clearance although blood flow may be limited by vascular access and cardiovascular status.

Removal of plasma water (ultrafiltration) is achieved by applying a hydrostatic pressure gradient across the dialysis membrane. The rate of water removal is determined primarily by the pressure gradient, but also depends on the permeability and surface area of the membrane. The pressure gradient is increased by raising the pressure on the blood side (by increasing the resistance to blood outflow) or by applying a negative pressure on the dialysate side of the membrane.

Vascular access is achieved using either a percutaneous double-lumen central venous catheter or an

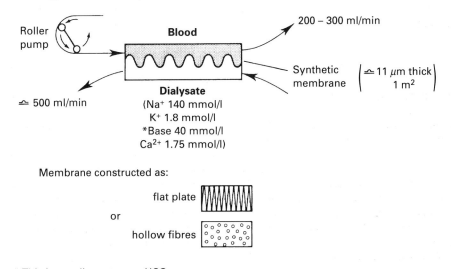

Fig. 12.2 Principles of haemodialysis.

arterio-venous (A-V) shunt created, for example, between the radial artery and the cephalic vein or the posterior tibial artery and the long saphenous vein. The rates of flow through A-V shunts are usually less than can be achieved via large-bore venous catheters.

Anticoagulation is usually achieved by administering heparin as a low-dose infusion (500–1000 u/hour) or as a bolus injection of 70–100 u/kg followed by smaller doses every 1–3 hours.

Haemodialysis is performed intermittently for periods of 4–6 hours either on alternate days or daily.

Indications. Because haemodialysis is a more efficient technique than PD, and corrects the metabolic disturbances more rapidly, it is traditionally the preferred method for the hypercatabolic patient. It can also be used when there are contraindications to PD such as intra-abdominal pathology. Other advantages of haemodialysis include early mobilization of the patient between sessions and a lower risk of infection.

Complications. The incidence of *bleeding* due to heparinization is small, but invasive procedures should be avoided just before, during or immediately after haemodialysis. Significant bleeding usually only arises in those with pre-existing pathology such as peptic ulceration or a coagulopathy. In those particularly at risk (e.g. patients who have recently had a cerebrovascular accident or a severe head injury) in whom haemodialysis is essential, anticoagulation with prostacyclin may be a safer alternative, although this is expensive and may cause hypotension. 'Regional heparinization', in which protamine is infused into the blood returning to the patient, has been recommended, but this is a difficult technique and a low-dose heparin infusion is probably equally effective.

The major disadvantage of haemodialysis is *hypotension*. This is most marked when attempts are made to remove large volumes of fluid by ultrafiltration, especially in those with cardiovascular instability or autonomic dysfunction. The cause has not yet been established, but it is thought that the combination of a non-sterile dialysate, a cuprophane membrane and acetate as the base in the dialysate solution in some way prevents the normal vasoconstrictor response to hypovolaemia (Shaldon *et al.*, 1983; Bradley *et al.*, 1990). If simultaneous dialysis and ultrafiltration leads to cardiovascular instability, the ultrafiltration can be performed as a separate procedure (Bradley *et al.*, 1990), either on different days or sequentially on the same day. In ARF outcome has been shown to be worse in patients treated using a cuprophane membrane, which induces complement and activates the lipoxygenase pathway, than in those dialysed with a biocompatible polyacrylonitrile membrane (Schiffl *et al.*, 1994).

Dialysis disequilibrium is related to the rapid onset of hypo-osmolality and causes headache, nausea, vomiting, cramps, restlessness, hypotension, and, when severe, seizures and coma. The syndrome is thought to be caused by cerebral oedema induced by a fall in plasma osmolality in the absence of changes in intracellular osmolality.

Hypoxaemia can be precipitated by microembolization of aggregated leucocytes and diffusion of carbon dioxide into the dialysate leading to hypoventilation.

Other problems of haemodialysis include the removal of water-soluble drugs and vitamins, and difficulties related to vascular access.

Haemofiltration

Haemofiltration relies on massive convection (see **Fig. 12.1**) of plasma water across a porous membrane and its replacement with an electrolyte solution. Solutes are removed only in proportion to their concentration in plasma, and large volumes of ultrafiltrate must therefore be produced to control uraemia and hyperkalaemia. Membranes may be made of polysulfone, polyamide or polyacrylonitrile, configured either as hollow fibres or flat plates. Current evidence favours the use of parallel-plate filters made of polyacrylonitrile, which have a low flow resistance (Yohay *et al.*, 1992) and are associated with greater diffusive clearances of small molecular weight molecules compared to hollow fibre dialysis. The pores in the membrane only allow the passage of molecules with molecular weights of up to about 30,000; therefore, albumin and other proteins are not lost from the circulation.

When performed *intermittently* (**Fig. 12.3**), a pumped flow rate of 400 ml/min can produce approximately 30 litres of ultrafiltrate in about four hours. This technique is particularly effective in the treatment of diuretic-resistant fluid overload in patients with or without renal failure since large amounts of fluid can be removed without significantly altering osmolality, and acetate uptake is avoided. Hypotension is uncommon during isolated ultrafiltration, probably because the integrity of the peripheral vascular responses to hypovolaemia is not disrupted by dialysis (Bradley *et al.*, 1990). The length of each session is determined by the volume of ultrafiltrate required to control uraemia, while the volume of infusate used to replace the fluid loss is adjusted to achieve the appropriate fluid balance.

Continuous haemofiltration. These techniques provide gradual continuous fluid removal and blood purification, thereby avoiding haemodynamic disturbances and disequilibrium. They are therefore well tolerated by critically ill patients with cardiovascular or respiratory instability. Additional fluid loads such as parenteral nutrition are easily accommodated, there is considerable flexibility in achieving the desired fluid balance and blood chemistry is well controlled. Continuous tech-

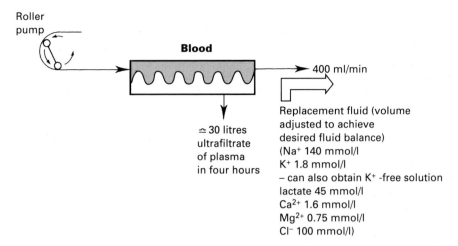

Roller pump

Blood

400 ml/min

$\simeq$ 30 litres ultrafiltrate of plasma in four hours

Replacement fluid (volume adjusted to achieve desired fluid balance)
(Na^+ 140 mmol/l
K^+ 1.8 mmol/l
– can also obtain K^+-free solution
lactate 45 mmol/l
Ca^{2+} 1.6 mmol/l
Mg^{2+} 0.75 mmol/l
Cl^- 100 mmol/l)

Fig. 12.3 Principles of intermittent haemofiltration.

niques also avoid the need for dedicated dialysis staff and can be used in neonatal and paediatric patients, as well as in adults. Occasionally they are useful in patients without renal failure who are fluid overloaded or receiving large volumes of fluid. Finally, continuous haemofiltration has been shown to remove inflammatory mediators such as the cytokines (Bellomo *et al.*, 1993), from the circulation of patients with sepsis, septic shock and adult respiratory distress syndrome (ARDS), an observation that should encourage the early use of these techniques in such patients.

Continuous   arterio-venous   haemofiltration (CAVH) . This entails the creation of an A-V shunt or percutaneous cannulation of the femoral artery and vein, the haemofilter being positioned between the arterial and venous limbs of a simple extracorporeal circuit without pumps. CAVH has been shown to be a safe and effective technique in critically ill septic patients with ARF (Ossenkoppele *et al.*, 1985).

The ultrafiltration rate and solute clearance is determined by the balance between the hydrostatic and oncotic transmembrane pressure gradients. Blood flow through the filter and the hydrostatic pressure generated is dependent primarily on the patient's systemic blood pressure, but is also influenced by blood viscosity and the quality of vascular access. Adequate filtration rates can usually be achieved with mean arterial blood pressures above 50-70 mm Hg. Larger, shorter, more centrally positioned cannulae are associated with higher filtration rates and many therefore prefer percutaneous cannulation of the femoral vessels to creation of an A-V shunt using the smaller distal vessels of the arm or leg. There is, however, an increased risk of vascular damage and infection with femoral cannulation; also patient movement can obstruct blood flow and this may restrict mobilization.

The hydrostatic pressure gradient can be increased by adjusting the height of the ultrafiltration column. By raising the filter and placing the collecting system on the floor the negative gravitational pressure can be increased by 0.74 mm Hg for every 1 cm of additional column height. This effect can be maximized by elevating the patient's bed. Venous back pressure (e.g. due to poor venous access or raised intrathoracic pressure) decreases flow through the filter and predisposes to clotting.

When conditions are optimal, flow rates through the filter may be sufficient to produce as much as 15-20 litres of ultrafiltrate per day. This volume can be reduced, if necessary, by applying a gate clamp to the collecting system tubing. The volume removed as ultrafiltrate is then replaced with blood, plasma, nutrients and crystalloid replacement fluid to achieve the desired fluid balance. Upstream (pre-dilutional) administration of replacement fluid has the advantage of reducing oncotic pressure and viscosity, thereby increasing clearance and reducing the risk of clotting.

In patients without a bleeding diathesis; anticoagulation can be achieved with a bolus of 15-20 u/kg of heparin followed by a maintenance infusion into the arterial side of the filter to maintain the activated partial thromboplastin time (APTT) at approximately 45 seconds. Alternatively, and certainly in those with a coagulopathy, thrombocytopenia or an increased risk of haemorrhagic complications, heparin can be administered as a low-dose continuous pre-filter infusion at a rate of 5-10 u/kg/h. It has been suggested that the use of *prostacyclin* (2-3 ng/kg/min) in combination with *low-dose heparin* (250 u/h) may limit platelet activation, prolong the life of the filter and reduce the risk of bleeding. In those who develop heparin-induced thrombocytopenia and in other high-risk cases, prostacyclin may be used alone in a dose of 2.5-5 ng/kg/min. Experience with low molecular weight heparin is at present limited.

(a)

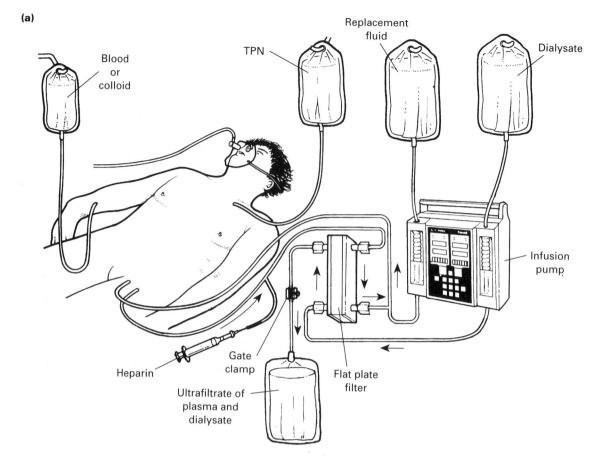

Fig. 12.4 (a) Continuous arterio-venous haemofiltration with dialysis (CAVHD).

Continuous A-V haemofiltration with dialysis (CAVHD) (**Fig. 12.4a**) (Stevens *et al.*, 1988). In catabolic critically ill patients biochemical control with CAVH may only be achieved by exchanging very large volumes of fluid, up to 20–40 l/day, or by using supplemental intermittent haemodialysis (Ossenkoppele *et al.*, 1985). CAVHD, which combines diffusion with convection to produce more effective biochemical control, is therefore preferred in catabolic patients, when systemic blood pressure is low and when vascular access is suboptimal.

Dialysate, usually warmed to 37°C, is administered countercurrent to blood flow using an infusion pump at a rate of 1 l/h. Provided blood flow is greater than dialysate flow there should be complete equilibration of small solutes across the membrane. Creatinine clearances range between approximately 13 and 20 ml/min. Solute transfer from dialysate to blood also occurs and the composition of the dialysate can be altered by adding bicarbonate to correct acidosis or potassium to control hypokalaemia.

Continuous veno-venous haemofiltration (CVVH) (**Fig. 12.4b**). Pump-driven haemofiltration allows better control of ultrafiltration, especially in those with poor vascular access and hypotension. CVVH may be associated with improved survival compared to CAVH, perhaps because the larger volumes of ultrafiltrate produced clear toxins and mediators from the circulation (Storck *et al.*, 1991). The increased complexity related to the inclusion of a pump in the circuit does not seem to result in increased complications or an increase in nursing staff requirements. Indeed the use of a single venous cannula appears to reduce the incidence of access-related complications. A dialysis component can be added (CVVHD) to improve biochemical control with only a minimal further increase in complexity. CVVHD is currently considered by many to be the technique of choice for managing ARF in the critically ill.

Complications of continuous haemofiltration. The relative ease with which CAVH(D) and CVVH(D) can be instituted belies the fact that they are potentially extremely dangerous, labour-intensive techniques that require considerable expertise. In particular there is an ever-present danger of serious errors in fluid and electrolyte balance. Complications related to vascular access include infection, thrombosis, haemorrhage and aneur-

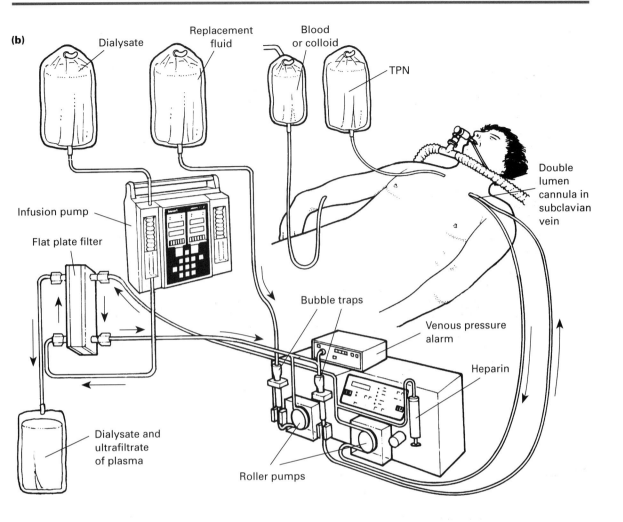

Fig. 12.4 (b) Continuous veno-venous haemodialfiltration (CVVHD).

ysm formation. It is important to consider the potential for continuous haemofiltration/dialysis to profoundly alter the pharmacokinetics of drugs administered to patients with renal failure.

NUTRITIONAL SUPPORT

The provision of adequate nutritional support is essential (see also Chapter 10). Hyperalimentation may reduce mortality rates, particularly in high-risk patients with infectious or haemorrhagic complications, and may even shorten the period of impaired renal function (Abel *et al.*, 1973). In general, patients should receive appropriate quantities of protein and energy, either enterally or parenterally, regardless of the amount of fluid and nitrogen required. Dialysis or haemofiltration should then be used to prevent fluid overload and control uraemia. There is some evidence to suggest that the

use of continuous haemofiltration to facilitate parenteral nutrition with a high-protein feed leads to improved survival in surgical ARF (Bartlett *et al.*, 1986).

CAVHD is associated with significant losses of non-urea nitrogen across the filter, while the use of a glucose-containing dialysate provides an important source of carbohydrate (Bellomo *et al.*, 1991). It may therefore be appropriate to increase the nitrogen content of feeds given to patients on continuous haemofiltration. Lipids are not removed during CAVHD and do not appear to be trapped in the filter.

GENERAL MANAGEMENT CONSIDERATIONS

Patients with ARF are extremely susceptible to infection. Meticulous mouth care is required to prevent oral candidiasis and, in those who are essentially anuric, the urethral catheter should be removed to minimize the risk of urinary tract infection. Careful adjustment of drug doses, particularly H_2-receptor antagonists and antibiotics, has already been mentioned. If possible, the patient should be weighed daily to assess fluid balance, although in practice this can be difficult in intensive care patients. Finally, it is clearly essential to treat the underlying condition (e.g. by performing a laparotomy in those with intra-abdominal infection) since ARF rarely recovers in the presence of persistent sepsis.

Diuretic phase

In patients with ATN, kidney function will normally recover spontaneously. This is heralded by the onset of a diuresis, usually 5–20 days after the initial insult, although in some cases this may occur within 48 hours or be delayed for up to 8–10 weeks.

Initially, the GFR remains relatively low; consequently blood urea and creatinine levels may continue to rise for a few days after the onset of a diuresis. Because tubular function is still impaired, the patient may lose large quantities of sodium, potassium and water, as well as phosphate and magnesium, although in some cases the diuresis may simply represent mobilization of accumulated solutes and water. Urinary losses must therefore be closely monitored; as an approximate guide, half the total fluid and electrolytes excreted should be replaced. Frequent careful assessment of each individual is, however, essential to avoid water and electrolyte (particularly potassium) depletion on the one hand, or persistent polyuria due to excessive fluid administration on the other.

Non-oliguric ARF (Anderson *et al.*, 1977)

Non-oliguric ARF probably represents a less severe form of vasomotor nephropathy in which the GFR is maintained at approximately 2–5 ml/min, urine continues to be produced and the urinary sodium concentration is approximately 50 mmol/l. This form of ARF is becoming more common, possibly due to the use of dopamine and diuretics as well as the increasing number of cases of tubular necrosis induced by toxic drugs. Dialysis is required less frequently or not at all, complications (gastrointestinal bleeding, sepsis, acidosis, and neurological disturbances) are reduced, recovery is more rapid and the mortality is lower.

Management of some specific types of ARF

RHABDOMYOLYSIS

The urine output must be maintained at more than 1.5–2 ml/kg/h by aggressive volume loading and the adminis-

tration of mannitol. Loop diuretics should be avoided since they have the theoretical disadvantage of acidifying the urine. The urine should be maintained alkaline by the systemic administration of sodium bicarbonate to prevent precipitation of myoglobin in the renal tubules.

ACUTE INTERSTITIAL NEPHRITIS

When nephritis is due to an acute hypersensitivity reaction to a drug, removal of the offending agent may prevent further deterioration in renal function. Recovery can, however, be slow and incomplete, although the administration of corticosteroids usually encourages recovery.

HYPERURICAEMIC ARF

Treatment consists of rehydration and haemodialysis, followed by alkalinization and the administration of allopurinol.

ARF DUE TO GLOMERULAR DISEASE

Most cases of *acute crescentic glomerulonephritis* progress rapidly and inexorably to end-stage renal failure. This is also generally the case in *Goodpasture's syndrome*, although high-dose steroids, immunosuppressants and plasma exchange may be beneficial. Although the combination of these measures can usually rapidly control pulmonary haemorrhage, the outcome of the renal lesion is clearly related to the severity of renal impairment at presentation. In over half of the patients, glomerular basement membrane antibody had disappeared from the circulation at two months, and this appears to be permanent (Lockwood *et al.*, 1981).

VASCULAR ARF

Acute renal artery occlusion requires immediate surgery or fibrinolytic therapy, followed by heparinization. In acute renal vein thrombosis, the patient should be heparinized and/or receive streptokinase.

ARF DUE TO OBSTRUCTION

The extent of renal parenchymal damage is related to the duration, degree and site of the obstruction, as well as the presence of infection. It is therefore imperative to relieve the obstruction as quickly as possible, although urinary tract instrumentation or surgery may be complicated by bacteraemia, endotoxaemia and septic shock. Surgery can be preceded by dialysis. Following relief of the obstruction there may be a massive diuresis, primarily due to defective tubular function, but also as a result of the accumulation of urea and other osmotically active molecules.

PROGNOSIS OF ARF (Kleinknecht et al., 1972; McMurray et al., 1978; Cameron, 1986, Barton et al., 1993)

The final outcome of ARF depends on the aetiology; mortality rates range from approximately 35-60% in medical, surgical or trauma patients, 0-30% in those cases related to obstetric disasters, and 75% or more in burns patients. When renal failure is the only problem, mortality rates may be as low as 8%, but in the remainder (i.e. those patients likely to require intensive care), the average mortality is higher than 60%. The presence of sepsis, particularly intra-abdominal sepsis, also adversely affects the prognosis, but age does not. Another factor affecting outcome is the site of surgery, mortality rates being particularly high following gastro-intestinal surgery, especially when the bowel rather than the stomach is involved (Cameron, 1986).

Although the overall mortality may have improved only slightly, if at all, over the last 25 years or so, this may be partly explained by changes in the type of patients being treated. Improvements in resuscitation, evacuation of casualties and surgical techniques have resulted in the survival of more seriously ill patients, while there has been a reduction in the number of obstetric patients with ARF (who have the best prognosis) and an increase in those associated with generalized sepsis, liver failure and cardiac arrest. Recently an overall mortality of 53% was reported in a large series of intensive care patients with ARF treated by continuous haemofiltration, and there was evidence that survival rates increased during the course of the study (Barton et al., 1993). It is worth noting that most patients now die as a result of the precipitating cause, rather than as a direct result of the renal failure.

In patients who do recover, tubular lesions usually heal completely and histological appearances may be normal 3-4 weeks after the insult. There is usually no obvious residual renal impairment and kidney function has normally recovered to about 80% of normal after one year.

REFERENCES

Abel RM, Beck CH, Abbott WM et al. (1973) Improved survival from acute renal failure after treatment with intravenous essential L-amino acids and glucose. Results of a prospective, double-blind study. New England Journal of Medicine 288: 695-699.

Anderson RJ, Linas SL, Berns AS et al. (1977) Non-oliguric acute renal failure. New England Journal of Medicine 296: 1134-1138.

Badr KF, Kelley VE, Rennke HG & Brenner BM (1986) Roles for thromboxane A₂ and leukotrienes in endotoxin-induced acute renal failure. Kidney International 30: 474-480.

Baldwin L, Henderson A & Hickman P (1994) Effect of post-operative low-dose dopamine on renal function after elective major vascular surgery. Annals of Internal Medicine 120: 744-747.

Barry KG, Cohen A, Knochel JP et al. (1961) Mannitol infusion II: the prevention of acute functional renal failure during resection of an aneurysm of the abdominal aorta. New England Journal of Medicine 264: 967-971.

Bartlett RH, Mault JR, Dechert RE, Palmer J, Swartz RD & Port FK (1986) Continuous arteriovenous hemofiltration: improved survival in surgical acute renal failure? Surgery 100: 400-408.

Barton IK, Hilton PJ, Taub NA et al. (1993) Acute renal failure treated by haemofiltration: factors affecting outcome. Quarterly Journal of Medicine 86: 81-90.

Bellomo R, Martin H, Parkin G, Love J, Kearley Y & Boyce N (1991) Continuous arteriovenous haemodiafiltration in the critically ill: influence on major nutrient balances. Intensive Care Medicine 17: 399-402.

Bellomo R, Tipping P & Boyce N (1993) Continuous veno-venous hemofiltration with dialysis removes cytokines from the circulaton of septic patients. Critical Care Medicine 21: 522-526.

Birch AG, Zakheim RM, Jones LG & Barger AC (1967) Redistribution of renal blood flow produced by furosemide and ethacrynic acid. Circulation Research 21: 869-878.

Bradley JR, Evans DB & Cowley AJ (1990) Comparison of vascular tone during combined haemodialysis with ultrafiltration and during ultrafiltration followed by haemodialysis: a possible mechanism for dialysis hypotension. British Medical Journal 300: 1312.

Brezis M, Rosen S, Silva P & Epstein FH (1984) Transport activity modifies thick ascending limb damage in the isolated perfused kidney. Kidney International 25: 65-72.

Brezis M, Rosen S, Stoff JS, Spokes K, Silva P & Epstein FH (1986) Inhibition of prostaglandin synthesis in rat kidney perfused with and without erythrocytes: implication for analgesic nephropathy. Mineral and Electrolyte Metabolism 12: 326-332.

Cameron JS (1986) Acute renal failure in the intensive care unit today. Intensive Care Medicine 12: 64-70.

Cox JW, Baehler RW, Sharma H et al. (1974) Studies of the mechanism of oliguria in a model of unilateral acute renal failure. Journal of Clinical Investigation 53: 1546-1558.

Cronin RE, De Torrente A, Miller PD et al. (1978) Pathogenic mechanisms in early norepinephrine-induced acute renal failure: functional and histological correlates of protection. Kidney International 14: 115-125.

Dawson JL (1964) Jaundice and anoxic renal damage: protective effect of mannitol. *British Medical Journal* **i**: 810-811.

De Torrente A, Miller PD, Cronin RE *et al.* (1978) Effects of furosemide and acetylcholine in norepinephrine-induced acute renal failure. *American Journal of Physiology* **235**: F131-F136.

Flores J, DiBona DR, Beck CH & Leaf A (1972) The role of cell swelling in ischemic renal damage and the protective effect of hypertonic solute. *Journal of Clinical Investigation* **51**: 118-126.

Gerber JG (1983) Role of prostaglandins in the hemodynamic and tubular effects of furosemide. *Federation Proceedings* **42**: 1707-1710.

Henderson IS, Beattie TJ & Kennedy AC (1980) Dopamine hydrochloride in oliguric states. *Lancet* **ii**: 827-828.

Hinshaw LB, Bradley GM & Carlson CH (1959) Effect of endotoxin on renal function in the dog. *American Journal of Physiology* **196**: 1127-1131.

Johnston PA, Bernard DB, Donohoe JF, Perrin NS & Levinsky NG (1979) Effect of volume expansion on hemodynamics of the hypoperfused rat kidney. *Journal of Clinical Investigation* **64**: 550-558.

Kleinknecht D, Jungers P, Chanard J, Barbanel C & Ganeval D (1972) Uremic and non-uremic complications in acute renal failure: evaluation of early and frequent dialysis on prognosis. *Kidney International* **1**: 190-196.

Kleinknecht D, Grunfeld JP, Gomez PC, Moreau JF & Gardia-Torres R (1973) Diagnostic procedures and long-term prognosis in bilateral renal cortical necrosis. *Kidney International* **4**: 390-400.

Kleinknecht D, Ganeval D, Gonzales-Duque LA & Fermanian J (1976) Furosemide in acute oliguric renal failure. A controlled trial. *Nephron* **17**: 51-58.

Kron IL, Harman PK & Nolan SP (1984) The measurement of intra-abdominal pressure as a criterion for abdominal re-exploration. *Annals of Surgery* **199**: 28-30.

Lindner A (1983) Synergism of dopamine and furosemide in diuretic-resistant, oliguric acute renal failure. *Nephron* **33**: 121-126.

Lindsay RM, Moorthy AV, Koens F & Linton AL (1975) Platelet function in dialyzed and non-dialyzed patients with chronic renal failure. *Clinical Nephrology* **4**: 52-57.

Lockwood CM, Pusey CD, Rees AJ & Peters DK (1981) Plasma exchange in the treatment of immune complex disease. *Clinics in Immunology and Allergy* **1**: 433-455.

Lucas CE, Zito JG, Carter KM, Cortez A & Stebner FC (1977) Questionable value of furosemide in preventing renal failure. *Surgery* **82**: 314-320.

Luke RG, Linton AL, Briggs JD & Kennedy AC (1965) Mannitol therapy in acute renal failure. *Lancet* **i**: 980-982.

MacAllister R & Vallance P (1994) Nitric oxide in essential and renal hypertension. *Journal of the American Society of Nephrology* **5**: 1057-1065.

McDonald RH, Goldberg LI, McNay JL & Tuttle EP Jr (1964) Effects of dopamine in man: augmentation of sodium excretion, glomerular filtration rate and renal plasma flow. *Journal of Clinical Investigation* **43**: 1116-1124.

McMurray SD, Luft FC, Maxwell DR *et al.* (1978) Prevailing patterns and predictor variables in patients with acute tubular necrosis. *Archives of Internal Medicine* **138**: 950-955.

Minuth AN, Terrell JB Jr & Suki WN (1976) Acute renal failure: a study of the course and prognosis of 104 patients and of the role of furosemide. *American Journal of Medical Science* **271**: 317-324.

Munn J, Tooley M, Bolsin S, Hronek I, Lowson S & Willcox J (1993) Effect of metoclopramide on renal vascular resistance index and renal function in patients receiving a low-dose infusion of dopamine. *British Journal of Anaesthesia* **71**: 379-382.

Myers BD & Moran SM (1986) Hemodynamically mediated acute renal failure. *New England Journal of Medicine* **314**: 97-105.

Ossenkoppele GJ, Van der Meulen J, Bronsveld W & Thijs LG (1985) Continuous arteriovenous hemofiltration as an adjunctive therapy for septic shock. *Critical Care Medicine* **13**: 102-104.

Parker S, Carlon GC, Isaacs M, Howland WS & Kahn RC (1981) Dopamine administration in oliguria and oliguric renal failure. *Critical Care Medicine* **9**: 630-632.

Polson RJ, Park GR, Lindrop MJ, Farman JV, Calne RY & Williams R (1987) The prevention of renal impairment in patients undergoing orthotopic liver grafting by infusion of low dose dopamine. *Anaesthesia* **42**: 15-19.

Reubi FC, Vorburger C & Tuckman J (1973) Renal distribution volumes of indocyanine green, [^{15}Cr]EDTA, and ^{24}Na in man during acute renal failure after shock. Implications for the pathogenesis of anuria. *Journal of Clinical Investigation* **52**: 223-235.

Shaldon S, Baldamus CA, Koch KM & Lysaght MJ (1983) Of sodium symptomatology and syllogism. *Blood Purification* **1**: 16-24.

Schiff H, Lang SM, König A, Strasser T, Haider MC & Held E (1994) Biocomptible membranes in acute renal failure: prospective case-controlled study. *Lancet* **344**: 570-572.

Shusterman N, Strom BL, Murray TG *et al.* (1987) Risk factors and outcome of hospital-acquired acute renal failure. Clinical epidemiologic study. *American Journal of Medicine* **83**: 65-71.

Stevens PE, Riley B, Davies SP, Gower PE, Brown EA & Kox W (1988) Continuous arteriovenous haemodialysis in critically ill patients. *Lancet* **ii**: 150-152.

Storck M, Hartl WH, Zimmerer E & Inthorn D (1991) Comparison of pump-driven and spontaneous continuous haemofiltration in postoperative acute renal failure. *Lancet* **337**: 452-455.

Thompson BT & Cockrill BA (1994) Renal-dose dopamine: a siren song? *Lancet* **344**: 7-8.

Wilkinson SP, Blendis LM & Williams R (1974) Frequency and type of renal and electrolyte disorders in fulminant hepatic failure. *British Medical Journal* **i**: 186-189.

Woolley JL, Barker GR, Jacobsen WK *et al.* (1988) Effect of the calcium entry blocker verapamil on renal ischemia. *Critical Care Medicine* **16**: 48-51.

Yohay DA, Butterly DW, Schwab SJ & Quarles LD (1992) Continuous arteriovenous hemodialysis: effect of dialyzer geometry. *Kidney International* **42**: 448-451.

13 Acute Liver Failure

TYPES OF ACUTE LIVER FAILURE

Fulminant hepatic failure

Fulminant hepatic failure (FHF) has been defined as a clinical syndrome developing as a result of massive necrosis of liver cells or any other sudden and severe impairment of hepatic function (Trey & Davidson, 1970). This definition includes the stipulation that there should be no history or evidence of pre-existing liver disease and that the signs of encephalopathy should appear within eight weeks of the onset of illness.

Late-onset hepatic failure

Late-onset hepatic failure can be diagnosed when the onset of encephalopathy is delayed to 8–26 weeks from the onset of symptoms. It may represent part of the spectrum of acute non-A, non-B viral hepatitis occurring in an older age group (Gimson & Williams, 1983). In general, bilirubin levels are less elevated and the prothrombin time less prolonged than in FHF, while the liver is small and ascites may be present.

Recently, in an attempt to standardize the nomenclature a new terminology has been proposed. This is based on the interval between jaundice and encephalopathy, the terms *hyperacute*, *acute* or *subacute liver failure* being applied depending on whether this interval is 0–7 days, 8–28 days or 29 days to 12 weeks respectively (O'Grady *et al.*, 1993). In this classification, in contrast to Trey & Davidson's original definition, cases with pre-existing symptomless chronic liver disease are included. This new terminology has not, however, received universal approval (Bernuau & Benhamou, 1993).

Acute-on-chronic liver failure

Acute-on-chronic liver failure occurs when an acute illness causes decompensation of pre-existing chronic liver disease. Usually the chronic liver impairment is related to hepatic cirrhosis (e.g. alcoholic, primary biliary, post-necrotic, sclerosing cholangitis), but is occasionally due to chronic active, or alcoholic, hepatitis, and is sometimes associated with infiltrative processes such as neoplasia or metabolic disorders.

Ischaemic/hypoxic hepatocellular damage

Ischaemic/hypoxic hepatocellular damage can occur in acute or chronic cardiac failure as well as following an episode of severe shock (haemorrhage, septic or cardiogenic) or hepatic vascular occlusion. It is now a very rare complication of cardiac surgery. In these cases there may be hepatomegaly and a marked rise in transaminases (> 1000 u/l) with a prolonged prothrombin time, but bilirubin levels are usually only moderately elevated. FHF is, however, rare following ischaemic liver damage and when it does occur the prognosis is poor.

CAUSES OF LIVER DYSFUNCTION IN CRITICAL ILLNESS

The causes of liver dysfunction in critical illness include:

- liver impairment associated with multiple organ failure (see Chapter 4);
- drug-induced liver damage;
- fatty infiltration of the liver precipitated by high calorie total parenteral nutrition (TPN);
- 'benign' postoperative cholestasis.

The latter may be due to a reduced ability to transport conjugated bilirubin and is usually associated with an increased bilirubin load (e.g. massive blood transfusion, resolving haematomas). Despite its name, mortality may be as high as 50%.

FULMINANT HEPATIC FAILURE

Causes (Table 13.1)

The most common cause of FHF in the UK is *paracetamol* hepatotoxicity, which in one series accounted for

48% of cases. *Viral hepatitis* was responsible for 37%, with hepatitis A being diagnosed in 32% and hepatitis B in 24% (Gimson & Williams, 1983). Other infective causes of FHF include hepatitis D (always occurs as a co-infection in those with hepatitis B, most often in drug abusers or following transfusion), hepatitis C virus (implicated in sporadic fulminant disease only rarely), a small group with non-A, non-B, non-C viral hepatitis (may be due to hepatitis E, although not so far in the UK), and *yellow fever. Epstein–Barr virus, cytomegalovirus, herpes simplex viruses* 1 and 2, and *varicella zoster* cause liver failure only rarely, but may contribute to the death of immunocompromised patients. Outside the UK, viral hepatitis is the most frequent cause of FHF accounting for about 70% of cases, while drug-induced liver failure is slightly less common. As well as paracetamol hepatotoxicity, idiosyncratic reactions to *antituberculosis drugs* (especially isoniazid), *monoamine oxidase inhibitors, tetracycline, sodium valproate* and *methyldopa* can cause FHF.

Severe hepatic necrosis may also occasionally follow *halothane* anaesthesia; the incidence is higher in females, the elderly and the obese, and is increased by multiple exposure. In addition, approximately 20% of patients undergoing repeated halothane anaesthesia have been found to have less severe forms of liver injury (Wright *et al.*, 1975).

FHF occurring during *pregnancy* (Williams & Ede, 1981) may be related to viral hepatitis or acute fatty liver. Severe hepatic dysfunction may also occasionally be related to toxaemia of pregnancy (HELLP syndrome, see Chapter 17) and can be caused by localized or systemic disseminated intravascular coagulation (DIC).

Poisoning with carbon tetrachloride, yellow phosphorus, mushrooms (*Amanita phalloides*) and alcohol can also be complicated by the development of FHF, while in children and young adults it is worth remembering that *Wilson's disease* can present acutely, although usually there is evidence of underlying chronic liver disease (chronic active hepatitis, cirrhosis). *Reye's syndrome* and *galactosaemia* may also cause FHF.

Mechanisms of FHF

VIRAL HEPATITIS

It is unclear why only some of those with *viral hepatitis* develop FHF while in others the infection pursues a more benign course. Hepatitis B virus has no direct cytopathic effect and the onset of massive hepatocellular necrosis does not appear to be related either to the strain of virus or the size of the inoculum. There is, however, some evidence to suggest that those who develop liver failure produce an enhanced immune response to all three antigenic determinants of the virus and that the excess antibody leads to the formation of immune complexes. The latter may then obstruct hepatic sinusoids and cause ischaemic necrosis of liver cells. It has also been suggested that activation of the host's immune responses with liberation of proinflammatory cytokines, may contribute to liver injury in viral hepatitis. In contrast, cellular damage following hepatitis A or non-A non-B infection is probably due to a direct cytopathic effect of the virus and in these cases it is likely that an impaired immune response contributes to the fulminant course.

HALOTHANE HEPATITIS

The exact mechanism of *halothane-induced FHF* remains unclear (Editorial, 1986). Nevertheless, it is known that in the presence of local hypoxia, halothane is metabolized in the liver by the reductive pathway to produce unstable radicals, which can damage liver cells. This hepatotoxicity may be enhanced when the hepatic microsomal enzyme cytochrome P-450 has been induced by previous exposure to drugs such as phenobarbitone or halothane itself. A number of features of halothane-associated FHF suggest that a hypersensitivity reaction is involved. For example, the syndrome is rare, it occurs after more than one exposure, and in many patients there is a history of a previous adverse reaction to halothane anaesthesia. It has been suggested, therefore, that FHF due to exposure to halothane is precipi-

Table 13.1 Causes of fulminant hepatic failure.

Infections	Viral hepatitis (Type A, Type B, Type C, Type D, Type E)
	Yellow fever
Poisons/chemicals	Paracetamol
	Halothane
	Monoamine oxidase inhibitors
	Tetracycline
	Sodium valproate
	Methyldopa
	Isoniazid
	Ethanol
	Phosphorus
	Carbon tetrachloride
	Amanita phalloides
Ischaemia	Shock
	Hepatic vascular occlusion
	Cardiac surgery
Miscellaneous	Fatty liver of pregnancy
	Reye's syndrome
	Wilson's disease
	Galactosaemia

tated by a hypersensitivity reaction to liver cell components rendered antigenic by interaction with halothane
or one of its metabolites. However, although a specific
halothane-related antibody can be detected in a proportion of patients, this is not always the case and it
seems that in some instances hepatitis attributed to halothane is in fact related to a viral infection (Neuberger *et
al.*, 1983), possibly exacerbated by the immunosuppression that can follow surgery and anaesthesia. It is also
possible that the antibody to 'halothane-altered hepatocytes' may arise as a secondary response to hepatocellular damage, rather than being the cause of cellular
destruction.

DRUG- AND TOXIN-INDUCED HEPATOTOXICITY

It is now known that hepatocellular damage following
paracetamol overdose is related to the production of a
toxic metabolite of paracetamol, which accumulates
when hepatic glutathione has been overwhelmed
(Black, 1980), but individuals vary considerably in their
susceptibility to liver damage induced by this agent. Paracetamol toxicity is dose dependent, but its effects are
exaggerated by drugs that induce cytochrome P-450 and
starvation and especially by alcohol. Therefore,
alcoholics taking therapeutic doses of paracetamol are
at risk of developing FHF, particularly after an episode
of 'binge' drinking. A number of specific antidotes are
available and management of paracetamol overdose is
discussed further in Chapter 18. In other drug- or toxin-
related causes of FHF, there is direct interference with
cellular metabolism.

Pathological changes in FHF

In FHF there is massive coagulative necrosis of liver cells
throughout the hepatic lobule, often with preservation
of the reticular framework, although ultimately the normal reticulin architecture of the lobule collapses. In viral
FHF the initial injury involves the periportal region, but
then spreads to encompass all zones. In contrast, drug-
induced injury and ischaemic damage begin around the
central vein and spread rapidly to involve the periportal
region. Severe fatty degeneration with accumulation of
microventricular fat in intact cells is seen in FHF associated with pregnancy, Reye's syndrome and tetracycline
administration.

Clinical features, investigations and
diagnosis (Tables 13.2 and 13.3)

The clinical features of FHF are largely attributable to
failure of the normal functions of the liver (synthesis,
storage and detoxification).

Table 13.2 Clinical features of fulminant hepatic failure.

Encephalopathy **Cerebral oedema**	
Jaundice	
Hepatic foetor	

Coagulopathy and bleeding	Reduced synthesis of clotting factors
	Thrombocytopenia
	Upper gastrointestinal haemorrhage
	Haemorrhage from nasopharynx,
	    respiratory tract, into
	    retroperitoneal space

Metabolic disturbances	Hypoglycaemia Metabolic alkalosis Lactic acidosis
Electrolyte disturbances	Hypokalaemia Hyponatraemia Hypernatraemia (unusual) Hypomagnesaemia Hypocalcaemia Hypophosphataemia
Cardiovascular dysfunction	Hypotension Vasodilatation Increased cardiac output Maldistribution of microcirculatory flow Increased capillary permeability
Respiratory dysfunction	Hyperventilation Intrapulmonary shunts Adult respiratory distress syndrome Pulmonary aspiration Atelectasis Bronchopneumonia
Impaired host defences and sepsis	Bacteraemia Spontaneous bacterial peritonitis Pneumonia Urinary tract infections
Renal dysfunction	Prerenal Acute tubular necrosis Hepatorenal syndrome
Pancreatitis	
Rare complications	Myocarditis Atypical pneumonia Aplastic anaemia Transverse myelitis Peripheral neuropathy

Table 13.3 Investigations in fulminant hepatic failure.	
Daily	Bilirubin, alkaline phosphatase, aminotransferases Haemoglobin, white blood count Prothrombin time, platelet count Urea, creatinine, sodium, potassium, magnesium Total protein, albumin, calcium, phosphate Chest radiograph, ECG
More frequently	Blood sugar Blood gases Acid–base
When indicated	Cultures of blood, urine, sputum, intravascular cannulae ECG, CT scan Ammonia levels Liver biopsy
To establish aetiology	Serological investigations for viral hepatitis Drug screen (especially paracetamol) Plasma caeruloplasmin concentration and urinary copper excretion for Wilson's disease

HEPATIC ENCEPHALOPATHY

The syndrome of FHF is characterized by an encephalopathy, which presents as an acute mental disturbance in the absence of signs of chronic liver disease. Usually this progresses over several days, but deep coma may develop in just a few hours. Occasionally the evolution of the disease is prolonged over several months (late-onset hepatic failure or subacute liver failure). Often, the initial changes are subtle (e.g. a change in personality, lack of attention to personal detail, perhaps with euphoria or depression and some slowing of mentation). Later, the patient may become confused and begin to behave inappropriately. Drowsiness is a prominent feature and some patients will sleep continually, although at this stage they can be roused. Difficulty with writing and an inability to reproduce shapes (e.g. a star) accurately are characteristic (*constructional apraxia*), and these skills can be tested repeatedly in order to follow the patient's progress. A 'flapping' tremor (*asterixis*) can often be demonstrated at this stage and is associated with a rigid facies, muscle stiffness and dysarthria. Many patients will then lose consciousness and progress to deep coma with hypertonia, decerebrate and/or decorticate posturing and disturbances of vital reflexes. Traditionally, hepatic encephalopathy is classified clinically into four grades as shown in **Table 13.4**. In practice, however, this classification is complicated by spontaneous fluctuations in coma grade and the necessity to administer sedatives to patients who are aggressive or to enable invasive procedures to be performed.

The *electroencephalographic (EEG) changes* (**Fig. 13.1**) correlate with the degree of cerebral dysfunction and although not necessary to establish the diagnosis, serial EEGs can be performed, together with regular clinical assessment of the grade of encephalopathy, in order to follow the patient's progress.

OTHER CLINICAL FEATURES

In the early stages, the liver may be palpable, although later in the illness it becomes small. Signs of chronic liver disease such as palmar erythema, spider naevi, splenomegaly and ascites are usually absent, but when FHF follows the more protracted course typical of non-A non-B hepatitis, both spider naevi and ascites may occur. In some cases, the patient may present with abdominal pain suggestive of an 'acute abdomen'.

The signs of encephalopathy are usually accompanied

Table 13.4 Hepatic encephalopathy.			
Grade	**Mental state**	**Asterixis**	**Electroencephalogram**
Grade I	Fluctuant mild confusion, euphoria, slowed mentation, disordered sleep rhythm	None	Normal
Grade II	Increasing drowsiness and inappropriate behaviour	Present	Becomes abnormal
Grade III	Severe confusion, semi-stuporose, but rousable and responsive to simple commands	Present if patient can cooperate	Always abnormal
Grade IV	Comatose, but may respond to painful stimuli	Lacking	Always abnormal

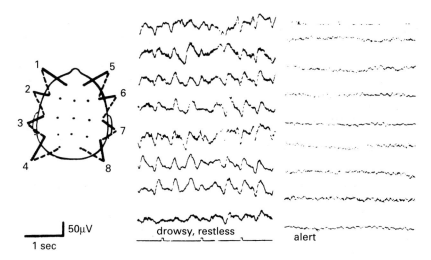

50μV

1 sec

drowsy, restless

alert

Fig. 13.1 Electroencephalographic changes in hepatic coma. High-voltage slow waves with some triphasic components best seen at the front of the head.

by rapidly increasing *jaundice* and a characteristic *'hepatic foetor',* an unpleasant sweetish smell due to exhalation of mercaptans. The rise in serum bilirubin concentration is associated with the appearance of bilirubin and its breakdown products in the urine. The diagnosis may, however, be difficult if the mental disturbance precedes the development of clinical jaundice. This occurs particularly in children with FHF and in adults who have taken a paracetamol overdose.

Serum aminotransferase levels are initially nearly always markedly elevated, often to more than 2000 u/l, but the alkaline phosphatase level is usually only moderately raised. Serum albumin, because of its long half-life, generally remains normal until later in the illness. A fall in aminotransferase levels despite increasing hyperbilirubinaemia indicates total destruction of liver cells and is associated with a very poor prognosis. Plasma levels of α-fetoprotein, pre-albumin and factor V, as well as the prothrombin time, have been used as prognostic indicators (see below). Blood ammonia levels are usually increased.

Bleeding

Patients with FHF invariably develop a severe *coagulopathy.* The prothrombin time is always markedly prolonged, reflecting reduced hepatic synthesis of clotting factors (V, VII, IX and X). Later this may be compounded by a fall in fibrinogen levels. The production of factors VIII, XI and XII may also be impaired. The prothrombin time is a useful guide to the progress of FHF.

Thrombocytopenia is common and may be due to hypersplenism, bone marrow depression or DIC. Functional platelet abnormalities have also been described in association with morphological changes; platelet adhesion is increased, but aggregation decreased. The platelet count tends to decrease progressively during the course of FHF and is lower in those who die.

Upper gastrointestinal haemorrhage is a potentially lethal complication of FHF and may be related to oesophagitis, gastric erosions or duodenal ulceration. Acute portal hypertension commonly develops after about three weeks and may result in variceal haemorrhage. Bleeding may also occur from the nasopharynx, the respiratory tract or into the retroperitoneal space. Intracerebral haemorrhage is unusual.

Metabolic disturbances

Hypoglycaemia is common and may be due to raised plasma insulin levels combined with a failure of hepatic gluconeogenesis. The development of a *metabolic alkalosis* is probably related to hypokalaemia and defective urea synthesis. In the later stages of FHF a *lactic acidosis* develops in over 50% of patients, reflecting both anaerobic metabolism and reduced clearance of lactate.

Electrolyte disturbances

In the absence of renal failure there is a marked tendency to *hypokalaemia* due to inadequate potassium intake, vomiting and secondary hyperaldosteronism. *Hypomagnesaemia* can be precipitated by the excessive use of diuretics. *Hyponatraemia* is also common, especially later in the course of FHF and is due to re-distribution of sodium into the cells combined with increased renal retention of water. *Hypernatraemia*, on the other hand, is unusual but can be precipitated by the sodium load in transfusions of fresh frozen plasma (FFP) or human albumin solution (HAS) and is some-times exacerbated by dehydration due to hypergly-caemia or diuretic administration. *Hypocalcaemia* may occur. *Hypophosphataemia* is common and may lead to a reduction in red cell 2,3-diphosphoglycerate con-centration and a decrease in oxygen availability (see Chapter 2).

Cardiovascular dysfunction

Hypotension is common, even in the absence of haem-orrhage or obvious sepsis, and is associated with a poor prognosis. The *peripheral resistance is low and cardiac output is usually increased*. Even when blood pressure is normal, severe tissue hypoxia may be present, as evid-enced by a metabolic acidosis and raised blood lactate levels. Furthermore, there is an inverse correlation between the mixed venous lactate concentration and both the systemic vascular resistance and the oxygen extraction ratio, suggesting that *vasodilation* is associ-ated with *maldistribution of microcirculatory flow* and tissue hypoxia (Bihari *et al.*, 1985). There is also a gen-eralized *increase in capillary permeability* leading to hypovolaemia and interstitial oedema. It has been postu-lated that the hyperdynamic circulation that is character-istic of liver failure may be related to induction of nitric oxide (NO) synthase, possibly in response to endotoxae-mia (Vallance & Moncada, 1991).

Arrhythmias are also common and may be related to hypoxia, acid–base disturbances or electrolyte abnor-malities. In one series, ectopic beats occurred in 20% of cases and heart block or bradycardia in 18%. ST segment and T wave abnormalities were seen in one-third (Weston *et al.*, 1976).

Respiratory dysfunction

A respiratory alkalosis due to hyperventilation is com-mon in the early stages of FHF (Record *et al.*, 1975) and may be a result of stimulation of the respiratory centre by toxins or an intracellular acidosis. Later, hypoxic depression of the respiratory centre may supervene and sudden unexpected *respiratory arrest* may occur, in some cases related to severe intracranial hypertension.

Many patients with FHF will be *hypoxaemic* and this may be due to intrapulmonary shunts (associated with diffuse dilatation of the pulmonary vasculature and, in some cases, pleural spider naevi) or pulmonary oedema. The commonest abnormality is *non-cardiogenic pul-monary oedema* (adult respiratory distress syndrome—ARDS, see Chapter 6), which occurred in 37 of a series of 100 patients with FHF reported by Trewby *et al.* (1978), and is associated with cerebral oedema. These authors were unable to demonstrate any correlation between the onset of ARDS and the presence of endo-toxaemia, hypoalbuminaemia or renal failure. It has been suggested that precapillary arteriolar dilatation dis-rupts pulmonary capillaries by exposing them to an increased hydrostatic pressure, but it seems more likely that the development of ARDS is simply a manifestation of the generalized increase in capillary permeability.

The presence of ascites may contribute to respiratory difficulty. Respiratory dysfunction may also be related to *pulmonary aspiration, atelectasis* or *bronchopneu-monia*.

Impaired host defences and sepsis

A number of abnormalities have been identified that contribute to the increased susceptibility of patients with FHF to infection. These include a *deficiency of complement* factors involved in both the classical and alternative pathways (Wyke *et al.*, 1980), a *reduced chemoattractant activity* of patients' sera for normal polymorphonuclear leucocytes (Wyke *et al.*, 1982a) and a *reduction in plasma fibronectin levels* (Gonzalez-Calvin *et al.*, 1982). Recently it has been suggested that decreased hepatic production of hepatocyte growth factor-like/macrophage-stimulating protein might cause impaired Kupffer cell phagocytosis in FHF (Harrison *et al.*, 1994). Consequently, bacteraemia is relatively com-mon and is most often due to Gram-positive organisms (mainly streptococci and *Staphylococcus aureus*), whereas *Escherichia coli* is the commonest type of Gram-negative organism isolated (Wyke *et al.*, 1982b). Common sites of infection include bacterial peritonitis, pneumonia and urinary tract infections. Line sepsis, cholangitis and endocarditis also occur. Fungal infec-tions are sometimes seen.

Renal dysfunction

Renal impairment is common in patients with FHF. Pre-renal factors such as gastrointestinal haemorrhage or excessive diuretic administration are frequently implic-ated. Acute tubular necrosis (ATN) may be precipitated by hypotension, sepsis or the administration of nephro-toxic drugs.

Hepatorenal syndrome (Epstein, 1992). This can be defined as renal failure occurring in patients with liver failure in the absence of clinical, laboratory or anatomical evidence of other possible causes. Renal impairment is considered to be *functional* since:

- pathological lesions are minimal and inconsistent;
- normal function returns if the liver recovers;
- kidneys from patients with hepatorenal syndrome function normally after transplantation into recipients with normal liver function (Koppel *et al.*, 1969);
- renal function recovers when patients with hepatorenal syndrome undergo successful liver transplantation (Gonwa *et al.*, 1991).

The pathogenesis of hepatorenal syndrome remains obscure, but renal dysfunction appears to be related to intense intrarenal vasoconstriction with preferential cortical ischaemia and reduced glomerular filtration. The factors responsible for these changes have not yet been fully elucidated, but possibilities include:

- activation of the renin–angiotensin system;
- increased sympathetic nervous system activity;
- alterations in the balance between vasodilator prostaglandins and vasoconstrictor thromboxanes;
- a relative impairment of renal kallikrein production.

Recent evidence has raised the possibility that the *endothelins* are involved in the pathogenesis of the hepatorenal syndrome (Moore *et al.*, 1992).

Since renal tubular function is preserved in the face of a reduced GFR, the capacity for sodium reabsorption and urine concentration is relatively normal. In contrast to ATN, therefore, urine sodium is low (< 10 mmol/l), urine osmolality is high (> 1000 mosm/kg) and the urine:plasma creatinine ratio is higher than 10. These changes cannot be reversed by volume replacement. Blood urea may be deceptively low because of the reduced capacity of the liver to metabolize ammonia to urea. The prognosis of hepatorenal syndrome is poor, with mortality rates exceeding 90%.

Pancreatitis

Haemorrhagic pancreatitis may develop in as many as 20–30% of patients with FHF and should be suspected in those with cardiovascular instability or hypocalaemia.

Rare complications

Rare complications include myocarditis, atypical pneumonia, aplastic anaemia, transverse myelitis and peripheral neuropathy.

Establishing the cause of FHF

The likely cause of FHF can often be ascertained from a careful history.

Hepatitis B infection is associated with intravenous drug abuse, blood transfusion and inoculation injuries, while *hepatitis A* arises from ingestion of contaminated food or water and often occurs in epidemics. The hepatitis B virus may also be spread via contaminated acupuncture needles, by tattooing and by close personal contact (e.g. sexual intercourse, particularly in homosexuals).

Serological investigations should include hepatitis A IgM antibody, hepatitis B core antigen antibody (HBcAb), hepatitis B surface antigen (HBsAg) and hepatitis B e antigen (HBeAg), as well as hepatitis C and D antibodies.

There may be a history of drug ingestion (intentional, with or without suicidal intent, or accidental) or exposure to poisons or chemicals. Appropriate *drug screening*, especially for paracetamol, should then be performed.

Halothane hepatitis should be suspected when the signs of hepatocellular necrosis (see earlier in this chapter), often accompanied by fever and chills, develop within two weeks of exposure.

Acute fatty liver of pregnancy usually presents as nausea, repeated vomiting and abdominal pain between the thirtieth and thirty-eighth week of gestation.

When *Wilson's disease* is suspected, plasma caeruloplasmin levels and urinary copper excretion should be determined.

Liver biopsy is indicated only very occasionally to exclude underlying cirrhosis or malignancy.

Pathogenesis of encephalopathy (Crossley *et al.*, 1983)

Reductions in cerebral energy production, abnormal neurotransmitter function, direct effects on neuronal membranes or, most likely, a combination of these factors, are thought to be responsible for the disturbance of neurotransmission that precipitates hepatic encephalopathy. These abnormalities are in turn largely related to the accumulation of toxic substances normally metabolized by the liver. Although there are many similarities between the clinical and biochemical features of encephalopathy in FHF and chronic liver impairment, there are also a number of respects in which they differ; in particular, cerebral oedema is a common and important complication of FHF, but is extremely rare in chronic liver disease. In both cases, the disturbance of cerebral function is often exacerbated by:

- hypoglycaemia;
- alterations in acid–base homeostasis;
- fluid and electrolyte abnormalities;
- hypoxia and hypercarbia.

In addition, patients with acute liver failure are very sensitive to the effects of analgesics and sedatives, not only because of impaired drug metabolism, but also because of increased cerebral sensitivity and changes in plasma protein binding.

Examples of recognized toxins that accumulate in liver failure include:

- ammonia;
- fatty acids;
- mercaptans (derived from methionine);
- phenols;
- various aromatic amino acids.

Although bile acids are also retained, it seems unlikely that these play a major role in the production of encephalopathy.

Blood levels of *ammonia* and short-chain *fatty acids* are elevated in hepatic failure and both can produce coma, although there is a poor correlation between the blood ammonia concentration and the degree of coma. Moreover, it is difficult to reconcile the central nervous system depression that characterizes hepatic encephalopathy with the neuroexcitatory properties of ammonia. The *mercaptans* are well-recognized cerebral toxins and can induce reversible coma (Zieve *et al.*, 1974), and it has been proposed that they may exert a synergistic effect with both ammonia and free fatty acids (Zieve *et al.*, 1974). One suggested mechanism of action for these toxins and *phenols* is inhibition of Na^+/K^+ ATPase on the neuronal membrane. This could impair membrane repolarization and might also disrupt the integrity of the blood–brain barrier.

It has also been suggested that *middle molecular weight substances* may contribute to the development of encephalopathy (Bloch *et al.*, 1978). These have been identified in the serum of patients with FHF as well as in chronic encephalopathy and can inhibit leucocyte sodium transport (Sewell *et al.*, 1982). There is evidence that this occurs within the brain where it could interfere with neurotransmission and might contribute to the formation of cerebral oedema by increasing intracellular sodium content (Seda *et al.*, 1984). This hypothesis is supported by the finding that haemodialysis with a polyacrylonitrile membrane (which is permeable to larger solutes than the standard cuprophane membrane) can improve encephalopathy in FHF and that haemofiltration (which removes middle molecules) can be associated with an increased level of consciousness (Matsubara *et al.*, 1990). These latter authors suggest that the combination of continuous haemofiltration and plasma exchange may provide a means of supporting patients awaiting liver transplantation.

The serum *amino acid* profile is abnormal in both chronic liver impairment and FHF. In patients with chronic liver disease and superimposed acute insults, there is an increase in blood levels of the aromatic amino acids and a reduction in the concentrations of the branched-chain amino acids (Rosen *et al.*, 1977). This abnormality is probably the result of increased catabolism as well as impaired liver function. Circulating levels of aromatic amino acids are also markedly increased in FHF, but in this situation the concentration of branched-chain amino acids is normal (Rosen *et al.*, 1977). It is thought that this altered amino acid profile is caused by massive hepatocellular necrosis with release of amino acids into the circulation and that catabolism plays a less important role. The high circulating levels of aromatic amino acids combined with their enhanced uptake by active carrier systems and disruption of the blood–brain barrier could lead to increased intracerebral concentrations of phenylalanine, tyrosine and tryptophan. The excess tyrosine might then be converted to *octopamine*, while phenylalanine could be metabolized first to phenylethylamine and then *phenylethanolamine*. These substances are thought to act as weak (or *'false'*) *neurotransmitters*, displacing some of the normal transmitter compounds such as dopamine and noradrenaline. Furthermore, tryptophan can be converted into the inhibitory neurotransmitter serotonin, and the intracerebral formation of normal excitatory transmitters may be reduced by competition for enzyme systems. Finally, ammonia stimulates brain glutamine synthesis, which results in a rapid exchange of brain glutamine for neutral plasma amino acids; this provides a possible link between the neurotoxicity of ammonia and the false neurotransmitter hypothesis (James *et al.*, 1979).

There is, however, some evidence against the false transmitter theory, and a number of other mechanisms have been postulated. For example, it has been suggested that in FHF blood levels of γ-aminobutyric acid (GABA)-like compounds are markedly increased, probably because of reduced hepatic metabolism. In addition, the number of postsynaptic binding sites for GABA in the brain is increased (Schafer & Jones, 1982). Since the blood–brain barrier is disrupted in FHF, the concentration of GABA-like compounds within the brain could rise, thereby contributing to neural inhibition. The increase in GABA binding sites may also partly explain the enhanced sensitivity of these patients to sedatives. Postsynaptic GABA receptors are coupled to benzodiazepine receptors and there is now evidence that in a subpopulation of patients with FHF, GABA-ergic neurotransmission is enhanced by elevated levels of benzodiazepine receptor agonist ligands, perhaps derived from the patient's diet or enteric flora (Basile *et al.*, 1991; Editorial, 1991; Mullen, 1991). This hypothesis is supported by the observation that benzodiazepine receptor antagonists can improve conscious level in hepatic encephalopathy (Grimm *et al.*, 1988).

CEREBRAL OEDEMA

Cerebral oedema has been demonstrated in post-mortem studies of patients dying with FHF (Silk *et al.*, 1977) and is probably present in over 80% of patients with grade IV encephalopathy. The cause remains uncertain but the permeability of the blood–brain barrier may be increased by circulating toxins (vasogenic oedema), and inhibition of Na^+/K^+ ATPase may lead to intracellular accumulation of sodium and water (cytotoxic oedema) (Seda *et al.*, 1984). The osmotic effects of glutamine and primary injury to astrocytes may also contribute to cerebral damage (Editorial, 1991). In contrast to many other conditions associated with intracranial hypertension, cerebral blood flow is usually reduced in FHF.

Management (Table 13.5)

GENERAL ASPECTS

In the great majority of those who survive an episode of FHF, liver architecture returns essentially to normal and the development of cirrhosis is very unusual (Karvountzis *et al.*, 1974). Aggressive management of FHF is therefore based on the premise that if the patient is supported through the acute illness, regeneration of the liver will be associated with complete recovery. Currently, there is some support for the hypothesis that a number of hepatocytes survive the initial insult, but are functionally impaired by persisting ischaemia/hypoxia, perhaps related in part to vascular obstruction. Reversal of haemodynamic and respiratory abnormalities is therefore a fundamental aspect of supportive care for the patient with FHF. It is likely, however, that at least in some cases, hepatic necrosis will be so extensive that liver regeneration is not possible.

Patients with FHF should be admitted to an intensive care unit as soon as their conscious level deteriorates and should then, if possible, be transferred to a specialist centre once they have been resuscitated and stabilized. Successful management then depends largely on the quality of supportive care combined with an awareness of the potential complications, so that they can be either prevented or recognized early and treated appropriately.

PRECAUTIONS AGAINST CROSS-INFECTION

All intensive care unit staff should be vaccinated against hepatitis B virus. In the event of an inoculation injury

or permucosal exposure to blood or high-risk body fluids, those whose immune status is unknown should receive hepatitis B immune globulin as soon as possible. They should then be tested for HBsAb and, if negative, vaccination should be started immediately. Following exposure to hepatitis A virus a single intramuscular dose of immune globulin should be given as soon as possible.

Measures to prevent cross-infection and minimize the dangers to staff should be instituted in all cases of viral hepatitis or when the aetiology of liver failure is uncertain. Initially all cases of FHF should be considered to be infectious. Particular care is required when handling blood, urine or faeces, and it is most important to avoid contamination of conjunctivae, cuts or abrasions, as well as self-inoculation. Safe practice for handling sharps includes:

- discard immediately into approved containers;
- never resheath a needle;
- do not leave needles on syringes;
- never overfill a sharps box;
- do not leave loose sharps on trolleys or towels following procedures.

Saliva and tears are also potentially infective. Staff should wear an impermeable apron and gloves when performing medical or nursing procedures; masks and protective goggles should be used when the risk of conjunctival inoculation is considered to be high. Frequent handwashing is essential; cuts and abrasions should be covered with a waterproof dressing. Because staff are frequently unaware that a particular patient is carrying a blood-borne virus it is now recommended that these safe practices should be adopted universally (*universal precautions*).

Excreta should be disposed of immediately. Hypochlorite is the disinfectant of choice, and a hypochlorite detergent (1000 parts per million) should be used for cleaning the bed area and equipment. Contaminated items, excreta and laboratory specimens should be clearly labelled as high risk. Automated analysers should be similarly labelled.

HYPOGLYCAEMIA

Blood sugar levels should be determined at least two-hourly. Hypoglycaemia can be avoided by giving a continuous intravenous infusion of 10% or 20% dextrose, supplemented as necessary by bolus doses of 50 ml 50% dextrose, to maintain the blood sugar level above 4 mmol/l. There is also, however, a danger of precipitating hyperglycaemia because of impaired glucose uptake by the liver and this may be associated with lactic acidosis.

Table 13.5 Management of fulminant hepatic failure.

Monitoring	Temperature
	ECG
	Intra-arterial pressure
	Central venous pressure
In selected cases	Pulmonary artery catheterization
	Cardiac output
	Oxygen delivery (DO_2), oxygen consumption ($\dot{V}O_2$), lactate
	Intracranial pressure
	Cerebral function monitor
Cardiovascular system	Expand circulating volume (colloids—albumin, fresh frozen plasma; blood)
	Inotropes and vasopressors (dopamine, noradrenaline, adrenaline)
	Treat arrhythmias conventionally
Respiratory support	Secure airway
	Protect lungs from aspiration
	Avoid hypoxia and hypercarbia
	Treat respiratory muscle fatigue
	Endotracheal intubation $\pm$ continuous positive airways pressure (CPAP)
	Mechanical ventilation $\pm$ positive end-expiratory pressure (PEEP)
Renal dysfunction	Prevent renal failure (volume replacement, optimize cardiac output and blood pressure)
	Continuous haemofiltration
Cerebral oedema	Mannitol $\pm$ frusemide
	Hyperventilation (beware excessive cerebral vasoconstriction)
	Thiopentone
Encephalopathy	Correct precipitating factors
	Avoid sedatives
	Treat convulsions
	Limit or eliminate protein intake
	If suspect blood in gastrointestinal tract, give enema (e.g. 80 ml magnesium sulphate in 50% solution w/v) 2–3 times a day until no melaena
	Lactulose 60 ml followed by 30 ml 8-hrly, PO or NG
Hypoglycaemia	Continuous intravenous infusion 10–20% dextrose
	Intravenous boluses of 50% dextrose as required to maintain blood sugar > 4 mmol/l
Bleeding	Fresh frozen plasma for active bleeding
	Platelets if platelet count $< 50,000 \times 10^6$ cells/l
	Fresh frozen plasma and platelets before invasive procedures
	Vitamin K 10 mg daily
	H_2-receptor blockade in all cases
Fluids and electrolytes	Large quantities intravenous potassium chloride
	Restrict sodium intake to < 50 mmol/day
	Hydration with dextrose solutions
Liver transplantation	
Precautions to minimize risk of cross-infection	

NUTRITION

Nutritional support, other than 10% or 20% dextrose, is impractical and unnecessary during the acute phase. Later feeding may be instituted, preferably via the enteral route.

BLEEDING

Prophylactic correction of the clotting factor deficiency with infusions of fresh frozen plasma (FFP) does not appear to influence the overall mortality and may precipitate sodium overload and possibly DIC. Administration of FFP is indicated in those with active bleeding. Platelet transfusions are rarely indicated, but should be given if the platelet count is less than $50,000 \times 10^6$ cells/l. FFP and platelets should also be given prior to surgical procedures and vascular cannulation. Vitamin K, 10 mg, should be administered daily, although this generally has little demonstrable effect. Blood losses should be replaced as indicated.

Upper gastrointestinal haemorrhage can be virtually eliminated if gastric pH is maintained above 5 by the administration of an H_2-receptor antagonist (Macdougall *et al.*, 1977) (see also Chapter 10).

ELECTROLYTE DISTURBANCES

Large quantities of intravenous potassium chloride are usually required to correct hypokalaemia. Sodium intake should be restricted to less than 50 mmol/day. Hydration should be maintained with 5%, 10% or 20% dextrose as required to maintain blood sugar levels above 4 mmol/l.

CARDIOVASCULAR SUPPORT

Adequate expansion of the circulating volume with colloid and blood as indicated is essential, guided by the central venous pressure (CVP), the urine output and, in some cases, the pulmonary artery occlusion pressure (PAOP). If this fails to restore the blood pressure, one should not hesitate to use inotropes or vasopressors since in the presence of raised intracranial pressure (ICP), hypotension can precipitate cerebral ischaemia. Dopamine is often chosen initially, although high doses may be necessary to produce some vasoconstriction and reverse hypotension. Many now recommend the use of noradrenaline to restore the systemic vascular resistance, while others suggest that adrenaline is a suitable agent. If more than moderate doses of dopamine are required, pulmonary artery catheterization is indicated. Administration of acetylcysteine to patients with FHF

has been shown to increase cardiac output, oxygen delivery (DO_2), oxygen extraction and oxygen consumption ($\dot{V}O_2$). Despite a fall in systemic resistance, blood pressure also increased (Harrison *et al.*, 1991). The authors suggested that these effects might account for the improved survival associated with delayed administration of acetylcysteine to patients with paracetamol-induced FHF and postulated that they might be due to stimulation of NO production in the microcirculation.

RESPIRATORY SUPPORT

Control of the airway and protection of the lungs from aspiration of blood or stomach contents is essential, and these patients should be intubated early—certainly as soon as the airway protective reflexes are depressed. Continuous positive airways pressure (CPAP) can be used to maintain adequate oxygenation in spontaneously breathing patients. Hypercarbia and hypoxaemia should be avoided by early institution of mechanical ventilation, although it is important to remember that the institution of intermittent positive pressure ventilation (IPPV) may be associated with a marked reduction in hepatic perfusion if cardiac output is allowed to fall. Mechanical ventilation is also indicated when there is evidence of respiratory muscle fatigue (see Chapters 6 and 7). In those with refractory hypoxaemia, positive end-expiratory pressure (PEEP) may be required and the underlying pulmonary abnormality should be treated as outlined in Chapter 6.

RENAL SUPPORT

Even though the development of renal failure is not necessarily related to the severity of liver impairment (e.g. ATN may occur without encephalopathy), its onset is associated with an extremely high mortality. Prevention of renal failure is therefore of paramount importance, and some recommend a low-dose dopamine infusion in all cases of FHF (but see Chapter 12). Maintenance of an adequate circulating volume, blood pressure and cardiac output is essential. Continuous haemofiltration is indicated for those with established renal failure or resistant fluid overload.

PREVENTION OF INFECTION

Because bacteraemia usually occurs within 48 hours of the onset of grade IV coma, and may be associated with a deterioration in liver function, broad-spectrum antibiotic prophylaxis has been recommended when patients develop grade III coma. Benzylpenicillin is usually combined with tobramycin or a third-generation cephalosporin. This practice is, however, controversial.

CEREBRAL OEDEMA

CT scanning is an unreliable means of detecting cerebral oedema in FHF, although it may demonstrate the focal intracranial lesions that sometimes accompany acute liver failure.

Although monitoring ICP can assist in the early detection and rational treatment of intracranial hypertension, some authorities feel that the complications, in particular bleeding and deterioration during transfer to and from the operating theatre, outweigh the benefits. In many transplantation centres, however, ICP monitoring is used to guide the treatment of perioperative intracranial hypertension. It has also been suggested that a cerebral perfusion pressure persistently less than 40 mm Hg despite aggressive treatment should preclude transplantation, although recently it has been reported that four patients with FHF survived neurologically intact despite persistent intracranial hypertension (> 35 mm Hg for 24-38 hours) refractory to standard therapy associated with a cerebral perfusion pressure of less than 50 mm Hg for 2-72 hours (Davies *et al.*, 1994). In the absence of ICP monitoring, intracranial hypertension should be suspected and treated if the pupils dilate or become unequal, react sluggishly or cease to react to light, and in the presence of decorticate/decerebrate posturing, hyperventilation, profuse sweating, opisthotonos or hypertension. Papilloedema is unusual.

The administration of steroids is of no value in controlling the cerebral oedema associated with FHF, but mannitol is extremely effective in reducing ICP and may improve survival in those with intracranial hypertension (Canalese *et al.*, 1982). Frusemide administration may be required to maintain the osmotic gradient and to allow transfusions of FFP, platelets and blood while avoiding hypervolaemia. In those with renal failure, continuous haemofiltration may create 'space' for the administration of mannitol. Other measures to control intracranial hypertension can be instituted as outlined in Chapter 14, although hyperventilation may further reduce the already subnormal cerebral blood flow. Thiopentone may be useful in the treatment of raised ICP associated with FHF (Forbes *et al.*, 1989).

ENCEPHALOPATHY

Identifiable precipitating factors, such as fluid and electrolyte disturbances, hypoxaemia, hypercarbia, hypoglycaemia and acid–base disturbances must be corrected. Sedatives and analgesics may also precipitate or exacer-bate coma, as well as hypotension, and should in general be avoided. If sedation is essential, small doses of a benzodiazepine are recommended. Alternatives include promethazine, chlormethiazole or phenobarbitone. Convulsions are relatively common and should be treated aggressively (see Chapter 14); under these circumstances, it is usually necessary to paralyse and ventilate the patient.

Although it is traditional to institute measures designed to minimize the nitrogenous load absorbed from the bowel, this practice is based on the observable improvement produced in chronic hepatic encephalopathy and there are no controlled data to suggest that such treatment is beneficial in FHF. Nevertheless, it is conventional to limit protein intake to less than 40 g/day in patients with stage I and II encephalopathy and withdraw protein from the diet of those in stage III and IV encephalopathy. If blood is suspected in the gastrointestinal tract, the bowel is emptied with an enema (e.g. 80 ml magnesium sulphate in 50% solution w/v) repeated 2-3 times a day until there is no melaena. Lactulose is also given in a starting dose of 60 ml, followed by 30 ml 8-hourly or more frequently, in order to produce two soft bowel motions a day. It is not necessary to produce diarrhoea. Lactulose is a non-absorbable synthetic disaccharide that is not metabolized in the small bowel. It is hydrolysed in the colon to lactic and acetic acid, thereby causing a fermentative diarrhoea, and may act by trapping ammonia in the bowel by virtue of the fall in pH of the colonic contents. A second-generation disaccharide (lactitol) is available in more convenient powder form and is more palatable than lactulose, while being equally effective in chronic stable encephalopathy. Oral neomycin, 1 g 6-hourly, can be used to sterilize the bowel, but because significant amounts of this drug are absorbed, there is a risk of ototoxicity in those with renal impairment and many centres have now discontinued its routine prescription.

It has been suggested that manipulation of the abnormal plasma amino acid profile by intravenous infusion of branched-chain amino acids might be beneficial in hepatic encephalopathy, although controlled studies have not demonstrated any benefit.

TEMPORARY LIVER SUPPORT

Temporary liver support is based on the principle that removal of the toxins that accumulate in FHF may prevent the development of cerebral oedema and provide a more favourable environment for hepatic regeneration (Zieve *et al.*, 1985).

Initially, techniques were used that were designed to replace some of the synthetic functions of the liver as well as remove the accumulated toxins. These included exchange transfusions or plasmapheresis, cross-circulation with healthy volunteers or patients in irreversible coma, and extracorporeal perfusion of isolated animal (or human) livers. Cross-circulation with healthy humans is, of course, only applicable to those with FHF of non-infectious origin and even then exposes the volunteer to significant risk; its use has been abandoned.

Although these techniques can produce temporary improvements in the patient's conscious level, there is no evidence that they influence long-term survival; they are also expensive, technically demanding and difficult to perform on a daily basis. Temporary liver support has therefore been largely abandoned, although it has recently been suggested that the use of *ex vivo* pig liver perfusion should be reconsidered for selected patients with otherwise untreatable acute liver failure (Chari *et al.*, 1994).

ARTIFICIAL LIVER SUPPORT

Because these techniques of liver support only remove toxins, important substances normally produced by the liver (e.g. clotting factors), may have to be replaced by appropriate intravenous infusions.

Charcoal haemoperfusion was used with considerable enthusiasm in the past. Activated charcoal adsorbs a wide range of water-soluble substances, including those of middle molecular weight. In an early study remarkable results were obtained by instituting charcoal haemoperfusion early (i.e. in grade III encephalopathy) (Gimson *et al.*, 1982), but more recent evidence from a large study suggests that this technique does not significantly influence the overall survival of patients in either grade III or IV hepatic encephalopathy (O'Grady *et al.*, 1988).

Haemodialysis with a polyacrylonitrile membrane allows a more rapid transfer of middle molecular weight substances than is possible with a standard cuprophane membrane, and also removes compounds of higher molecular weight. Although initially survival rates were reported improved (Silk *et al.*, 1977), this technique is no longer used.

At present the use of artificial liver support cannot therefore be generally recommended except possibly as part of a research programme within specialist units. Recently, however, it has been reported that a combination of total hepatectomy and extracorporeal liver support (a charcoal filter and a hollow-fibre module seeded with porcine hepatocytes) can control cerebral oedema and maintain patients alive and neurologically intact until an organ becomes available for transplantation (Rozga *et al.*, 1993).

INSULIN AND GLUCAGON INFUSIONS

Attempts to stimulate hepatic regeneration by administering a combination of insulin and glucagon were associated with reduced survival (Harrison *et al.*, 1990).

PROSTAGLANDIN E

Although preliminary evidence suggested that administration of prostaglandin E might improve survival in FHF (Sinclair *et al.*, 1989), this has not been confirmed by controlled studies (Lee, 1993).

HUMAN HEPATOCYTE GROWTH FACTOR

In the future it may prove possible to stimulate the rapid regeneration of hepatocytes by administering appropriate growth factors (Lee, 1993).

LIVER TRANSPLANTATION

Liver transplantation is an effective treatment for FHF (Emond *et al.*, 1989), with one-year survival rates ranging from about 50% to approximately 75%. Some have confined orthotopic liver transplantation to those with grade IV encephalopathy, although by this stage there is often associated cerebral oedema, which almost certainly increases the risks, while others have proposed that transplantation is the best option for all patients with FHF. To improve patient selection and increase the time available for obtaining a donor organ, criteria have been devised (**Table 13.6**) that can be used to assist

Table 13.6 Suggested criteria for liver transplantation in fulminant hepatic failure (From O'Grady *et al.*, 1989).

Paracetamol

pH < 7.30 (irrespective of grade of encephalopathy)
or
Prothrombin time > 100 s and creatinine > 300 μmol/l in patients with grade III or IV encephalopathy

Non-paracetamol

Prothrombin time > 100 s (irrespective of grade of encephalopathy)
or Any three of the following (irrespective of grade of encephalopathy)

    Age < 10 or > 40 years
    Aetiology—non A non B hepatitis, halothane hepatitis, idiosyncratic drug reaction
    Duration of jaundice before onset of encephalopathy > 7 days
Prothrombin time > 50 s
Serum bilirubin > 300 μmol/l

early identification of those patients with a poor prognosis who are most likely to benefit from transplantation, preferably before the development of advanced encephalopathy or other complications that could adversely effect the outcome (O'Grady *et al.*, 1989). More recently, liver transplantation has been shown to have a limited, but definite role in the management of patients with paracetamol-induced FHF, selected according to these criteria (O'Grady *et al.*, 1991). Before proceeding to transplantation it is important to assess whether the function of other organs, especially the brain, is preserved, whether infection is present, and whether the underlying disease is likely to recur in the graft (Lee, 1993).

Orthotopic liver transplantation does, however, suffer from a number of disadvantages: in particular, it is a major surgical procedure associated with considerable blood loss and if the graft does not function the patient either dies or must be retransplanted immediately. In addition, in those with acute liver failure in whom there is a possibility of spontaneous recovery of liver function, removal of the native liver obviates any chance of such an outcome. These considerations have led to the concept of auxiliary liver transplantation (ALT) in which healthy liver tissue is placed somewhere in the body while the native liver is left *in situ* (Terpstra, 1993). The successful use of ALT has recently been reported in a child with subacute liver failure. The native liver, which was 90% necrotic at the time of transplantation, regained normal histological features within three months. The auxiliary graft was then removed and immunosuppressive therapy stopped (Boudjema *et al.*, 1993).

Prognosis

The mortality of FHF remains high and this condition therefore represents an important challenge because, although rare, it is a disease that affects young people and from which those who survive will make a complete recovery.

Although overall survival rates in patients with FHF are less than 20%, the individual prognosis is very dependent on the aetiology of the hepatocellular damage. In a large series of patients treated between 1973 and 1985, for example, mortality rates varied from 55% for hepatitis A, 65% for paracetemol-induced hepatic necrosis and 76% for hepatitis B, to as high as 85% for reactions to drugs (including halothane) and more than 90% for non A non B hepatitis (O'Grady *et al.*, 1989). Survival is also influenced by the delay between the onset of jaundice and the development of encephalopathy. Using their proposed new classification the group from King's College Hospital found that survival was 36% in those with hyperacute liver failure, despite the fact that all progressed to grade IV coma and 69% had evidence of cerebral oedema. Those with acute liver failure also had a high incidence of cerebral oedema (56%), but only 7% survived and only 14% of those with subacute hepatic failure survived (O'Grady *et al.*, 1993).

There is some evidence that mortality has fallen over the last 15–20 years, almost certainly largely as a result of improvements in the standards of general intensive care rather than specific interventions, and survival rates of 67% for hepatitis A, 53% for paracetamol-induced FHF and 39% for hepatitis B have been reported (O'Grady *et al.*, 1989).

Prognosis is also influenced by the age of the patient, the grade of encephalopathy, the bilirubin level and the creatinine concentration. Serum aminotransferases are of no value in assessing the prognosis, but the prothrombin time at presentation and the direction and rapidity of its change, as well as the peak level, provide a reasonable guide to the likely outcome. The presence of a metabolic acidosis is associated with an extremely poor prognosis, and the longer the duration of jaundice before the onset of encephalopathy, the higher the mortality. The relative importance of these variables seems to depend on whether or not FHF was precipitated by paracetamol (see **Table 13.6**). Not surprisingly the prognosis is better when the coma has an identifiable precipitating cause such as the administration of sedatives. Clearly the development of serious complications such as respiratory failure, renal failure, hypotension, convulsions or haemorrhage will adversely affect the outcome.

Causes of death

In one series of 132 consecutive patients in grade IV encephalopathy, autopsy was performed in 96 of the 105 who died. In only 25 of these was death considered to be solely attributable to massive hepatic necrosis. In 36% of cases, cerebral oedema was considered to be the main contributory factor, while in 28 patients, death was due to major gastrointestinal haemorrhage and, in 12, sepsis was a contributory factor. Most importantly, in 10 of these patients, liver function appeared to be improving at the time of death, suggesting that if these major complications could have been prevented or successfully treated, a number of patients might have survived (Gazzard *et al.*, 1975).

ACUTE DECOMPENSATION OF CHRONIC LIVER DISEASE

Acute decompensation of chronic cirrhosis requiring admission to the intensive care unit is most often the result of shock, usually related to gastrointestinal haemorrhage. Other precipitating factors include infection (particularly with *E. coli* and spontaneous bacterial peritonitis), alcohol, sedative or hepatotoxic drugs, increased dietary protein, metabolic disturbances (especially hypokalaemic alkalosis caused by the excessive use of diuretics), constipation, anaesthesia and surgery. Most patients have portal hypertension with portal–systemic collaterals (shunts), which allow circulating toxins to bypass the liver and contribute to the development of portal–systemic encephalopathy.

Clinical features

Acute decompensation of chronic liver disease is characterized by *jaundice* and *encephalopathy*. *Ascites* is common and is almost invariable in those with bleeding varices or advanced encephalopathy. Other signs of chronicity such as *palmar erythema* and *spider naevi* are usual. The encephalopathy tends to develop more gradually than in FHF and cerebral oedema is rare.

The prognosis for those who develop the features of FHF is extremely poor, partly because there is little potential for hepatic regeneration. Survival is also unusual in those who need respiratory support.

Management

Patients in whom there is thought to be a reversible component and those being considered for transplantation should be admitted for intensive care.

Measures to reduce the absorption of nitrogenous compounds from the bowel should be instituted and combined with general supportive care as outlined above for FHF. Infection must be identified and treated appropriately.

The management of gastrointestinal haemorrhage is discussed in Chapter 15.

Diagnostic paracentesis should be performed to exclude spontaneous bacterial peritonitis, which occurs in 4–15% of cirrhotic patients with ascites. Broad-spectrum antibiotics should be given if there are more than 250×10^6 neutrophils/l of fluid, if organisms are identified on a Gram stain or if organisms are cultured. The antibiotic regimen can be altered appropriately when sensitivities are available.

Control of ascites involves salt and water restriction (e.g. sodium intake < 50 mmol/day or even < 20 mmol/day) combined with administration of diuretics (e.g. frusemide 40 mg combined with amiloride 5 mg daily). There is, however, a danger of sodium depletion with excessive diuretic administration and, traditionally, rapid mobilization of ascitic fluid is avoided. Nevertheless, when severe ascites is causing respiratory embarrassment, paracentesis of up to 3–5 l/day can be performed and appears to be safe. It can be accompanied by intravenous administration of albumin solutions. Ultrafiltration or insertion of a Levine shunt may be of value in resistant cases.

REFERENCES

Basile AS, Hughes RD, Harrison PM, *et al.* (1991) Elevated brain concentrations of 1,4 benzodiazepines in fulminant hepatic failure. *New England Journal of Medicine* **325**: 473–478.

Bernau J & Benhamou JP (1993) Classifying acute liver failure. *Lancet* **342**: 252–253.

Bihari D, Gimson AES, Lindridge J & Williams R (1985) Lactic acidosis in fulminant hepatic failure. Some aspects of pathogenesis and prognosis. *Journal of Hepatology* **1**: 405–416.

Black M (1980) Acetaminophen hepatotoxicity. *Gastroenterology* **78**: 382–392.

Bloch P, Delorme ML, Rapin JR, *et al.* (1978) Reversible modifications of brain neurotransmitters of the brain in experimental acute hepatic coma. *Surgery, Gynecology and Obstetrics* **146**: 551–558.

Boudjema K, Jaeck D, Simeoni U, Bientz J, Chenard MP & Brunot P (1993) Temporary auxiliary liver transplantation for subacute liver failure in a child. *Lancet* **342**: 778–779.

Canalese J, Gimson AES, Davis C *et al.* (1982) Controlled trial of dexamethasone and mannitol for the cerebral oedema of fulminant hepatic failure. *Gut* **23**: 625–629.

Chari RS, Collins BH, Magee JC *et al.* (1994) Brief report: treatment of hepatic failure with *ex vivo* pig-liver perfusion fol-

lowed by liver transplantation. *New England Journal of Medicine* **331**: 234–237.

Crossley IR, Wardle EN & Williams R (1983) Biochemical mechanisms of hepatic encephalopathy. *Clinical Science* **64**: 247–252.

Davies MH, Mutimer D, Lowes J, Elias E & Neuberger J (1994) Recovery despite impaired cerebral perfusion in fulminant hepatic failure. *Lancet* **343**: 1329–1330.

Editorial (1986) Halothane associated liver damage. *Lancet* **i**: 1251–1252.

Editorial (1991) The brain in fulminant hepatic failure. *Lancet* **338**: 156–157.

Emond JC, Aran PP, Whitington PF, Broelsch CE & Baker AL (1989) Liver transplantation in the management of fulminant hepatic failure. *Gastroenterology* **96**: 1583–1588.

Epstein M (1992) The hepatorenal syndrome—newer perspectives. *New England Journal of Medicine* **327**: 1810–1811.

Forbes A, Alexander GJ, O'Grady JG *et al.* (1989) Thiopental infusion in the treatment of intracranial hypertension complicating fulminant hepatic failure. *Hepatology* **10**: 306–310.

Gazzard BG, Portmann B, Murray-Lyon IM & Williams R (1975) Causes of death in fulminant hepatic failure and relationship to quantitative histological assessment of parenchymal damage. *Quarterly Journal of Medicine* **44**: 615-626.

Gimson AES & Williams R (1983) Acute hepatic failure: aetiological factors, pathogenic mechanisms and treatment. In: Thomas HC & MacSween RNM (eds), *Recent Advances in Hepatology*, Vol. 1, pp. 57-69. Edinburgh: Churchill Livingstone.

Gimson AES, Braude S, Mellon J, Canalese J & Williams R (1982) Earlier charcoal haemoperfusion in fulminant hepatic failure. *Lancet* **ii**: 681-683.

Gonzalez Calvin J, Scully MF, Sanger Y et al. (1982) Fibronectin in fulminant hepatic failure. *British Medical Journal* **285**: 1231-1232.

Gonwa TA, Morris CA, Goldstein RM, Husberg BS & Klintmalm GB (1991) Long-term survival and renal function following liver transplantation in patients with and without hepatorenal syndrome—experience in 300 patients. *Transplantation* **51**: 428-430.

Grimm G, Ferenci P, Katzenschlager R, et al. (1988) Improvement of hepatic encephalopathy treated with flumazenil. *Lancet* **ii**: 1392-1394.

Harrison PM, Hughes RD, Forbes A et al. (1990) Failure of insulin and glucagon infusion to stimulate liver regeneration in fulminant hepatic failure. *Journal of Hepatology* **10**: 332-336.

Harrison PM, Wendon JA, Gimson AES, Alexander GJM & Williams R (1991) Improvement by acetylcysteine of hemodynamics and oxygen transport in fulminant hepatic failure. *New England Journal of Medicine* **324**: 1852-1857.

Harrison P, Degen SJF, Williams R & Farzaneh F (1994) Hepatic expression of hepatocyte-growth-factor-like/macrophage-stimulating protein mRNA in fulminant hepatic failure. *Lancet* **344**: 27-28.

James JH, Ziparo V, Jeppsson B & Fischer JE (1979) Hyperammonaemia, plasma aminoacid imbalance, and blood-brain aminoacid transport: a unified theory of portal-systemic encephalopathy. *Lancet* **ii**: 772-775.

Karvountzis GG, Redeker AG & Peters RL (1974) Long-term follow-up studies of patients surviving fulminant viral hepatitis. *Gastroenterology* **67**: 870-877.

Koppel MH, Coburn JW, Mims MM et al. (1969) Transplantation of cadaveric kidneys from patients with hepatorenal syndrome. Evidence for the functional nature of renal failure in advanced liver disease. *New England Journal of Medicine* **280**: 1367-1371.

Lee WM (1993) Acute liver failure. *New England Journal of Medicine* **329**: 1862-1872.

Macdougall BRD, Bailey RJ & Williams R (1977) H_2-receptor antagonists and antacids in the prevention of acute gastrointestinal haemorrhage in fulminant hepatic failure. Two controlled trials. *Lancet* **i**: 617-619.

Matsubara S, Okabe K, Ouchi K, Miyazaki Y, Yajima Y, Suzuki H, Otsuki M & Matsuno S (1990) Continuous removal of middle molecules by hemofiltration in patients with acute liver failure. *Critical Care Medicine* **18**: 1331-1338.

Moore K, Wendon J, Frazer M, Karani J, Williams R & Badr K (1992) Plasma endothelin immunoreactivity in liver disease and the hepatorenal syndrome. *New England Journal of Medicine* **327**: 1774-1778.

Mullen KD (1991) Benzodiazepine compounds and hepatic

encephalopathy. *New England Journal of Medicine* **325**: 509-511.

Neuberger J, Gimson AES, Davis M & Williams R (1983) Specific serological markers in the diagnosis of fulminant hepatic failure associated with halothane anaesthesia. *British Journal of Anaesthesia* **55**: 15-19.

O'Grady JG, Gimson AE, O'Brien CJ et al. (1988) Controlled trials of charcoal haemoperfusion and prognostic factors in fulminant hepatic failure. *Gastroenterology* **94**: 1186-1192.

O'Grady JG, Alexander GJM, Hayllar KM & Williams R (1989) Early indications of prognosis in fulminant hepatic failure. *Gastroenterology* **97**: 439-445.

O'Grady JG, Wendon J, Tan KC, Potter D, Cottam S, Cohen AT, Gimson AES & Williams R (1991) Liver transplantation after paracetamol overdose. *British Medical Journal* **303**: 221-223.

O'Grady JG, Schalm SW & Williams R (1993) Acute liver failure: redefining the syndromes. *Lancet* **342**: 273-275.

Record CO, Iles RA, Cohen RD & Williams R (1975) Acid-base and metabolic disturbances in fulminant hepatic failure. *Gut* **16**: 144-149.

Rosen HM, Yoshimura M, Hodgman JM & Fisher JE (1977) Plasma amino acid patterns in hepatic encephalopathy of differing etiology. *Gastroenterology* **72**: 483-487.

Rozga J, Podesta L, LePage E, Hoffman A, Morsiani E, Sher L, Woolf GM, Makowka L & Demetriou AA (1993) Control of cerebral oedema by total hepatectomy and extracorporeal liver support in fulminant hepatic failure. *Lancet* **342**: 898-899.

Schafer DF & Jones EA (1982) Hepatic encephalopathy and the γ-aminobutyric acid neurotransmitter system. *Lancet* **i**: 18-20.

Seda HWM, Hughes RD, Gove CD & Williams R (1984) Inhibition of rat brain Na^+/K^+-ATPase activity by serum from patients with fulminant hepatic failure. *Hepatology* **4**: 74-79.

Sewell RB, Hughes RD, Poston L & Williams R (1982) Effects of serum from patients with fulminant hepatic failure on leucocyte sodium transport. *Clinical Science* **63**: 237-242.

Silk DBA, Trewby PN, Chase RA et al. (1977) Treatment of fulminant hepatic failure by polyacrylonitrile-membrane haemodialysis. *Lancet* **ii**: 1-3.

Sinclair SB, Greig PD, Blendis LM et al. (1989) Biochemical and clinical response of fulminant viral hepatitis to administration of prostaglandin E. A preliminary report. *Journal of Clinical Investigation* **84**: 1063-1069.

Terpstra OT (1993) Auxiliary liver grafting: a new concept in liver transplantation. *Lancet* **342**: 758.

Trewby PN, Warren R, Contini S et al. (1978) The incidence and pathophysiology of pulmonary edema in fulminant hepatic failure. *Gastroenterology* **74**: 859-865.

Trey C & Davidson CS (1970) The management of fulminant hepatic failure. In: Popper H & Schaffner F (eds), *Progress in Liver Diseases*, Vol. 3, pp. 282-298. New York: Grune and Stratton.

Vallance P & Moncada S (1991) Hyperdynamic circulation in cirrhosis: a role for nitric oxide? *Lancet* **337**: 776-778.

Weston MJ, Talbot IC, Horoworth PJN et al. (1976) Frequency of arrhythmias and other cardiac abnormalities in fulminant hepatic failure. *British Heart Journal* **38**: 1179-1188.

Williams R & Ede RJ (1981) Hepatitis in pregnancy. *British Medical Journal* **283**: 1074-1075 (Editorial).

Wright R, Eade OE, Chisholm M *et al*. (1975) Controlled prospective study of the effect on liver function of multiple exposures to halothane. *Lancet* **i**: 817-820.

Wyke RJ, Rajkovic IA, Eddleston ALWF & Williams R (1980) Defective opsonisation and complement deficiency in serum from patients with fulminant hepatic failure. *Gut* **21**: 643-649.

Wyke RJ, Yousif-Kadaru AGM, Rajkovic IA, Eddleston ALWF & Williams R (1982a) Serum stimulatory activity and polymorphonuclear leucocyte movement in patients with fulminant hepatic failure. *Clinical and Experimental Immunology* **50**: 442-449.

Wyke RJ, Canalese JC, Gimson AES & Williams R (1982b) Bacteraemia in patients with fulminant hepatic failure. *Liver* **2**: 45-52.

Zieve L, Doizaki WM & Zieve FJ (1974) Synergism between mercaptans and ammonia or fatty acids in the production of coma: a possible role for mercaptans in the pathogenesis of hepatic coma. *Journal of Laboratory and Clinical Medicine* **83**: 16-28.

Zieve L, Shekleton M, Lyftogt C & Draves K (1985) Ammonia, octanoate and a mercaptan depress regeneration of normal rat liver after partial hepatectomy. *Hepatology* **5**: 28-31.

14 Neurological Disorders

HEAD INJURIES AND RAISED INTRACRANIAL PRESSURE

Introduction

Severe head injury is the commonest cause of raised intracranial pressure (ICP) requiring intensive therapy; this section is concerned with the management of such cases. Often the same principles can be applied to those with elevated ICP due to other causes. This includes not only patients with meningoencephalitis and spontaneous intracranial haemorrhage, but also a number of other causes of intracranial hypertension such as fulminant hepatic failure (FHF) (see Chapter 13), near-drowning (see Chapter 9), eclampsia (see Chapter 17) and Reye's syndrome.

Each year, approximately 15 individuals per 100,000 of the population will require intensive hospital treatment for a head injury, and the annual death rate in Great Britain is about 9/100,000 of the population, approximately four of these dying before they reach hospital (Jennett & MacMillan, 1981). The prognosis of those with severe head injury (comatose for more than 6 hours) who do survive to reach hospital remains poor; mortality varies between 40 and 50%, less than one-quarter are likely to make a good recovery, and many of those who survive to leave hospital will be permanently disabled (the prevalence of major disability after head injury in Britain is estimated at 150/100,000 of the population). Head injuries account for about 30% of all accidental deaths, and cause 15% of all deaths in the 15–24 year age group (Jennett & MacMillan, 1981).

Fortunately, there has been a progressive decline in the number of deaths ascribed to head injury since 1967 (Jennett & MacMillan, 1981), probably partly related to the introduction of a variety of road safety measures such as seat belt legislation and penalties against those who drink and drive, and this is a continuing trend. Nevertheless, avoidable factors have been identified in as many as 74% of those who talk before dying of head injury, and in 54% of cases these were considered to have undoubtedly contributed to death (Rose et al., 1977). Since approximately 46% of the deaths attributable to head injury occur outside hospital (Jennett &

MacMillan, 1981), a few from avoidable airway problems, and others arrive at hospital with partially obstructed airways or having inhaled gastric contents, improved management at the roadside and during transfer might contribute to a reduction in both the mortality and the morbidity of these cases. Furthermore, resuscitation at referring hospitals is often inadequate and many patients arriving at neurosurgical centres are hypoxic with partially obstructed airways and/or hypotensive. In one series, airway obstruction and systemic hypotension were identified in 25% and 21% of cases respectively (Rose et al., 1977), and it has been shown that initial systemic hypotension is associated with a 50% increase in mortality (Chesnut et al., 1993). Finally, delayed recognition and treatment of complications, particularly intracranial haematomas, was the commonest avoidable factor and was most often due to delayed transfer from the primary surgical ward to the neurosurgical unit (Rose et al., 1977).

Pathophysiology (Table 14.1)

At the time of injury, a variable amount of *primary cerebral damage* is sustained, which is largely irreversible, for example lacerations, contusions (bruising most commonly involves the frontal and temporal poles) and diffuse axonal injury. The latter is due to shearing or rotational forces in high kinetic energy, acceleration/deceleration injuries, and on microscopy is characterized by the presence of 'retraction balls'. Lesser degrees of stretch injury with reversible loss of function are responsible for the transient cerebral disturbance known as 'concussion'. *Secondary brain damage*, caused by neuronal ischaemia and/or hypoxia is, however an important and potentially preventable cause of mortality and residual disability (Adams et al., 1980). This is associated with episodes of inadequate cerebral perfusion (focal or diffuse), which may be caused by traumatic arterial disruption, cerebral vasospasm, vascular distortion, raised ICP or hypotension. Arterial hypoxaemia and anaemia may also contribute to the brain injury. The release of endogenous mediators such as the eicosanoids (see Chapter 4), entry of free calcium into cells and the production of free radicals may be involved in the development of vasogenic oedema, vasoparesis and secondary cerebral damage.

Table 14.1 Mechanisms of cerebral damage following head injury.

Primary cerebral damage

Lacerations

Contusions

Diffuse axonal injury

Secondary cerebral damage

Inadequate cerebral perfusion
  Traumatic arterial disruption
  Cerebral vasospasm
  Vascular distortion
  Intracranial hypertension
  Hypotension

Arterial hypoxaemia

Anaemia

Release of mediators

CHANGES IN CEREBRAL BLOOD FLOW

Cerebral perfusion pressure

Cerebral blood flow (CBF) is dependent on the difference between the mean arterial blood pressure (MAP) and the mean intracranial pressure (ICP)—the *cerebral perfusion pressure* (CPP). When CPP falls below a critical level, conventionally 60 mm Hg (the lower limit for autoregulation in normal brain), it is likely that cerebral blood flow will fall; there is then a danger of ischaemic cerebral damage. Electrical abnormalities indicative of cerebral ischaemia are detectable when CPP falls below approximately 25–30 mm Hg, or regional cortical blood flow values are less than 20 ml/min/100 g brain tissue. Nevertheless, perfusion pressures of this order can be tolerated for several minutes, provided effective measures to restore CBF are instituted immediately (Prior, 1985). In practice, the calculated value for CPP is derived from the overall ICP and therefore only provides a guide to the adequacy of global cerebral perfusion. In reality, pressures may be much higher locally in areas of contusion, intracerebral haemorrhage and deep to haematomas. These are only reflected as a measurable rise in ICP when the increased pressure has been dissipated by brain shifts. Moreover, MAP recorded from a systemic artery is not necessarily an accurate reflection of the pressure within intracranial vessels. Therefore, critical reductions in perfusion may occur locally in the most seriously damaged areas of brain even when overall CPP is apparently adequate. Finally, ischaemic lesions are frequently identified in the arterial boundary zones where perfusion is always most precarious.

Autoregulation

The normal cerebral circulation autoregulates, maintaining cerebral blood flow constant over a wide range of perfusion pressure (**Fig. 14.1**). This is an intrinsic property of the smooth muscle in the walls of the cerebral arterioles and is independent of their nerve supply. Diseased vessels such as those with atheroma lose the ability to autoregulate, while in patients with hypertension both the lower and upper limits for autoregulation are often elevated. In drug-induced hypotension,

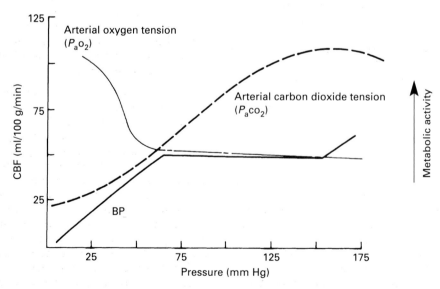

Fig. 14.1 Factors influencing cerebral blood flow (CBF). From McDowall (1976), with permission.

CBF remains constant at lower pressures than usual. Regional loss of autoregulation is common in comatose head-injured patients, while hemispheric impairment of autoregulation occurs less frequently (Cold & Jensen, 1978). In these circumstances, flow is directly related to pressure. Even when autoregulation is intact, the response of the cerebral vessels is delayed by 1.5–2 min so that sudden increases in blood pressure may nevertheless produce surges of intracranial hypertension. Autoregulation is gradually restored over a period of about five days (Cold & Jensen, 1978).

Influence of cerebral oxygen requirements

CBF is normally closely matched to cerebral oxygen requirements. In comatose head-injured patients, however, wide variations in CBF may occur, despite a consistent reduction in the cerebral metabolic rate for oxygen (CMR_{O_2}). In one study, for example, 55% of patients exhibited transient *cerebral hyperaemia* (defined as a normal or increased CBF in the presence of a reduced CMR_{O_2}), while in 45% flows were subnormal (Obrist *et al.*, 1984). In addition, there was little or no evidence of ischaemia in the latter group; rather, they exhibited the normal coupling of CBF and CMR_{O_2}. This hyperaemia is probably caused by a loss of vasomotor tone with impaired autoregulation and seems to be at least partly related to the cerebrospinal fluid (CSF) lactic acidosis that can occur in head-injured patients.

Influence of blood gas tensions

Hypercarbia increases the concentration of hydrogen ions in the interstitial spaces, causing cerebral vasodilatation, loss of autoregulation and a rise in CBF (see **Fig. 14.1**); *severe hypoxaemia* with an arterial oxygen tension (P_aO_2) of less than 8 kPa (60 mm Hg) also increases CBF (see **Fig. 14.1**), possibly by a direct effect or via chemoreceptor stimulation and neurogenic influences. Finally, it is important to remember that most inhalational anaesthetic agents cause cerebral vasodilatation.

Steal and reverse steal

The phenomena of 'steal' and 'reverse steal,' which cause local alterations in the distribution of CBF, are also relevant to the management of head-injured patients. Vessels in damaged areas of brain are often relatively unresponsive to the factors that normally influence vascular tone and simply respond passively to alterations in perfusion pressure. In contrast, vessels in intact brain react normally to such stimuli. Hypercarbia will therefore cause dilatation of responsive vessels, diverting blood flow away from areas of cerebral damage and possibly precipitating ischaemia ('steal'). Conversely, hypocarbia will increase flow and hydrostatic pressure in damaged vessels, and this may potentiate oedema formation as well as increase pressure in injured areas of brain ('reverse steal').

Intracranial pressure

The rise in ICP that can occur following severe head injury may be caused by:

- intracranial haemorrhage;
- an increase in intracranial blood volume;
- cerebral oedema;
- a combination of these.

Alterations in *intracranial blood volume*, associated with the loss of cerebrovascular tone and hyperaemia mentioned previously, are probably largely responsible for intracranial hypertension occurring in the early stages of head injury and for phasic changes in ICP (see below). In one study, there was a highly significant association between hyperaemia and the presence of intracranial hypertension (ICP > 20 mm Hg) (Obrist *et al.*, 1984).

Cerebral oedema develops later and may be vasogenic or cytotoxic (non-vasogenic).

- *Vasogenic oedema* is related to loss of capillary integrity exacerbated by vasodilatation, either locally in areas of contusion or globally; it is associated with a massive increase in capillary hydrostatic pressure and extravasation of protein-rich fluid into the interstitial spaces. This generates pressure gradients and the oedema then spreads, mostly through the white matter, to produce more generalized swelling.
- *Cytotoxic oedema* is intracellular and is related to a failure of cellular energy metabolism due to ischaemic/hypoxic injury.

Not only do haematomas and oedema cause intracranial hypertension, which may be associated with global reductions in cerebral perfusion and local impairment of the microcirculation, but they also produce 'brain shifts' and 'herniation' (**Fig. 14.2**). Unilateral mass lesions above the tentorium cause lateral distortion of the brain with local increases in pressure and impaired perfusion. Initially, the relatively rigid falx cerebri acts as a barrier to mass movements, but eventually brain may herniate beneath this structure, damaging the corpus callosum. If the supratentorial pressures exceed approximately 40 mm Hg, uncal transtentorial herniation, or 'coning', may occur jeopardizing brain stem perfusion and compressing the third cranial nerve. Initial pupillary constriction is followed by dilatation

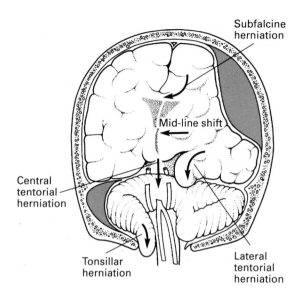

Fig. 14.2 Brain shifts and herniation in response to an intracranial haematoma.

and absent responses to light. Herniation of the cerebellar tonsil(s) may occur through the foramen magnum and the brain stem itself may be forced downwards. These brain shifts cause vascular distortion and ischaemic cerebral injury.

Intracranial compliance

It is important to appreciate the relationship between the volume of the contents of the skull and the ICP–the 'intracranial compliance curve' (**Fig. 14.3**). As intracranial volume increases, there is at first only a gradual rise in ICP because of a compensatory reduction in the

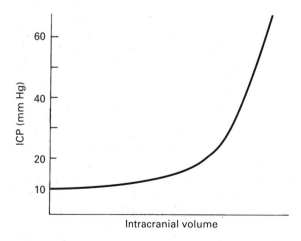

Fig. 14.3 Intracranial compliance curve. (ICP, intracranial pressure.)

volume of blood and CSF within the skull. The CSF is displaced largely into the spinal compartment, where a reduction in the volume of blood within the extradural venous plexuses prevents local increases in pressure. If intracranial volume continues to increase, however, intracranial compliance falls progressively until further compensation is impossible and ICP rises rapidly. In addition, when intracranial compliance is reduced, stimuli such as coughing, physiotherapy and endotracheal intubation, which normally cause only small transient increases in ICP, produce more pronounced and sustained intracranial hypertension.

Immediate care (see also Chapter 9) (**Table 14.2**)

The quality of the immediate care received by a head-injured patient, both outside and following admission to hospital, can profoundly influence the final outcome. This is well illustrated by the reduction in mortality from head injury that followed the introduction of trained paramedics and a helicopter transfer service in San Diego (Klauber *et al.*, 1985).

The *airway* must be secured and protected, if necessary by endotracheal intubation (**Table 14.3**) and, because patients in traumatic coma are frequently hypoxic (Miller *et al.*, 1981), supplemental *oxygen* should always be given. In some cases, immediate institution of *positive pressure ventilation* will be necessary to control the arterial carbon dioxide tension (P_aCO_2) and reduce acute severe intracranial hypertension. It must be assumed that the stomach is full and the cervical spine unstable. During laryngoscopy, the head and neck should therefore be stabilized by an assistant or using sandbags and a rapid sequence induction performed. Increases in ICP should be prevented or minimized by ensuring adequate oxygenation and prior hyperventilation and by administering sufficient intravenous anaesthetic agent and muscle relaxant.

Hypotension, which is nearly always the result of hypovolaemia, must be avoided. Restoration of an adequate blood pressure must be achieved as rapidly as possible with intravenous volume replacement, and occasionally inotropes.

At this stage, intravenous *mannitol* can be administered to control intracranial hypertension. A *urinary catheter* is then required and the stomach should be emptied using an *orogastric tube* (the nasal route can only be used when a basal skull fracture has been excluded). The patient should not be transferred or undergo investigations until adequate resuscitation has been completed, and even then should always be accompanied by a suitably qualified doctor.

Table 14.2 Management of severe head injuries.

IMMEDIATE CARE

Secure and protect airway
Administer oxygen
Consider positive pressure ventilation
Restore blood pressure
Consider intravenous mannitol
Pass orogastric tube
Insert urinary catheter

INTENSIVE CARE MANAGEMENT

Monitoring
    Intracranial pressure
    Jugular bulb venous oxygenation
    Near-infrared spectroscopy
    Cerebral function monitor
    Evoked potentials
    EEG

Prevention of ischaemic/hypoxic injury and brain shifts

Control blood pressure

Control intracranial pressure
    Reduce intracranial blood volume
        Mechanical ventilation
        Sedation
        Ensure unobstructed cerebral venous drainage
    Control cerebral oedema
        Osmotic diuretic (e.g. mannitol)
        Loop diuretic (e.g. frusemide)
    Other measures
        Remove bone flap
        Excise injured brain tissues
        Remove CSF via intraventricular catheter

Control seizure activity

Additional measures (e.g. calcium entry blockers, free radical scavengers)

General measures
    Peptic ulcer prophylaxis
    Prophylaxis for thromboembolic complications
    Antibiotics
    Physiotherapy
    Nutritional support
Management of pulmonary dysfunction
Management of diabetes insipidus, inappropriate antidiuretic hormone (ADH) secretion
Management of coagulopathy

Table 14.3 Indications for endotracheal intubation in patients with severe head injury.

Absent gag reflex
Airway protection (e.g. oropharyngeal bleeding, facial fractures)
To allow mechanical ventilation
To allow hyperventilation when patient is deteriorating due to intracranial hypertension

History, examination and investigations

Enquiries should be made about the circumstances of the injury and retrieval, the occurrence of seizures and the possibility of intoxication, as well as pre-existing medical problems and medications.

Other injuries must be excluded, which in the uncon-scious patient will often require peritoneal lavage (see Chapter 9). Scalp lacerations, bruising and abrasions suggest an underlying fracture, while ecchymoses behind the ears (Battle's sign) or around the eyes are suggestive of a basal skull fracture.

Skull radiographs should be obtained in those with:

- neurological signs or symptoms;
- leakage of CSF or blood from the nose or ear;
- suspected penetrating injury;
- pronounced bruising or swelling of the scalp.

They may reveal linear or depressed fractures; occasionally midline shift of a calcified pineal gland is seen on the antero–posterior film.

Linear fractures can cause haemorrhage from torn extradural vessels, and the presence of a skull fracture is associated with an increased risk of intracranial haematoma (Mendelow *et al.*, 1983), while those with depressed fractures may develop intracranial infection if untreated. Sometimes, there is leakage of CSF through fracture sites and this may be seen as clear fluid trickling from the nose or ear. A positive test for sugar using a Dextrostix will confirm that the fluid is indeed CSF. *Cervical spine radiographs* should also be obtained at this time.

Head-injured patients who remain comatose follow-ing resuscitation in hospital should be investigated as soon as possible by *computed axial tomography* (CT scan), and in such patients it is reasonable to forego the skull radiograph. The opportunity may be taken to scan the cervical spine. The CT scan may demonstrate cerebral swelling and reveal and localize intracranial haematomas (**Fig. 14.4**). Compression of the ventricles may also be visible on CT scan and suggests significantly raised ICP (**Fig. 14.5**), while midline shift is seen in the presence of significant unilateral mass lesions (see **Fig. 14.4**). Areas of ischaemic infarction, contusions and intracranial air may also be revealed. The absence of an intracranial haematoma on the initial scan does not exclude the possibility that this complication will develop subsequently, particularly if the scan is per-formed soon after injury. Consequently, frequent neurological assessment, monitoring of ICP and repeat scans may be required to ensure that delayed intra-cranial haemorrhage is not missed.

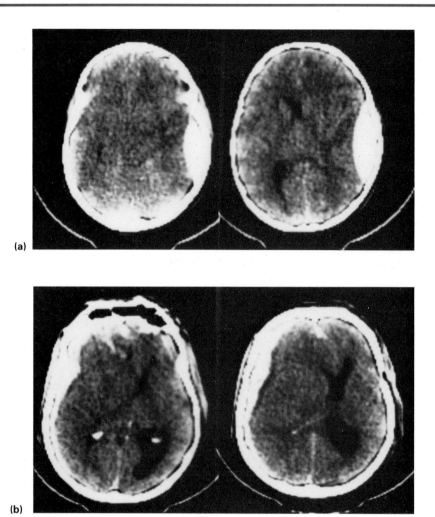

Fig. 14.4 Intracranial haematomata demonstrated by computed axial tomography. (a) Acute extradural haematoma: biconvex high attenuation collection with associated ipsilateral ventricular compression from oedema. (b) Acute subdural haematoma: high attenuation collection concave outer and convex inner margin, and marked midline shift. (Courtesy of Dr K. Hall.)

The place of *magnetic resonance imaging* (MRI) in the management of head injuries is uncertain, not least because of the logistical difficulties in supporting and monitoring patients during the procedure. MRI may be more sensitive than CT scanning for the detection of small extracerebral haematomas not requiring surgery, non-haemorrhagic contusions and ischaemic areas, while CT scanning is superior for detecting intracranial air, intraventricular and subarachnoid blood, and foreign bodies, as well as for measuring bone depression. CT scanning remains the procedure of choice for the investigation of head injuries.

The *electrocardiogram* may reveal bizarre ST segment, T wave changes such as those shown in **Fig. 14.6**.

Monitoring

CLINICAL

In the unsedated patient, a clinical assessment of neurological status is possible. The *level of consciousness* can be graded according to whether the patient is alert and orientated, drowsy but rousable, and whether they obey simple commands or react to painful stimuli. A more sophisticated assessment is possible using the *Glasgow coma scale*. This scoring system was, however, designed primarily to allow meaningful comparisons between the results obtained in different centres and with alternative treatment regimens; therefore, although it is undoubtedly valuable for research, when used in

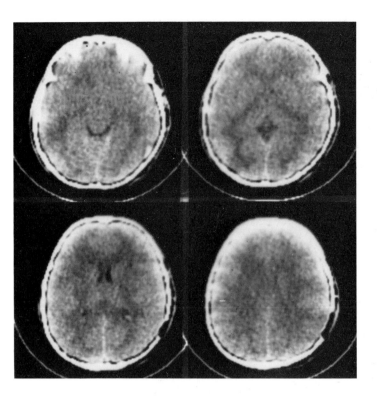

Fig. 14.5 Diffuse cerebral swelling in a patient with severe head injury. Note the ventricular compression. (Courtesy of Dr K. Hall.)

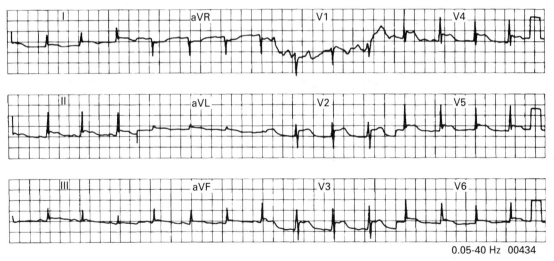

0.05-40 Hz 00434

Fig. 14.6 Electrocardiogram recorded from a patient in traumatic coma showing ST segment/T wave abnormalities.

isolation it is insufficiently sensitive for clinical use. *Localizing signs*, such as weakness and hypertonicity of the limbs on one side of the body, should also be sought, and the size and reactivity of the *pupils* assessed. Pupillary signs are late indicators of intra-cranial compression and the aim should always be to detect deterioration before such changes occur. Papil-loedema is uncommon in the acute phase of a head injury.

Patients who develop an extradural haematoma, usu-ally due to laceration of a middle meningeal artery or vein, may present with a deteriorating conscious level following a *'lucid' interval*. Subdural haematomas, on the other hand, are usually seen in those with a severe head injury and laceration of the brain, while intra-cerebral haemorrhage is a feature of penetrating or very severe closed injuries.

INTRACRANIAL PRESSURE MONITORING

Because head-injured patients admitted to the intensive care unit for controlled ventilation are usually sedated and paralysed, the clinical signs of rising ICP and neurological deterioration, except the haemodynamic and late pupillary changes, are masked. Most intensive care clinicians, but not all neurosurgeons, therefore believe that it is important to measure ICP, both as a guide to therapy aimed at its control and to detect increasing intracranial compression. If there is a sustained rise in ICP resistant to treatment, a repeat CT scan may reveal an intracranial haematoma requiring evacuation. Furthermore, ICP monitoring enables nurses, physiotherapists and medical staff to assess the effects of procedures on intracranial dynamics. Suggested indications for ICP monitoring include:

- the need for mechanical ventilation;
- Glasgow coma score of less than 8;
- the presence of a small haematoma seen on CT scan;
- following decompressive surgery.

Techniques for monitoring ICP

ICP may be monitored most sensitively and accurately by introducing a fluid-filled catheter into a lateral ventricle, although this may be difficult in those in whom the ventricles are compressed by cerebral swelling. There is also a risk of introducing infection. An *intraventricular catheter* does, however, enable the clinician to remove CSF in order to control ICP. Alternatives include a *hollow 'bolt'*, which can be threaded into the skull to measure subdural pressure, and *catheter tip transducers* or fluid-filled *catheters inserted subdurally*. *Extradural measurements* have been abandoned because of their extremely poor correlation with intraventricular pressures. Even subdural pressures often differ significantly from intraventricular measurements, tending to underestimate, especially when ICP is high. Recently a miniaturized fibre-optic catheter-tip device has been introduced that can be inserted to a depth of 1 cm into the brain to measure *intraparenchymal pressure*. This 'Camino' subdural screw reads slightly higher than ventricular pressure, but is perhaps the best alternative to catheterization of the ventricles. Progressive zero drift, which cannot be detected or corrected, is a problem during longer-term monitoring with these devices.

Interpretation

Correct interpretation of ICP recordings depends on an appreciation of the *intracranial compliance curve* (see

Fig. 14.3). Even during the initial phase of intracranial volume expansion, compensation is not perfect and ICP in fact rises from a normal value of less than 10 mm Hg to about 25 mm Hg. Above this level, there is a danger of decompensation, and an ICP of less than 25 mm Hg is therefore often used as a target for treatment aimed at controlling intracranial hypertension (Moss *et al.*, 1983). There is, however, some evidence that outcome may be improved by controlling ICP to lower values (e.g. 16 mm Hg). In addition, it must be recognized that the absolute value of the ICP provides only an approximate guide to the degree of cerebral compression.

Intracranial compliance can be assessed by injecting a small volume of fluid into the ventricles (no longer recommended) or can be inferred from the response of the ICP to stimuli such as endotracheal suction (an increase in ICP of more than 15 mm Hg during the latter manoeuvre indicates that intracranial compliance is markedly reduced). Also as intracranial compliance falls, there is an increase in the amplitude of the fluctuations in ICP, which occur in phase with the pulse and with ventilation. This is a valuable sign of intracranial compression. Finally, large (60–80 mm Hg) spontaneous increases in ICP lasting about 20 minutes *('A' waves)* as well as rhythmic oscillations at 0.5–2 cycles/min *('B' waves)* and fluctuations related to blood pressure at about 6/min *('C' waves)*, all suggest that intracranial compliance is markedly reduced.

Relationship between intracranial pressure and outcome

It has been shown that in patients who are unable to obey simple commands, but who do not have an intracranial haematoma, any increase in ICP to above 10 mm Hg is associated with a worse outcome. In those with mass lesions, however, only an ICP above 40 mm Hg on admission was associated with a poor outcome (Miller *et al.*, 1977). The presence of A waves is associated with a mortality of about 60%, but B and C waves do not seem to imply a worse prognosis (Moss *et al.*, 1983). This relationship between ICP and outcome does not necessarily imply that intracranial hypertension is directly responsible for death, nor that reducing ICP will alter mortality; rather, it is likely that the level of ICP is a reflection of the degree of cerebral damage.

JUGULAR BULB VENOUS OXYGEN SATURATION AND CONTENT (Dearden, 1991)

A thin radiopaque catheter can be inserted percutaneously into the internal jugular vein and passed retrogradely until it lies high in the jugular bulb. Simultaneous sampling of jugular venous and systemic arterial blood allows determination of the cerebral arteriovenous oxygen content difference ($C_{a-J}O_2$). The jugular bulb oxygen saturation (S_JO_2), and the jugular venous lactate level can also be determined. (The normal $C_{a-J}O_2$ in adults is around 7 ml O_2/100 ml and the normal S_JO_2 is 54-75%.) Fibre-optic catheters allow continuous S_JO_2 monitoring *in vivo*. If CBF is also determined (e.g. using the intravenous [133]xenon method) cerebral oxygen consumption (CMRo$_2$) can be calculated.

Interpretation

A low C_{a-JO2} and/or a high S_JO_2 indicate that cerebral oxygen supply exceeds demand (e.g. when CBF is increased due to loss of autoregulation or when cerebral metabolism is reduced by administering hypnotics). Conversely a fall in S_JO_2 and/or a high $C_{a-J}O_2$ indicate that cerebral oxygen supply is inadequate, perhaps because CPP and therefore CBF are low or CMRo$_2$ is increased (e.g. by seizure activity).

Determination of $C_{a-J}O_2$ and S_JO_2 can be used clinically to detect episodes of global ischaemia and to assist the selection of the most appropriate therapy for ICP reduction (see later in this chapter), it has also been suggested that these measurements can provide prognostic information. It is important to appreciate that jugular venous oxygenation is only a reflection of the global balance between cerebral oxygen supply and demand; it will not necessarily detect episodes of regional cerebral ischaemia.

NEAR-INFRARED SPECTROSCOPY

Near-infrared light penetrates the skull and during transmission through or reflection from brain tissue, undergoes wavelength changes, which are dependent on the relative concentrations of oxygenated and deoxygenated haemoglobin. In the future this technique may allow continuous non-invasive monitoring of the adequacy of cerebral oxygen supply.

NEUROPHYSIOLOGICAL MONITORING (Prior, 1985)

A number of neurophysiological techniques can be used to assess the functional state of the nervous system in patients with severe head injury.

Conventional bedside EEGs can be recorded at intervals to obtain diagnostic and prognostic information. They may reveal the presence of seizure activity, can suggest hypoxic/ischaemic damage and will localize any dysfunction as well as indicate its severity and progress. The use of conventional EEGs for continuous monitoring of intensive care patients is, however, both expensive and impractical. Some form of data reduction is required to monitor the EEG for prolonged periods automatically and to produce information that can be readily interpreted by clinicians after simple instruction.

In critically ill patients, the fundamental requirement is to monitor the serial EEG changes that accompany depression and recovery of neuronal function; these are similar whatever their aetiology (drugs, anaesthesia, hypothermia or hypoxia/ischaemia). Depression of neuronal function is accompanied by a reduction in the overall level of cortical electrical activity until electrical silence occurs. The most significant early warning of deterioration is the appearance of *'burst suppression'* activity (i.e. the breaking up of previously continuous EEG waves by increasingly long periods of electrical silence). The associated EEG *frequency changes* are more complex and less consistent, although there is a general tendency for frequencies to decrease. Both frequency and time domain analyses have been used to extract and display the most clinically relevant features of the EEG. Time domain analyses involve processing the EEG as a continuous signal (e.g. voltage plotted against time), whereas a frequency domain analysis averages the potentials present during a time period ('epoch') and then plots frequency against another variable such as power. Because the frequency plots provide no time information, serial plots are conventionally displayed sequentially in the *'compressed spectral array'* (**Fig. 14.7**).

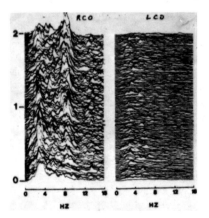

Fig. 14.7 Compressed spectral array recording from right and left centro-occipital regions showing interhemisphere asymmetry. Note the relative lack of activity from the left hemisphere recording compared with the large waves over a relatively wide frequency range on the right. The persistent reduction of left-sided activity in this patient, four days after a head injury, suggests that contusion has led to some permanent left hemisphere damage. (Unpublished data of A. Bricolo and S. Turazzi, reproduced with permission.)

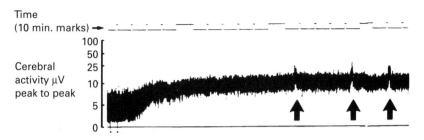

Fig. 14.8 Recording of cortical electrical activity obtained using the cerebral function monitor. Activity increases as the patient emerges from a period of heavy sedation. Seizure discharges are then seen and are indicated by the arrows.

Frequency domain analysis

A number of instruments are available that will perform this type of analysis. Although such techniques provide detailed information regarding frequency alterations, the output is relatively complex and difficult to interpret (see **Fig. 14.7**). In addition, it is possible to miss isolated events of short duration such as a brief seizure discharge, or the periods of electrical silence that are characteristic of 'burst suppression.' Frequency-based the EEG data are therefore most useful for the detection of subtle changes that may occur, for example, during sleep or with light levels of anaesthesia.

Time domain analysis

For a more generally applicable monitoring system, a recording of the voltage range and the amount of activity is a better indication of the brain's energy output.

Continuous monitoring of the EEG can be performed, for example, using the *cerebral function monitor* (CFM). This is a relatively simple, robust, portable apparatus. It produces a continuous filtered and compressed paper trace of cortical electrical activity at 6–30 cm/hr. This is recorded from two electrodes, which are generally positioned over the parietal region on either side, while a third electrode is placed in the midline to help

rejection of interference. The recording electrodes are positioned close to the arterial boundary zones, which are particularly vulnerable to reductions in cerebral perfusion, to maximize their sensitivity to ischaemic events.

The CFM will detect subclinical seizure discharges and status epilepticus (**Fig. 14.8**). Episodes of profound cerebral ischaemia are associated with reductions in CFM voltage (**Fig. 14.9**) and, if not rapidly corrected, cortical activity is permanently extinguished (**Fig. 14.10**). The extent of depression of the CFM can be used as a guide to the level of sedation achieved with intravenous anaesthetic agents (**Fig. 14.11**). Thus, depression of the baseline of the CFM trace to below 5 μV is generally equivalent to a 'burst suppression' pattern seen on the conventional EEG and indicates that $CMRO_2$ is maximally reduced. Under these circumstances, increasing the level of sedation is unlikely to produce further significant decreases in CBF and ICP (Bingham *et al.*, 1985).

Finally, the CFM recording can provide an indication of prognosis. If the trace is variable and responsive to noxious stimuli (**Fig. 14.12**) or sleep-like, a good outcome is likely provided further episodes of cerebral ischaemia and major brain shifts are avoided. If the tracing is monotonous with the loss of the normal variability and responses to pain, the majority of survivors will be vegetative, while near or total absence of electrical activity (provided this is not due to heavy sedation or hypothermia) is invariably associated with death.

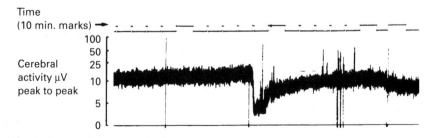

Fig. 14.9 A brief episode of profound cerebral ischaemia occurring in a patient with severe head injury. Rapid institution of measures to improve cerebral oxygenation is associated with partial recovery of cortical electrical activity.

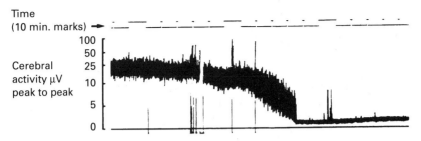

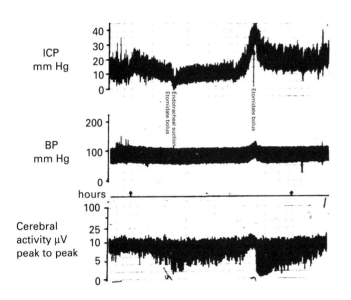

Fig. 14.10 In this cardiac surgery patient, postoperative failure of cerebral perfusion culminates in permanent extinction of cortical electrical activity.

Fig. 14.11 The effects of administering bolus doses of the intravenous anaesthetic agent etomidate (0.2 mg/kg) on intracranial pressure (ICP), systemic blood pressure (BP) and cortical electrical activity as recorded by the cerebral function monitor (CFM). Etomidate administration reduces ICP on both occasions and this is associated with a fall in the baseline of the CFM trace to below 5 μV. There is also a small reduction in systemic blood pressure. There is no increase in ICP following endotracheal suction subsequent to the first bolus dose of etomidate.

Combined time and frequency domain analysis

An example of this type of analysis is the *cerebral function analysing monitor* (CFAM). This records the amplitude of electrical activity as a mean, together with the 90th and 10th percentile values, as well as peaks and troughs that exceed these. In addition, frequency analysis is provided as the percentage of power falling into the traditional frequency bands (beta, alpha, theta and delta). It seems unlikely that this has any advantage over the CFM in routine clinical practice.

Evoked potentials (**Fig. 14.13**)

Averaged evoked potentials to external sensory stimuli (visual, auditory and somatosensory) also provide useful prognostic information. They are particularly valuable in traumatic coma because the short latency brain stem components of the auditory and somatosensory responses are unaffected by heavy sedation or anaesthesia, even when the EEG has been rendered isoelectric, and they can assess the functional integrity of

lower pathways. They are, however, affected by hypothermia. The most useful are the somatosensory evoked potentials, which are obtained by electrical stimulation at a peripheral site (e.g. the median nerve). Auditory brain stem (click) stimuli may also give valuable information. Provided a peripheral response is obtained, though this may not be possible (e.g. if the eyes or ears have sustained direct traumatic damage), the conduction time through the brain stem to the appropriate cortical site can be measured. Major asymmetries or absence of potentials are associated with serious neurological deficits, vegetative survival or death. Delayed central somatosensory conduction times may indicate a transient functional disturbance (e.g. due to white matter oedema).

Management

Intensive care management of severe head injuries is primarily concerned with the prevention of secondary ischaemic/hypoxic cerebral insults and minimizing brain shifts. This is based on maintaining adequate

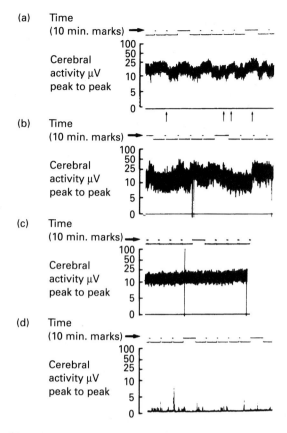

Fig. 14.12 Prognostic information can be derived from the cerebral function monitor (CFM) recording in patients with severe head injury. (a) Variable and responsive trace or (b) sleeplike—a good outcome is likely, provided further episodes of cerebral ischaemia and major brain shifts are avoided. (c) Monotonous trace—the majority of survivors will be vegetative. (d) Near or total absence of electrical activity— provided this is not due to heavy sedation or hypothermia, this is invariably associated with death.

cerebral perfusion by controlling ICP, reducing brain swelling and optimizing systemic blood pressure. Cerebral metabolic demands should also be minimized and in this respect it is particularly important to control seizure activity and reduce fever.

BLOOD PRESSURE CONTROL

Hypotension will usually respond to expansion of the circulating volume with blood or colloid guided by central venous pressure (CVP) measurements. In a few complicated cases (e.g. those with multiple injuries, adult respiratory distress syndrome or pre-existing cardiac disease), pulmonary artery catheterization is indicated. In those who fail to respond to intravenous colloids, inotropic support should be instituted. Dopamine

can be used initially but, if this fails, adrenaline, with its more potent vasoconstrictor activity, may be more effective. The aim should be to maintain an MAP higher than 80 mm Hg (or a systolic pressure greater than 110 mm Hg) while avoiding excessively high blood pressures, which because of impaired autoregulation may directly injure the capillary bed. In some patients the hyperadrenergic state that can follow severe head injury causes extreme hypertension, but specific treatment (e.g. with an intravenous β-blocker) should only be used when all other measures (sedation, control of intracranial hypertension) have failed. Vasodilators may cause catastrophic falls in CPP and should be avoided.

REDUCTION OF INTRACRANIAL PRESSURE

Intracranial pressure can be reduced by decreasing intracranial blood volume, reducing cerebral oedema or both.

Reducing intracranial blood volume

Intracranial blood volume is reduced largely by manipulating CBF. Because this produces relatively small alterations in intracranial volume, the change in intracranial pressure is greatest when cerebral compliance is markedly reduced.

Mechanical ventilation. There is no conclusive evidence that the routine use of intermittent positive pressure ventilation (IPPV), with or without induced hypocarbia, affects outcome in those with severe head injury, and in view of the acknowledged difficulties involved in assessing the value of alternative treatments in these patients, its use is likely to remain controversial. Nevertheless, because of the effects of alterations in blood gas tensions on cerebral vascular tone, including the 'steal' phenomenon, which may be induced by a rising P_aCO_2 (see earlier in this chapter) and because hypoxaemia can precipitate neuronal damage in marginally ischaemic areas, it is *clearly essential to avoid both hypercarbia and hypoxaemia*. It is therefore universally accepted that maintenance of a patent airway with adequate ventilation and oxygenation is vital. This may require tracheal intubation and, in some cases, controlled ventilation. It is also generally agreed that artificial ventilation should be instituted in head-injured patients who are hypoventilating or have respiratory arrhythmia, and in those with pulmonary dysfunction (see later). Patients who remain hypoxaemic despite administration of supplemental oxygen should also be ventilated, and severely hypoxic patients may benefit from IPPV with positive end-expiratory pressure (PEEP)

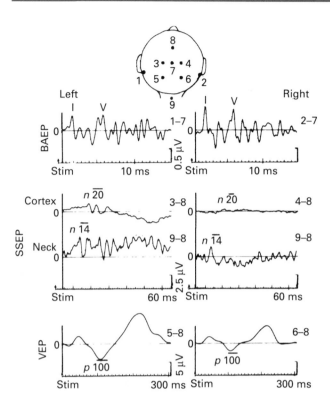

Fig. 14.13 Averaged sensory evoked potentials in traumatic coma. Brain stem auditory evoked potentials (BAEP), somatosensory potentials over second cervical vertebra and contralateral somatosensory cortex following median nerve stimulation at the wrist (SSEP) and visual evoked potentials to binocular flash stimulation (VEP). Note slight delay of BAEP wave I on the right, but otherwise normal BAEP, depressed cortical SSEP and reduced amplitude VEP over the right hemisphere. Six weeks later the patient was conscious and active, but with a left hemiparesis. stim, stimulation. From Prior (1985), with permission.

(see Chapter 7). The application of PEEP is unlikely to increase ICP unless $P_a\text{CO}_2$ is allowed to rise; certainly application of PEEP up to 10 cm H_2O is entirely safe, provided ICP is monitored and is preferable to allowing the patient to remain hypoxaemic. Some head-injured patients will hyperventilate in response to an increased CSF hydrogen ion concentration caused by cerebral ischaemia, and many authorities recommend that IPPV should also be instituted in those cases. Other suggested indications for controlled ventilation include spontaneous flexor or extensor posturing, failure to respond to painful stimuli, convulsions and significant intracranial hypertension (e.g. ICP > 25 mm Hg) (Moss *et al.*, 1983) (**Table 14.4**).

Potential advantages of controlled ventilation for patients in traumatic coma include:

- avoidance of fluctuations in blood gas tensions;
- abolition of the work of breathing;
- greater cardiovascular stability;
- sedatives and analgesic drugs can be administered without the risk of precipitating hypercarbia.

Elective hyperventilation can be used to induce hypocarbia, thereby achieving a reduction in CBF and ICP. The fall in ICP is, however, often relatively short-lived because interstitial pH, and therefore cerebrovascular tone, approaches control levels after about four hours and is at its previous value within 12–24 hours. Although it is not certain that these time relations apply

in those with head injury, it would seem that hyperventilation is of most benefit as a means of rapidly reducing acutely raised ICP. Other possible benefits of induced hypocarbia include the 'inverse steal' phenomenon, which might increase blood flow to damaged areas of brain, and correction of cerebral tissue acidosis, which may increase neuronal survival and improve autoregulation. On the other hand, excessive hypocarbia may produce a massive increase in blood flow through damaged areas of brain and this could enhance oedema formation, precipitate intracerebral haemorrhage and produce local pressure effects. Furthermore, vasoconstriction could precipitate cerebral ischaemia.

Currently it is difficult to make firm recommendations, but it would seem reasonable to aim routinely to achieve only moderate hypocarbia ($P_a\text{CO}_2$ not less than 4 kPa), thereby avoiding the dangers of extreme cerebral vasoconstriction, and to reserve aggressive hyperventilation ($P_a\text{CO}_2$ not less than 3.3 kPa) for those in whom other methods of controlling ICP have failed.

It has been suggested that hyperventilation should be used more selectively in the management of traumatic coma since in those in whom CBF is already reduced, such treatment is more likely to precipitate brain ischaemia. Conversely, patients with hyperaemia, who remain particularly responsive to alterations in arterial carbon dioxide tension, will probably benefit from hyperventilation and are at least risk of developing cerebral ischaemia (Obrist *et al.*, 1984). Determination of

Table 14.4 Some suggested indications for intermittent positive pressure ventilation (IPPV) in head-injured patients.

Coma with inadequate airway protection, but unable to tolerate endotracheal tube without sedation/paralysis
Spontaneous extensor posturing
Spontaneous flexor posturing
No response to pain
Repeated convulsions
Spontaneous hyperventilation with arterial carbon dioxide tension (P_aCO_2) < 3.5 kPa (25 mm Hg)
Arterial oxygen tension (P_aO_2) < 10.0 kPa (75 mm Hg) on air or $P_aO_2 < 13$ kPa (100 mm Hg) on supplemental oxygen
$P_aCO_2 > 6.0$ kPa (45 mm Hg)
Underventilating or showing respiratory arrhythmia in the acute phase
Associated pathology (e.g. chest injury, respiratory pathology) for which IPPV is indicated
Persistent hyperpyrexia unresponsive to conventional therapy
An intracranial pressure (ICP) of more than 25 mm Hg for greater than 25% of a 30-minute period (others suggest a mean ICP persistently > 15 mm Hg)

the $C_{a-j}O_2$ (see earlier in this chapter) enables patients with hyperaemia to be identified, and cerebral ischaemia precipitated by excessive hyperventilation can be detected as a reduction in S_jO_2.

When used to control intracranial hypertension, hyperventilation should be continued until ICP has stabilized at less than 15 mm Hg for 24–72 hrs, and to avoid a rebound increase in ICP, P_aCO_2 must be allowed to rise slowly. If there are associated respiratory problems, IPPV will have to be continued until they resolve.

Some authorities go so far as to recommend IPPV for all unconscious head-injury patients. Others consider that in many cases the risks of IPPV and sedation (loss of the signs of neurological deterioration, increased risk of pulmonary complications, dangers of tracheostomy and long-term intubation) outweigh the benefits, and it has been claimed that the extensive unselective use of controlled ventilation may be associated with a worse outcome (Jennett *et al.*, 1980). Others believe that the selective use of controlled ventilation can improve outcome in those with diffuse brain injury (Moss *et al.*, 1983).

Sedation. Sedation is commonly achieved by administering a continuous intravenous infusion of a *benzodiazepine* such as midazolam, usually accompanied by an *opiate* infusion to provide analgesia. *Muscle relaxants* are often given, usually as a continuous infusion, to minimize the increases in intrathoracic pressure that may otherwise occur in response to positive pressure ventilation and physiotherapy, as well as to prevent coughing and resisting the ventilator. It should be noted that continuous infusions of benzodiazepines, including midazolam, may be associated with prolonged recovery times and that such treatment has little intrinsic effect on ICP. Recent evidence suggests that early routine paralysis does not improve outcome from severe head injury and may be detrimental because intensive care stay is prolonged and the incidence of extracranial complications, especially pneumonia, is increased (Hsiang *et al.*, 1994). It would seem sensible to reserve prolonged neuromuscular blockade for those with resistent intracranial hypertension.

A number of *anaesthetic induction agents* can be administered as continuous intravenous infusions to provide a constant controllable level of sedation. In addition, most have been shown to decrease CBF, probably secondary to a reduction in $CMRO_2$. (An important exception is ketamine, which causes hypertension and a rise in ICP.) It is also possible that the reduction in $CMRO_2$ will protect relatively ischaemic areas of brain from further damage, and seizure activity may be controlled. A disadvantage of all intravenous anaesthetics is that they produce a variable degree of cardiovascular depression and can thereby adversely affect CPP (Prior *et al.*, 1983). Bolus doses of intravenous anaesthetic agents can also be used to rapidly reduce acutely raised ICP and to prevent surges in ICP in response to noxious stimuli such as physiotherapy and endotracheal suction (see **Fig. 14.11**) (Prior *et al.*, 1983). This is most effective when combined with muscle relaxation (White *et al.*, 1982). Associated hypotension can on occasions cause worrying reductions in CPP (Prior *et al.*, 1983), although attenuation of the rise in ICP may in itself be beneficial by minimizing intracranial pressure gradients and brain shifts. A beneficial response to the administration of an intravenous anaesthetic agent (a significant reduction in ICP associated with a rise in CPP) is most likely when the baseline voltage of the CFM is greater than 5 μV, the cardiovascular system is stable, the circulating volume is adequate and in the presence of significant intracranial hypertension (ICP >25 mm Hg) (Bingham *et al.*, 1985).

Of all the intravenous anaesthetic agents, *barbiturates* have received most attention, but their use in traumatic coma remains controversial. Although they can undoubtedly control intracranial hypertension and may redistribute blood flow to ischaemic areas as well as abolish seizure activity, the reduction in ICP is often transient and their effects on functional neurological outcome are unclear. Furthermore, barbiturates are particularly potent cardiovascular depressants and continuous infusions may have to be accompanied by the administration of inotropic agents to maintain haemodynamic stability. Pulmonary artery catheterization is then often indicated. A further disadvantage of the barbiturates is that they are redistributed to fat stores and as a consequence their sedative effect may persist for some time (at least 48 hours) after the infusion has been discontinued. Neurological assessment, and in particular examination of brain stem function, must therefore be considerably delayed. Prophylactic barbiturate therapy does not influence the incidence or duration of raised ICP, neither does it seem to affect outcome (Ward et al., 1985); most would suggest that barbiturates should only be used, if at all, when other methods have failed to control severe intracranial hypertension. In this small subset of head-injured patients, high-dose barbiturates seem to be effective adjunctive therapy for the control of ICP and there is some suggestion that outcome may be improved (Eisenberg et al., 1988). Barbiturate therapy is likely to be most effective in those with hyperaemia and retained carbon dioxide reactivity (Dearden, 1991).

In the past, the short-acting intravenous anaesthetic agents *althesin* and *etomidate* were used in a number of centres for sedation and control of ICP in traumatic coma (Moss et al., 1983; Prior et al., 1983). These agents caused less cardiovascular depression than barbiturates and recovery was relatively rapid once the infusion had been discontinued. Neither of these drugs is now available for prolonged intravenous infusion, but *propofol*, which also has a more rapid metabolic clearance, appears to be a useful alternative to the barbiturates (Farling et al., 1989).

Cerebral venous drainage. Clearly, intracranial blood volume will rise if cerebral venous drainage is impeded. The potential value of adequate muscle relaxation as a means of minimizing venous pressures has already been mentioned. In addition, the tapes securing the endotracheal or tracheostomy tube must not constrict the neck veins and the patient's head should be centrally positioned. Traditionally, the head is elevated to reduce ICP, but the response of ICP and intracranial compliance to alterations in head position appears to be variable and it has been recommended that the optimal position should be determined for each patient individually (Ropper et al., 1982).

Control of cerebral oedema

Increases in capillary hydrostatic pressure will exacerbate oedema formation. Control of CBF and systemic blood pressure therefore has the additional theoretical advantage of minimizing cerebral oedema. Most clinicians also restrict intravenous administration of crystalloid solutions (e.g. to 20 ml/kg/day of 0.18% saline in dextrose 4%).

Diuretics. The fall in ICP that can follow the administration of an *osmotic diuretic* is probably largely due to a reduction in brain water secondary to the creation of an osmotic gradient between the intravascular and interstitial spaces. In brain-injured patients, administration of *mannitol* has been shown to reduce cerebral white matter water content (Nath & Galbraith, 1986) and this is associated with a reduction in ICP, an increased CPP and improved CBF. The maximum effect is seen 10–20 minutes after the infusion, but is often transient; its duration depends on the rate at which the gradient is dissipated as osmotically active molecules diffuse into brain tissue, and this in turn is influenced by the integrity of the blood–brain barrier. Fluid might therefore be removed predominantly from normal areas of brain, and this could accentuate brain shift. In addition, repeated doses are usually progressively less effective and eventually the increasing concentration of osmotically active molecules in the interstitial space may actually enhance oedema formation—the *'rebound phenomenon'*. It has also been suggested that the reduction in ICP produced by mannitol is due largely to cerebral vasoconstriction, possibly as a compensatory response to an increase in CBF produced by the fall in blood viscosity (Muizelaar et al., 1983). The latter mechanism would explain the early (within a few minutes) reduction in ICP that can follow the administration of mannitol.

Overzealous use of mannitol may precipitate dehydration, electrolyte disturbances and overexpansion of the intravascular compartment. The latter is particularly liable to occur in patients with impaired renal function and will be especially dangerous in the presence of heart disease. Hypovolaemia as well as fluid and electrolyte disturbances can compromise renal function and may be associated with a metabolic acidosis.

To reduce the risk of rebound and fluid overload, the volume of osmotic agent administered should be carefully controlled. If a patient is deteriorating rapidly in the early stages following a head injury, 20% mannitol can be given in a dose of 0.3–1.0 g/kg. Subsequently 20% mannitol, 0.3–0.5 g/kg, should be administered not more often than every six hours, and then only if the ICP is unacceptably high. If on any occasion intracranial hypertension fails to respond, there is no diuresis or the plasma osmolality rises to more than 320 mosm/l, further mannitol should be withheld. If the serum osmolality is allowed to rise to more than 350 mosm/l there is a risk of serious cellular damage.

Mannitol is not recommended as a means of reducing ICP in patients with post-traumatic hyperaemia since the expansion of the circulating volume and fall in viscosity may further increase CBF. Mannitol is most effective when pressure autoregulation is preserved and is superior to barbiturates when $C_{a-j}O_2$ is normal (Dearden, 1991). It is also particularly useful as a means of controlling ICP before surgery. Diuretics should be used cautiously in those with vascular lesions and in the elderly because decompression may encourage further intracranial bleeding.

If osmotic diuretics and heavy sedation fail to control ICP, it may be worth trying the effect of a *loop diuretic* such as frusemide. This may enhance and prolong the reduction in ICP produced by mannitol (Pollay *et al.*, 1983).

Steroids. Steroids (e.g. dexamethasone, 10 mg initially, then 4 mg 6-hourly) are no longer recommended to control the cerebral oedema associated with severe head injury. Although they are thought to reduce the swelling surrounding a space-occupying lesion such as a cerebral metastasis, they are ineffective in controlling intracranial hypertension, and do not improve outcome following severe head injury (Cooper *et al.*, 1979; Braakman *et al.*, 1983). Complications include salt and water retention and an increase in both the incidence and severity of infectious complications (De Maria *et al.*, 1985). If steroids are used, they should be discontinued gradually to avoid a rebound increase in oedema.

Other measures to control intracranial hypertension. In resistant cases, intracranial hypertension may only be controlled by *removal of a bone flap* or by *excising damaged areas of brain*. Not only does this allow further expansion of brain substance, but the latter manoeuvre may remove a potential source of oedema fluid.

Finally, if an intraventricular catheter is *in situ*, CSF can be removed intermittently or continuously into a drainage system, although this is unlikely to reduce oedema in brain tissue.

REVERSAL OF METABOLIC ABNORMALITIES

Calcium entry blockers may prove useful in the treatment of post-traumatic vasospasm (Compton *et al.*, 1990), and their effectiveness might be enhanced by the addition of a *glutamate release blocker* such as baclofen. The roles of *free radical scavengers* and specific measures to *reverse cerebral lactic acidosis* are not yet clear.

CONTROL OF SEIZURE ACTIVITY

Most recommend prophylactic administration of phenytoin (100 mg 8-hrly intravenously or orally, preceded by a loading dose of 15 mg/kg infused at a rate not exceeding 50 mg/min). If fitting occurs despite this, intravenous diazepam or clonazepam should be given. Occasionally a thiopentone infusion may be required. Alternative anticonvulsants such as sodium valproate are sometimes prescribed.

GENERAL MEASURES

Peptic ulcer prophylaxis

Peptic ulcer prophylaxis should be instituted in all head injuries (see Chapter 10).

Antibiotics

Ampicillin and flucloxacillin are usually prescribed for patients with a CSF leak or an ICP monitoring device *in situ*, and also post-craniotomy.

Physiotherapy

Head-injured patients require expert physiotherapy, not only to prevent and treat pulmonary complications, but also to prevent contractions and to assist rehabilitation.

Nutritional support

Severe head injury is associated with a hypermetabolic state and in some cases the metabolic rate may increase by as much as 40–100%. This leads to a marked negative nitrogen balance and dramatic weight loss. Patients are hyperdynamic with increased $\dot{V}O_2$ and $\dot{V}CO_2$. The greatest increase in $\dot{V}O_2$ is seen in those with brain stem involvement, possibly related to increases in catecholamine levels. Fever, agitation and the release of mediators, such as cortisol and interleukin-1 may also be involved in the production of the hypermetabolic state.

Nutritional support is therefore vital and should be started early, preferably within 48 hours. As always the enteral route is preferred, but peripheral or total parenteral nutrition (TPN) may be required (see Chapter 10).

PULMONARY DYSFUNCTION

The alveolar–arterial oxygen difference ($C_{A-a}O_2$) is increased in more than 85% of patients with severe head injury. Specific causes include:

- neurogenic pulmonary oedema;

- prolonged respiratory depression or apnoea leading to atelectasis;
- airway obstruction;
- lung contusion;
- aspiration pneumonitis;
- fat embolism;
- nosocomial pneumonia.

In many patients, however, the cause of the pulmonary dysfunction is not obvious and it has been suggested that in such cases ventilation/perfusion (V/Q) mismatch (possibly related to hypothalamic injury), microemboli and depletion of surfactant may contribute to impaired gas exchange. This may represent a spectrum of lung injury associated with cerebral damage of which neurogenic pulmonary oedema is the extreme example.

Neurogenic pulmonary oedema (Editorial, 1985)

In 1918, Moutier published a series of cases of rapidly fatal pulmonary oedema occurring in soldiers who had suffered severe head injury. More recently, pulmonary oedema has been reported in battle casualties in Vietnam who died almost immediately following a major head injury (Simmons *et al.*, 1969). Neurogenic pulmonary oedema is less common in civilian head injuries except in young patients who have sustained massive and usually rapidly fatal brain damage. Pulmonary oedema associated with intracranial pathology has also been described in patients with subarachnoid haemorrhage, cerebral emboli, cerebral tumours and cysts, and chronically raised ICP.

Mechanisms. Neurogenic pulmonary oedema develops extremely rapidly, is particularly associated with hypothalamic lesions and does not occur in the presence of cervical cord transection. It is thought to be related to acute hypothalamic dysfunction with medullary ischaemia and brain stem distortion causing a *massive sympathetic discharge*. It seems that initially this produces marked vasoconstriction and a dramatic rise in pulmonary and systemic arterial pressures, with a fall in cardiac output. As a consequence, there is a shift of circulating volume, pulmonary venous constriction and a rise in pulmonary capillary pressure. The transient, but massive, increase in pulmonary capillary pressure disrupts the endothelium, producing a 'permeability' oedema, which persists even though intravascular pressures rapidly return to normal. Other causes of increased capillary permeability such as microemboli may also be implicated.

Management. Management is supportive and consists of IPPV, with or without PEEP, together with aggressive therapy to reduce ICP. (Mannitol should probably be avoided. It is preferable to use loop diuretics, ventricular drainage, an intravenous anaesthetic agent or surgical decompression). Vasodilatation (e.g. using α-blockers, sodium nitroprusside (SNP), chlorpromazine or labetalol may be beneficial, although associated hypotension might jeopardize cerebral perfusion and these agents can reverse hypoxic pulmonary vasoconstriction. It has been suggested that isoprenaline is the inotrope of choice in these patients because it produces both systemic and pulmonary vasodilatation, and also increases cardiac output. Despite these measures, mortality in neurogenic pulmonary oedema remains high, mainly because of the severity of the associated brain injury.

Pulmonary embolism

There is a considerable risk of deep vein thrombosis in head-injured patients as a result of hypercoagulability and reduced muscular activity. The incidence has been estimated at 30–40%, with fatal pulmonary embolism occurring in 2–3%. Because of the dangers of anticoagulation, initial prevention is with compression stockings or pneumatic boots.

OTHER COMPLICATIONS

Diabetes insipidus (see later in this chapter and Chapter 16) is a relatively common complication of severe head injury, but the syndrome of *inappropriate antidiuretic hormone (ADH)* secretion (see Chapter 16) is unusual.

Coagulopathies, particularly disseminated intravascular coagulation (DIC), can complicate head injury and must be managed aggressively to reduce the risk of intracranial haemorrhage.

Prognosis of severe head injury

The Glasgow outcome scale (Jennett & Bond, 1975) can be used to assess recovery from severe head injury in terms of five broad categories (**Table 14.5**). Although

Table 14.5 Outcome after brain damage (Glasgow outcome scale).

Dead
Persistent vegetative state—Awake, but non-sentient
Severe disability—Conscious, but dependent
Moderate disability—Independent, but disabled
Good recovery—Non-disabling sequelae

some patients may continue to improve for up to a year or even longer after their injury, the majority reach their ultimate outcome category within three months, and 90% fail to improve further beyond six months. When outcome from severe head injury (GCS ≤ 8 for at least six hours) is assessed at six months, the overall mortality is in the region of 40-50%, about 25% will make a good recovery, around 17% will be moderately disabled, and 12-17% will be severely disabled or vegetative (Jennett et al., 1980, Gennarelli et al., 1982). Outcome is related to the Glasgow coma score, the age of the patient (Moss et al., 1983) and the nature of the intracranial lesion (Gennarelli et al., 1982). Prognosis is worst in those with acute subdural haematomas, while epidural haematomas and diffuse injury with coma lasting less than 24 hours are associated with a much better outcome (Genarelli et al., 1982).

It is important to appreciate, however, that even those who are categorized as having made a 'good recovery' may experience considerable difficulties as a result of personality and cognitive changes. In some cases, mental disturbances such as anxiety, depression, fatigue, slowness of thinking and personality disorders are disabling and can be quite devastating for patients and their families. More comprehensive psychosocial evaluation of the outcome of head injury is possible using scales such as the Glasgow Assessment Schedule (Editorial, 1986).

BRAIN DEATH AND IRREVERSIBLE CEREBRAL DAMAGE

Brain stem death (Conference of Royal Medical Colleges and Faculties of the United Kingdom, 1976; Jennett, 1982)

If the brain stem is destroyed, consciousness is lost and spontaneous respiration ceases. Independent existence is then impossible and in the absence of therapeutic intervention, cardiac arrest rapidly supervenes. 'Brain stem death' is therefore now considered to be a definition of death itself. With the advent of artificial ventilation, it became possible to support such a dead patient temporarily, although in all cases cardiovascular failure eventually develops and progresses to cardiac standstill. To continue to support such a patient artificially is therefore futile. Furthermore, it needlessly prolongs the distress to both relatives and staff, is undignified for the patient, and is an inefficient and uneconomical use of resources. It is therefore desirable to discontinue artificial ventilation once the diagnosis of brain stem death has been established. Before considering such a diagnosis it is essential that certain preconditions and exclusions are fulfilled.

PRECONDITIONS

The preconditions for diagnosing brain stem death are as follows.

- The patient is in *apnoeic coma* (i.e. unresponsive and on a ventilator, with no spontaneous respiratory efforts).
- *Irremediable structural brain damage* due to a disorder that can cause brain stem death has been diagnosed with certainty (e.g. head injury, intracranial haemorrhage).

EXCLUSIONS

Exclusions for diagnosing brain stem death are as follows.

- The possibility that unresponsive apnoea is the result of *poisons, sedative drugs* or *neuromuscular blocking agents* must be excluded. The drug history should be carefully reviewed and adequate time allowed for the persistence of drug effects to be excluded. A nerve stimulator may be used to ensure that the patient is not paralysed. Blood and urine should be tested for the presence of drugs if there is any doubt.
- *Hypothermia* must be excluded as a cause of coma. It is recommended that the central body temperature should be more than 35°C.
- There must be no significant *metabolic or endocrine disturbance* that could produce or contribute to coma or cause it to persist. There should be no profound abnormality of the plasma electrolytes, acid-base balance or blood glucose levels.

ASSESSMENT OF BRAIN STEM FUNCTION

It is then necessary to establish that all brain stem reflexes are absent. *(The tests should not be performed in the presence of seizures or abnormal postures.)*

- The *pupils* should be fixed and unresponsive to bright light. Both direct and consensual light reflexes should be examined. (Difficulty in interpretation may be experienced when there has been direct trauma to the eye and/or optic nerve, and if topical mydriatics have been used.) Pupil size is irrelevant, although most often they will be dilated.
- *Corneal reflexes* should be absent. (Again, there may be difficulty when the eyelids are bruised and oedematous due to trauma.)
- *Oculocephalic reflexes* should be absent (i.e. when the head is rotated from side to side, the eyes move with the head and therefore remain stationary relative to the orbit). In a comatose patient whose brain stem

is intact, the eyes will rotate relative to the orbit (i.e. doll's eye movements are present).

- *Vestibulo-ocular reflexes* should be absent ('caloric testing'). If 20 ml of ice-cold water is slowly instilled into the external auditory meatus it will stimulate the tympanic membrane. If the patient's brain stem is intact, reflex eye movements will occur within 20–30 seconds, provided that access to the tympanic membrane is not prevented (e.g. by blood or wax in the meatus). This should be checked by direct inspection. It should be remembered that gentamicin can cause end-organ poisoning, and central pathways may be impaired by drugs. Severe trauma may prevent caloric testing on one side or the other.
- There should be *no motor responses within the cranial nerve territory* to painful stimuli applied centrally or peripherally. Spinal reflexes may be present.
- There must be no *gag or cough reflexes* in response to pharyngeal, laryngeal or tracheal stimulation.
- *Spontaneous respiration* should be absent. This test is crucial to the diagnosis of brain stem death. The patient should be ventilated with 5% carbon dioxide in 95% oxygen for ten minutes and then disconnected from the ventilator for a further ten minutes. Oxygenation is maintained by insufflation with 100% oxygen at high flows via a catheter placed in the endotracheal tube. The patient is observed for any signs of spontaneous respiratory efforts. A blood gas sample should be obtained during this period to ensure that the P_aCO_2 is sufficiently high to stimulate spontaneous respiration (> 6.7 kPa, 50 mm Hg). It must be remembered that a few patients with severe chronic obstructive pulmonary disease (COPD) are dependent on a hypoxic drive to respiration.

In the UK, it is not considered necessary to perform confirmatory tests such as *EEG* and *carotid angiography* since these may be misleading.

The examination should be performed by two doctors a minimum of six hours after the onset of coma, or if due to cardiac arrest, at least 24 hours after restoration of an adequate circulation. The tests should be performed on two separate occasions, the interval between the two being agreed by all the staff involved. The doctors should be either the consultant in charge of the case and one other (clinically independent of the first and registered for more than five years), or the consultant's deputy, provided he or she has been registered at least five years and has adequate appropriate experience, and one other. Neither should be a member of the transplant team. A neurologist should be consulted if the underlying diagnosis is in doubt.

Organ donation

As a result of advances in immunosuppression, surgical technique and intensive care, transplantation of cadaveric organs is now a highly successful treatment for patients with end-stage organ failure. Unfortunately there is a persistent shortfall of organs for transplantation, and this, combined in some instances with inadequate facilities and organizational difficulties, has meant that the number of transplants performed has consistently failed to match the demand. Clearly, therefore, every effort must be made to maximize organ retrieval rates from suitable brain stem-dead (BSD) patients. Suggested measures have included further publicity to increase the proportion of cases where consent is obtained, increased discussion to allow multiple rather than limited organ retrieval, required discussion with the transplant coordinator and the avoidance of non-procurement of suitable organs by improved organization of retrieval teams and the provision of adequate facilities in transplant units. The likely impact of introducing required request or 'opting out' legislation is less certain (Gore et al., 1989).

Although it has been shown that the number of donors can be substantially increased by transferring patients with lethal cerebrovascular accidents and incipient BSD from general wards to the intensive care unit for mechanical ventilation until BSD is confirmed (Feest et al., 1990), this practice raises a number of legal and ethical issues and is associated with a variety of practical difficulties (Hinds & Collins, 1996).

CARE OF THE MULTIPLE ORGAN DONOR

Because of the shortage of donors, retrieval of multiple organs, which can be performed without jeopardizing the function of individual organs, should now be the objective in all suitable BSD patients. In such cases, assiduous supportive treatment is essential to prevent deterioration of initially suitable donors as this will both increase donation rates and improve graft survival and function (Timmins & Hinds, 1991). Complications related to the profound physiological consequences of BSD are common and include:

- hypotension;
- requirement for multiple transfusions;
- diabetes insipidus;
- DIC;
- arrhythmias;
- pulmonary oedema;
- hypoxia;
- acidosis;
- seizures.

Since these complications may jeopardize organ function, potential donors should be carefully monitored and corrective measures instituted early.

Haemodynamic support

The most frequent complication of BSD is hypotension, which may be caused by peripheral vasodilatation, myocardial depression or both. Initially hypotension should be treated with aggressive fluid resuscitation, but in those who fail to respond there should be no hesitation in instituting inotropic support. Most recommend dopamine initially because of its effects on the splanchnic circulation, but dobutamine may be used in those who fail to respond to a moderate dose of dopamine and when specifically indicated (e.g. in patients with cardiac failure due to myocardial contusion). In some cases it may be appropriate to administer noradrenaline for short periods to counteract profound vasodilatation and maintain blood pressure during fluid resuscitation. Adrenaline may also be useful in those with refractory hypotension. Pulmonary artery catheterization is justified in difficult cases to guide volume replacement and selection of the most appropriate inotrope.

Endocrine disorders

Brain stem death can precipitate a variety of endocrine disturbances. Deficiency of antidiuretic hormone (*diabetes insipidus*, see Chapter 16) leads to an inappropriate diuresis, hypovolaemia, hyperosmolality and hypernatraemia. The diagnosis is confirmed by demonstrating a high plasma osmolality associated with a low urine osmolality. Treatment initially involves replacing measured urine volume and electrolyte losses with appropriate fluids. Hypernatraemia must be avoided by using hypotonic solutions (e.g. 5% dextrose) with added electrolytes guided by plasma levels and urinary losses. It should be remembered that colloidal solutions given to maintain the circulating volume contain considerable quantities of sodium. Treatment with *vasopressin* is controversial since it causes a dose-dependent vasoconstriction, which may be associated with a higher incidence of acute tubular necrosis and a reduced graft survival rate. Nevertheless, most currently favour the use of very low doses of vasopressin in patients with a massive diuresis.

Circulating levels of *thyroid hormones* such as triiodothyronine (T_3) are reduced following BSD and it has been suggested that this may be responsible for reduced aerobic metabolism and a deterioration in myocardial function. Currently, however, T_3 supplementation is not recommended.

Cortisol and *insulin* levels also fall after brain death and hyperglycaemia is therefore common, often exacerbated by increased catecholamine levels and the administration of large volumes of glucose-containing fluids to replace urinary losses.

Temperature control

Temperature regulation is markedly impaired after BSD because of a reduction in heat production secondary to a fall in metabolic rate, loss of muscular activity and peripheral vasodilatation. Profound hypothermia can decrease cardiac performance and precipitate a coagulopathy, and BSD cannot be diagnosed if the core temperature is less than 35°C. Body temperature should therefore be maintained by using increased insulation and active warming.

CRITERIA FOR ORGAN DONATION

BSD must have been established (see above) and the consent of the next of kin and the coroner must have been obtained.

Kidney

The criteria for selecting a suitable kidney donor are shown in **Table 14.6**. Renal perfusion must be maintained before organ donation by appropriate expansion of the circulating volume and, if necessary, a dopamine infusion. Arterial oxygenation, ventilation, body temperature, acid–base status and electrolyte balance must all be maintained. In addition, blood samples should be obtained for screening for hepatitis antigen and HIV, blood group determination and tissue typing. The kidneys must be removed by a surgeon who has examined the donor and is satisfied with the diagnosis of BSD. The procedure must be performed under full operating conditions in theatre.

Heart and heart–lung

The criteria for selecting a suitable donor are shown in **Table 14.6**. Investigations and management are as for kidney donors but, in addition, a chest radiograph and 12-lead ECG should be obtained. Occasionally coronary arteriography will be requested.

Liver

Most suitable kidney donors are also suitable liver donors. There should be no history of drug or alcohol abuse.

Cornea

All adults are suitable donors provided there is no history of eye disease, intraocular surgery, syphilis, hepa-

Table 14.6 Guidelines for the selection of suitable donors.(If there is any doubt the local transplant coordinator should be contacted early for advice on donor/individual organ suitability.)

Kidney

Brain stem dead
2–70-years-old
Adequately perfused and hydrated
Artificially ventilated

Free from:
      hepatitis antigen and HIV
      malignant disease (except primary brain tumour)
      systemic infection
      chronic urinary tract infection (acute urinary tract
         infection related to catheterization is not a
         contraindication)
      renal disease

The following are not necessarily contraindications:
      diabetes
      pneumonia
      hypertension
      hypotension

Heart or heart–lung

Brain stem dead
Preferably under 50 years old
Adequately perfused and hydrated
Artificially ventilated

Free from:
      hepatitis antigen and HIV
      malignant disease (except primary brain tumour)
      systemic infection
      diabetes mellitus
      ischaemic heart disease
      cardiac murmurs

No family history of heart disease
No history of heavy smoking
In male donors over 35 years old and female donors over 40
      years old, coronary angiograms may rarely be requested by
      the transplant team.

titis, HIV infection or postinfectious polyneuritis. The eyes can be removed up to 24 hours after cardiorespiratory arrest, but preferably within 1 hour.

Irreversible cerebral damage

Once the diagnosis of BSD has been firmly established, there is no ethical dilemma involved in discontinuing mechanical ventilation. A much more difficult problem arises when the brain stem remains intact, but the cerebral cortex ceases to function, either because of direct ischaemic/hypoxic damage (e.g. following cardiac arrest) or because of severe disruption of the white matter, such as may occur following head injury. These patients may breathe adequately unaided and can survive for long periods in a *persistent vegetative state*. Most would now accept that treatment other than basic medical and nursing care is inappropriate under these circumstances. An even more difficult ethical dilemma is presented by the patient who is severely disabled, but better than vegetative, and there is as yet no consensus on the correct management of such cases (see also Chapters 1 and 8).

STATUS EPILEPTICUS

Status epilepticus is a common medical emergency that can be defined as *persistent or recurrent motor seizures without intervening periods of consciousness*. The interval between fits is usually in the order of 5-15 minutes. The term can also be applied to continuous seizures lasting at least 30 minutes, even when consciousness is not impaired.

Clinical presentation

Major (or grand mal) status epilepticus presents with typical tonic and clonic convulsions involving the whole body. Sometimes, however, exhaustion or structural lesions within the central nervous system (CNS), partially terminate the convulsions, which may then become purely clonic or asymmetrical. In some cases, the location of the seizures varies, while in others the only manifestations are loss of consciousness with spasmodic twitching or flickering of the eyelids. These *modified forms* of status epilepticus are commonly encountered in critically ill patients.

In *partial status epilepticus*, there is repetitive focal twitching, but this may sometimes become secondarily generalized with loss of consciousness. Some patients suffer a particularly prolonged 'grand mal' seizure in which the protracted clonic and tonic phases can cause extreme hypoventilation and hypoxaemia. In others, there are frequent convulsive episodes, but consciousness is regained between seizures. Treatment is nevertheless equally urgent.

Unremitting myoclonic jerks may occur in isolation and are almost exclusively related to degenerative, hypoxic, toxic or metabolic encephalopathies. The twitching may be generalized or localized, rhythmic or disorganized, infrequent or occurring in bursts. They may arise spontaneously or be triggered by external stimuli.

Causes and precipitating factors

Status epilepticus is unusual in patients with *chronic epilepsy*, but may be precipitated by:

- trauma;
- lack of sleep;
- fasting;
- excessive alcohol;
- intercurrent infection;
- failure to take antiepileptic medication;
- interference with the absorption or metabolism of antiepileptic medication (liver failure, renal failure, pregnancy, interaction with other drugs).

When patients with *no previous history of epilepsy* present in status epilepticus, an underlying cause should be suspected. There are many possibilities, including:

- head injury;
- post-craniotomy;
- cerebral tumour (primary or secondary);
- brain abscess;
- cerebrovascular thrombosis or haemorrhage;
- meningitis;
- fat embolism;
- toxins;
- withdrawal syndromes;
- ischaemic cerebral damage;
- hypoglycaemia;
- water intoxication;
- extreme dehydration.

Pathophysiology

Major prolonged seizures can cause significant brain damage. Not only are the metabolic requirements of discharging neurones increased, but their oxygen supply is often impaired. Hypoxaemia may be caused by airway obstruction, apnoeic episodes or an aspiration pneumonitis, while CBF can be decreased by hypotension and cardiac arrhythmias. Hypercarbia and the accumulation of lactic acid produce an intracerebral acidosis. ICP rises and in the most severe cases cerebral oedema may develop as a consequence of impaired autoregulation, venous congestion, neuronal hypoxia and an increase in the permeability of the blood–brain barrier.

Initially, patients in status epilepticus are usually hyperglycaemic, but later blood sugar levels may be low. A lactic acidosis develops in severe cases. In some patients, life-threatening autonomic dysfunction supervenes with hyperthermia, excessive sweating, dehydration, hypertension and, later, hypotension. The violent muscular contractions may produce myolysis, myoglobinuria and, in some cases, renal failure.

Management (Delgado-Escueta *et al.*, 1982) (Table 14.7)

Seizure activity must be controlled immediately and vital functions preserved. Remedial underlying disorders must be identified and treated.

GENERAL ASPECTS

The patient must be *protected from injury*, without using excessive restraint, and should be placed in the *lateral position*. The *airway* must be cleared and, if it is available, *oxygen* should be administered. Tracheal intubation may be required to secure the airway and

Table 14.7 Management of status epilepticus.

Immediate measures	
Protect patient from injury	
Place patient in lateral position	
Secure and protect airway	
Administer oxygen	
Establish venous access	
Restore blood pressure	

General measures	
Correct	Fluid and electrolyte abnormalities
	Hyper-/hypoglycaemia
	Hypocalcaemia
	Hypomagnesaemia
	Persistent acidosis
Control hyperpyrexia	
Treat cerebral oedema	
Prevent acute renal failure	
When indicated	Mechanical ventilation
	Administer muscle relaxants

Administer anticonvulsants	
Benzodiazepines	Diazepam
	Clonazepam
Phenytoin	
Thiopentone	In those who fail to respond to a benzodiazepine and phenytoin
Phenobarbitone	In selected cases
Sodium valproate	
Propofol	
Vigabatrin	
Chlormethiazole	

protect the lungs from aspiration; in these cases, the nasal route is preferred since this avoids the danger of the patient biting on the tube. An intravenous infusion should be established and at this time blood can be obtained for determination of anticonvulsant levels, blood glucose, urea and electrolytes, and a full blood count. If necessary, the circulating volume is then expanded to *restore the systemic blood pressure*.

Abnormalities of *fluid and electrolyte balance*, as well as *hyperglycaemia, hypoglycaemia, hypocalcaemia* and *hypomagnesaemia*, must be corrected. The *acidosis* usually resolves spontaneously, but may require correction if it persists. It is important to avoid fluid overload in those receiving a continuous infusion of anticonvulsant. *Hyperpyrexia* can exacerbate cerebral damage and should be vigorously treated with fanning, tepid sponging, axillary ice packs and nasogastric or rectal antipyretics.

Mechanical ventilation is indicated if there is:

- respiratory depression (often induced by large doses of anticonvulsant);
- refractory hypoxaemia;
- increasing acidosis;
- cerebral oedema;
- hyperpyrexia:
- if the seizures are not controlled within 50-60 minutes.

Muscle relaxation may be required in those with prolonged uncontrolled seizures, but it is then essential to monitor the EEG (e.g. by using a CFM) to detect continued seizure activity. Because in some cases subclinical seizure activity may not be detected by the CFM, a formal EEG should be performed at intervals.

It may be reasonable to administer mannitol to those with prolonged status in whom *cerebral oedema* is suspected. Attempts to prevent *acute renal failure* in those with DIC and/or myoglobinuria may involve fluid loading, alkalinization of the urine and the administration of mannitol, frusemide and 'low-dose' dopamine (see Chapter 12).

ANTICONVULSANTS

Convulsive status should not be allowed to continue; if it persists for more than 60 minutes, severe permanent brain damage may occur. Specific treatment is therefore urgent and should be instituted as soon as the airway has been secured and intravenous access has been established.

Benzodiazepines

Intravenous *diazepam* is rapidly effective in most forms of status and is the first-line treatment. Repeated boluses or an infusion are required to maintain the effect and in protracted status the efficacy of these agents may decline progressively. In adults, 10-20 mg of diazepam can be given intravenously over a few minutes, followed by a continuous infusion (50 mg in 500 ml 5% dextrose initially at 40 ml/h). Diazepam should not be given intramuscularly since absorption is erratic and slow.

Clonazepam is an effective alternative to diazepam, initially as a bolus of 0.25-0.5 mg to a total of 5 mg intravenously, followed by an infusion at 2-3 mg/12 hours. Clonazepam is, however, a more potent respiratory depressant than diazepam.

The role of the more rapidly metabolized midazolam is unclear, but it may be effective both as a bolus and as an infusion.

Phenytoin (diphenylhydantoin)

Phenytoin is additive with diazepam. A single loading dose to a total of 15 mg/kg can be given slowly intravenously (50 mg/min diluted in 0.9% saline). Although the onset of effect may be delayed for 20-30 minutes, serum levels are maintained in the therapeutic range for 24 hours. Some authorities recommend that phenytoin should be given simultaneously with the first dose of diazepam. The main danger is myocardial toxicity. The loading dose should be followed by a daily dose of 200-500 mg. The serum phenytoin level should be monitored.

Barbiturates

Thiopentone is an effective anticonvulsant at doses lower than those normally required to induce anaesthesia. Nevertheless, there is a risk of cardiovascular and respiratory depression, and endotracheal intubation is necessary. Many patients will require IPPV. Thiopentone is indicated when the patient fails to respond to diazepam and phenytoin and should be given as an initial bolus of 1-3 mg/kg intravenously. This should be followed by a continuous infusion titrated to control seizure activity; this may require more than 3 mg/min in some cases. Blood thiopentone levels should be monitored.

Phenobarbitone can be given intravenously or intramuscularly and has a slower onset of action. It can be used as an adjunct at a later stage.

Sodium valproate

Sodium valproate can be given nasogastrically, rectally or intravenously. It causes little respiratory depression and is more effective in focal and complex partial epilepsy.

Vigabatrin

Vigabatrin is a new antiepileptic which may be useful at a later stage in the management of tonic, clonic and partial seizures.

Propofol

This intravenous anaesthetic agent has been reported to be effective in controlling status epilepticus. It has the advantage of rapid clearance once the infusion is discontinued.

Chlormethiazole

Chlormethiazole is an effective anticonvulsant and is occasionally used for the treatment of refractory status epilepticus. It must be given as a continuous infusion, initially 40–120 mg/min then at 4–8 mg/min according to response.

INVESTIGATIONS

Further investigations may include a CT scan to identify intracranial space-occupying lesions, and a lumbar puncture when meningoencephalitis, subarachnoid haemorrhage or an intracranial abscess is suspected. An EEG can identify and localize seizure activity and may assist in the diagnosis of the underlying disorder.

Prognosis

Currently, mortality rates are in the region of 10–15%. Outcome is related to the nature of the underlying structural lesion and the speed with which seizures are terminated.

TETANUS (Kerr, 1979)

The advent of effective prophylactic immunization has virtually eliminated tetanus in the developed world. In these countries, this condition now occurs mainly in those who have failed to maintain an adequate level of immunity. In Britain for example, 13–17 cases are notified each year. On the other hand, tetanus is common in most developing countries, where several hundred thousand die of this disease every year, many of the victims being neonates and young children. In Europe, the disease occurs most frequently in women and in the elderly. Often, the site of entry is a trivial wound, which in some cases may even be invisible. In others, the organism gains access via varicose ulcers, areas of ischaemic gangrene (particularly in diabetics) or following intra-abdominal, pelvic or obstetric surgery. In developing countries, uterine and neonatal tetanus are relatively frequent, as is tetanus associated with injuries to the feet.

Pathogenesis

Tetanus is caused by *Clostridium tetani*, an anaerobic Gram-positive spore-bearing bacillus found mainly in cultivated soil and as an inhabitant of the lower gastrointestinal tract. This organism produces a potent exotoxin *(tetanospasmin)*, which is responsible for the clinical manifestations of the disease. Exotoxin travels from the site of infection to the spinal cord, mainly via the perineurium of motor nerves, but also sometimes within autonomic and sensory nerve fibres, at a rate of approximately 75 mm/day. It then accumulates preferentially in the ipsilateral ventral root of the spinal cord where it passes into the presynaptic terminals of the inhibitory spinal interneurones and blocks release of the transmitter substances γ-aminobutyric acid (GABA) and glycine. Gamma motor neurones, interneurones and gamma segments of the medulla are therefore disinhibited and discharge spontaneously. Simultaneous contraction of both agonist and antagonist muscle groups produces the characteristic spasms.

Clinical features and investigations

The incubation period for tetanus varies from 4 to 15 days and tends to be shorter in the more severe cases. Nevertheless, severe attacks can also occur following a long incubation period. Investigations are generally unhelpful in identifying cases of tetanus and the diagnosis is made clinically. The majority of patients present with classical trismus ('lockjaw'). Initially, there is only some slight difficulty in opening the mouth, but this may progress until the patient is unable to eat and develops a characteristic 'risus sardonicus'. Dysphagia may also be present at this stage. More unusual presentations include *cephalic tetanus*, in which a wound in the head and neck region is associated with local cranial nerve involvement, or *local tetanus*, where spasms are confined to the injured area. The differential diagnosis includes local causes of trismus (e.g. an abscess), hysteria and dystonic reactions to phenothiazines.

All these forms of tetanus may then progress at a variable rate through the various grades of severity. Usually, the paroxysms gradually become more generalized to involve the muscles of the neck, the trunk and, to a lesser extent, the limbs. During contractions, the neck may become rigid and hyperextended, while spasm of the paravertebral muscles can produce a marked lumbar lordosis (*opisthotonos*). Ventilation may be seriously impaired and respiratory arrest can occur, either due to involvement of the thoracic and abdominal musculature or because of glottic spasm. In addition, swallowing becomes impossible and this contributes to the risk of asphyxia. Limb involvement usually consists of tonic spasms, occurring particularly on the same side as the offending wound.

In severe cases, there may be continuous, but fluctuating, *overactivity of the sympathetic nervous system* (Kerr *et al.*, 1968). This is associated with profuse sweating, salivation, paroxysmal hypertension, tachycardia, arrhythmias, vasoconstriction, pyrexia and gastrointestinal stasis. Occasionally, dangerous episodes of bradycardia and hypotension occur, either spontaneously or in response to stimuli such as endotracheal suction, and these may culminate in cardiac arrest. The signs of autonomic dysfunction usually develop 2–4 days after the patient first requires muscle relaxants and resolve within 7–10 days.

Material from wounds should be Gram stained and cultured anaerobically for *C. tetani*, which can be identified in about one-third of cases.

Table 14.8 Management of tetanus.

Eradication of infection

Incise, clean, lay open and debride wound

Antibiotics	Benzypenicillin *or*
	Erythromycin
	Tetracycline
	Metronidazole

Neutralize toxin

Booster dose of tetanus toxoid in those previously immunized

Passive immunization with tetanus immunoglobulin of human origin and first dose of tetanus toxoid in those who have not previously been immunized

Passive immunization with tetanus immunoglobulin of human origin in all patients with established tetanus

Intensive care

Isolated trismus	Avoid disturbance (no oral fluids, no gastric tube)
	Sedate (diazepam)
	Close observation
Generalized tetanus	Tracheal intubation (thiopentone and suxamethonium)
	Sedation
	Muscle relaxation
	Treat autonomic disturbances
	Ensure adequate hydration
	Nutritional support
	Subcutaneous heparin

Management (Table 14.8)

ERADICATION OF INFECTION

The source of infection is identified in only about two-thirds of tetanus cases and many appear very trivial (e.g. an ingrowing toenail). Nevertheless, potentially infected wounds must be incised, cleaned and laid open, and all the dead tissue excised. Frequently, if even apparently minor puncture sites are explored, a deep-seated necrotic area will be found, often surrounding a foreign body. When tetanus develops following an abortion, dilatation and curettage or a hysterectomy should be performed, while in cases associated with limb ischaemia, amputation may be required.

Benzylpenicillin (penicillin G) should be administered in a dose of 3.6–7.2 g/day or more for at least one week. Erythromycin or tetracycline can be used as an alternative in those allergic to penicillin, and there is some evidence that metronidazole is equally or even more effective than penicillin. Hyperbaric oxygen is probably of little value.

NEUTRALIZATION OF TOXIN

Patients at risk of developing tetanus who have previously been immunized should receive a *booster dose of tetanus toxoid*. Such active immunization must be combined with thorough wound debridement and antibiotic prophylaxis, as outlined above. The rare at-risk patient who has never been vaccinated will require *passive immunization* with *tetanus immunoglobulin of human origin (HTIG)*, as well as the first dose of tetanus toxoid. Most authorities recommend that patients with established tetanus should be passively immunized with HTIG administered intravenously or intramuscularly. This may reduce the mortality, possibly by neutralizing circulating toxin, thereby preventing relapse or further deterioration. Others consider that systemic passive immunization is unhelpful in the established case since toxin is already fixed within the spinal cord; for this reason, intrathecal administration has been reported as being more efficacious but is not routinely recommended.

INTENSIVE CARE

All patients with tetanus should be admitted to an intensive care unit for observation, assessment and treatment. The priorities are to control the spasms, prevent aspiration and/or asphyxia by endotracheal intubation or tracheostomy and avoid complications. Those with *isolated trismus* should be disturbed as little as possible to avoid precipitating a paroxysm. In particular, oral fluids should not be permitted, nor should a nasogastric tube be passed since both can precipitate laryngeal spasm. Sedatives, preferably diazepam, should be given to control muscle spasms, and the patient should be closely observed. Facilities for emergency intubation must be immediately available at the bedside.

Patients with *generalized tetanus* will require tracheal intubation (using thiopentone and suxamethonium to avoid laryngospasm during intubation) followed by early tracheostomy combined with sedation to control spasms. *Diazepam* has excellent muscle relaxant properties with minimal cardiovascular effects, and is the sedative of choice in this situation. It can be administered as a continuous intravenous infusion, although it is important to remember that active metabolites of diazepam are cumulative. If this fails, *intravenous opiates* can be added to the regimen. *Barbiturates* (e.g. an intravenous dose of thiopentone followed by regular phenobarbitone) may also be effective. All these agents can cause respiratory depression; therefore, controlled ventilation is often required. *Chlorpromazine*, which produces some α-adrenergic blockade, may also prove valuable.

If this regimen is unsuccessful (spasms lasting more than 15–20 seconds persist), the patient should be paralysed, preferably using a continuous infusion of a *nondepolarizing muscle relaxant*. Pancuronium has been used most frequently, but atracurium or vecuronium may prove to be suitable alternatives. Because neuromuscular blockade and IPPV may have to be maintained for 15–20 days, this is a potentially hazardous technique and should only be used in those unresponsive to alternative measures.

Autonomic disturbances are minimized by heavy sedation (a combination of diazepam, amylobarbitone and promazine, with diazepam as the mainstay of treatment, has been recommended) and the use of adrenergic blocking agents. β-blockers can be used to control tachycardias, and labetalol is often effective. Episodes of hypotension may resolve if the patient is stimulated (e.g. by endotracheal suction, vigorous passive limb movements or allowing the P_aCO_2 to rise).

General measures

The general principles of managing the immobile ventilated intensive care patient are outlined in Chapter 10.

Patients with tetanus lose relatively large quantities of salt and water as a result of excessive sweating and salivation. These losses are difficult to quantify and careful daily assessment of *fluid and electrolyte balance* is particularly important. Tetanus patients are often hypovolaemic when first seen, and this may be unmasked by sedation and/or IPPV; rapid *volume expansion* is then required. *Nutritional support* can usually be provided via the enteral route, but constipation can be a problem and paralytic ileus may occur in those receiving muscle relaxants. Occasionally, therefore, parenteral feeding is necessary. *Prophylactic subcutaneous heparin* should be given to all patients.

Prognosis

The acute phase of tetanus persists for 3–4 weeks, and complete recovery may take up to a further four weeks. The disease is most severe during the first week, plateaus during the second and wanes in the third. Provided patients receive extensive rehabilitation, a full recovery without neurological sequelae can be anticipated. Some patients, however, will have sustained crush fractures of one or more vertebral bodies as a result of their spasms.

In one series of adult patients with tetanus, the mortality rate was 11% and the majority of deaths (38.4%) were related to unexpected cardiac arrest (Trujillo *et al.*, 1980). With improved recognition and treatment of autonomic disturbances, however, nosocomial infections, particularly pneumonia, are becoming the leading cause of death. Other causes of death include pulmonary embolism and complications of tracheostomy. Occasionally, severe generalized tetanus develops extremely rapidly with continuous spasms, high fever, hypertension and tachycardia. In such cases, death usually follows within 24–48 hours due to major circulatory disturbances.

MYASTHENIA GRAVIS (Scadding & Havard, 1981)

Myasthenia gravis is relatively rare, with an incidence of approximately 1 in 30,000. It is commonest in young females, two-thirds of all cases being women, with a peak onset in the twenties. Men tend to develop the disease later in life, and most of those who present when more than 50 years of age are males.

Pathogenesis

Myasthenia gravis is an *autoimmune disorder* in which there is a reduction in the effective number of acetylcholine receptors at skeletal muscle motor end plates. In many patients (87–93% of cases), antibodies to these receptors can be detected, and although there is a poor correlation between absolute antibody levels and the severity of the disease, they are almost certainly important in the pathogenesis of myasthenia gravis. Antibodies to striated muscle are detected in approximately one-third of patients with myasthenia, usually in those with a thymic tumour, but are also found in association with thymic tumours in the absence of muscle weakness. It is therefore unlikely that their presence is of pathogenic significance.

In 75% of cases, there is histological evidence of a thymic abnormality, usually germinal centre hyperplasia, but in about 10% there is a thymoma, the majority of which are benign.

Clinical features

The *muscle weakness* in myasthenia gravis is typically exacerbated by exertion and improved by rest. It has a characteristic distribution affecting, in descending order of frequency, the extra-ocular, bulbar, neck, limb girdle, distal limb and trunk muscles. Some patients complain of *fatigue* rather than weakness, and in some the disease remains confined to the eye muscles. *Other autoimmune disorders* such as thyroid disease and pernicious anaemia are significantly associated with myasthenia gravis and there is an increased frequency in certain HLA subgroups.

A number of myasthenic syndromes have been described and may be encountered on the intensive care unit when such a patient fails to breathe following an anaesthetic during which muscle relaxants were used. For example, the *Eaton–Lambert syndrome* (Lambert *et al.*, 1956) occurs in association with small-cell bronchial carcinoma and is characterized by muscle weakness with aching and stiffness which, in contrast to true myasthenia, improves on exertion and spares the ocular and bulbar muscles. Nevertheless, these patients are also exquisitely sensitive to non-depolarizing muscle relaxants, and anticholinesterases have little beneficial effect. Oral guanidine and steroids may improve muscle strength, and plasma exchange may be effective.

Investigations

EDROPHONIUM TEST

The diagnosis of myasthenia gravis can be established and the adequacy of treatment assessed using an intravenous test dose of the short-acting anticholinesterase *edrophonium*. To perform this test an intravenous cannula should be inserted, the ECG should be monitored continuously and atropine should be available to counteract bradycardia. Facilities for resuscitation should also be available. An indicator of muscle function, appropriate for the particular patient, should be chosen for assessment before and after edrophonium. Usually, the most severely affected muscle group is selected. Therefore, if extra-ocular muscle weakness is most prominent, eye movement and/or diplopia can be evaluated, while straight arm raising time can be used for those with predominantly limb involvement. Many of the patients admitted to the intensive care unit will have respiratory muscle weakness and in these cases *forced vital capacity* provides an excellent objective indicator of the response to an anticholinesterase. Edrophonium should be administered slowly intravenously, initially in a dose of 2 mg, followed one minute later by a further 8 mg, provided no adverse effects are seen. Muscle function should be assessed one and ten minutes later.

ELECTROMYOGRAPHY

Electromyography shows characteristic changes in 90% of patients with generalized myasthenia gravis, as well as in many of those with only ocular symptoms.

Treatment (Table 14.9)

ANTICHOLINESTERASES

Oral *pyridostigmine bromide* (60 mg tablets) is the treatment of choice; initially, 60 mg four times daily, and then gradually increased to achieve the optimal response. If required, pyridostigmine can be taken dur-

Table 14.9 Management of myasthenia gravis.

Treatment	
Anticholinesterase	Pyridostigmine bromide
	Neostigmine
Anticholinergics	
Immunosuppressants	Steroids
	Azathioprine
Plasma exchange	
Thymectomy	
Intensive care	
Myasthenic or cholinergic crisis	May require mechanical ventilation
	Anticholinergics may be required
	Physiotherapy
Management post-thymectomy	

ing the night, but the maximum dose is 20 tablets a day. In difficult cases, pyridostigmine can be combined with *neostigmine* (15 mg tablets), which has a more rapid onset of action and can therefore be particularly useful first thing in the morning. It may not be possible to abolish muscle weakness completely, and if the dose of anticholinesterase is progressively increased in an attempt to achieve complete relief of symptoms a 'cholinergic crisis' may be precipitated.

ANTICHOLINERGICS

Anticholinergics may be required to control side-effects such as salivation, lachrymation, colic and diarrhoea. In general, however, these drugs are best avoided in the routine management of myasthenia since they may mask the onset of a cholinergic crisis.

IMMUNOSUPPRESSANTS

Corticosteroids may be useful in those who fail to improve following thymectomy or preoperatively in the most seriously ill patients. They are also valuable in ocular myasthenia and in those who are unsuitable for surgery. The administration of corticosteroids may be associated with an initial, sometimes severe, deterioration and any improvement may not be apparent for several weeks. Corticosteroids can precipitate hypokalaemia by increasing urinary potassium excretion, and this can exacerbate the muscle weakness. Plasma potassium levels should be maintained in the upper normal range.

Azathioprine can be used in those with severe myasthenia unresponsive to other measures, but can also produce an initial deterioration. Improvement may be delayed for up to 6-12 weeks, and is maximal at 6-15 months. Azathioprine can cause bone marrow depression and liver dysfunction. Frequently a combination of corticosteroids and azathioprine is used.

PLASMA EXCHANGE (Behan & Behan, 1987)

In some patients, plasma exchange produces a dramatic, but temporary improvement. There is controversy about the mechanism of this beneficial effect because there is no direct relationship between the severity of the disease and the specific antibody titre and because the procedure may be effective in those with no detectable antibody. Exchange is usually performed on five successive days, the maximum response is normally seen at 7-10 days and improvement persists for about one month. Plasma exchange can be a useful technique for managing acute problems (e.g. severe acute myasthenia

during the perioperative period) or to allow weaning from ventilatory support. Azathioprine can be used to prevent a rebound increase in antibody levels.

THYMECTOMY

Early thymectomy produces a more rapid onset of remission and a lower mortality than medical therapy and is now the recommended treatment for virtually all patients. The explanation for this improvement is unclear, although it is known that cell-mediated immunity, which is expressed through the T lymphocyte system and is dependent on the thymus, plays a role in the pathogenesis of myasthenia gravis and that antibody levels fall following thymectomy. Thymectomy or radiotherapy can also be used to treat thymoma, but the prognosis is worse in these cases and radiotherapy may be associated with a deterioration in the myasthenia.

INTENSIVE CARE

As a result of improvements in the medical management of myasthenia, respiratory support is required less frequently, although an increasing number of patients are admitted for postoperative care following thymectomy.

Management of myasthenic and cholinergic crises

Deterioration sufficient to necessitate admission to an intensive care unit may be precipitated by:

- treatment with corticosteroids, azathioprine or radiotherapy;
- hormonal changes (such as occur during menstruation or pregnancy and in thyrotoxicosis);
- intercurrent infection;
- surgery;
- various drugs—respiratory depressants, diuretics (probably as a result of hypokalaemia), aminoglycosides (which can inhibit acetylcholine release), laxatives (which can decrease the absorption of anticholinesterases), antiarrhythmics such as procainamide, lignocaine, propranolol and quinidine, as well as the quinine present in tonic water (which reduce the excitability of muscle membrane and probably also inhibit neuromuscular transmission).

It may be difficult to distinguish between an *exacerbation of myasthenia* and a *cholinergic crisis*; both can result in respiratory failure, bulbar palsy and virtually complete paralysis. In a cholinergic crisis, respiratory difficulty may be exacerbated by excessive secretions. In severe cases, immediate tracheal intubation and mechanical ventilation will be required, while in others an edrophonium test (see above) can be performed to establish the aetiology of the crisis.

The indications for instituting mechanical ventilation and for weaning patients with myasthenia and other neuromuscular causes of ventilatory failure are discussed in Chapters 6 and 7. Ventilatory function assessed by the forced vital capacity (FVC) is the best guide to the ability to wean from controlled ventilation, while the adequacy of bulbar muscle function largely determines the timing of extubation and the need for a tracheostomy.

When mechanical ventilation has been initiated, anticholinesterases should be withdrawn and reintroduced 24-48 hours later, if necessary guided by the response to edrophonium. Some believe that a period without anticholinesterase therapy allows the motor end-plate to regain its sensitivity, but the evidence for this is scanty. If the response to anticholinesterases is unsatisfactory, the use of plasma exchange with or without azathioprine or corticosteroids should be considered.

Secretions must be controlled with frequent physiotherapy and, if necessary, anticholinergics; some patients will require a tracheostomy, particularly if bulbar muscles are involved. Plasma potassium and magnesium levels should be maintained in the high normal range and adverse drug effects (see earlier in this section) must be avoided.

Subcutaneous heparin should be administered as prophylaxis against thromboembolic complications.

Management post-thymectomy

The appropriate management for patients admitted to intensive care following thymectomy depends on the severity and distribution of their preoperative muscle weakness. Therefore, mild myasthenics without respiratory or bulbar muscle involvement may be extubated immediately. Those with more severe disease will require elective postoperative ventilation until respiratory function is adequate (FVC > 10-15 ml/kg). The endotracheal tube should remain in place until both respiratory and bulbar muscle function are considered to be satisfactory and the risk of unexpected deterioration is minimal (i.e. approximately 48 hours postoperatively). Nasal endotracheal tubes are generally preferred in these cases because they are more easily tolerated by the alert patient. Some centres have rigid protocols for postoperative care following thymectomy; others adjust their treatment regimen to suit the individual patient.

ACUTE INFLAMMATORY POLYRADICULONEUROPATHY (Ropper, 1992)

In 1916, Guillain, Barré and Strohl described two cases of paralysis with muscle tenderness and areflexia associated with a high protein content, but normal white cell count, in the CSF. Both patients eventually recovered. Landry had previously described a similar case in 1859, although he had not obtained CSF, and the condition should therefore properly be called the Landry–Guillain–Barré–Strohl syndrome. However, common practice is to omit the names of both Landry and Strohl from this eponym. The term *acute inflammatory polyneuropathy* (AIP) encompasses this well-known syndrome as well as other causes of acute polyneuritis not associated with an identifiable preceding infection or CSF changes. Acute neuropathies due to toxic, metabolic or nutritional causes, as well as those associated with collagen diseases and vasculitis, are excluded from this definition.

Pathology

In some cases, cellular infiltrates consisting predominantly of lymphocytes are found throughout the peripheral nervous system in association with segmental demyelination. Many patients, however, will exhibit demyelination without obvious lymphocytic infiltration and in these cases the disease is probably largely antibody-mediated. In a few cases, there is an axonal neuropathy (Winer, 1992). Only Schwann cell-derived myelin is attacked, while that originating from oligodendrocytes within the CNS is spared. The inflammatory response is most marked in the nerve roots and the condition may therefore more correctly be called an acute demyelinating inflammatory polyradiculoneuropathy (ADIP). Although motor involvement is clinically most conspicuous, the dorsal roots, dorsal root ganglia and the ventral roots are also affected. Raised antibody titres against myelin have been identified in patients with AIP and a peripheral nervous system protein known as myelin neuritogenic protein may be an important autoantigen. The pathogenesis of this disease may therefore be either cross-antigenicity between the infecting organism and the myelin sheath, or the organism itself may be incorporated into and persist within the myelin sheath. An alternative explanation is that the precipitating infection inhibits the suppressor cells that normally prevent the development of autoimmune phenomena.

Clinical features

The frequency of AIP is approximately 1.6/1,000,000 of the population/year. The sex incidence is equal, with a slight preponderance of cases between the ages of 16 and 25 years. A *precipitating event* can be identified in approximately two-thirds of cases, often a minor respiratory tract infection or gastrointestinal upset. AIP is particularly associated with cytomegalovirus, Epstein–Barr virus and campylobacter infections, but probably can also follow *Mycoplasma* or even bacterial infections as well as immunization and surgery.

Weakness is normally distal initially and may be asymmetrical, but *ascending paralysis* often progresses rapidly to involve proximal muscle groups, including the respiratory and bulbar muscles. Although motor involvement predominates, sensory symptoms such as paraesthesiae and numbness are common, and marked sensory loss is occasionally seen. In some cases, *muscle pain and tenderness* is severe, while sphincter function is usually preserved. Sometimes, a patient will present with *cranial nerve involvement*; for example, the combination of ophthalmoplegia, ataxia and areflexia is a well-recognized variant of AIP. The presence of muscle fibrillation indicates complete denervation and suggests that recovery will be delayed or incomplete.

The autonomic nervous system may also be involved in AIP (Lichtenfeld, 1971), most commonly in those with extensive disease or cranial nerve involvement. The manifestations of the *autonomic neuropathy* are complex and can be lethal. Sinus tachycardia is a common feature and may be punctuated by periods of profound bradycardia or even asystole occurring either spontaneously or in response to stimulating procedures such as tracheal suction. These episodes are often accompanied by sweating and flushing. Blood pressure is unstable and prolonged periods of hypertension may occur. These are associated with vasoconstriction and may be interspersed with episodes of hypotension, with or without tachycardia. Associated ECG abnormalities include flattening of T waves, ST segment depression, an increased QRS voltage, left axis deviation and prolongation of the Q-T interval. Gastrointestinal disturbances may also occur, as may profuse sweating and salivation. Hallucinations are sometimes associated with these autonomic disturbances.

The *differential diagnosis* includes:

- porphyria;
- diphtheria;
- heavy metal poisoning;
- volatile solvent abuse;
- other toxic neuropathies;
- poliomyelitis;
- botulism;
- hysteria.

ADIP must also be distinguished from the chronic form (CDIP), which follows a more insidious course with progressive deterioration or stepwise relapses and is not usually preceded by an infection.

Investigations

An *elevated CSF total protein* concentration (> 0.4 g/l), with a normal white cell content (< 10/ml) is characteristic of the Guillain–Barré syndrome, but is not invariable in AIP. The CSF protein content is elevated in more than 90% of those with Guillain–Barré syndrome within one week of the onset of symptoms. *Nerve conduction studies* may demonstrate reduced conduction velocities and prolonged distal latencies.

Management (Table 14.10)

SPECIFIC TREATMENT

Immunosuppressants

In a small controlled study the administration of prednisolone to patients with AIP appeared to delay recovery as well as increase the incidence of residual disability and relapse (Hughes *et al.*, 1978). Preliminary results from a larger trial also suggest that high-dose methylprednisolone is ineffective in Guillain–Barré syndrome (Hughes, 1991). Steroids and other immunosuppressant agents (e.g. azathioprine and cyclophosphamide) are therefore no longer recommended in AIP.

Plasma exchange

Current evidence supports the use of plasma exchange in the more severe cases of Guillain–Barré syndrome, particularly those who become bedbound or require mechanical ventilation, provided treatment is instituted within 1-2 weeks of the onset of the disease (Winer, 1992). Although overall mortality is not affected, plasma exchange reduces the likelihood of patients requiring mechanical ventilation, decreases the time to onset of motor recovery, to weaning from ventilatory support and to walking, and also shortens hospital stay (French

---

Table 14.10 Management of Guillain–Barré syndrome.

Specific treatment

Plasma exchange
Immune globulin

Intensive care

Mechanical ventilation
Control of autonomic neuropathy
Pain control
Prevent complications

Co-operative Group on Plasma Exchange in Guillain-Barré Syndrome, 1987; The Guillain-Barré Syndrome Study Group, 1985). The incidence of complications also seems to be reduced, possibly due to a reduction in the duration and severity of the acute phase. Moreover in the long term more treated patients recover full muscle strength at one year (French Cooperative Group on Plasma Exchange in Guillain-Barré Syndrome, 1987).

A suitable protocol is to remove approximately one plasma volume per exchange (40–50 ml/kg) for 3–5 exchanges over a period of 7–14 days (Behan and Behan, 1987). Plasma exchange is not recommended in those with infectious complications. It is not an entirely innocuous procedure and should only be performed when experienced staff are available. Complications may occur in as many as half of those treated, and a mortality rate of 3/10,000 procedures has been reported (Behan & Behan, 1987).

Although the mechanism for the beneficial effect of plasma exchange in Guillain-Barré syndrome remains uncertain, it is assumed to be related to removal of a humoral demyelinating factor. Its efficacy does not seem to depend on the administration of immunoglobulins or complement fractions as replacement fluid since the use of either fresh frozen plasma (FFP) or diluted albumin are equally effective (French Cooperative Group on Plasma Exchange in Guillain-Barré Syndrome, 1987).

Immune globulin

Recent evidence suggests that intravenous immune globulin is an effective, safe and easy to use treatment for Guillain-Barré syndrome with obvious practical advantages when compared to plasma exchange (Van der Meche et al., 1992).

INTENSIVE CARE

Mechanical ventilation

About 20–30% of patients with Guillain-Barré syndrome will require mechanical ventilation. Respiratory and bulbar muscle function must be closely monitored so that controlled ventilation can be instituted before lung function deteriorates or respiratory arrest supervenes. The FVC should be measured at least twice a day in all cases, and more frequently in those who develop respiratory muscle weakness. As well as the absolute value of FVC, the speed with which ventilatory impairment progresses influences the decision to intervene. If lung function is also impaired (e.g. due to recurrent aspiration or secondary pneumonia) the patient may require artificial ventilation before the FVC has fallen below the conventional 10–15 ml/kg. Mechanical ventilation

should also be considered if the patient complains of breathlessness and must be instituted immediately if the P_aCO_2 is elevated. The presence of abdominal paradox (indrawing of the abdominal wall during inspiration) and respiratory difficulty when supine are indicative of significant diaphragm weakness. Nasotracheal intubation is more easily tolerated by awake patients and is therefore preferred in those with AIP. Tracheostomy should be performed early.

Management of autonomic neuropathy

Autonomic disturbances can be minimized by achieving and maintaining an adequate circulating volume, by ensuring satisfactory oxygenation, especially during endotracheal suction, and by adequate sedation. Suxamethonium should be avoided when intubating patients with AIP. β-blockade can be used to control episodes of hypertension and tachycardia, although high doses may be required. Chlorpromazine and phentolamine have also been used as antihypertensives. Insertion of a pacemaker should be considered in those with significant bradycardia and is essential if the patient has an episode of asystole. Atropine may alleviate the situation until the pacemaker is in place. Because severe autonomic disturbances can occur suddenly and unexpectedly, some routinely administer regular atropine and a β-blocking agent to all patients with AIP who require intensive care. Others simply treat the haemodynamic abnormalities appropriately as they arise.

Pain control

Limb pains are common and may be severe, particularly during passive movements. Administration of quinine, non-steroidal anti-inflammatory drugs (NSAIDs) and tricyclics may control the pain, but opiates are often required. Nasogastric methadone has been recommended and even epidural opiates have been suggested if the pain is very severe.

Prevention of complications

Potentially lethal complications of AIP include:

● thromboembolism;
● pulmonary infection;
● gastrointestinal haemorrhage.

These complications are theoretically preventable. Prophylactic subcutaneous heparin and frequent passive limb movement minimize the risk of deep vein thrombosis and pulmonary embolism. Antacid prophylaxis (see Chapter 10) and measures to reduce the risk of aspiration, atelectasis and pulmonary infection are also important aspects of the care of patients with severe AIP. Patients with paralytic ileus may require parenteral nutrition. Psychological disturbances should be prevented or managed as outlined in Chapter 10. Excellent nursing care and physiotherapy are essential for a successful outcome.

Prognosis

Evolution of the disease is usually complete within three weeks, but the speed of recovery is variable. Some improvement is generally seen within a few days of the period of maximum disability, but sometimes several weeks elapse before recovery begins. About half the survivors will have improved substantially within 3-6 months, and 60% will have completely recovered within one year. Approximately 16% will have a significant permanent residual handicap, while about 3% develop a chronic or relapsing course. The latter patients are distinguished by having a higher prevalence of certain HLA antigens and responding to immunosuppression (Winer, 1992). It is possible to achieve an overall mortality rate of around 5% or less. A poor outcome is associated with more rapidly progressive disease, the need for mechanical ventilation, the presence of small distally evoked muscle action potentials and older age (Winer, 1992).

CRITICAL ILLNESS NEUROPATHY
(Zochodne *et al.*, 1987)

Criticial illness neuropathy is a recently recognized acquired neuropathy that usually occurs in association with persistent sepsis and multiple organ dysfunction syndrome (MODS). It is thought to develop in at least half of those who remain septic for more than two weeks, and the longer the patient remains on the unit the more severe the neuropathy becomes.

Critical illness neuropathy is characterized by a primary axonal degeneration involving both motor and, to a lesser extent, sensory nerves, which is confined to the peripheral nervous system and leads to weakness and muscle wasting with evidence of denervation. Clinically the initial manifestation is often difficulty weaning the patient from respiratory support as the sepsis and MODS resolve. There is muscle wasting, the limbs are weak and flaccid, and deep tendon reflexes are reduced or absent. Cranial muscles are relatively spared.

Nerve conduction studies confirm axonal loss. The amplitude of the motor and sensory compound action potentials are reduced, but conduction velocities are relatively preserved. Fibrillation potentials may be seen on needle electromyography. The CSF protein concentration is normal or minimally elevated. These findings differentiate critical illness neuropathy from Guillain-Barré syndrome in which nerve conduction studies show evidence of demyelination and the CSF protein is usually high.

The cause of critical illness neuropathy is not known and there is no specific treatment. With resolution of the underlying sepsis and MODS, complete recovery can be anticipated in 1-6 months, although weaning from respiratory support and rehabilitation are likely to be prolonged.

REFERENCES

Adams JH, Graham DI, Scott G, Parker LS & Doyle D (1980) Brain damage in fatal non-missile head injury. *Journal of Clinical Pathology* **33**: 1132-1145.

Behan PO & Behan WMH (1987) Plasma exchange in neurological diseases, *British Medical Journal* **295**: 283-284.

Bingham RM, Procaccio F, Prior PF & Hinds CJ (1985) Cerebral electrical activity influences the effects of etomidate on cerebral perfusion pressure in traumatic coma. *British Journal of Anaesthesia* **57**: 843-848.

Braakman R, Schouten HJA, Blaauw–Van-Dishoeck M & Minderhoud JM (1983) Megadose steroids in severe head injury. Results of a prospective double-blind clinical trial. *Journal of Neurosurgery* **58**: 326-330.

Chesnut RM, Marshall LF, Klauber MR, *et al.* (1993) The role of secondary brain injury in determining outcome from severe head injury. *Journal of Trauma* **34**: 216-222.

Cold GE & Jensen FT (1978) Cerebral autoregulation in unconscious patients with brain injury. *Acta Anesthesiologica Scandinavica* **22**: 270-280.

Compton JS, Lee T, Jones NR, Waddell G & Teddy PJ (1990) A double-blind placebo controlled trial of the calcium entry blocking drug, nicardipine, in the treatment of vasospasm following severe head injury. *British Journal of Neurosurgery* **4**: 9-15.

Conference of Royal Medical Colleges and their Faculties of the United Kingdom (1976) Diagnosis of brain death. *British Medical Journal* **ii**: 1187-1188.

Cooper PR, Moody S, Kemp Clark W *et al.* (1979) Dexamethasone and severe head injury. A prospective double-blind study. *Journal of Neurosurgery* **51**: 307-316.

Dearden NM (1991) Jugular bulb venous oxygen saturation in the management of severe head injury. *Current Opinion in Anaesthesiology* **4**: 279-286.

Delgado-Escueta AV, Wasterlain C, Treiman DM & Porter RJ (1982) Current concepts in neurology: management of status epilepticus. *New England Journal of Medicine* **306**: 1337-1340.

DeMaria EJ, Reichman W, Kenney PR, Armitage JM & Gann DS

(1985) Septic complications of corticosteroid administration after central nervous system trauma. *Annals of Surgery* **202**: 248-252.

Editorial (1985) Neurogenic pulmonary oedema. *Lancet* **i**: 1430-1431.

Editorial (1986) Psychosocial outcome of head injury. *Lancet* **i**: 1361-1362.

Eisenberg HM, Frankowski RF, Contant CF, Marshall LF, Walker MD, and The Comprehensive Central Nervous System Trauma Centres (1988) High-dose barbiturate control of elevated intracranial pressure in patients with severe head injury. *Journal of Neurosurgery* **69**: 15-23.

Farling PA, Johnston JR & Coppel DL (1989) Propofol infusion for sedation of patients with head injury in intensive care. A preliminary report. *Anaesthesia* **44**: 222-226.

Feest TG, Riad HN, Collins CH, Golby MGS, Nicholls AJ & Hamad SN (1990) Protocol for increasing organ donation after cerebrovascular deaths in a district general hospital. *Lancet* **335**: 1133-1135.

French Cooperative Group on Plasma Exchange in Guillain-Barré syndrome (1987) Efficiency of plasma exchange in Guillain-Barré syndrome: role of replacement fluids. *Annals of Neurology* **22**: 753-761.

Gennarelli TA, Spielman GM, Langfitt TW *et al.* (1982) Influence of the type of intracranial lesion on outcome from severe head injury. *Journal of Neurosurgery* **56**: 26-32.

Gore SM, Hinds CJ & Rutherford AJ (1989) Organ donation from intensive care units in England: first report. *British Medical Journal* **299**: 1193-1197.

The Guillain-Barré Syndrome Study Group (1985) Plasmapheresis and acute Guillain-Barré syndrome. *Neurology* **35**: 1096-1104.

Guillain G, Barré JA & Strohl A (1916) Sur un syndrome de radicu lo-nivrite avec hyperalbuminose du liquide encphalorachidien sans réaction céllulaire. *Bulletins et memoires de la Société Médicale des Hopitaux de Paris* **40**: 1462-1470 (translated *Archives of Neurology* (1968) **18**: 450-452).

Hinds CJ & Collins C (1996) Ethical issues of organ donation. In: Tinker J, Brown D, Sibbald WJ (eds) *Critical Care: Standards, Audit and Ethics*. London, Arnold, pp. 350-359.

Hsiang JK, Chesnut RM, Crisp CB, Klauber MR, Blunt BA & Marshall LF (1994) Early, routine paralysis for intracranial pressure control in severe head injury: is it necessary? *Critical Care Medicine* **22**: 1471-1476.

Hughes RAC (1991) Ineffectiveness of high dose intravenous methylprednisolone in Guillain-Barré syndrome. *Lancet* **338**: 1142.

Hughes RAC, Newsom-Davis JM, Perkin GD & Pierce M (1978) Controlled trial of prednisolone in acute polyneuropathy. *Lancet* **ii**: 750-753.

Jennett B (1982) Brain death. *Intensive Care Medicine* **8**: 1-3.

Jennett B & Bond M (1975) Assessment of outcome after severe brain damage. *Lancet* **i**: 480-484.

Jennett B & MacMillan R (1981) Epidemiology of head injury. *British Medical Journal* **282**: 101-104.

Jennett B, Teasdale G, Fry J *et al.* (1980) Treatment for severe head injury. *Journal of Neurology, Neurosurgery and Psychiatry* **43**: 289-295.

Kerr J (1979) Current topics in tetanus. *Intensive Care Medicine* **5**: 105-110.

Kerr JH, Corbett JL, Prys-Roberts C, Smith AC & Spalding JMK (1968) Involvement of the sympathetic nervous system in tetanus. Studies on 82 cases. *Lancet* **ii**: 236-241.

Klauber MR, Marshall LF, Toole BM, Knowlton SL & Bowers SA (1985) Cause of decline in head-injury mortality rate in San Diego County, California. *Journal of Neurosurgery* **62**: 528-531.

Lambert EH, Eaton LM & Rooke ED (1956) Defect of neuromuscular conduction associated with malignant neoplasms. *American Journal of Physiology* **187**: 612-613.

Lichtenfeld P (1971) Autonomic dysfunction in the Guillain-Barré syndrome. *American Journal of Medicine* **50**: 772-780.

McDowall DG (1976) Neurosurgical anaesthesia and intensive care. In: Hewer CL & Atkinson RS (eds) *Recent Advances in Anaesthesia and Analgesia* 12. Edinburgh: Churchill Livingstone, pp. 16-43.

Mendelow AD, Teasdale G, Jennett B *et al.* (1983) Risks of intracranial haematoma in head injured adults. *British Medical Journal* **287**: 1173-1176.

Miller JD, Becker DP, Ward JD *et al.* (1977) Significance of intracranial hypertension in severe head injury. *Journal of Neurosurgery* **47**: 503-516.

Miller JD, Butterworth JF, Gudeman SK *et al.* (1981) Further experience in the management of severe head injury. *Journal of Neurosurgery* **54**: 289-299.

Moss E, Gibson JS, McDowall DG & Gibson RM (1983) Intensive management of severe head injuries. *Anaesthesia* **38**: 214-225.

Moutier F (1918) Hypertension et mort par oedème pulmonaire aigu chez les blessés cranio-encéphaliques. *Presse Medicale* **26**: 108-109.

Muizelaar JP, Wei EP, Kontos HA & Becker DP (1983) Mannitol causes compensatory cerebral vasoconstriction and vasodilation to blood viscosity changes. *Journal of Neurosurgery* **59**: 822-828.

Nath F & Galbraith S (1986) The effect of mannitol on cerebral white matter water content. *Journal of Neurosurgery* **65**: 41-43.

Obrist WD, Langfitt TW, Jaggi JL, Cruz J & Gennarelli TA (1984) Cerebral blood flow and metabolism in comatose patients with acute head injury. Relationship to intracranial hypertension. *Journal of Neurosurgery* **61**: 241-253.

Pollay M, Fallenwider C, Roberts PA & Stevens FA (1983) Effect of mannitol and furosemide on blood-brain osmotic gradient and intracranial pressure. *Journal of Neurosurgery* **59**: 945-950.

Prior PF (1985) EEG monitoring and evoked potentials in brain ischaemia. *British Journal of Anaesthesia* **57**: 63-81.

Prior JGL, Hinds CJ, Williams J & Prior PF (1983) The use of etomidate in the management of severe head injury. *Intensive Care Medicine* **9**: 313-320.

Ropper AH (1992) The Guillain-Barré syndrome. *New England Journal of Medicine* **326**: 1130-1136.

Ropper AH, O'Rourke D & Kennedy SK (1982) Head position, intracranial pressure, and compliance. *Neurology* **32**: 1288-1291.

Rose J, Valtonen S & Jennett B (1977) Avoidable factors contributing to death after head injury. *British Medical Journal* **ii**: 615-618.

Scadding GK & Havard CWH (1981) Pathogenesis and treatment of myasthenia gravis. *British Medical Journal* **283**: 1008-1012.

Simmons RL, Martin AM Jr, Heisterkamp CA 3rd & Ducker TB (1969) Respiratory insufficiency in combat casualties. II. Pulmonary edema following head injury. *Annals of Surgery* **170**: 39-44.

Timmins AC and Hinds CJ (1991) Management of the multiple-organ donor. *Current Opinion in Anaesthesiology* **4**: 287-292.

Trujillo MJ, Castillo A, España JV, Guevara P & Egañez H (1980) Tetanus in the adult: intensive care and management experience with 233 cases. *Critical Care Medicine* **8**: 419-423.

Van der Meché FGA, Schmitz PIM & The Dutch Guillain-Barré Study Group (1992) A randomized trial comparing intravenous immune globulin and plasma exchange in Guillain-Barré syndrome. *New England Journal of Medicine* **326**: 1123-1129.

Ward JD, Becker DP, Miller JD *et al.* (1985) Failure of prophylactic barbiturate coma in the treatment of severe head injury. *Journal of Neurosurgery* **62**: 383-388.

White PF, Schlobohm RM, Pitts LH & Landauer JM (1982) A randomized study of drugs for preventing increases in intracranial pressure during endotracheal suction. *Anesthesiology* **57**: 242-244.

Winer J (1992) Guillain-Barré syndrome revisited. Pathogenesis still unknown. *British Medical Journal* **304**: 65-66.

Zochodne DW, Bolton CF, Wells GA, Gilbert JJ, Hahn AF, Brown JD & Sibbald WA (1987) Critical illness polyneuropathy. A complication of sepsis and multiple organ failure. *Brain* **110**: 819-841.

15 Gastrointestinal Disorders

Not only may dysfunction of organs perfused by splanchnic vessels contribute significantly to the development and lethality of multiple organ failure (see Chapter 4), but primary pathology involving the gastrointestinal tract is a frequent cause of critical illness.

GASTROINTESTINAL HAEMORRHAGE

Acute gastrointestinal bleeding is an important cause of in-hospital morbidity and mortality. In the intensive care unit, gastrointestinal haemorrhage may be encountered under two circumstances:

- patients who initially present with massive upper or lower gastrointestinal haemorrhage;
- critically ill patients, often with multisystem involvement, in whom gastrointestinal haemorrhage develops as a secondary complication.

Upper gastrointestinal haemorrhage

CAUSES

The commonest causes of upper gastrointestinal haemorrhage are:

- peptic ulceration;
- gastritis and gastric erosions;
- stress ulceration;
- oesophagitis;
- oesophageal varices.

In the National American Society of Gastrointestinal Endoscopy (ASGE) survey of upper gastrointestinal bleeding, for example, duodenal ulcer, gastric erosions, gastric ulcer and oesophagitis accounted for 70% of the lesions identified (Silverstein *et al.*, 1981). Certain lesions are more common in particular categories of patients. For example, *angiodysplasia* of the stomach and duodenum is the most common cause of acute or recurrent bleeding in patients with chronic renal failure, while patients with aortic grafts may bleed from *aortoenteric fistulae*, and in cirrhotics a high percentage of bleeding originates from *varices*, although in up to 30% of cases bleeding is from a non-variceal site, such as *Mallory-Weiss* tears or *peptic ulceration*.

CLINICAL PRESENTATION

Most commonly patients present with *haematemesis* and *melaena*, combined, when bleeding is severe, with signs and symptoms of *shock* including anxiety, sweating, dizziness, pallor and confusion (see Chapter 4). Haematemesis occurs in about one half to two-thirds of patients with upper gastrointestinal haemorrhage, and melaena is seen in around two-thirds of cases. Although bright-red rectal bleeding is almost always a sign of colonic haemorrhage, upper gastrointestinal bleeding may result in the passage of maroon-coloured stools when large quantities of blood in the gastrointestinal tract increase intestinal motility.

The presence of *pain* may suggest peptic ulceration, pancreatitis or biliary disease, while a history of protracted retching and *vomiting* raises the possibility of Mallory-Weiss syndrome (gastric or gastro-oesophageal tear). *Dysphagia, anorexia* and *weight loss* may suggest the diagnosis of carcinoma, and in those who have previously undergone aortoiliac reconstructive surgery, bleeding may be due to an aortoenteric fistula. Finally, a meticulous drug history, including the use of anticoagulants, salicylates and alcohol, should always be taken.

PHYSICAL EXAMINATION

Physical examination should include an assessment of the severity of blood loss and the patient's physiological response to haemorrhage and resuscitation. The patient should also be examined for clues as to the source of bleeding such as hepatosplenomegaly, epigastric tenderness and wasting. The stigmata of alcoholic liver disease should be sought, as should the mucocutaneous changes of diseases known to be associated with gastrointestinal haemorrhage (hereditary haemorrhagic telangiectasia, Ehlers-Danlos syndrome and Peutz-Jeghers syndrome).

INVESTIGATIONS (Table 15.1)

Initial evaluation of patients with suspected gastrointestinal haemorrhage, including those with rectal bleeding not clearly due to lower gastrointestinal haemorrhage, should include *placement of a nasogastric tube*. Only rarely (< 1% of cases) does upper gastrointestinal haemorrhage occur without a positive bloody nasogastric aspirate, usually when there is active bleeding from the duodenum without reflux into the stomach.

Initial laboratory investigations should include haemoglobin and haematocrit determinations together with a request for cross-matching. Stool and gastric aspirates may be tested for blood if not obviously bloody. A full blood count and electrolyte determinations together with liver function tests and coagulation studies are essential in all patients. Routine chest and abdominal radiographs should be obtained. Because silent myocardial infarction may complicate significant gastrointestinal bleeding, an electrocardiogram is indicated in older patients.

Table 15.1 Management of upper gastrointestinal haemorrhage.

Resuscitation:

Rapidly restore circulating volume	Large-bore intravenous access In selected cases monitor central venous pressure Pulmonary artery catheterization may be indicated
Supplemental oxygen	

Investigations

	Pass nasogastric tube and perform gastric lavage Haemoglobin concentration/ haematocrit Test stool and gastric aspirate for blood if not obviously bloody Urea and electrolytes Coagulation studies Liver function tests Chest and abdominal radiographs Endoscopy Angiography

Continued management

Blood transfusion to maintain haematocrit at about 30% Fresh frozen plasma, platelets and clotting factor concentrates as indicated	Consider surgery in those patients with ongoing or haemodynamically important bleeding

---

Endoscopy

In the majority of patients the site of bleeding is most likely to be identified by endoscopy, which may provide clues as to the source of haemorrhage even when the stomach cannot be entirely cleared of blood. Measures must be taken to avoid aspiration in those with a full stomach, including the avoidance of excessive sedation, as well as ensuring the availability of adequate suctioning apparatus and skilled assistance. In some instances endotracheal intubation may be required before endoscopy can proceed.

The timing of endoscopy is important. All resuscitative measures should have been instituted and the patient should be stable before the procedure is begun. An exception may be made in those with massive haemorrhage who require an immediate life-saving procedure. In stable patients who continue to bleed, endoscopy should be performed as soon as possible to determine the most appropriate intervention.

When bleeding has stopped or has been easily controlled by general supportive measures, endoscopy can be performed as a semi-elective procedure, although its value in such patients has been questioned (Dronfield *et al.*, 1984; Peterson *et al.*, 1981). Specific endoscopic signs may, however, be helpful in predicting the likelihood that an ulcer will rebleed. For example, when an actively bleeding ulcer is seen at endoscopy, haemorrhage will cease spontaneously in only 20–30% of cases. The finding of a nonbleeding 'visible vessel' ('*sentinel clot*' or *pigmented protuberance*) in an ulcer base is also associated with an increased risk of recurrent haemorrhage. Endoscopic findings that suggest that the risk of rebleeding is low (< 10%) include ulcers with a clean base or containing flat pigmented spots (Kovacs & Jensen, 1987). The size and location of the ulcer may also influence the risk of rebleeding; ulcers located on the posterior wall of the duodenal bulb and those larger than 1 cm in diameter have an increased chance of rebleeding (Branicki *et al.*, 1990).

Angiography

When endoscopy fails to locate the source of haemorrhage in a patient who continues to bleed angiography may be indicated (Allison *et al.*, 1982). Emergency angiography allows localization of the bleeding site and subsequent administration of vasopressin or embolization (see later in this chapter). When angiography is not immediately available or the patient is in danger of exsanguinating, emergency surgery is indicated to control bleeding.

MANAGEMENT (see **Table 15.1**)

When a patient presents with gastrointestinal bleeding, the primary initial consideration is resuscitation and haemodynamic stabilization, rapid restoration of the patient's vascular volume being of paramount importance. Large-bore intravenous access should be established and consideration given to central venous and urinary catheterization in patients who are shocked, in the elderly and in those with significant cardiopulmonary disease. Pulmonary artery catheterization is occasionally indicated. Pending cross-matching of blood, volume losses should be replaced with crystalloid or colloidal solutions. Supplemental oxygen should be given in all cases (see also Chapter 4).

A nasogastric tube should be passed and the stomach lavaged with tap water. Gastric lavage helps to determine the severity and activity of bleeding, and also facilitates endoscopic examination.

No absolute rules exist to guide blood transfusion. In general, a haematocrit value of 30% is a reasonable goal. Packed red blood cells are sufficient to meet transfusion requirements in most cases. Fresh frozen plasma, platelets and clotting factor concentrates may be required. Patients with ongoing or haemodynamically important bleeding require a surgical opinion.

PROGNOSIS

Using broad categories of diseases a large survey of patients with gastrointestinal bleeding demonstrated that mortality increased in relation to the number of associated conditions and increasing age (Silverstein *et al.*, 1981). Also a number of readily identifiable presenting features are associated with an increased mortality. For example, patients who report red haematemesis, with or without melaena or coffee-grounds emesis with melaena have a higher mortality rate than those presenting with melaena alone. In general there is a correlation between the aspiration of red blood from the nasogastric tube and a poor outcome. Haemorrhage occurring as a complication of hospitalization and associated with hypotension is also associated with a greatly increased mortality rate compared with bleeding in the absence of hypotension or tachycardia. A haematocrit less than 30% or a haemoglobin less than 8 g/dl on presentation is associated with a worse outcome, although the increase in risk is less than that associated with hypotension. Perhaps the best predictor of mortality is continued bleeding after admission. The ASGE survey reported a mortality rate of 34% in patients with upper gastrointestinal bleeding requiring transfusion of 10 or more units of blood (Silverstein *et al.*, 1981).

SPECIFIC CAUSES OF UPPER GASTROINTESTINAL HAEMORRHAGE

Gastrointestinal haemorrhage from oesophageal varices (Ganger, 1992)

The presentation of patients with bleeding varices is often not substantially different from that of patients with upper gastrointestinal haemorrhage of other aetiologies. Sometimes, however, variceal haemorrhage is characterized by its *sudden onset* and *massive quantity* in the *absence of upper abdominal pain*. Occasionally, *painless melaena* for several days may be the only sign.

On physical examination, signs of chronic liver disease and/or portal hypertension may be present, but do not of course confirm the diagnosis of variceal bleeding. Endoscopic studies have demonstrated that even in those with documented varices, bleeding may be from other causes in a significant proportion of cases (Pitcher, 1977).

The general approach to managing a patient with variceal bleeding differs little from that described above, although it is important to note that these patients may have disorders of acid–base balance, coagulation, blood glucose levels, fluid status and conscious level as a result of associated liver disease (see Chapter 13).

Specific medical therapy (**Table 15.2**) for variceal haemorrhage may include:

- vasopressin;
- somatostatin analogues;
- balloon tamponade;
- injection sclerotherapy;
- invasive radiological procedures including transjugular intrahepatic portosystemic shunting (TIPS);
- surgery.

Vasopressin. This lowers portal venous pressure by causing splanchnic arteriolar constriction. The initial intravenous infusion rate is usually 0.3 u/minute and may be increased to 0.6 u/minute if there is no response. Generally this agent can be expected to control bleeding in 40–70% of patients. Unfortunately rebleeding is common and there is no evidence that vasopressin alone reduces mortality (Hussey, 1985). Significant complications of vasopressin can occur at any dose. Common side-effects include bradycardia and hypertension. Vasopressin also reduces coronary blood flow and cardiac output; global tissue oxygen delivery can be decreased significantly (Berk *et al.*, 1979) and some would therefore recommend cardiac output monitoring. Vasopressin is relatively contraindicated in patients with severe coronary artery, cerebrovascular or peripheral vascular disease. Glyceryl trinitrate or nitroprusside can be administered with vasopressin to ameliorate the adverse effects of vasoconstriction (Groszman *et al.*, 1982).

Table 15.2 Management of variceal bleeding.	
Active variceal bleeding	
Resuscitation	
Pharmacological therapy	Intravenous infusion of vasopressin (can combine with glyceryl trinitrate or nitroprusside) or somatostatin analogue
Endoscopic sclerotherapy or band ligation	
If bleeding continues	
Repeat sclerotherapy or banding	
Consider balloon tamponade	
Consider transjugular intrahepatic portosystemic shunting (TIPS)	
Consider oesophageal transection	
Long-term obliteration of oesophageal varices	
Endoscopic sclerotherapy or band ligation	
β-blockade	
Recurrent variceal bleeding	
TIPS	
Consider portosystemic shunt	
Consider transplantation	
Gastric varices	
Attempt endoscopic therapy	
TIPS	
Portosystemic shunt	

Somatostatin. Somatostatin or its analogues have also been used for bleeding from variceal (Kravetz *et al.*, 1984) and non-variceal sources (Magnusson *et al.*, 1985). Somatostatin decreases both splanchnic blood flow and gastric acid secretion.

Endoscopic sclerosis. This involves injecting the varices with a sclerosing agent (e.g. ethanolamine) during endoscopy. Originally the procedure was performed via a rigid Negus oesophagoscope under general anaesthesia. Endoscopic sclerosis can now be performed with a flexible endoscope, although neither approach is suitable for the treatment of gastric varices. Complications include:

● oesophageal motility disturbances;
● oesophageal ulceration;
● oesophageal stenosis;
● oesophageal perforation;
● decreased lower oesophageal sphincter pressures.

Injection therapy controls bleeding in a significant number of patients with variceal haemorrhage (Copenhagen Esophageal Varices Sclerotherapy Project, 1984), and one year survival may be improved by sclerotherapy when compared with standard medical therapy (MacDougall *et al.*, 1982). Whether sclerotherapy is the treatment of choice for all patients with bleeding varices remains unclear (Cello *et al.*, 1984; Sung *et al.* 1993). Injection sclerotherapy controls acute variceal haemorrhage in 90–95% of patients, usually with a single injection treatment (70%) (Terblanche *et al.*, 1989). Nevertheless 30% require more than one injection, and it is recommended that patients who continue to bleed despite two emergency injections should have their variceal haemorrhage temporarily controlled by balloon tamponade and then undergo a surgical shunt or operative oesophageal transection.

Endoscopic variceal ligation or banding, a technique first reported in 1990 (Goff, 1990) may also prove valuable in this situation. A prospective randomized controlled comparison of oesophageal variceal banding and emergency injection sclerotherapy has now been published (Stiegmann *et al.*, 1992). The two treatments were equally effective in controlling variceal bleeding, but ligation was associated with fewer treatment-related complications and a lower mortality.

Balloon tamponade. This is indicated if vasopressin therapy fails. A variety of balloons are available including the *Sengstaken–Blakemore* tube, which incorporates a 300 ml gastric balloon, a 45–60 ml oesophageal balloon and gastric aspiration ports. The *Patten–Johnson (Minnesota)* quadruple tube is a modification of the Sengstaken–Blakemore tube and has an additional port for suctioning the secretions that usually accumulate above the oesophageal balloon.

Balloon tamponade should only be used in an intensive care unit; the majority of patients require tracheal intubation to prevent aspiration of secretions and many also require mechanical ventilation. Complications of balloon tamponade include *oesophageal rupture* and *pulmonary aspiration* (Pitcher, 1971). The danger of rupture and/or ulceration can be minimized by carefully monitoring the balloon position and pressure, endeavouring to control bleeding with the gastric balloon only and limiting the duration of its use to 24 hours.

Although balloon tamponade has been reported to be effective in controlling haemorrhage in 40–90% of patients, rebleeding is unfortunately common. Balloon tamponade, like vasopressin, is usually only a temporary measure until definitive treatment can be undertaken.

Invasive radiological procedures. Portosystemic shunting was formerly achieved only by major surgery. TIPS is a new non-operative interventional radiological technique that may prove to be useful in those with persistent bleeding. A catheter is passed into the hepatic vein via the jugular vein and a tract is opened into a major portal branch with a rigid needle followed by a guide wire. The tract is dilated with an angioplasty balloon catheter and patency is maintained by an expandable metal stent (Ring *et al.*, 1992). TIPS has been successfully used in poor-risk patients with a low rate of subsequent encephalopathy. Its long-term use requires further evaluation and comparison with injection sclerotherapy in controlled trials.

Surgical procedures. Surgical procedures such as *variceal ligation* (e.g. transoesophageal stapling) or *emergency decompressive procedures* (e.g. portocaval shunting) can effectively control variceal bleeding.

Regardless of the specific treatment used to control haemorrhage, hepatic encephalopathy secondary to the increased intestinal protein load is common in those patients with compromised hepatic function (see Chapter 13).

Bleeding peptic ulcer (Laine & Peterson, 1994)
(Table 15.3)

Patients with bleeding peptic ulcer should initially be managed and resuscitated as outlined above.

Pharmacological therapy. Haemorrhage may be controlled by decreasing gastric blood flow, increasing gastric pH or stabilizing the clot. A variety of agents have been studied.

H_2-receptor antagonists have been extensively studied. Although pooled data indicated that rates of rebleeding and emergency surgery may be reduced and survival improved by H_2-receptor blockade (Collins & Langman,

1985), a recent randomized placebo-controlled trial failed to show any influence of the H_2-receptor antagonist famotidine on morbidity or mortality of bleeding from peptic ulcer (Walt *et al.*, 1992). To date, the most potent inhibitor of gastric acid secretion is the substituted benzimidazole *omeprazole*, which is a proton pump inhibitor. Unfortunately, promising initial results (Brunner & Chang, 1990) with this agent have not been confirmed in a recent double-blind trial (Daneshmend *et al.*, 1992). Neither antacids nor sucralfate have a place in the initial management of acute upper gastrointestinal haemorrhage.

Somatostatin is a potent inhibitor of gastric acid secretion and reduces splanchnic blood flow. Several large randomized trials (Magnusson *et al.*, 1985; Christiansen *et al.*, 1989) have evaluated its use in ulcer haemorrhage as either the natural hormone or its commercially available long-acting analogue *octreotide*. Overall there are few published data to support a role for somatostatin in the treatment of ulcer haemorrhage. Similarly no trials have documented the efficacy of *vasopressin* in ulcer haemorrhage.

The antifibrinolytic agent, *tranexamic acid* decreased mortality in a randomized controlled trial, despite having no effect on the rates of rebleeding or surgery (Barer *et al.*, 1983). A second study reported that this agent significantly reduced both the number of treated patients requiring blood transfusion and the proportion who required emergency surgery (van Holstein *et al.*, 1987). There was a high rate of thrombophlebitic complications in those given tranexamic acid and since the rate of recurrent bleeding was not significantly reduced, this agent is not currently widely used.

Endoscopic techniques. The two most extensively studied endoscopic means of achieving haemostasis of bleeding ulcers are *thermal coagulation and injection therapy*. The former may be accomplished by laser, monopolar, bipolar, or multipolar electrocautery and by heater probe. A National Institutes of Health (NIH) consensus statement concluded that the two most promising forms of endoscopic haemostatic therapy are the heater probe and bipolar electrocautery (NIH Consensus Conference, 1989). Injection therapy is the simplest and least expensive means of achieving haemostasis. A variety of solutions, both sclerosants and vasoactive agents, have been used to control haemorrhage by a combination of thrombosis, inflammation and sclerosis.

As mentioned above, the single most important determinant of outcome in those with gastrointestinal haemorrhage originating from ulcer disease is whether bleeding persists or recurs (Branicki *et al.*, 1990). A recent meta-analysis of the various randomized trials of endoscopic therapy for ulcer bleeding concluded that survival is markedly improved largely through a reduction in the rate of recurrent bleeding, but also

---

Table 15.3 Management of bleeding peptic ulcer.

Pharmacological treatment
    H_2-receptor antagonists
    Omeprazole
    (Somatostatin/octreotide)
    (Vasopressin)
    (Tranexamic acid)

Endoscopic techniques
    Thermal coagulation
    Injection therapy

Arteriography

Surgery

because fewer patients need emergency surgery (Sacks *et al.*, 1990).

Surgery (Cochran, 1993). Surgical intervention has long been a mainstay of therapy for bleeding ulcers, although the precise indications for surgery, its timing and the relative merits of the various procedures remain controversial. There is, however, no question that immediate operative intervention, with or without previous endoscopy, is the procedure of choice for exsanguinating haemorrhage. Conversely, emergency surgery has little role in the management of ulcers that have been found endoscopically to have a low risk of rebleeding.

For bleeding gastric ulcer most authors recommend gastric resection with or without vagotomy (Welch *et al.*, 1986), although others have suggested that simple oversewing may be equally effective (McGuire & Horsley, 1986). Truncal vagotomy with antrectomy or pyloroplasty is currently the operative treatment of choice for bleeding duodenal ulcer.

Arteriography. This procedure has a limited though well-defined role in the management of massive bleeding in patients who are poor surgical risks. In such cases over 50% of bleeding ulcers can be controlled by embolization of the bleeding artery. Procedural complications such as gastric necrosis can, however, be life-threatening (Liebermann *et al.*, 1984).

Acute gastric erosions (Durham & Shapiro, 1991)

Gastritis or multiple acute gastric erosions may cause bleeding:

- in patients who ingest substances that irritate the gastric mucosa such as non-steroidal anti-inflammatory drugs (NSAIDs) or alcohol;
- as a complication of critical illness—'*stress ulceration*' (see Chapter 10).

The incidence of stress-related gastric mucosal injury increased from the 1950s and through the 1970s, as did the recognition of this clinical entity. Initially it was considered to be a surgical disease occurring in patients with trauma, shock, sepsis, severe burns or central nervous system injury. It is now appreciated, however, that stress-induced injury to the gastric mucosa may also be seen in medical patients in the intensive care unit. The ageing population as well as the increasing number of critically ill patients with multiple organ failure has led to an increase in the number of patients susceptible to stress-related gastric mucosal injury.

Pathogenesis. The presence of acid and pepsin in the stomach lumen are prerequisites for the development of stress ulceration. The major inciting events impair the mechanisms that normally preserve the integrity of the gastric mucosa and may include:

- a reduction in mucosal blood flow;
- impaired production of gastric mucus;
- a decrease in the pH gradient from the gastric lumen to the intracellular space;
- a disturbed acid–base balance;
- a reduction in mucosal prostaglandins;
- impaired epithelial cell renewal.

Mucosal injury may be enhanced by:

- reflux of bile acids from the duodenum;
- uraemia.

Cushing's ulcers are associated with markedly elevated circulating gastrin levels with very high acid production and their pathogenesis may be peculiar to patients with intracranial pathology.

Pathology. Initially there is submucosal haemorrhage, which results in gastric petechiae or areas of haemorrhagic gastritis. Microscopic erosions then develop followed by ulceration superficial to the submucosa. Multiple asymptomatic superficial lesions occur in the areas of functioning oxyntic gland mucosa (i.e. the fundus and midbody of the stomach). The lesions do not extend through the mucosa and bleeding arises from the superficial capillaries. There is no fibrous base or intense inflammatory reaction. This contrasts with peptic ulcer disease in which the lesions are few in number, are more commonly located in non-acid-producing areas, penetrate deeply beneath the mucosa, are associated with chronic inflammatory changes and can cause massive bleeding from a large single vessel.

Diagnosis and clinical course. Patients should be monitored for stress-related gastric bleeding. This can be accomplished by the placement of a nasogastric tube. Endoscopy can be used to define the source if active bleeding develops.

Between 75 and 100% of intensive care patients have endoscopic evidence of gastric injury within 24–48 hours of admission. Approximately 20% of these patients will develop bleeding, which may be overt or occult, but in only 2–5% will this be clinically significant (Shuman *et al.*, 1987). The ultimate prognosis depends upon correcting the underlying disease.

Prevention. Prevention is discussed in Chapter 10.

Management of acute haemorrhage from stress ulcers. Occasionally stress ulcers may give rise to life-threatening gastric bleeding. Following *effective resuscitation*, patients should undergo *emergency endoscopy* to define the source. *Therapeutic endoscopy* with coagulation probes is less helpful when there are multiple bleeding points. *H_2-receptor blockers* and *sucralfate* should be administered if not already prescribed, otherwise the addition of *omeprazole* or *misoprostol* may prove beneficial.

In cases of massive bleeding, *emergency arteriography* can be performed. *Selective embolization* of the left gastric artery may then control the bleeding. Alternatively an *intra-arterial infusion of vasopressin* for 48–72 hours at a dosage of 0.2–0.4 units/minute may be used.

Surgery plays a limited role because of the diffuse nature of the bleeding. Furthermore, there is no consensus as to which operation should be performed. Vagotomy and pyloroplasty and subtotal and total gastrectomy are all associated with a high mortality and rebleeding is common except when a total gastrectomy is performed.

Lower gastrointestinal haemorrhage

CAUSES

Lower gastrointestinal haemorrhage is most common in the elderly (Boley *et al.*, 1981). Causes include:

- colorectal carcinoma;
- colonic polyps;
- ischaemic colitis;
- inflammatory bowel disease;
- diverticular disease;
- colonic vascular ectasias (angiodysplasia).

Diverticular bleeding is arterial and thought to be due to erosion of an arteriole at the base of a single diverticulum by a faecolith. *Vascular ectasias* are degenerative lesions associated with ageing. It is believed that they result from repeated partial low-grade obstruction of the colonic submucosal veins, especially where they pierce the muscular layer of the colon (Boley *et al.*, 1979). The obstruction causes dilatation and tortuosity of the vein and subsequently of the arterio–capillary–venular unit with the development of a small arteriovenous communication. Bleeding from vascular ectasias is characteristically recurrent and may stop spontaneously.

CLINICAL PRESENTATION

Both the rate and the pattern of bleeding depends on the underlying cause. Bleeding from diverticulosis, for example, is usually acute and severe and in most patients occurs without preceding symptoms. On the other hand, approximately one-quarter of patients with ectatic bleeding have had previous melaena or anaemia due to blood loss.

INVESTIGATIONS (**Table 15.4**)

Every patient should undergo immediate *nasogastric aspiration* to exclude upper gastrointestinal haemorrhage. The most suitable investigation for a patient with suspected lower gastrointestinal haemorrhage is usually dictated by the rate of bleeding. Massive bleeding may preclude any direct examination other than *rigid sigmoidoscopy*. If large quantities of blood are originating from a source above the sigmoidoscope, *angiography* should be undertaken to localize the site of bleeding. The value of angiography is not, however, confined to those with massive haemorrhage since it is capable of detecting active bleeding at rates as low as 0.5–1.0 ml/min. Selective angiography can be performed not only for diagnostic purposes, but also therapeutically. Vasoconstrictors such as vasopressin may be administered intra-arterially at the time of angiography, and bleeding vessels can be selectively embolized with autologous clot, gelfoam emboli or metal spring coils. *Barium examinations* should not be performed before angiography as this may mask the angiographic findings.

When bleeding is not severe, *colonoscopy* can be performed after sigmoidoscopy. The advantage of colon-

---

Table 15.4 Management of lower gastrointestinal haemorrhage.

Investigations

Nasogastric aspiration (to exclude upper gastrointestinal haemorrhage)

Rigid sigmoidoscopy

Colonoscopy

Angiography

Administration of an intravascular tracer

Treatment

Selective angiography
    Vasopressin
    Embolization

Colonoscopy
    Injection (sclerosant, adrenaline)
    Cautery
    Laser coagulation
    Polypectomy

Surgery

oscopy under these circumstances is that individual lesions such as angiodysplasia or a bleeding diverticulum can often be identified. Even if a specific lesion cannot be seen, the general area of bleeding can frequently be ascertained. Furthermore, it may be possible to control the bleeding with injection (adrenaline, sclerosant), cautery, laser coagulation or polypectomy.

In patients with intermittent or small volume bleeding, angiography may be negative and in such cases *administration of an intravascular tracer* such as ^{99m}technetium (Tc)-labelled red blood cells, has been recommended. With the gastrointestinal scintiscan the patient can then be monitored for gastrointestinal bleeding for as long as 24 hours after a single injection (Markisz *et al.*, 1982). In many institutions this examination is used in preference to arteriography in those with lower gastrointestinal bleeding.

MANAGEMENT (see **Table 15.4**)

Patients with lower gastrointestinal haemorrhage should initially be managed and resuscitated as outlined earlier.

Diverticular haemorrhage

Despite the large number of diverticula often found in the left or sigmoid colon, the source of bleeding is most frequently a single diverticulum in the right colon. Although diverticular haemorrhage is often severe, bleeding either stops spontaneously or is controlled with medical therapy in over three-quarters of patients. Fewer than 10% of patients with diverticular bleeding require operative treatment and only rarely is emergency intervention indicated (Giacchino *et al.*, 1979).

Bleeding from vascular ectasias

Similarly, bleeding from vascular ectasias is characteristically recurrent and may stop spontaneously. Otherwise patients may require colonoscopy and coagulation biopsy (Howard *et al.*, 1982). Bleeding that fails to stop with general measures may respond to an intra-arterial infusion of vasopressin following angiographic diagnosis. Patients whose bleeding continues or recurs are candidates for either segmental colectomy or hemicolectomy.

ABDOMINAL EMERGENCIES

Abdominal emergencies arising in hospital

The clinical features, management and prognosis of abdominal crises developing *de novo* in an in-patient

are distinctly different from those of the acute abdomen typically seen in the Accident and Emergency Department. It is also important to appreciate that despite their differing aetiologies and anatomy, all major gastrointestinal emergencies may be complicated by the development of endotoxaemia/bacteraemia and peritonitis. Subsequent deterioration may then be related to dissemination of the inflammatory response and, in the most severe cases, progression to multiple organ dysfunction (see Chapter 4). Since many of these conditions are amenable to surgery, the advice of an experienced surgeon is essential.

CAUSES

Patients recovering from major abdominal, orthopaedic, cardiovascular or thoracic procedures may develop intra-abdominal catastrophes either primarily or secondary to specific surgical complications. *Perforated peptic ulcer, diverticulitis, appendicitis* and *acalculous cholecystitis* can all complicate extensive surgery (Devine *et al.*, 1984), while *pancreatitis* can be precipitated by any intra-abdominal procedure, but most often complicates renal transplantation, cardiopulmonary bypass or endoscopic retrograde cholangiopancreatography (ERCP). *Intestinal or colonic ileus* can occur after spinal fractures, trauma, burns or myocardial infarction, and may also be caused by sepsis, metabolic disturbances or medications (especially opiates). Mural thrombosis complicating cardiac arrhythmias or recent myocardial infarction may embolize to the mesenteric vessels causing *acute ischaemia and bowel infarction*. Low cardiac output states such as congestive heart failure, myocardial infarction, hypovolaemia, and arrhythmias can also produce *bowel ischaemia* (see also Chapter 4).

CLINICAL PRESENTATION AND DIAGNOSIS

It is important to enquire about all medications, as well as to obtain a history of all previous medical conditions and surgical procedures. Often a change in vital signs such as an increased pulse rate or the development of metabolic acidosis may be the only indication of an intra-abdominal problem. Vague abdominal discomfort, distension, loss of appetite and oliguria are important indications that all is not well. Bowel obstruction, ileus and gastric dilatation may not be accompanied by vomiting in an unconscious, sedated and ventilated patient in whom the only signs may be frequent small episodes of regurgitation or failure to absorb enteral feed.

On physical examination such a patient may not grimace on palpation and peritonitis may be masked by a flaccid distended abdominal wall. Radiological and laboratory investigations are essential to avoid missing a treatable abdominal catastrophe. Sometimes an abdominal tap of patients who are suspected of having necrotic bowel may produce foul-smelling blood-stained fluid and therefore hasten surgery.

Gastroduodenal emergencies

PERFORATED ULCER

Clinical features

Perforation of a duodenal ulcer is a common cause of *sudden, severe abdominal pain*. In the majority of patients there will be no history of previous symptoms compatible with peptic ulcer disease. Perforation may occur at any age, but the peak incidence is between the ages of 20 and 40 years. Patients in whom perforation complicates treatment with steroids or NSAIDs are usually older and may present with minimal symptoms and signs.

A patient with a perforated ulcer will *lie still* and take *shallow breaths* to avoid exacerbating abdominal pain. The abdomen is *board-like* on palpation, although older patients and those on steroids may not exhibit peritonism. *Liver dullness may be lost* because of free air between the liver and the chest wall. *Bowel sounds will be absent* after a few hours.

Diagnosis

The most important investigation is an *erect plain chest radiograph* and an upright or left lateral *decubitus view of the abdomen*; in the majority of cases this will demonstrate free air within the abdominal cavity.

Management

A perforated peptic ulcer is a surgical emergency and demands immediate attention. A *nasogastric tube* should be inserted; *antibiotics, fluid resuscitation* and *surgery* are indicated. In the presence of concurrent medical illness, sepsis or perforation existing for more than 48 hours, a simple closure is the most prudent course. In stable patients with pre-existing ulcer disease proximal to the duodenum, resection of ulcers and vagotomy is generally preferred.

Intestinal emergencies

SMALL BOWEL OBSTRUCTION

Clinical features

The diagnosis of small bowel obstruction is suggested by:

- cramping abdominal pain;
- vomiting;
- constipation;
- varying degrees of abdominal distension.

Physical examination may also yield clues to the aetiology of bowel obstruction. In adults, the most common causes are:

- adhesions from previous surgery;
- herniation;
- volvulus;
- intussusception;
- Crohn's disease;
- Malignancy.

Investigations

The confirmatory diagnostic investigations are plain and decubitus *abdominal radiographs*. *Contrast studies with barium* are performed only to distinguish mechanical obstruction from paralytic ileus and partial from complete bowel obstruction and in those patients in whom therapy will be changed if the cause is known (e.g. Crohn's disease, irradiation enteritis or extrinsic pressure from abscesses).

Management

Initial management should consist of *intravenous fluids, correction of electrolyte disturbances* and *gastric decompression*. Controversy exists as to whether decompression is best performed by a long intestinal tube or nasogastric tube. Most surgeons prefer a nasogastric tube (Brolin, 1983).

Indications for *surgery* in a patient with small bowel obstruction are:

- persistent abdominal tenderness;
- pain after decompression;
- failure to improve clinically 12–24 hours after successful decompression;
- the presence of tachycardia and fever.

A longer period of decompression and observation may be indicated in patients recovering from surgery since under these circumstances it is frequently difficult to differentiate bowel obstruction from prolonged ileus.

INTESTINAL ISCHAEMIA

Causes

Acute occlusion of the superior mesenteric artery is usually due to an *embolus* originating from the heart. The superior mesenteric artery is more susceptible to embolism than the inferior because of its larger lumen and more direct origin from the aorta. Intestinal ischaemia may also be related to *low cardiac output, spontaneous thrombosis* or *systemic embolism.*

Mesenteric venous thrombosis may be idiopathic or may evolve as a result of an intra-abdominal catastrophe such as appendicitis, diverticulitis, abscess or pancreatitis. It may also complicate hypercoagulable states such as polycythaemia rubra vera and the use of oral contraceptives.

Clinical features

Small and large bowel embolism cause *severe pain* that is unrelieved by narcotics and is out of proportion to the physical findings. More peripheral emboli cause less severe pain and their presence may not be detected until there are *peritoneal signs of infarction* or vital signs deteriorate. Ischaemia due to low cardiac output may be precipitated by congestive heart failure, cardiac arrhythmias, acute myocardial infarction and severe hypovolaemia, while sepsis/septic shock may be associated with mucosal hypoxia despite a high cardiac output (see Chapter 4).

Management

Following effective resuscitation and administration of *antibiotics*, gangrenous bowel must be *resected*. In some cases when large segments of intestine are involved and its viability is questionable the patient may be re-explored 24 hours later, by which time demarcation may be more obvious. Treatment in the meantime is directed towards correcting the primary cause, except if there is extensive infarction or the prognosis of the underlying disease is hopeless when continued aggressive therapy may be inappropriate. In a few cases angiography performed as soon as possible after the onset of abdominal pain may allow the surgeon to *revascularize the intestine*, thereby avoiding irreversible necrosis.

Prognosis

Mortality approaches 90%, but may be decreased by early diagnosis.

ISCHAEMIC COLITIS

Causes

Ischaemic colitis may follow surgical procedures, but can also present *de novo*. Primary colonic ischaemia

due to vascular disease usually affects the splenic flexure where the collateral circulation is most precarious. Embolic ischaemic colitis is unusual (see earlier). Interruption of the inferior mesenteric artery and its collateral vessels may follow abdominal aortic aneurysmectomy or resection of the left hemicolon.

Clinical features and diagnosis

Clinical features include *abdominal distension, burgundy-coloured stools* and *tenesmus*. Although in some cases the condition is self-limiting, in others ischaemia may progress to necrosis with *peritonitis, fever, leucocytosis, sepsis, shock,* and *metabolic acidosis.* In the early stages a plain radiograph of the abdomen may show 'thumb printing' of the oedematous mucosa. *Proctoscopy* or *colonoscopy* may confirm oedematous, dusky, necrotic mucosa.

Management

Although in some instances management can be expectant with *bowel rest* and *antibiotics*, *resection* of the affected area and proximal colostomy/ileostomy is essential if the patient demonstrates peritonism. The most seriously ill patients may present with septic shock as a consequence of faecal peritonitis; they will require fluid resuscitation and, usually, inotrope administration perioperatively.

COLONIC PSEUDO-OBSTRUCTION

Clinical features

In colonic pseudo-obstruction there is dilatation of the colon in the absence of a mechanical cause. Pseudo-obstruction may be seen following operations in the retroperitoneal area such as vascular and orthopaedic surgery, as well as in debilitated medical patients and those with electrolyte imbalance. The diagnosis is suggested by extreme abdominal distension, which can be seen to involve the whole colon including the rectum on abdominal radiography. The greatest danger is perforation of the caecum, which is associated with a 50% mortality (Strodel & Brothers, 1989).

Management

If the colon is not greatly distended treatment should include:

- intestinal decompression by nasogastric tube, rectal tube or colonoscopy;
- discontinuation of narcotics and sedatives if possible;
- correction of metabolic imbalance and electrolyte disturbances.

If the colon is markedly distended and the patient has pain and tenderness, raising the possibility of imminent perforation, *caecostomy* is the preferred method of decompression. If perforation has occurred, a *limited right hemicolectomy* with construction of an ileostomy and a mucous fistula is advised.

Biliary tract emergencies

ACUTE ACALCULOUS CHOLECYSTITIS
(Williamson, 1988)

Detection of sepsis originating from the gall bladder (calculous or acalculous cholecystitis) is particularly difficult in critically ill patients who are sedated and unresponsive and often have multiple organ dysfunction syndrome (MODS).

Aetiology

A variety of factors have been implicated (Howard, 1981) including:

- burns;
- trauma;
- previous surgery;
- sepsis;
- shock;
- multiple transfusions;
- prolonged ventilation;
- opiate sedation;
- long-term parenteral nutrition.

Biliary sludge is commonly found in these patients and is composed of calcium bilirubinate with an increased proportion of unconjugated bilirubin. The precise role of sludge in the development of acalculous cholecystitis is, however, unclear.

Pathogenesis

A combination of the above factors may lead to *ischaemia* and *necrosis of the gall bladder mucosa*, which may then become secondarily infected.

Clinical presentation

Clinical and laboratory features are similar to those of calculous cholecystitis and include:

- fever;
- pain;
- vomiting;
- tender right upper quadrant mass on abdominal examination;
- a raised white cell count;
- elevated bilirubin;
- raised alkaline phosphatase.

Investigations

Ultrasound scanning and *cholescintigraphy* are widely used in the diagnosis of cholecystitis. Ultrasound findings of diagnostic significance in acalculous cholecystitis include:

- thickening of the gall bladder wall to 5 mm or more (in the absence of hypoalbuminaemia);
- transverse gallbladder diameter of 5 cm or more;
- a sonolucent layer within the gall bladder wall;
- sediment or sludge within the gall bladder lumen;
- pericholecystic fluid collections.

Treatment

Open cholecystectomy or *cholecystostomy* may be performed, but *percutaneous cholecystostomy* is less invasive, and may be useful in critically ill patients (Lee *et al.*, 1991).

Acute pancreatitis

CAUSES

The most common associated aetiological factor is *gallstones*, although most patients with cholelithiasis never develop evidence of pancreatitis. *Alcohol*, the other major associated factor, causes predominantly chronic damage to the pancreas and it is usually only after several years that a minority of alcoholics develop acute pancreatitis. At least 30 other causes of pancreatitis have been identified encompassing an array of anatomical and metabolic abnormalities, drugs, toxins and infections. The substantial number of cases labelled as *'idiopathic'* serves to emphasize the lack of understanding of the causes of this disease.

PATHOGENESIS (Barry, 1988)

Pancreatitis is believed to be due to autodigestion by activated enzymes within the gland. *Duodenopancreatic reflux* may be a common factor underlying many of the aetiological associations since duodenal contents contain enzymes capable of activating proenzymes in the pancreas. They would normally also contain bacteria, raising the possibility that pancreatic infection is a triggering event.

The factors that determine whether a given attack will be mild or severe are also incompletely understood. Clinical and experimental evidence suggests that the degree of protease activation early in the course of the disease is a key factor in determining the outcome. In severe cases dissemination of the inflammatory response is associated with the development of systemic inflammatory response syndrome (SIRS), sepsis and multiple organ dysfunction syndrome (MODS) (see Chapter 4).

CLINICAL FEATURES

Patients with pancreatitis frequently describe *abdominal pain* that is central, radiates to the back and is eased by sitting forward. *Nausea and vomiting* is an invariable accompaniment to the pain. There may be a history of heavy alcohol intake. It is important to take a detailed drug history.

On examination the patient is usually agitated with *epigastric tenderness*. Pleural effusions may be suspected from examination of the chest. Retroperitoneal haemorrhage is evidenced by a grey discoloration in the flanks (*Grey Turner's sign*) or in the umbilicus (*Cullen's sign*). The abdomen is usually distended due to an associated *ileus*. The differential diagnosis includes perforated bowel, cholecystitis, bowel obstruction, renal colic, myocardial infarction pneumonia and ketoacidosis.

The clinical course of severe acute pancreatitis consists of two distinct phases.

- An early toxaemic phase characterized by a disseminated inflammatory response with marked fluid shifts related to the systemic release of activated enzymes and toxic substances from the pancreas. This phase may be complicated by multiple organ failure (Balldin, 1987) (see Chapter 4—SIRS and MODS).
- A late necrotic phase. Intra-abdominal necrosis creates a culture medium for bacterial invasion from the digestive tract leading to local and systemic septic complications (Beger *et al.*, 1986) (see Chapter 4).

Eleven clinical features identified by Ranson (Ranson *et al.*, 1976) correlate with morbidity, length of stay in intensive care and eventual mortality. The following five can be assessed on admission:

- age greater than 55 years;
- blood glucose greater than 11 mmol/l;
- white blood cell count greater than 16,000/mm³;
- serum lactate dehydrogenase (LDH) greater than 350 u/l;

- serum aspartate aminotransferase greater than 120 u/l.

The other six features are evaluated within 48 hours of admission:

- serum calcium level less than 2 mmol/l;
- arterial oxygen tension (P_aO_2) less than 8 kPa (60 mm Hg);
- base deficit greater than 4 mmol/l;
- blood urea increase greater than 2 mmol/l;
- haematocrit fall greater than 10%;
- fluid sequestration greater than 6 litres.

Fewer than three of the criteria correlate with the benign form of pancreatitis. Patients with three or more of the criteria, those who need monitoring during large-volume fluid administration, patients who require ventilatory support, and those with metabolic imbalance, renal insufficiency, cardiovascular instability and impending multiple organ dysfunction should be admitted to intensive care.

Patients who have undergone pancreatic surgery may also be admitted for postoperative care.

INVESTIGATIONS (Table 15.5)

The diagnosis of acute pancreatitis depends on documenting a raised serum amylase (> 1000 u) in a patient with compatible clinical features.

Computerized tomography (CT) of the abdomen is the best means of visualizing the pancreas. It may suggest the cause of the attack (e.g. gallstones, fatty infiltration of the liver if related to alcohol or liver metastases) (London *et al.*, 1989). The severity of pan-

Table 15.5 Management of acute severe pancreatitis.
Investigations
Serum amylase
Computerized tomography (CT) scan
Abdominal ultrasound
General principles of management
Nasogastric intubation
Parenteral nutrition
Control symptoms (e.g. pain, nausea and vomiting)
Prevent and treat vital organ dysfunction
Endoscopy
Endoscopic retrograde cholangiopancreatography (ERCP)
Peritoneal lavage
Surgery

creatitis can also be inferred from the extent of pancreatic enlargement and the presence of peripancreatic inflammatory changes as well as from the number and location of fluid collections. Not all patients with acute pancreatitis, however, require a CT scan since documentation of pancreatic or peripancreatic necrosis (nonperfused areas) or pseudocysts does not by itself influence treatment. Nevertheless contrast-enhanced CT remains the most valuable investigation for evaluating patients in the second week of acute pancreatitis. Pancreatic necrosis with accompanying fever and leucocytosis is an indication for CT-guided fine needle aspiration and microbiological examination of the aspirate. The finding of intrapancreatic gas pockets increases the likelihood of identifying infected pancreatic necrosis.

Abdominal ultrasound will readily identify gallstones. Visualization of the pancreas by ultrasonography in acute disease is, however, usually limited by overlying bowel gas caused by associated ileus.

MANAGEMENT (see **Table 15.5**)

The general principles include:

- metabolic and nutritional support;
- avoidance of enteral feeding and drainage of the stomach;
- control of symptoms (e.g. pain, nausea and vomiting);
- prevention and treatment of vital organ dysfunction (e.g. mechanical ventilation, inotropic support and blood purification).

Endoscopy

The role of early endoscopy for detecting common bile duct stones, sphincterotomy and stone extraction has been evaluated in two controlled clinical trials (Neoptolemos *et al.*, 1988; Fan *et al.*, 1993). Although there was no convincing evidence that the severity of the disease was moderated, many centres still proceed with ERCP in those patients in whom gallstones are thought to be an aetiological factor.

Adjunctive therapy

Although as mentioned above many of the systemic effects of pancreatitis are mediated through kinins found in the peritoneal exudate, there is no evidence to support the administration of antiproteases or inhibition of pancreatic exocrine secretions (e.g. with somatostatin and its long-acting analogues).

Peritoneal lavage

Early and prolonged peritoneal lavage may reduce both the frequency and mortality from pancreatic sepsis (Ranson & Berman, 1990) although this finding is in contradistinction to those of earlier studies (Mayer *et al.*, 1985).

Surgery

Since many cases of acute pancreatitis are due to gallstones, and because passage of stones through the ampulla is thought to be an important initiating event, there has been a long-standing interest in the potential role of *early biliary tract surgery* in arresting progression of acute pancreatitis secondary to gallstones. Despite initial enthusiasm, a controlled study (Kelly & Wagner, 1988) concluded that cholecystectomy and common bile duct exploration within 48 hours of diagnosis was associated with a prohibitive morbidity and mortality.

Major pancreatic resection has become obsolete except in a very few cases of total pancreatic necrosis because of the technical difficulty, as well as the high morbidity and mortality. Instead a surgical approach similar to that for advanced peritonitis (*planned relaparotomies, prolonged peritoneal lavage and open packing of wounds*) may be required in those patients with pancreatic necrosis. Infection of pancreatic necrosis occurs in 40–70% of patients and can be confirmed or excluded by percutaneous aspiration guided by ultrasound or CT, followed by culture and Gram stain. Infected pancreatic necrosis should be removed by *surgical debridement* (Rattner *et al.*, 1992). Once necrosis develops the ultimate outcome is determined by the amount of pancreatic and extrapancreatic necrosis, the presence of bacterial contamination, and perhaps most importantly, the general condition of the patient.

The optimum treatment of *sterile necrosis* continues to be debated (Rattner *et al.*, 1992) and it is unclear whether surgical debridement improves the outcome for those who are unstable, demonstrate signs of raised intra-abdominal pressure or exhibit a significant systemic inflammatory response. There are three main surgical approaches to debridement of pancreatic necrosis (Penninckx *et al.*, 1992):

- necrosectomy and continuous lavage of the lesser sac (Beger *et al.*, 1988);
- blunt debridement with open packing of the resulting cavity and wound (D'Egidio & Schein, 1991);
- blunt debridement with closed packing and closed-system suction catheters.

With all these techniques the thoroughness of the

initial debridement is the most important determinant of the need for subsequent re-explorations and survival. Since infection is clearly associated with mortality in necrotizing pancreatitis, control of bacterial and fungal colonization of devitalized tissue is essential. Prophylactic antibiotics do not prevent infection, but may promote selection of resistant organisms. An Italian cooperative trial suggested that prophylactic imipenem reduced the rate of infection in pancreatic necrosis, but surprisingly this was not associated with a reduction in mortality (Pederzoli et al., 1993).

It is becoming generally accepted that early surgical management of acute pancreatitis should be limited to patients with unrelenting diffuse peritonitis and multiple organ failure after two or three days of intensive non-operative management. Ideally surgery should be postponed to the second or third week in order to allow sequestrectomy of necrotic pancreas and facilitate debridement. In some patients earlier surgical intervention will be necessary to ameliorate the cardiovascular, pulmonary and renal effects of raised intra-abdominal pressure.

PROGNOSIS

Acute pancreatitis is associated with major local or systemic complications in 20% of patients, half of whom will die with conventional supportive treatment. Pancreatic infection is the commonest cause of death, sterile necrosis being much less often associated with a fatal outcome: 60% of patients with infected necrosis die compared to 6% of patients with sterile necrosis (Beger et al., 1986).

REFERENCES

Allison DJ, Hemingway AP & Cunningham DA (1982) Angiography in gastrointestinal bleeding. *Lancet* **2**: 30-33.

Balldin G (1987) Release of vasoactive substances in ascites and blood in acute pancreatitis. In: Beger HG, Buchler M (eds) *Acute Pancreatitis: research and clinical management.* Springer-Verlag, Berlin, Heidelberg, New York, pp. 63-70.

Barer D, Ogilivie A, Henry D et al. (1983) Cimetidine and tranexamic acid in treatment of acute upper-gastrointestinal-tract bleeding. *New England Journal of Medicine* **308**: 1571-1575.

Barry RE (1988) The pathogenesis of acute pancreatitis. *British Medical Journal* **296**: 589.

Beger HG, Bittner R, Block S & Buchler M (1986) Bacterial contamination of pancreatic necrosis. A prospective clinical study. *Gastroenterology* **91**: 433-438.

Beger HG, Buchler M, Bittner R, Block S, Nevalainen T & Roscher E (1988) Necrosectomy and postoperative local lavage in necrotizing pancreatitis. *British Journal of Surgery* **75**: 207-212.

Berk JL, Hagen JF & Freid VJ (1979) The effect of vasopressin on oxygen availability. *Annals of Surgery* **189**: 439-441.

Boley SJ, DiBiase A, Brandt LJ & Sammartano RJ (1979) Lower intestinal bleeding in the elderly. *Annals of Surgery* **137**: 57-64.

Boley SJ, Brandt LJ & Frank MS (1981) Severe lower intestinal bleeding: diagnosis and treatment. *Clinical Gastroenterology* **10**: 65-91.

Branicki FJ, Boey J, Fok PJ et al. (1990) Bleeding duodenal ulcer: a prospective evaluation of risk factors for rebleeding and death. *Annals of Surgery* **211**: 411-418.

Brolin RE (1983) The role of gastrointestinal tube decompression in the treatment of mechanical intestinal obstruction. *Annals of Surgery* **49**: 131-137.

Brunner G & Chang J (1990) Intravenous therapy with high doses of ranitidine and omeprazole in critically ill patients with bleeding peptic ulcerations of the upper intestinal tract: an open randomized trial. *Digestion* **45**: 217-225.

Cello JP, Grendell JH, Crass RA, Trunkey DD, Cobb EE & Heil-bron DC (1984) Endoscopic sclerotherapy versus portacaval shunt in patients with severe cirrhosis and variceal hemorrhage. *New England Journal of Medicine* **311**: 1589-1594.

Christiansen J, Otterjan R & Von-Arx F (1989) Placebo-controlled trial with the somatostatin analogue SMS 201-995 in peptic ulcer bleeding. *Gastroenterology* **97**: 568-574.

Cochran TA (1993) Bleeding peptic ulcer: surgical therapy. *Gastroenterology Clinics of North America* **22**: 751-778.

Collins R & Langman M (1985) Treatment with histamine H$_2$ antagonists in acute upper gastrointestinal hemorrhage. Implications of randomised trials. *New England Journal of Medicine* **313**: 660-666.

Copenhagen Esophageal Varices Sclerotherapy Project (1984) Sclerotherapy after first variceal haemorrhage in cirrhosis. A randomized multicenter trial. *New England Journal of Medicine* **311**: 1594-1600.

Daneshmend TK, Hawkey CJ, Langman MJS, Logan RFA, Long RG & Walt RP (1992) Omeprazole versus placebo for acute upper gastrointestinal bleeding: randomised double blind controlled trial. *British Medical Journal* **304**: 143-147.

D'Egidio A & Schein M (1991) Surgical strategies in the treatment of pancreatic necrosis and infection. *British Journal of Surgery* **78**: 133-137.

Devine RM, Farnell MB & Mucha P Jr (1984) Acute cholecystitis as a complication in surgical patients. *Archives of Surgery* **119**: 1389-1393.

Dronfield AW, Langman MJS, Atkinson M et al. (1984) Outcome of endoscopy and barium radiography for acute gastrointestinal bleeding: controlled trial in 1037 patients. *British Medical Journal* **284**: 545-548.

Durham RM & Shapiro MJ (1991) Stress gastritis revisited. *Surgical Clinics of North America* **71**: 791-810.

Fan S-T, Lai ECS, Mok FPT, Lo C-M, Zheng S-S & Wong J (1993) Early treatment of acute biliary pancreatitis by endoscopic papillotomy. *New England Journal of Medicine* **328**: 228-232.

Ganger DR (1992) Management of variceal bleeding. *Intensive and Critical Care Digest* **11**: 42-45.

Giacchino JL, Geis WP, Pickleman JR *et al.* (1979) Changing perspectives in massive lower intestinal haemorrhage. *Surgery* **86**: 368-376.

Goff JS (1990) Esophageal variceal ligation. *Canadian Journal of Gastroenterology* **4**: 639-642.

Groszmann RJ, Kravetz D, Bosch J *et al.* (1982) Nitroglycerin improves the haemodynamic response to vasopressin in portal hypertension. *Hepatology* **2**: 757-762.

Howard OM, Buchanan JD & Hunt RH (1982) Angiodysplasia of the colon. Experience of 26 cases. *Lancet* **2**: 16-19.

Howard RJ (1981) Acute acalculous cholecystitis. *American Journal of Surgery* **141**: 194-198.

Hussey KP (1985) Vasopressin therapy for upper gastrointestinal tract hemorrhage. Has its efficacy been proven? *Archives of Internal Medicine* **145**: 1263-1267.

Kelly TR & Wagner DS (1988) Gallstone pancreatitis: a prospective randomized trial of the timing of surgery. *Surgery* **104**: 600-605.

Kovacs TOG & Jensen DM (1987) Endoscopic control of gastroduodenal hemorrhage. *Annual Review of Medicine* **38**: 267-277.

Kravetz D, Bosch J, Teres J *et al.* (1984) Comparison of intravenous somatostatin and vasopressin infusions in treatment of acute variceal hemorrhage. *Hepatology* **4**: 442-446.

Laine L & Peterson WL (1994) Bleeding peptic ulcer. *New England Journal of Medicine* **331**: 717-727.

Lee MJ, Saini S, Brink JA *et al.* (1991) Treatment of critically ill patients with sepsis of unknown cause. Value of percutaneous cholecystectomy. *American Journal of Radiology* **156**: 1163-1166.

Liebermann DA, Keller FS, Katon RM & Rosch J (1984) Arterial embolization for massive upper gastrointestinal tract bleeding in poor surgical candidates. *Gastroenterology* **86**: 876-885.

London NJM, Neopotolemos JP, Lavelle J, Bailey I & James D (1989) Serial computed tomography scanning in acute pancreatitis: a prospective study. *Gut* **30**: 397-403.

MacDougall BR, Westaby D, Theodossi A, Dawson JL & Williams R (1982) Increased long-term survival in variceal haemorrhage using injection sclerotherapy. Results of a controlled trial. *Lancet* **1**: 124-127.

McGuire HH Jr & Horsley JS 3rd (1986) Emergency operations for gastric and duodenal ulcers in high risk patients. *Annals of Surgery* **203**: 551-557.

Magnusson, I, Ihre T, Johansson C *et al.* (1985) Randomised double blind trial of somatostatin in the treatment of massive upper gastrointestinal haemorrhage. *Gut* **26**: 221-226.

Markisz JA, Font D, Royal HD *et al.* (1982) An evaluation of ^{99m}Tc-labeled red cell scintigraphy for the detection and localization of gastrointestinal bleeding sites. *Gastroenterology* **83**: 394-398.

Mayer AD, McMahon MJ, Corfield AP *et al.* (1985) Controlled clinical trial of peritoneal lavage for the treatment of severe acute pancreatitis. *New England Journal of Medicine* **312**: 399-404.

NIH Consensus Development Conference (1989) Therapeutic endoscopy and bleeding ulcers. *Journal of the American Medical Association* **262**: 1369-1372.

Neoptolemos JP, Carr-Locke DL, James D, London NJ, Bailey IA & Fossard DP (1988) Controlled trial of urgent endoscopic retrograde cholangiopancreatography and endoscopic sphincterotomy versus conservative treatment for acute pancreatitis due to gallstones. *Lancet* **ii**: 979-983.

Pederzoli P, Bassi C, Vesentini S & Campedelli A (1993) A randomized multicenter clinical trial of antibiotic prophylaxis of septic complications in acute necrotizing pancreatitis with imipenem. *Surgical Gynecology and Obstetrics* **176**: 480-483.

Penninckx F, Filez L & Kerremans R (1992) Abdominal controversies in the ICU patient. *Ballière's Clinical Anaesthesiology* **6**: 327-348.

Peterson WL, Barnett CC, Smith HJ *et al.* (1981) Routine early endoscopy in upper gastrointestinal tract bleeding; a randomized controlled trial. *New England Journal of Medicine* **304**: 925-929.

Pingleton SK & Hadzima SK (1983) Enteral alimentation and gastrointestinal bleeding in mechanically ventilated patients. *Critical Care Medicine* **11**: 13-16.

Pitcher JL (1971) Safety and effectiveness of the modified Sengstaken-Blakemore tube: a prospective study. *Gastroenterology* **61**: 291-298.

Pitcher JL (1977) Variceal hemorrhage among patients with varices and upper gastrointestinal haemorrhage. *Southern Medical Journal* **70**: 1183-1185.

Ranson JH & Berman RS (1990) Long peritoneal lavage decreases pancreatic sepsis in acute pancreatitis. *Annals of Surgery* **211**: 708-718.

Ranson JHC, Rifkind JM & Turner JW (1976) Prognostic signs and non-operative peritoneal lavage in acute pancreatitis. *Surgery, Gynecology and Obstetrics* **143**: 209-219.

Rattner DW, Legermate DA, Lee MJ, Mueller PR & Warshaw AL (1992) Early surgical debridement of symptomatic pancreatic necrosis is beneficial irrespective of infection. *American Journal of Surgery* **163**: 105-110.

Ring EJ, Lake JR, Roberts JP *et al.* (1992) Using transjugular intrahepatic portosystemic shunts to control variceal bleeding before liver transplantation. *Annals of Internal Medicine* **116**: 304-309.

Sacks HS, Chalmers TC, Blum AL, Berrier J & Pagano D (1990) Endoscopic haemostasis. An effective therapy for bleeding peptic ulcers. *Journal of the American Medical Association* **264**: 494-499.

Shuman RB, Schuster DP & Zuckerman GR (1987) Prophylactic therapy for stress ulcer bleeding: a reappraisal. *Annals of Internal Medicine* **106**: 562-567.

Silverstein FE, Gilbert DA, Tedesco FJ *et al.* (1981) The national ASGE survey on upper gastrointestinal bleeding. *Gastrointestinal Endoscopy* **27**: 73-102.

Stiegmann GV, Goff JS, Michaeltz-Onody PA, Korula J, Lieberman D, Saeed ZA, Reveille M, Sun JH & Lowenstein SR (1992) Endoscopic sclerotherapy as compared with endoscopic ligation for bleeding esophageal varices. *New England Journal of Medicine* **326**: 1527-1532.

Strodel WE & Brothers T (1989) Colonic decompression of pseudo-obstruction and volvulus. *Surgical Clinics of North America* **69**: 1327-1335.

Sung JJY, Chung SCS, Lai CW *et al.* (1993) Octreotide infusion or emergency sclerotherapy for variceal haemorrhage. *Lancet* **ii**: 637-641.

Terblanche J, Burroughs AK & Hobbs KEF (1989) Controversies in the management of bleeding oesophageal varices. *New England Journal of Medicine* **320**: 1393-1398, 1469-1475.

von Holstein CCS, Eriksson SBS & Kallen R (1987) Tranexamic acid as an aid to reducing blood transfusion requirements in gastric and duodenal bleeding. *British Medical Journal* **294**: 7-10.

Walt RP, Cottrell J, Mann SG, Freemantle NP & Langman MJS (1992) Continuous intravenous famotidine for haemorrhage from peptic ulcer. *Lancet* **340**: 1058-1062.

Welch CE, Rodkey GV, Von Ryall & Gryska P (1986) A thousand operations for ulcer disease. *Annals of Surgery* **204**: 454-467.

Williamson RCN (1988) Acalculous disease of the gall bladder. *Gut* **29**: 860-872.

16 Endocrine Emergencies

The involvement of intensive care specialists in the management of endocrine emergencies has led to the application of new techniques and clinical practice to conditions that in the past were managed exclusively by physicians on general wards. This has inevitably led to some controversy, particularly in the care of diabetic emergencies, which are the most frequently encountered acute endocrine disorders. Some are still reluctant to routinely admit such patients to an intensive care unit, despite the potential advantages of a high nurse:patient ratio, the availability of constant monitoring and ready access to repeated biochemical and blood gas analysis, together with the immediate availability of skilled medical staff.

DIABETES MELLITUS

Definition

Diabetes mellitus is a group of metabolic disorders characterized by hyperglycaemia due to an absolute or relative deficiency of insulin, together with a relative or absolute increase in glucagon concentration.

Normal physiology

In normal healthy individuals the blood glucose concentration is controlled within narrow limits, even after a meal when glucose may be stored in muscle or liver cells as glycogen, taken up into fat cells and converted into lipid, or metabolized via glycolysis to produce energy. This regulation is achieved by alterations in insulin secretion, which promote anabolic processes involving the storage of glucose, amino acids and fat, and corresponding changes in the counter-regulatory hormones, including glucagon, thyroid hormones, adrenaline, noradrenaline, cortisol and growth hormone. Glucose may subsequently be released from the liver by glycogenolysis or gluconeogenesis, and during prolonged fasting the body's energy needs are met by lipolysis and oxidation of fatty acids.

Types of diabetes mellitus

NON-INSULIN DEPENDENT DIABETES MELLITUS

Patients with non-insulin dependent diabetes mellitus (NIDDM) usually present over the age of 40 years. The tendency to develop NIDDM is strongly inherited (Lo et al., 1991), but the age at which the disease is manifest is influenced by body weight, diet, level of physical activity and intercurrent illness. Such patients do not require maintenance insulin treatment, at least initially. Their risk of myocardial infarction, intracerebral haemorrhage and peripheral vascular disease is much higher than in similarly aged non-diabetics.

INSULIN-DEPENDENT DIABETES MELLITUS

Patients with insulin-dependent diabetes mellitus (IDDM) have severe insulin deficiency as a result of pancreatic beta cell injury. The risk of developing IDDM is HLA-linked, and autoimmune processes with autoantibodies directed against antigens present in the islet cells play an important role in its pathogenesis (Bingley & Gale, 1991). About two-thirds of patients with IDDM present before 30 years of age.

Diabetic ketoacidosis

Diabetic ketoacidosis (DKA) is the most common endocrine emergency and occurs most frequently in patients with IDDM. In almost three-quarters of all cases it can be traced to one of three causes:

- newly developed IDDM;
- infection or intercurrent illness (e.g. myocardial infarction) in a known diabetic patient;
- a decrease in insulin dosage made by the physician or the patient.

Less frequently DKA may be precipitated by:

- trauma;.
- acute pancreatitis.

PATHOPHYSIOLOGY

The combination of insulin deficiency and excess production of stress hormones (e.g. adrenaline, cortisol) promotes accelerated hepatic glucose production via glycogen breakdown and unrestrained gluconeogenesis. Combined with the reduction in cellular uptake and use of glucose this leads to a rise in blood sugar levels, which precipitates glycosuria and an osmotic diuresis, with loss of water, sodium, potassium, phosphate and other electrolytes. Initially the loss of glucose in the urine limits the rise in blood sugar levels, while the fluid losses are replaced by drinking. Eventually, however, nausea and vomiting exacerbate dehydration and prevent adequate fluid intake. The same hormonal changes promote lipolysis with release of triglycerides and non-esterified fatty acids from fat cells. The fatty acids are metabolized to ketones in hepatic mitochondria and this contributes to the development of a metabolic acidosis.

CLINICAL FEATURES

When IDDM develops *de novo*, ketoacidosis is usually heralded by several days of *polyphagia, polydipsia* and *polyuria* followed by *weakness, anorexia* and finally *nausea and vomiting*. In those with established diabetes mellitus, however, ketoacidosis can develop in a matter of hours.

Examination reveals the *musty, fruity odour* of ketones on the breath. The patient may hyperventilate *(Kussmaul breathing)* in an attempt to compensate for progressive metabolic acidosis. There may be signs of severe *volume depletion. Abdominal pain*, a *board-like abdomen* and *rebound tenderness* may simulate intra-abdominal pathology. Examination of the lower limbs may reveal signs of *peripheral vascular insufficiency* and superimposed *infection*. Patients with infection are not necessarily febrile and may be mildly hypothermic.

Whenever diabetes mellitus is newly diagnosed the possibility that it might be secondary to another disorder (e.g. *Cushing's syndrome, acromegaly, phaeochromocytoma, thyrotoxicosis*) should be considered. *Pancreatic carcinoma* is a possibility in any patient with recent-onset diabetes mellitus associated with abdominal pain, jaundice and weight loss. *Drug therapy* (e.g. thiazide diuretics and steroids) and *parenteral or enteral feeding* may also reveal glucose intolerance.

Particular care should be taken to detect problems associated with the underlying diabetes (e.g. neuropathy, retinopathy and vascular insufficiency), as well as likely causative factors such as abscess, urinary tract infection, pneumonia or myocardial infarction.

DIAGNOSIS AND INVESTIGATIONS

The diagnosis of hyperglycaemia can be rapidly established by bedside testing, but must always be confirmed by laboratory analysis. Ketosis is diagnosed when urinalysis reveals ketones (++ or greater) or when undiluted plasma produces a positive result on bedside ketostix testing. A venous plasma concentration of bicarbonate less than 14 mmol/l or an anion gap ($[Na^+ + K^+] - [HCO_3^- + Cl^-]$) (see Chapter 5) greater than 20 provides confirmatory evidence. In this context an acidosis is defined as an arterial pH of less than 7.30.

A full blood count should be obtained, together with blood glucose, urea and electrolytes (specify chloride if out-of-hours) and plasma osmolality. Arterial blood should be analysed for acid–base status. Urinalysis should be undertaken and specimens of urine and blood sent for culture. A chest radiograph should be organized and an ECG recorded. Since multiple investigations are likely to be required, results should be carefully recorded in the notes or on a flow chart. It is important to remember that a neutrophil leucocytosis is common in diabetic patients with DKA and does not necessarily indicate infection, while a low or normal temperature does not rule out infection. Furthermore, the serum amylase may be spuriously elevated. The differential diagnosis in an unconscious patient should include alcohol or drug intoxication, intracerebral or subarachnoid haemorrhage, and meningitis.

MANAGEMENT

Resuscitation phase (Table 16.1)

DKA is a medical emergency associated with significant morbidity and mortality (Tunbridge, 1981). Corrective measures must not be delayed and should start in the Accident and Emergency Department (Foster & McGarry, 1983). Normal resuscitative priorities apply to diabetic emergencies as for all critically ill patients. Oxygen should be administered to an unobstructed airway, respiratory function should be assessed, and adequate intravenous fluids must be administered immediately to restore vital signs. Because cardiovascular function may be impaired in diabetic patients (autonomic neuropathy, coronary artery disease, cardiomyopathy), measurement of central venous pressure (CVP), and in some cases pulmonary artery occlusion pressure (PAOP), may be indicated in hypotensive diabetic patients with DKA, particularly those over 60 years of age. Urine output may be a misleading guide to haemodynamic function because of the osmotic diuresis induced by the high sugar load. Specific management of the patient with DKA involves:

● controlled rehydration;

Table 16.1 Guidelines for the management of diabetic ketoacidosis in the resuscitation phase.

Confirm the diagnosis

Capillary blood glucose level
Measure ketones in urine/blood

Take blood

Glucose, sodium, potassium, plasma osmolality
Urea, bicarbonate, chloride
Amylase
Full blood count
Blood cultures
Cardiac enzymes
Arterial blood gas analysis

Intravenous fluids

Large volumes of 0.9% saline are usually required. For example:

    1 litre in 30 minutes then
    1 litre in 1 hour then
    1 litre in 2 hours then
    1 litre every 4 hours

Potassium replacement (e.g. potassium chloride 20–30 mmol/hour, not more than 80 mmol/hour)

History and examination

Precipitating cause
    ? Stopping insulin
    ? Infection
    ? Myocardial infarction
    ? Drug therapy
Assessment of dehydration
    Blood pressure
    Capillary filling
    Peripheral cyanosis
    Peripheral temperature
    Reduced tissue turgor
Underlying disorders
    Cardiac disease
    Renal impairment

Table 16.1 (*continued*).

Insulin

6–10 units/hour intravenously

Further investigations

Chest radiograph
Electrocardiogram
Urinalysis
Mid-stream urine specimen

Other measures

Supplemental oxygen in all cases
Nasogastric tube
Coma position if stuporose
Urinary catheter
Blood/plasma expander for persistent hypotension
Heparin 5000 units subcutaneously twice daily in the obese, the elderly, in comatose or severely dehydrated patients and in those with a coincidental haemoglobinopathy
Consider central venous pressure measurement or pulmonary artery catheterization in those who are hypotensive or at risk of developing pulmonary oedema
Consider bicarbonate if pH less than 7.0
Consider antibiotics

Reassess

Hourly capillary blood glucose
Hourly assessment of circulating volume
Two-hourly sodium and potassium levels
Two-hourly arterial blood gas analysis
Record results on flow chart

- provision of insulin and potassium;
- the avoidance of complications (e.g. hypoglycaemia, hypokalaemia).

Fluid replacement. The admission of unstable diabetics into intensive therapy units has led to considerable debate regarding the management of volume replacement and rehydration. Particular controversy has surrounded the relative merits of crystalloids or colloids (Hillman, 1987), 0.9% saline or 0.18% saline in dextrose 4% for rehydration, as well as the rate of fluid administration and the most sensitive means of detecting unwanted effects (e.g. the use of pulse oximetry to identify pulmonary flooding).

The average fluid deficit in patients with DKA is 6–10 litres. Although restoration of these losses is essential for reversing hyperglycaemia, acidosis and hypotension, injudicious administration of large volumes of crystalloid solutions may precipitate tissue oedema and worsen pulmonary gas exchange (Sprung *et al.*, 1980; Fein *et al.*, 1982). Nevertheless most would accept that immediate expansion of the circulating volume with plasma or whole blood is indicated if the patient is hypotensive. Although 0.9% saline should initially be infused in large volumes, a more cautious approach should be adopted in the elderly and in those with pre-existing cardiovascular or respiratory disease. Later 0.18% saline in dextrose 4% can be substituted for 0.9% saline if the plasma sodium exceeds 160 mmol/l. Persistent or recurrent hypotension and oliguria should be corrected with additional intravenous colloid solutions. In less severe cases and when there is no hypotension, 0.18% saline in dextrose 4% can be used as the initial fluid therapy.

Potassium. Patients with DKA are almost always potassium depleted due to a combination of osmotic diuresis, polydipsia and vomiting. Potassium levels are, however, usually elevated initially because of an acidosis-induced potassium shift from the intracellular to the extracellular space, but quickly fall when insulin is given and the acidosis is corrected. In most patients, therefore, intravenous potassium replacement (20–30 mmol of potassium chloride/hour) should be given when insulin treatment is started to prevent hypokalaemia. If the initial plasma potassium concentration is low, replacement can be given more rapidly, but generally not faster than 80 mmol/hour. Regular monitoring of electrolyte concentrations (e.g. every 2 hours) is essential during the initial phases of treatment.

Insulin. Various fixed 'low-dose' intravenous insulin regimens are used by most clinicians treating DKA. An initial infusion rate of 6–10 units insulin/hour may be given through a separate vein or by 'piggy-back' into the intravenous line carrying the replacement fluid. Adsorption of insulin to the plastic tubing of the giving set is not a problem in clinical practice.

Rapid alterations in blood glucose levels and pH can cause cerebral oedema (Hammond & Wallis, 1992) as changes in the cerebrospinal fluid lag behind those in the blood. Accordingly a reduction in blood glucose of not more than 5 mmol/l/hour is an appropriate target.

It is important to appreciate that the movement of glucose into the cells in response to insulin administration is accompanied by a shift of potassium from the extracellular to the intracellular space with potentially disastrous consequences if significant hypokalaemia supervenes. There is also a danger of precipitating hypoglycaemia, the clinical signs of which include *sweating, tachycardia, hypotension* and an *obtunded level of consciousness* (see later in this chapter).

Bicarbonate. Although severe metabolic acidosis has a number of adverse consequences, its rapid correction with bicarbonate is also associated with some risks including a reduction in tissue oxygen delivery and exacerbation of hypokalaemia (see also Chapter 4). In those with mild or moderate acidosis, the blood pH will usually normalize within a few hours without the need for bicarbonate administration. Severe acidosis, however, may impair myocardial contractility, diminish vascular responsiveness to pressor amines and predispose to cardiac arrhythmias. Therefore, bicarbonate should be reserved for patients with an initial pH of less than 7.0, and in such cases 8.4% sodium bicarbonate can be added to the dextrose saline used as replacement fluid or administered as 1.26% sodium bicarbonate solution, which is iso-osmolar with normal plasma.

Other measures. Because DKA may be associated with gastric atony, comatose or lethargic patients should have a *nasogastric tube* inserted to minimize the risk of aspiration of gastric contents.

Antibiotics should not be routinely prescribed, although in the most seriously ill patients broad-spectrum antibiotics may be considered according to local policy (see Chapter 11) following a careful search for infection, and after urine and blood cultures have been sent to the microbiology laboratory. Infections that are easily overlooked include:

- otitis media;
- mastoiditis;
- sinusitis;
- perirectal abscess.

Heparin (e.g. 5000 units subcutaneously twice daily) should be prescribed in comatose or severely dehydrated patients, the elderly, the obese and in those with coincidental haemoglobinopathy.

Monitoring phase (Table 16.2)

The post-resuscitation phases of DKA are generally not well managed unless a diabetic specialist is involved, and serious errors commonly occur about 24–48 hours after admission. Once the blood glucose level has fallen to less than 12 mmol/l, the 0.9% saline infusion can be changed for 0.18% saline in dextrose 4%, 5% dextrose or 10% dextrose 1 litre 6-hourly, with continued intravenous potassium and an insulin infusion adjusted to maintain the blood glucose in the range 10–

Table 16.2 Guidelines for the management of diabetic ketoacidosis in the monitoring phase (blood glucose < 12 mmol/l).

Change fluids (e.g. to 1 litre 0.18% saline in dextrose 4%, 5% dextrose or 10% dextrose as required to maintain blood glucose concentrations, with 20 mmols potassium chloride per litre 6-hourly)

Continue intravenous insulin infusion for 24 hours after clearance of ketonuria. Change fixed-dose to a variable-dose regimen, for example:

Blood glucose (mmol/l)	Insulin infusion rate (units/h)
0–3.5	0
3.6–6.0	1
6.1–9.0	2
9.1–12.0	3
12.1–16.0	4
16.1–20.0	5
20.1 or above	6 (call doctor)

15 mmol/litre. This regimen should be continued for 24 hours after clearance of ketonuria, even if the patient is well recovered clinically. Acidosis sufficient to require bicarbonate administration is extremely unlikely during this phase.

Recovery phase (Table 16.3)

When the ketoacidosis has resolved for more than 24 hours and there is no doubt that the patient is able to eat and drink normally, established patients can usually resume their previous insulin therapy, while new patients can be managed using actrapid insulin subcutaneously at least 8-hourly. Intravenous insulin has a very short half-life and an *insulin infusion should never be discontinued without giving a depot subcutaneous dose.* This is one of the most common dangerous mistakes made during the management of such patients. Arrangements should be made to provide patient education and follow-up through the local Diabetic Nurse Specialist.

Hyperosmolar non-ketotic diabetic emergencies

Hyperosmolar non-ketotic (HONK) decompensation of diabetes mellitus is characterized by:

- extreme hyperglycaemia;
- hyperosmolality;
- severe dehydration, but minimal acidosis (Arieff & Carroll, 1972).

PATHOPHYSIOLOGY

Residual insulin secretion probably determines whether a patient presents with DKA or with a HONK state.

Table 16.3 Guidelines for the management of diabetic ketoacidosis in the recovery phase
(ketoacidosis resolved for more than 24 hours and there is no doubt that the patient is able to eat and drink normally).

Stop all intravenous fluid therapy. The insulin infusion should not be stopped before subcutaneous (s.c.) insulin has been started.

Start regular pre-meal subcutaneous insulin 3 or 4 times daily (24 hour total dose of insulin should be equal to the previous 24 hours' insulin consumption) or resume previous insulin regimen

---

Arrange patient education and follow-up

Those who develop HONK usually have sufficient insulin to inhibit unrestrained ketogenesis, but not to prevent hyperglycaemia. Initially, compensation for polyuria may be achieved by increased oral intake of water and this may in turn lead to hyponatraemia. Later, however, increased oral intake fails to keep pace with the continued urinary losses, particularly during the night. Hypernatraemia, hyperglycaemia and hyperosmolality combine to diminish conscious level and eventually the patient becomes comatose.

CAUSES

As in DKA, decompensation is often precipitated by stressful stimuli such as *infection* or *surgery*. *Drug administration* can also precipitate hyperosmolar crisis; potassium-losing diuretics (hypokalaemia decreases insulin secretion), phenytoin (directly inhibits insulin secretion) and glucocorticoids (increased gluconeogenesis and peripheral insulin antagonism) have all been implicated in this regard. *Cerebrovascular accidents* and *subdural haematomas* must also be considered when searching for precipitating factors. In hospitalized patients, *hyperalimentation* or *infusion of concentrated glucose solutions* can cause hyperosmolar crisis.

CLINICAL PRESENTATION AND DIAGNOSIS

Most patients are middle-aged or elderly individuals with mild to moderate NIDDM or no previous history of diabetes mellitus.

Polyuria and *polydipsia* may be present, but are often not obvious in older, less alert patients. *Disturbances in consciousness* are common. Some patients present with *seizures* or *focal neurological deficits* including hemiparesis. The hyperventilation and abdominal pain seen in patients with DKA are unusual in HONK. *Mild renal insufficiency* is common.

The diagnosis of a HONK crisis is usually not difficult once the plasma glucose is measured and the plasma osmolality is determined. Serum sodium levels of 155–160 mmol/l are common.

MANAGEMENT **(Table 16.4)**

Initial measures

Oxygen should be administered to an unobstructed *airway*. *Ventilatory support* is occasionally required, particularly if pneumonia is implicated as a precipitating factor. Vital signs should be monitored and invasive cardiovascular monitoring instituted. A *nasogastric tube* and *urinary catheter* should be inserted. Many of those

---

Table 16.4 Guidelines for the management of hyperosmolar non-ketotic decompensation of diabetes mellitus.

Initial measures

Secure airway, administer oxygen
Mechanical ventilation may be required
Invasive cardiovascular monitoring
Pass nasogastric tube
Catheterize the bladder

Specific treatment

Rehydration	Synthetic gelatin combined with hypotonic saline or 5% dextrose
	Or 0.9% saline ($\frac{1}{3}$ to $\frac{1}{2}$ estimated fluid deficit in first 12 hours, approximately $\frac{2}{3}$ over next 12 hours and correct any remaining deficit over next 12 hours)
Potassium replacement	Deficits are generally less than in diabetic ketoacidosis (DKA)
Insulin	As in DKA except start with lower dose (e.g. 3 units/hour) and monitor blood glucose very closely

General measures

Must include subcutaneous heparin

---

who succumb have Gram-negative infection and this must be considered when searching for a precipitating factor or selecting antibiotic therapy in patients known to be infected.

Specific management

Therapy is directed at producing predictable gradual reductions in circulating and tissue glucose concentrations, which together with a fall in plasma sodium will lower plasma osmolality.

Fluid and electrolyte therapy. Overzealous intravascular resuscitation with large volumes of hypotonic crystalloid solutions such as 0.45% saline may promote generalized extracellular oedema. Pulmonary oedema will be associated with hypoxia, while cerebral oedema may produce life-threatening rises in intracranial pressure (Hammond & Wallis, 1992), and rapid falls in plasma sodium may precipitate acute myelinolysis (see Chapter 10). It has been suggested that careful expansion of the intravascular volume with synthetic gelatin solutions can produce slow and controlled falls in plasma and extracellular sodium concentrations when combined with hypotonic saline or 5% dextrose administration (Hillman, 1987) without significant risk of pulmonary oedema, acute myelinolysis or cerebral complications. Others give approximately one-third to one-half of the estimated fluid deficit in the first 12 hours as 0.9% saline, approximately two-thirds of the deficit over the next 12 hours as 0.9% saline, with repletion of any remaining

deficit in the following 12 hours also with 0.9% saline. Rehydration of these patients with 0.9% saline is usually associated with further rises in serum sodium concentrations as water leaves the vascular compartment to correct intracellular dehydration. This increase in serum sodium should be accepted as an inevitable consequence of correcting the intracellular environment and should not inhibit continued administration of 0.9% saline or synthetic gelatin solutions, provided plasma sodium levels do not exceed 165 mmol/l and there are no signs of peripheral or pulmonary oedema. In such cases further volume replacement should be guided by measurements of PAOP.

Potassium replacement is also necessary, but because acidosis is usually only mild, deficits are generally less than with DKA. Underlying renal disease when present also reduces urinary potassium losses.

Insulin. Insulin is administered as in DKA, although some patients with HONK are particularly sensitive to insulin and it may be safer to commence the infusion at 3 units/hr with very careful blood sugar monitoring for the first two or three hours. If the plasma glucose concentration fails to fall satisfactorily, the insulin infusion rate can be increased to 6 units per hour. The aim should be to avoid rapid changes and return the plasma glucose concentration to normal within 6–10 hours.

Immobile patients with hyperosmolar states are at significant risk of thromboembolism and should receive regular *subcutaneous heparin* (e.g. 5000 units 2–3 times daily).

Continued management. Diabetic patients should never be discharged from the intensive care unit or hospital without establishing the cause of the decompensation and initiating measures to prevent its recurrence. Survivors of HONK coma typically require long-term management of NIDDM.

PROGNOSIS

In some series the mortality rate for HONK coma is as high as 30–50% (Davidson, 1981). This reflects in part the coexistence of severe disease in elderly patients.

Perioperative management of the patient with diabetes mellitus (Husband *et al.*, 1986)

Diabetic patients may be admitted to intensive care units not only for management of an acute diabetic emergency but also as a consequence of an unrelated disorder (e.g. surgery, major trauma).

For the purposes of this discussion, surgery may be broadly divided into minor procedures, following which the patient is able to resume oral intake on the same day, or major interventions, which preclude oral intake in the early postoperative period. The latter inevitably includes thoracic, cardiac and neurosurgical operations, as well as major intra-abdominal procedures. Certain types of surgical procedure may precipitate particularly rapid and large fluctuations in blood sugar levels (e.g. when there are associated metabolic changes as may occur during hypothermic cardiopulmonary bypass and when surgery is performed as an emergency). Diabetic patients can also be categorized into three broad groups:

- diet-controlled NIDDM;
- oral hypoglycaemic controlled NIDDM;
- IDDM.

Using these definitions a straightforward scheme of perioperative management can be prepared such as that outlined in **Table 16.5**.

Hypoglycaemia

Hypoglycaemia is defined as a circulating blood sugar level less than 2 mmol/l. It is a potentially life-threatening emergency.

Table 16.5 Guidelines for the management of diabetic patients undergoing surgery.

Classification of diabetes mellitus	Minor surgery protocol	Major surgery protocol
Diet controlled (NIDDM) (Often middle-aged and overweight. Pathological process is one of peripheral insulin resistance.)	• Monitor blood sugar level (BSL). Normal stress response causes elevation of fasting BSL, but acidosis unlikely and therefore no intervention required.	• Monitor BSL. Normal stress response causes elevation of BSL thereby avoiding any possibility of hidden hypoglycaemia. Insulin may be required especially in those receiving parenteral nutrition.
Oral hypoglycaemic controlled (NIDDM) (May initially have been controlled by diet alone, but now require glibenclamide or metformin daily.)	• Omit oral hypoglycaemic agent the night before surgery and the morning of operation. • Schedule for morning theatre list and monitor BSL pre, per- and postoperatively. • Recommence therapy after first meal.	• Omit oral hypoglycaemic agent the night before surgery and the morning of operation. • Schedule for morning theatre list. • Monitor BSL perioperatively. • Potassium–insulin–glucose (PIG) regimen likely to be required postoperatively.
Insulin-dependent (IDDM) (Usually juvenile or middle-aged. Pathological process is absolute insulin insufficiency. Associated autonomic neuropathy and widespread vascular disorders possible.)	• Admit to hospital preoperatively and convert the patient from long-acting insulins to three times daily short-acting insulin. • Monitor BSL. • On the morning of surgery establish secure intravenous access and commence a PIG infusion at 1 ml/kg/h (P = 10 mmol potassium chloride, I = 10 units insulin, G = 500 ml 10% glucose). • Monitor BSL and potassium and adjust the PIG prescription accordingly. • Continue PIG until after first meal.	• Admit to hospital preoperatively and convert the patient from long-acting insulins to three times daily short-acting insulin. • Monitor BSL. • On the morning of surgery establish secure intravenous access and commence a PIG infusion at 1 ml/kg/h. • Monitor BSL and potassium and adjust the PIG prescription accordingly. • Continue PIG until after first meal.

CAUSES

Hypogylcaemia may occur as a complication of *insulin therapy, oral hypoglycaemic treatment* or *systemic disease*. While *intentional overdosage* with intravenous insulin or oral hypoglycaemic tablets may occur in those with suicidal intent, the more usual circumstances surrounding insulin-induced hypoglycaemia are *accidental* (e.g. complicating routine self-treatment in brittle diabetic subjects) or *iatrogenic* during management of DKA, hyperalimentation or diabetic patients undergoing surgery. Islet cell neoplasms of the pancreas *(insulinomas)* also present as recurrent hypoglycaemic episodes. Hypoglycaemia can also occur as a complication of:

- hepatic failure (see Chapter 13);
- hypothermia (see Chapter 19);
- hypopituitarism (see later in this chapter);
- Addisonian crisis (see later in this chapter);
- salicylate poisoning in children (see Chapter 18);
- Reye's syndrome.

Repeated hypoglycaemic episodes in a diabetic patient whose insulin dosage has been decreasing may indicate the development of renal insufficiency, adrenal failure or hypopituitarism.

CLINICAL FEATURES

Patients may complain of *weakness, lethargy, incoordination* and *confusion*. This may ultimately progress to *seizures* and *coma*. Rapid falls in blood sugar levels produce *adrenergic symptoms* such as tremulousness, sweating, palpitations and anxiety, which are attributable to the increased sympathetic drive. *Faintness* and *sweating* with *tachycardia, variable blood pressure* and *pupillary dilatation* are easily overlooked or mistaken for alternative pathologies. Measurement of blood glucose is therefore essential in any patient presenting with 'funny turns', hypothermia or altered consciousness.

It has been suggested recently that the warning signs of hypoglycaemia are less well appreciated by patients receiving human insulin than by those using animal insulins. This phenomenon, which is probably related to more rapid absorption of human insulin, has been extensively investigated, but no clear differences between the hypoglycaemic effects of human and animal insulin have emerged (Gale, 1989). It is also important to appreciate that loss of awareness of hypoglycaemia occurs over time in many diabetics, regardless of the type of insulin prescribed.

Hypoglycaemia from sulphonylureas is especially dangerous because glucose levels can be suppressed for hours or even days. Most hypoglycaemic episodes are due to chlorpropamide, which has a half-life in excess of 36 hours. Since chlorpropamide is excreted mainly unmetabolized by the kidney, co-existing renal insufficiency greatly prolongs its half-life and increases the risk of hypoglycaemia.

MANAGEMENT

Simultaneously with the usual resuscitative measures, any insulin infusion should be discontinued and *20 ml of 50% dextrose (or 50 ml 20% dextrose) injected intravenously*. This usually produces an immediate improvement in conscious level and vital signs. The circulating blood glucose level can then be maintained by the continuous administration of 10% or 20% dextrose. To avoid superficial thrombophlebitis concentrated dextrose solutions should be administered via a central vein.

Accidental or deliberate overdose with sulphonylureas can be refractory to an infusion of concentrated dextrose alone and may require the additional administration of *hydrocortisone, glucagon* or *diazoxide*. Glucocorticoids increase glucose levels by stimulating gluconeogenesis and antagonizing the effects of insulin, glucagon mobilizes glucose from hepatic glycogen stores and diazoxide acts directly on the pancreas to decrease insulin secretion. Haemodialysis is not helpful generally since sulphonylureas are protein bound.

Intentional overdosage with intravenous insulin injections may prove impossible to reverse, especially when there is significant delay in discovering the collapsed hypoglycaemic patient. Parenteral administration of insulin has, nevertheless, been successfully treated by surgical resection of the tissue into which the insulin was injected.

Malnourished alcoholic patients are susceptible to hypoglycaemia as a consequence of alcohol-induced suppression of gluconeogenesis. Furthermore, glucagon administration is usually not effective in reversing hypoglycaemia in such patients since liver glycogen stores are often depleted.

Prolonged coma despite treatment of hypoglycaemia should prompt consideration of other potential causes of unconsciousness such as hypoxic cerebral injury, intracerebral haemorrhage, drug or alcohol intoxication, meningitis or hypothermia.

Clearly whatever the aetiology of hypoglycaemia, subsequent treatment and investigations should be aimed at the primary disorder.

PROGNOSIS

The prognosis after severe prolonged hypoglycaemia depends on the duration of coma and corresponding cerebral injury.

THYROID EMERGENCIES

Thyroid crisis

CAUSES

Thyroid crisis is a life-threatening hypermetabolic condition. A precipitating event such as *infection, surgery* or other *intercurrent illness* can usually be identified. It may also follow *massive overdose of thyroid hormone preparations, radioiodine therapy* and the *administration of iodinated contrast dyes.*

CLINICAL PRESENTATION

In thyroid crisis, the characteristic features of hyperthyroidism are accentuated (Mackin *et al.*, 1974). Cardiovascular manifestations include *tachycardia, atrial fibrillation* and *heart block*. There is *profuse sweating, extreme irritability, tremor, nausea, vomiting* and *abdominal pain. Delirium* progresses to *coma or convulsions* in the most severe cases. Abnormalities of liver function and *jaundice* may also be seen. *Fever* is invariable and sets thyroid crisis apart from hyperthyroidism, but makes the distinction from sepsis extremely difficult. *Leucocytosis* is also well recognized in thyrotoxicosis even in the absence of infection.

Amphetamine overdose also resembles severe thyrotoxicosis and a toxicology screen should be undertaken when drug abuse is suspected, especially if the thyroid gland is not palpable. Phaeochromocytoma can also present in a similar fashion, but severe hypertension and paroxysmal attacks usually dominate the clinical presentation of this condition.

Blood should be collected for thyroid function tests before commencing therapy.

MANAGEMENT (Table 16.6)

In these extremely ill patients therapy for thyrotoxicosis must precede laboratory confirmation of the diagnosis. Treatment is aimed at decreasing the synthesis and secretion of thyroid hormone and countering the effects of thyroid hormone already in the circulation, as well as treating any precipitating illness.

General measures

Many patients are dehydrated and will require intravenous *fluid and electrolyte replacement*. A *cooling blanket* or *tepid sponging* can be used to decrease body temperature. Salicylates should not be used since they displace thyroid hormone from binding proteins and may worsen hypermetabolism. *Chlorpromazine* (25–50 mg intramuscularly) can be given to reduce agitation and anxiety and may also facilitate cooling. Standard antiarrhythmic drugs can be used, including digoxin for atrial fibrillation, after correction of hypokalaemia (see Chapter 8).

Table 16.6 Guidelines for the management of thyroid crisis.

General measures

Intravenous fluids
Cooling blanket and/or tepid sponging
Chlorpromazine (25–50 mg intramuscularly)
Treat arrhythmias

Specific treatment

Propylthiouracil (200 mg orally or ng 6-hrly)
Iodine preparations should be delayed for approximately 1 hour following the first dose of propylthiouracil eg:
      Potassium iodide (60 mg orally 8-hrly)
      Lugol's iodine (10 drops of a solution containing 130 mg of iodine/ml 12-hrly
      Sodium iodide (1 g intravenously)
      Radiographic contrast dyes

Lithium carbonate (initially 300 mg 6-hrly) can be used in those with iodine sensitivity

Propranolol (80 mg orally 8-hrly or 2 mg intravenously as required)

Guanethidine (10–20 mg orally 6-hrly) when β blockade is contraindicated

Dexamethasone (2 mg intravenously 6-hrly)

Plasmapharesis in severe, unresponsive cases

Specific management

Propylthiouracil (PTU) impedes formation of thyroid hormone and blocks peripheral conversion of thyroxine (T_4) to the metabolically active hormone triiodothyronine (T_3). 200 mg of PTU every 6 hours is recommended and can be given by nasogastric tube if the patient is unable to take oral medication.

The administration of *iodine*, which blocks the release of thyroid hormone should be delayed for approximately 1 hour following the first dose of PTU to minimize the possibility of massive hormone release following iodination. Traditional preparations include *potassium iodide* (60 mg orally three times daily), Lugol's iodine (use 10 drops of a solution containing 130 mg of iodine/ml diluted in milk or water twice daily), or *sodium iodide* (1 g intravenously). Recently the *radiographic contrast dyes* containing iodine have been used in place of traditional preparations. The cholecystographic contrast agent sodium ipodate (orografin), for example, is metabolized to yield large amounts of iodide, which is capable of inhibiting both thyroid hormone secretion and peripheral conversion of T_4 to T_3. Ipodate is administered in a 3 g oral daily dose (Burger & Philippe, 1992).

Lithium carbonate may be used to block thyroid hormone release in those with iodine sensitivity. There is a considerable risk of serious cardiovascular and central nervous system (CNS) side-effects because of the narrow therapeutic ratio. The initial dose of 300 mg 6-hrly should be adjusted to maintain plasma lithium levels of approximately 1 mmol/l. Lithium should be avoided in those with cardiac failure or renal insufficiency.

Propanolol (80 mg orally 8-hourly or 2 mg intravenously as required) blocks the sympathetic effects of thyroid hormone and is especially useful to reduce tachycardia (Hellman *et al.*, 1977). It impairs conversion of T_4 to T_3 and blocks sympathetic hyperactivity, which is responsible for many of the psychomotor and cardiovascular features of thyrotoxicosis. β-blockers are relatively contraindicated in patients with moderate or severe cardiac failure and should not be used in those with reversible airflow limitation. In these cases *guanethidine* (10–20 mg orally 6-hourly) can be administered cautiously. *Dexamethasone* 2 mg intravenously every six hours can also be used to reduce the conversion of T_4 to T_3.

The response to treatment can be monitored by observation of clinical signs (e.g. pulse, temperature and agitation) and by regular serum T_3 estimations.

In extreme cases unresponsive to conventional therapy *plasmapharesis* has been used.

PROGNOSIS

Thyroid crisis is associated with a mortality of 20–40%.

Myxoedema coma

Myxoedema coma is an extreme form of hypothyroidism associated with a high mortality.

CAUSES (Blum, 1972)

Frequent precipitating causes include:

- exposure to cold;
- surgery;
- trauma;
- infection;
- cerebrovascular accident;
- drug administration (e.g. chlorpromazine, narcotics, β-blockers).

Coma may be secondary to the metabolic deficit induced by profound hypothyroidism, carbon dioxide narcosis, accentuated effects of sedative drugs or hypoglycaemia.

CLINICAL PRESENTATION AND DIAGNOSIS

Myxoedema coma usually occurs in older patients with long-standing unrecognized primary thyroid disease (Lindberger, 1975) most commonly caused by autoimmune thyroiditis, radioiodine therapy or thyroidectomy. A failure of thyrotrophin (TSH) secretion due to pituitary disease is termed secondary hypothyroidism, while hypothalamic dysfunction is a tertiary disorder also associated with a low TSH level.

The classical manifestations of hypothyroidism are usually present and may include:

- previous thyroid disease or antithyroid medication, lithium or amiodarone therapy;
- a family history of thyroid or organ-specific autoimmune disease;
- characteristic facies;
- extreme bradycardia;
- hypotension;
- jeopardized respiratory performance including hypoventilation and upper airway obstruction by tongue enlargement;
- delayed or absent relaxation of the tendon reflexes;
- paralytic ileus and urinary retention;
- seizures and cerebellar signs.

Hypothermia and *hyponatraemia* secondary to diminished free water clearance are common. Occasionally the patient is *hypoglycaemic*. Routine investigations may also reveal a normocytic or megaloblastic *anaemia*. Raised *cardiac enzymes* (creatine phosphokinase, CPK; lactate dehydrogenase, LDH; aspartate aminotransferase, AST) may cause confusion with an acute myocardial infarction or reflect a cardiac event in a susceptible patient. In myxoedema coma, however, these enzymes may remain high for several days, unlike the acute transient changes seen after a myocardial infarction. An *ECG* is helpful in the differential diagnosis, typical changes in hypothyroidism include small voltages and a prolonged QT interval.

Thyroid function tests should be requested urgently together with a serum cortisol. Most commonly the tests reveal a primary thyroid disorder (low T_4, high TSH), but occasionally show secondary (pituitary) or tertiary (hypothalamic) hypothyroidism (low T_4, low TSH) with the possibility of additional adrenal insufficiency.

MANAGEMENT (**Table 16.7**)

General measures

Impaired myocardial performance and hypotension should be managed in accordance with the usual principles and patients with carbon dioxide retention may require ventilatory support. It must be remembered that these patients are particularly sensitive to CNS depressants. The mild hyponatraemia that is frequently present usually responds to fluid restriction (total input of around 500 ml in 24 hours). Generally hypertonic saline (50–100 ml of 5% sodium chloride) should be avoided unless the plasma sodium concentration is less than 110 mmol/l or the hyponatraemia precipitates convulsions. Intravenous glucose 10 or 20% may be infused to reverse hypoglycaemia. In those with mild to moderate hypothermia, gradual rewarming with a covering blanket is all that is required. The rapid increase in

body temperature that can be achieved with more active rewarming (see Chapter 19) may increase oxygen consumption, exacerbate hypoglycaemia and precipitate cardiovascular collapse.

Specific therapy

There are concerns that overzealous thyroid hormone replacement in myxoedema coma might also increase oxygen consumption and precipitate cardiovascular collapse (Chernow *et al.*, 1983). These authors recommend that T_3 is preferable to T_4 and that T_3 therapy should commence with a very low dose (2.5–5 μg twice daily) given intravenously.

Others are more cautious and recommend oral or nasogastric therapy. The dose of T_3 is increased in a stepwise fashion every 2–3 days (5, 10, 20 μg daily). Because thyroid replacement therapy can precipitate cardiac ischaemia and ventricular arrhythmias, continuous ECG monitoring is essential. In the most severe cases pulmonary artery catheterization is warranted. There is also a danger that co-existing adrenal insufficiency could decompensate into adrenal crisis as the metabolic rate increases with thyroid replacement. Corticosteroids should therefore be given as hydrocortisone 100 mg intramuscularly 8-hourly. Blood should be obtained for determination of plasma cortisol concentration before treatment since this will guide further administration of hydrocortisone.

Maintenance with T_4 is commenced by some immediately although the various regimens lack secure scientific justification and some switch to T_4 (50–100 μg/day) only when the dose of T_3 has been increased to at least 20 μg twice daily. The efficacy of therapy is gauged by repeated TSH estimations.

The sick euthyroid syndrome

More than 30 years ago Oppenheimer *et al.* (1963) first reported that thyroid function tests may be abnormal in seriously ill patients who do not have thyroid disease. The biochemical abnormality in this 'sick euthyroid syndrome' (SES) is thought to be due to a decrease in the concentration or activity of 5-deiodinase, which results in a decrease in the production of T_3 from T_4 and a reduction in the breakdown of reverse T_3 (rT_3) to T_2 (Felicetta & Sowers, 1987). Serum concentrations of free T_3 are therefore low whereas free rT_3 levels are elevated. Serum free T_4 concentrations are generally normal as are TSH levels. This combination of laboratory findings may be seen in as many as 70% of hospitalized patients (Kapstein *et al.*, 1982). The presence of severe SES is associated with a high mortality (Slag *et al.*, 1981).

Although it has been suggested that the SES is an

Table 16.7 Management of myxoedema coma.

General measures

Haemodynamic support
Mechanical ventilation may be indicated
Fluid restriction for hyponatraemia
Hypertonic saline rarely required
Intravenous glucose for hypoglycaemia
Gradual rewarming

Specific treatment

Triiodothyronine (T_3) 2.5 μg twice daily intravenously or nasogastrically/orally
Hydrocortisone 100 mg intramuscularly 8-hrly
Subsequently maintenance therapy with T_4 (50–100 μg daily)

adaptive response to severe illness that might lead to a useful reduction in metabolic rate (Burger *et al.*, 1976; Utiger, 1980), it seems unlikely that these changes are beneficial since their severity is closely related to a poor outcome. It has been reported that T_3 receptor expression is increased in patients with SES (Williams *et al.*, 1989), but not to the same extent as in those with chronic liver or renal disease. This suggests that cellular adaptation to low T_3 or T_4 concentrations can take some time and it is possible that in acutely ill intensive care patients such compensation may never take place.

In acutely ill patients it is important to distinguish SES from thyroid disease. An accurate history should be obtained and a thorough physical examination may reveal signs suggestive of hypothyroidism. In primary hypothyroidism TSH levels will be elevated and the TSH response to TRH is exaggerated, while in hypothyroidism due to hypothalamic/pituitary disorders, TSH is low. Once true hypothyroidism has been excluded the laboratory findings associated with SES are primarily of interest because of their prognostic significance.

Currently treatment of SES with thyroid hormone replacement is considered to be unnecessary, even though it has been suggested that the changes in circulating thyroid hormones may interfere with cellular oxygen uptake (Palazzo & Suter, 1991). Recovery is associated with a rapid return of thyroid function to normal (Baue *et al.*, 1984).

CALCIUM METABOLISM

Hypercalcaemia

CAUSES

The most frequent causes of hypercalcaemia are *primary hyperparathyroidism* and *malignancy*. The former results most commonly from a parathyroid adenoma or rarely a carcinoma. A parathyroid hormone-related protein (PTHrP), that shares the parathyroid hormone (PTH) receptor and has similar physiological actions to PTH has been identified in cases of malignancy-related hypercalcaemia (Broadus *et al.*, 1988). A number of less common causes have also been identified. Granulomatous diseases such as *sarcoidosis* and *tuberculosis* can be associated with unregulated production of 1 : 25 dihydroxy cholecalciferol. Drugs such as *thiazide diuretics* may also worsen coincidental hyperparathyroidism.

CLINICAL FEATURES

Symptoms may vary from *non-specific gastrointestinal complaints* to *acute mental changes* with drowsiness,

confusion, mania, psychosis and coma. *Pruritus* is a frequent accompaniment together with *polyuria* and *polydipsia*.

INVESTIGATIONS

The total serum calcium concentration is normally maintained within a narrow range (2.2–2.67 mmol/l). Since a large proportion of the total measured calcium is bound to serum proteins it is necessary to adjust for alterations in plasma albumin. An accepted correction factor is to add 0.02 mmol/l to the calcium level per gram of albumin below 40 g/l.

Hyperparathyroidism produces typical radiographic appearances in the hand with subperiosteal erosions and bone cysts. Long-standing hypercalcaemia can result in nephrocalcinosis and renal calculi, both of which may be visible on plain abdominal radiographs. Once the diagnosis has been made, a search for the cause of hypercalcaemia must be undertaken.

MANAGEMENT

Emergency management involves rehydration and the administration of agents that inhibit bone resorption.

- Plasma osmolality should be restored to within the normal range of 280–290 mosm/l with intravenous fluid administration (e.g. 0.9% saline).
- Biphosphonates inhibit bone resorption by binding to hydroxyapatite and inhibiting the dissolution of bone crystals (Davies & Heath, 1989). These slow effects take two or three days to decrease the serum calcium level and approximately one week to achieve the nadir (Bilezikian, 1992). The currently available agents include disodium etidronate 7.5 mg/kg intravenously over four hours, and repeated daily for 3 days, disodium pamidronate as a single 90 mg intravenous infusion over 24 hours or sodium clodronate 300 mg as an intravenous infusion over four hours, repeated daily for a maximum of 7–10 days.
- Calcitonin is a potent inhibitor of osteoclastic bone resorption and can rapidly lower serum calcium levels. It is given in a dose of 3–4 u/kg intravenously initially followed by 4 u/kg subcutaneously at 12–24-hour intervals.
- Plicamycin (an osteoclast RNA synthesis inhibitor) may be used when life-threatening complications seem imminent: 25 µg/kg should be administered intravenously in one litre of 0.9% saline over four hours daily for 3–4 days. Its longer term use may lead to bone marrow, renal and hepatic toxicity.
- Glucocorticoids such as hydrocortisone 100 mg 6-hourly by intramuscular injection or 60 mg of prednis-

olone orally have beneficial effects in hypercalcaemia due to vitamin D intoxication, granulomatous disorders and haematological malignancy, but are not effective in those with primary hyperparathyroidism or solid cancers (Percival *et al.*, 1984).

Hypocalcaemia

CAUSES

Hypoparathyroidism. Removal of all the parathyroid glands during thyroidectomy or of a single functional parathyroid adenoma during parathyroidectomy is likely to precipitate hypocalcaemia in the immediate postoperative period. In either event it is advisable to monitor the magnesium concentration as well as the calcium level since both the secretion of PTH and its activity are compromised by hypomagnesaemia.

Abnormal vitamin D metabolism. Disorders of vitamin D metabolism (e.g. impaired production of the active metabolite of vitamin D in renal disease and vitamin D-dependent rickets) cause hypocalcaemia, principally by reducing the absorption of calcium from the intestine and enhancing renal excretion.

Sequestration of calcium. Sudden sequestration of circulating calcium can occur in severe pancreatitis as a result of intra-abdominal saponification of fat. Muscle trauma with rhabdomyolysis, cytotoxic chemotherapy, malignant hyperthermia, rapid transfusion with citrated blood and severe burns may also precipitate hypocalcaemia.

CLINICAL PRESENTATION

General symptoms include *fatigue, irritability* and *anxiety.* Patients may give a history of circumoral and peripheral *paraesthesiae.* When the serum calcium falls below 2.0 mmol/l spontaneous indications of neuromuscular irritability such as *carpopedal spasm* may be observed. In addition, tapping the facial nerve may elicit the typical facial twitch that represents a *positive Chvostek's sign. Trousseau's sign* may be demonstrated by observing paraesthesiae and carpal spasm following inflation of a blood pressure cuff above the systolic pressure for 3 minutes. Characteristically adduction of the thumb precedes flexion of the metacarpophalangeal joints and extension of the interphalangeal joints, which is then followed by flexion of the wrist. Occasionally hypocalcaemia can precipitate *laryngeal spasm.* It is also a recognized cause of *seizures* and may contribute to the development of *cardiac failure* as well as con-*duction defects* involving delays in ventricular repolarization and lengthening of the QT interval.

MANAGEMENT

Continuous ECG monitoring is recommended during intravenous replacement therapy to detect the development of cardiac arrhythmias. The recommended dose is 10 ml of 10% calcium gluconate administered intravenously over ten minutes. This can be followed by 40 ml of 10% calcium gluconate in one litre of 0.9% saline solution infused over eight hours. The rate of administration should be guided by frequent serum calcium determinations. Once the patient has been stabilized, longer term maintenance therapy can be achieved with oral or nasogastric calcium supplements (1–2 g of elemental calcium/day) and 1 α-hydroxylated derivatives of vitamin D (e.g. alfacalcidol 1 μg/day) provided deficiency of vitamin D is confirmed. Hypomagnesaemia should also be corrected by infusing 1–5 mmol of magnesium sulphate over 10 minutes intravenously.

PHAEOCHROMOCYTOMA

Phaeochromocytoma is a rare cause of hypertension (< 1% of cases) although it is recognized that a significant number are still unsuspected clinically and are only diagnosed at post-mortem (Sutton *et al.*, 1981).

Pathology

Phaeochromocytomas arise from chromaffin cells, which are derivatives of neural crest tissue. Approximately 95% of these tumours are found in the abdomen, the vast majority (80%) in the adrenal gland. The most common extra-adrenal sites for phaeochromocytomas lie along the chain of sympathetic ganglia. A little less than 10% of phaeochromocytomas are malignant, although the presence of a phaeochromocytoma in an unusual location should suggest this possibility.

Clinical features (Ross & Griffith, 1989)

Although the *hypertension* associated with phaeochromocytoma is often sustained, even in these cases there may be marked *paroxysmal* increases in blood pressure. Other patients may only develop hypertension during an attack. Other features include headache, sweating and anxiety with palpitations and diarrhoea.

Although crises often occur spontaneously, they may be precipitated by certain drugs such as metoclopramide and foods containing tyramine such as beer. Some wines and cheeses may also precipitate an attack by directly stimulating the release of catecholamines from the tumour. Surgery, labour and delivery, deep palpation of the abdomen or micturition (in those with a bladder tumour) may also initiate an attack. *Hypotension* during a crisis should arouse suspicion of a *reduced cardiac output*, either as a result of catecholamine-induced myocardial damage or ventricular arrhythmias. Other life-threatening complications include *dissecting aneurysm, acute renal failure* and *stroke.*

There are several familial diseases associated with phaeochromocytoma. Multiple endocrine neoplasia Type II, for example, is a disorder characterized by medullary carcinoma of the thyroid, hyperparathyroidism and phaeochromocytoma. In patients with these disorders it is important to exclude a phaeochromocytoma before proceeding to parathyroidectomy or thyroid surgery. Other familial associations include neurofibromatosis (5% of patients), Von Hippel–Lindau disease and the Sturge–Weber syndrome.

Investigations

A full blood count may show an increased haematocrit, reflecting the volume contraction caused by constant α-adrenergic stimulation. Glucose tolerance may be impaired. Hypercalcaemia is also a recognized association and may be related to secretion of a PTH-like peptide. The diagnosis is confirmed by measuring plasma or urine catecholamine levels or collecting 24-hour urine samples in acid for vanillyl mandelic acid (VMA) estimation (Sheps *et al.*, 1990). The diagnosis is confirmed if the urine VMA excretion exceeds 8 mg in 24 hours. The tumour can then be located using computerized tomography (CT) scanning or magnetic resonance imaging (MRI) in conjunction with venous sampling for catecholamine measurements. Scanning with I^{131}-meta-iodobenzylguanidine produces specific uptake in sites of sympathetic activity.

Management

During a paroxysmal crisis continuous electrocardiographic and invasive blood pressure monitoring is recommended. Administration of *sodium nitroprusside* by infusion or *phentolamine* (1–5 mg boluses intravenously) will usually control the hypertensive surges. Tachycardia may be ameliorated by the simultaneous parenteral administration of *β-blocking agents* (e.g. oral propranolol 80 mg 8-hrly).

There is a significant risk of cardiac arrhythmias, especially numerous premature ventricular contractions, ventricular tachycardia or ventricular fibrillation, particularly in those with pre-existing heart disease.

Initial treatment should be with intravenous *lignocaine* as a 100 mg bolus followed by an infusion at 2–4 mg/min. In patients who fail to respond to lignocaine administration, propranolol should be given in a dosage of 2–10 mg intravenously as 1 mg increments every 4–5 min. If α stimulation remains unopposed β-blockers can paradoxically worsen hypertension during acute episodes and some authorities therefore believe that these agents should not be administered unless the patient has already received an α-blocking drug.

Severe hypotension can complicate acute therapy for a hypertensive crisis. Reducing or discontinuing the infusion of nitroprusside or phentolamine and expansion of the circulating volume is usually all that is required to restore the blood pressure. Treatment with vasoactive drugs such as adrenaline or noradrenaline should be avoided and may be ineffective because of adrenergic receptor 'down-regulation'.

Once the acute attack has been controlled, a long-acting α-adrenergic blocking agent such as phenoxybenzamine may be commenced at a dosage of 10 mg orally twice daily or 20 mg in 500 ml of 5% dextrose intravenously over 2 hours. The dosage is then increased by 10–20 mg/day until the usual dose of 1–2 mg/kg daily in two divided doses is reached.

Once the patient has been stabilized on maintenance therapy with phenoxybenzamine and circulating volume has been restored, further investigations can be undertaken. During the acute hypertensive crisis little consideration is usually given to biochemical confirmation of the diagnosis, although it is of course at this time that catecholamine secretion is at its highest.

ADRENAL CRISIS

Causes

Addisonian crisis is most commonly seen in patients with chronic untreated primary adrenal disease (Irvine & Barnes, 1972), although adrenal insufficiency may also be secondary to hypothalamic–pituitary disease. Whatever the cause, adrenal failure may present acutely or when an acute stressful episode, which may be major such as surgery or relatively minor such as gastroenteritis, precipitates rapid decompensation following a period of insidious deterioration. Adrenal failure may also occur when long-term corticosteroid therapy is discontinued (Schlaghecke *et al.*, 1992) and when treated patients fail to increase their glucocorticoid cover during an episode of major stress or illness. Adrenal haemorrhagic infarction due to bacteraemia is now rare except in children with meningococcaemia, although it may occasionally be seen in adults with staphylococcal or Gram-negative infections. Pituitary infarction may be associated with a sudden loss of adrenocorticotrophic hormone (ACTH) secretion and this may also precipitate an 'adrenal crisis'.

Clinical presentation

Nausea, vomiting, weight loss and *abdominal pain* are prominent in both the primary and secondary forms of adrenal insufficiency. *Hypotension, postural changes in blood pressure* and *dehydration* are often most prominent in those with primary adrenal crisis, whereas in secondary hypocortisolism due to hypothalamic–pituitary disease, mineralocorticoid secretion is maintained and signs of volume depletion are minimal. *Hyperpigmentation* due to high circulating levels of ACTH also helps to distinguish primary adrenal disease from hypothalamic–pituitary failure. In the final stages of adrenal apoplexy, *apathy, confusion* and *extreme weakness* develop, progressing to *shock* and, if unrecognized, death. The possibility of adrenocortical insufficiency should be considered in all shocked patients.

Laboratory investigations

Typical initial laboratory findings include *hyponatraemia* and *hyperkalaemia*. Hyponatraemia is due primarily to a diminished ability to excrete free water rather than mineralocorticoid deficiency. When adrenal failure occurs acutely, however, electrolyte levels may be normal. Fasting *hypoglycaemia* may occur since glucocorticoids are necessary for gluconeogenesis. Although *hypercalcaemia* may be seen, this is secondary to dehydration and requires no treatment. The blood count may show a mild to moderate normocytic normochromic anaemia with a neutropenia. Blood should be taken for basal cortisol and aldosterone estimations. Plasma ACTH is raised in Addison's disease and low in pituitary disease. In a severely ill patient a plasma cortisol less than 150 mmol/l is consistent with the diagnosis of adrenal insufficiency. An ACTH stimulation test can be performed later once the patient has recovered.

Management

Treatment must be instituted immediately following collection of blood samples for subsequent cortisol determination.

Intravenous hydrocortisone should be given as a 200 mg bolus followed by either an infusion of 200 mg over the next 16 hours or 100 mg intramuscularly every 6 hours. Once the precipitating event has resolved and the diagnosis has been confirmed corticosteroid doses can be tapered over the following 4 or 5 days to replacement levels (e.g. oral hydrocortisone 20 mg in the morning and 10 mg in the evening). Specific mineralocorticoid replacement will not be required until later because high-dose hydrocortisone possesses sufficient mineralocorticoid activity. Subsequently *fludrocortisone* replacement can be adjusted depending on postural symptoms, plasma electrolytes and renin activity. A typical dose range is 50–300 µg orally daily.

Fluid replacement should initially be with 0.18% saline in dextrose 4%. Usually 2–4 l will be required over the first 24 hours in patients with primary adrenal insufficiency, especially if vomiting complicates the presentation. In those with hypopituitarism the fluid deficit is less severe and rarely requires replacement with more than 1–2 l. If the patient is hypoglycaemic, an intravenous bolus of 50 ml of 50% dextrose should be given. Subsequently an infusion of a concentrated dextrose solution may be indicated. Invasive monitoring may be required to guide fluid management.

PITUITARY EMERGENCIES

Causes

Long-standing pituitary insufficiency may be associated with *pituitary tumours, infiltrative diseases* (e.g. granulomata) and *vascular lesions*. Pituitary failure can also occur following an acute insult such as *postpartum infarction* or *haemorrhage* or *infarction* of a *pituitary tumour*. Impairment of the control of vasopressin release from the posterior pituitary, as seen with severe intracranial hypertension following closed head injury, is by far the commonest cause of diabetes insipidus encountered on the intensive care unit (see Chapter 14).

Clinical presentation

Patients with hitherto undetected ACTH and TSH deficiency may *decompensate* in response to the stress of infection, trauma, surgery or sedation, particularly when they are currently being given or have recently received steroids. Some patients with pituitary failure present in *coma* preceded by a sudden onset of headache with visual impairment. In these cases the first indication that collapse may be related to an endocrine emergency is often the presence of clinical signs such as hypogonadism, galactorrhoea or characteristic appearances of the skin or hair such as those seen in myxoedema. *Hypothermia* is almost invariable and life-threatening *hypoglycaemia* can occur. Patients with posterior pituitary or hypothalamic diseases sometimes present with *diabetes insipidus*, with thirst, polyuria and nocturia being the main complaints.

Investigations

Once the patient has been resuscitated, a careful history and examination should be followed by baseline measurements of haemoglobin concentration, plasma electrolytes, urine and plasma osmolalities and glucose concentration. Circulating levels of cortisol, prolactin and growth hormone should be determined for definitive diagnosis. Thyroid function tests will also be required.

Management

Hydrocortisone (100 mg intravenously) should then be given followed by 100 mg intramuscularly 6-hourly pending detailed evaluation of the hypothalamo-pituitary–adrenal axis, including urgent CT scanning, and institution of appropriate replacement therapy with oral corticosteroids, T_4 and desmopressin as indicated.

REFERENCES

Arieff AI & Carroll HJ (1972) Nonketotic hyperosmolar coma with hyperglycemia. Clinical features, pathophysiology, renal function, acid–base balance, plasma–cerebrospinal fluid equilibria and effects of therapy in 37 cases. *Medicine* **51**: 73-94.

Baue AE, Gunther B, Hartl W, Ackenheil M & Heberer G (1984) Altered hormonal activity in severely ill patients after injury or sepsis. *Archives of Surgery* **119**: 1125-1132.

Bilezikian JP (1992) Management of acute hyperglycemia. *New England Journal of Medicine* **326**: 1196-1203.

Bingley PJ & Gale EAM (1991) Lessons from family studies. In: Harrison LC, Tait BD (eds), Genetics of diabetes Part I. *Baillière's Clinical Endocrinology and Metabolism* **5**: 261-283.

Blum M (1972) Myxoedema coma. *American Journal of the Medical Sciences* **264**: 432-443.

Broadus AE, Mangin M, Ikeda K, *et al*. (1988) Humoral hypercalcemia of cancer. Identification of a novel parathyroid hormone-like peptide. *New England Journal of Medicine* **319**: 556-563.

Burger A, Nicod P, Suter P, Vallotton MB, Vagenakis A & Braverman L (1976) Reduced active thyroid hormone levels in acute illness. *Lancet* **i**: 653-655.

Burger AG & Philippe J (1992) Thyroid emergencies. In: Burger AG, Philippe J (ed.) *Baillière's Endocrine Emergencies. Clinical Endocrinology and Metabolism* **6**: 77-93.

Chernow B, Burman KD, Johnson DL *et al*. (1983) T_3 may be a better agent than T_4 in the critically ill hypothyroid patient: evaluation of transport across the blood–brain barrier in a primate model. *Critical Care Medicine* **11**: 99-104.

Davidson MB (1981) Diabetic ketoacidosis and hyperosmolar nonketotic coma. In Davidson MB (ed). *Diabetes Mellitus: Diagnosis and Treatment*. New York, John Wiley and Sons, pp. 193-241.

Davies JRE & Heath DA (1989) Comparison of different dose regimes of aminohydroxyproplyidene-1, 1-bisphosphane (APD) in hypercalemia of malignancy. *British Journal of Clinical Pharmacology* **28**: 269-274.

Fein IA, Rackow EC, Sprung CL & Grodman R (1982) Relation of colloid osmotic pressure to arterial hypoxemia and cerebral edema during crystalloid volume loading of patients with diabetic ketoacidosis. *Annals of Internal Medicine* **96**: 570-575.

Felicetta J & Sowers J (1987) Endocrine changes with critical illness. *Critical Care Clinics* **5**: 855-869.

Foster DW & McGarry JD (1983) The metabolic derangements and treatment of diabetic ketoacidosis. *New England Journal of Medicine* **309**: 159-169.

Gale EAM (1989) Hypoglycaemia and human insulin. *Lancet* **ii**: 1264-1266.

Hammond P & Wallis S (1992) Cerebral oedema in diabetic ketoacidosis. *British Medical Journal* **305**: 203-204.

Hellman R, Kelly KL & Mason WD (1977) Propranolol for thyroid storm. *New England Journal of Medicine* **297**: 671-672.

Hillman K (1987) Fluid resuscitation in diabetic emergencies—a reappraisal. *Intensive Care Medicine* **13**: 4-8.

Husband DJ, Thai AC & Alberti KGMM (1986) Management of diabetes during surgery with glucose-insulin-potassium infusion. *Diabetic Medicine* **3**: 69-74.

Irvine WJ & Barnes EW (1972) Adrenocortical insufficiency. *Clinical Endocrinology and Metabolism* **1**: 549.

Kapstein EM, Weiner JM, Robinson WJ, Wheeler WS & Nicoloff JT (1982) Relationship of altered thyroid hormone indices to survival in non-thyroidal illness. *Clinical Endocrinology* **16**: 565-574.

Lindberger K (1975) Myxoedema coma. *Acta Medica Scandinavica* **198**: 87-90.

Lo SS, Tun RYM, Hawa M & Leslie RDG (1991) Studies of diabetic twins. *Diabetes/Metabolism Reviews* **7**: 223-238.

Mackin JF, Canary JJ & Pittman CS (1974) Thyroid storm and its management. *New England Journal of Medicine* **291**: 1396-1398.

Oppenheimer JH, Squef R, Surks MI & Hauer H (1963) Binding of thyroxine by serum proteins evaluated by equilibrium dialysis and electrophoretic techniques. Alterations in non-thyroidal illness. *Journal of Clinical Investigation* **42**: 1769-1782.

Palazzo MG & Suter PM (1991) Delivery dependent oxygen consumption in patients with septic shock: daily variations, relationship with outcome and the sick-euthyroid syndrome. *Intensive Care Medicine* **17**: 325-332.

Percival RC, Yates AJP, Gray RES, Neal FE, Forrest ARW & Kanis JA (1984) Role of glucocorticoids in management of malignant hypocalcaemia. *British Medical Journal* **289**: 287.

Ross EJ & Griffith DNW (1989) The clinical presentation of phaeochromocytoma. *Quarterly Journal of Medicine* **266**: 485-496.

Schlaghecke R, Kornely E, Santer RT & Ridderskamp P (1992) The effect of long term glucocorticoid therapy on pituitary-adrenal responses to exogenous corticotrophin-releasing hormone. *New England Journal of Medicine* **326**: 226–230.

Sheps SG, Jiang NS, Klee GG & van Heerden JA (1990) Recent developments in the diagnosis and treatment of phaeochromocytoma. *Mayo Clinic Proceedings* **65**: 88–95.

Slag MF, Morley JE, Elson MK, Crowson TW, Nuttall FQ & Shafer RB (1981) Hypothyroxinemia in critically ill patients as a predictor of high mortality. *Journal of the American Medical Association* **245**: 43–45.

Sprung Cl, Rackow EC & Fein IA (1980) Pulmonary edema: a complication of diabetic keotacidosis. *Chest* **77**: 687–688.

Sutton MG, Sheps SG & Lie JT (1981) Prevalence of clinically unsuspected phaeochromocytoma. Review of 50 year autopsy series. *Mayo Clinic Proceedings* **56**: 354–360.

Tunbridge WMG (1981) Factors contributing to deaths of diabetics under fifty years of age. On behalf of the Medical Services Study Group and British Diabetic Association. *Lancet* **i**: 569–572.

Utiger RD (1980) Decreased extrathyroidal triiodothyronine production in non-thyroidal illness: benefit or harm? *American Journal of Medicine* **69**: 807–810.

Williams GR, Franklyn JA, Neuberger JM & Sheppard MC (1989) Thyroid hormone receptor expression in the 'sick euthyroid' syndrome. *Lancet* **ii**: 1477–1481.

17 Obstetric Intensive Care

Critical illness in the obstetric population may occur coincidentally or as a consequence of pregnancy. There are also a variety of emergencies that may involve the pregnant woman such as trauma, haemorrhage, cardiopulmonary collapse and pulmonary embolism, as well as numerous medical conditions that carry an increased risk for the pregnant woman and her fetus (e.g. cardiopulmonary disease, diabetes mellitus and sickle cell disease).

In the UK reports from the Confidential Enquiries into Maternal Deaths in England and Wales have recorded the changing pattern of ultimately fatal illnesses complicating pregnancy since the triennial system of reporting began in 1952 (**Fig. 17.1**). Although most would agree that intensive care is now indicated for many of these life-threatening disorders, estimates of the incidence of intensive care admissions currently vary between 1-9 for every 1000 obstetric deliveries (Mabie & Sibai, 1990; Kilpatrick & Matnay, 1992). Admission policies and case mix clearly differ from city to city (Collop & Sahn, 1993), but it is generally accepted that women with life-threatening complications of pregnancy should be managed according to the same principles as any other patient with a similar condition.

PHYSIOLOGICAL ALTERATIONS IN PREGNANCY

Cardiac output begins to rise in the first trimester and increases progressively to peak at 30-50% of pre-existing levels at 32 weeks' gestation (de Swiet, 1980). This rise in cardiac output is due to increases in both heart rate and stroke volume.

Plasma volume expands by 40-50%, while red cell mass increases by only 20-30%, producing a dilutional 'physiological anaemia of pregnancy'.

The placental bed serves as a large arteriovenous shunt, which reduces total *systemic vascular resistance*. There is also arteriolar vasodilation, which may be related to endothelial release of prostacyclin and nitric oxide (NO), and/or to increased circulating levels of progesterone.

These changes in cardiac output and systemic vascular resistance are associated with increases in blood flow to the kidneys, the uterus, the breasts, and the skin. Mean arterial blood pressure (MAP) falls by 5-15 mm Hg during the second trimester, returning to near normal levels at term.

Similar alterations occur in the *pulmonary circulation*. There is vasodilation with an increased pulmon-

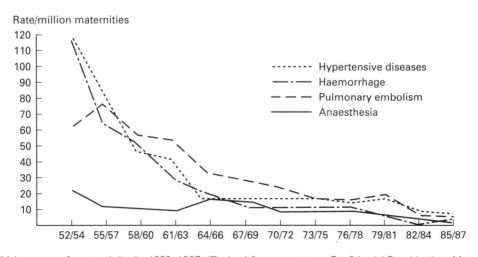

Fig. 17.1 Main causes of maternal deaths 1952–1987. (Derived from reports on Confidential Enquiries into Maternal Deaths in England and Wales.)

ary blood volume while mean pulmonary artery pressure and pulmonary artery occlusion pressure (PAOP) remain within the normal range. Nevertheless the capacity of the pulmonary circulation to compensate for a further increase in circulating volume is reduced and the pregnant patient therefore has an increased risk of developing pulmonary oedema.

Minute ventilation is increased by 50% during pregnancy and *tidal volume* (V_T) increases to a greater extent than *respiratory rate* (**Table 17.1**). Functional residual capacity (FRC) is decreased by about 20% with a fall in both expiratory reserve volume (ERV) and residual volume (RV). Total lung capacity (TLC) is, however, only marginally reduced. Oxygen consumption is increased by about 20%, with a further 60% increase during active labour. During late pregnancy mild hypoxaemia may occur, especially when the patient is supine, because of the reduction in FRC combined with the increased $\dot{V}_{O_2}$.

PRE-ECLAMPSIA

Pre-eclampsia is a condition unique to pregnancy and complicates approximately 15% of primigravid pregnancies. Eclampsia complicates severe pre-eclampsia and occurs in approximately 0.04% of deliveries. Pre-eclampsia and eclampsia are the commonest causes of maternal death in the developed countries (Redman, 1988).

Definitions

Pre-eclampsia is defined as the onset of *hypertension* with *proteinuria, oedema,* or both, at more than 20 weeks' gestation. Hypertension is defined as a rise in systolic blood pressure of more than 15 mm Hg or a blood pressure higher than 140/90 mm Hg on more than two occasions six hours apart. *Eclampsia* is the occurrence of *seizures* in a patient with pre-eclampsia.

Table 17.1 Respiratory changes in pregnancy.		
	Non-pregnant	**Pregnant** (at term)
Total lung capacity (TLC) (ml)	4200	↓ 4000
Tidal volume (V_T) (ml)	450	↑↑ 600
Inspiratory capacity (IC) (ml)	2500	↑ 2650
Expiratory reserve volume (ERV) (ml)	700	↓↓ 550
Residual volume (RV) (ml)	1000	↓↓ 800
Functional residual capacity (FRC) (ml)	1700	↓↓ 1350
Vital capacity (VC) (ml)	3200	→ 3200

Severe pre-eclampsia is diagnosed in the presence of one or more of the following:

● blood pressure higher than 160 mm Hg systolic or 110 mm Hg diastolic on two occasions more than 6 hours apart;
● proteinuria greater than 5 g/24 hours or 3–4+ on a dipstick;
● oliguria of less than 400 ml/24 hours;
● cerebral or visual disturbances;
● pulmonary oedema or cyanosis.

Chronic hypertension is diagnosed when the pre-pregnant blood pressure is known to be higher than 140/90 mm Hg or when hypertension is detected before 20 weeks' gestation. Pre-eclampsia is said to be superimposed on chronic hypertension when there is exacerbation of hypertension of more than 30 mm Hg systolic or 15 mm Hg diastolic combined with the appearance of significant proteinuria or generalized oedema. *Transient hypertension* during pregnancy may occur without other signs of pre-eclampsia.

Pathophysiology

The pathophysiological changes of pre-eclampsia suggest that organ dysfunction is largely related to reduced perfusion. Impaired perfusion of the kidney, liver, brain and intervillous spaces of the placenta can be demonstrated, and examination of retinal vessels, nail beds and conjunctivae provides direct evidence of *vasoconstriction*. This vasoconstriction is accompanied by a *reduced plasma volume* and *activation of the coagulation cascade*. In some cases these changes antedate clinically evident disease by several weeks (De Boer *et al.*, 1989).

Although there is some controversy about the changes in cardiac output in pre-eclampsia, the largest study of untreated cases found that *cardiac output was low to normal* (Wallenburg, 1988). This finding, in conjunction with documented hypertension, supports the suggestion that *increased systemic vascular resistance* is an important component of the clinical condition. Pre-eclampsia is also accompanied by a *low plasma volume, with reduced plasma renin* and *high atrial natriuretic peptide* concentrations (Malee *et al.*, 1992), suggesting that profound vasoconstriction reduces the intravascular capacity. The vasoconstriction and consequent reduction in organ perfusion are probably secondary to the increased sensitivity to circulating pressor agents that has been observed in women with pre-eclampsia.

At post-mortem, histological changes include *cerebral oedema, placental thrombotic lesions, pulmonary oedema* and a wide range of *hepatic abnormalities*. The electron microscopic changes observed in renal and placental vessels of women with pre-eclampsia and eclampsia reveal changes seen in no other form of hypertension. The glomerular capillary endothelial cells are greatly increased in size with electron-dense cytoplasmic inclusions that may occlude the capillary lumen (Spargo *et al.*, 1976). This *glomeruloendotheliosis* supports the concept that pre-eclampsia is a unique disorder of pregnancy in which vascular endothelial damage plays a central role.

Eclampsia complicates the severe clinical disorder, but not necessarily very high blood pressure, and is a reflection of neuromuscular hyperreactivity. It is usually accompanied by *cerebral oedema* and *intracranial haemorrhages*. The latter is consistently reported as the most common cause of death (Redman, 1988).

Aetiology

The aetiology of pre-eclamptic toxaemia (PET) and eclampsia is still poorly understood. It is now suggested that there is an autosomal recessive *genetic predisposition* to develop an immune response within the placenta. Epidemiological data and animal experiments indicate that *impaired placental perfusion*, frequently secondary to *abnormal implantation* is the initiating factor. It is proposed that blood-borne products originating from the poorly perfused fetoplacental unit affect the maternal circulation, primarily by activating vascular endothelial cells. In particular *prostacyclin* formation appears to be reduced and there is a relative rise in the circulating concentrations of the vasoconstrictor *thromboxane A_2*. There is also some preliminary evidence to suggest that a systemic disorder of *NO* production may be involved in the aetiology of hypertension and thrombocytopenia in pre-eclampsia (De Belder *et al.*, 1995). This leads to *endothelial damage, loss of plasma volume, platelet activation, intravascular coagulation* and *diminished organ perfusion*. Vasospasm and microthrombi may then exacerbate the deficient placental perfusion and further disturb endothelial cell function. This autoacceleration of the disorder is compatible with the clinical presentation of pre-eclampsia.

Clinical presentation

Although the combination of *hypertension, proteinuria, hyperreflexia* and *oedema* are well known, there are other presentations of pre-eclampsia. Three-quarters of all *eclamptic seizures* still occur in hospital and may occur for the first time in the post-partum period. Furthermore a group of patients has been recognized with the constellation of *haemolysis, elevated liver enzymes* and *low platelets* (HELLP syndrome) (Weinstein, 1982). Patients manifesting this syndrome usually present before term (< 36 weeks' gestation)

complaining of malaise, epigastric or right upper quadrant pain and nausea or vomiting. Some will have nonspecific viral syndrome-like symptoms, while hypertension and proteinuria may be absent or slight (Sibai, 1990). Any pregnant woman presenting with some or all of these symptoms should have a full blood count with platelet and liver enzyme determinations, irrespective of her blood pressure.

Management (Redman & Roberts, 1993)

OBSTETRIC MANAGEMENT

Once hypertension is under control, the optimum timing and mode of delivery must be discussed. When eclampsia develops before or during labour the outlook for mother and baby is worse the longer delivery is delayed.

MANAGEMENT AFTER DELIVERY (**Table 17.2**)

Pre-eclampsia/eclampsia appears to be the single most common condition requiring postpartum admission to an intensive care unit. Generally moderate haemodynamic instability is managed antenatally in the delivery unit by the anaesthetic and obstetric staff. Once the

Table 17.2 Guidelines for the post-delivery management of pre-eclampsia and eclampsia.

General measures

Sedation and analgesia
Mechanical ventilation in selected cases

Control of hypertension

Sympathetic antagonists
Vasodilators
      Hydralazine
      Sodium nitroprusside
Calcium channel blockers

Prevention of seizures

Phenytoin
Magnesium sulphate

Fluid balance

Restrict crystalloids
Careful expansion of circulating volume
Monitor central venous pressure (CVP) and, in selected cases, pulmonary artery occlusion pressure (PAOP)
Diurectics may be indicated (e.g. for pulmonary oedema)

patient has delivered, the specialized services associated with fetal assessment and delivery are no longer a priority (Kilpatrick & Matthay, 1992).

Following expeditious delivery of the baby, treatment should include:

- control of and prophylaxis against seizures;
- control of severe hypertension;
- assessment of oliguria.

Any patient with severe pre-eclampsia/eclampsia who has undergone Caesarean section should be returned to the intensive care unit. They should remain sedated and sometimes mechanically ventilated for approximately 12–24 hours, depending on their mental state, their level of irritability and the dosage of antihypertensives required. Sedation and analgesia are generally maintained with continuous infusions of an opiate and a benzodiazepine. Lateralizing signs or continued irritability post-Caesarean section are an indication for computerized tomography (CT) or magnetic resonance imaging (MRI) scanning.

Control of hypertension

It is recommended that postnatal patients are routinely admitted for high-dependency nursing care if they require intravenous antihypertensive medication by infusion. It is increasingly accepted that such therapy should be monitored by indwelling intra-arterial and central venous cannulae as in the non-pregnant population. Relative systolic hypertension and oliguria with documented high urinary osmolality may be tolerated in the early postpartum period. It is, however, advisable to treat diastolic blood pressures higher than 110 mm Hg to minimize the risk of intracranial haemorrhage. Crystalloid solutions should be restricted to 1.2 l/day and colloids should be administered if there is oliguria (< 0.5 ml/kg/h) associated with low cardiac filling pressures. A spontaneous diuresis heralds resolution of the condition. Indications for a pulmonary artery flotation catheter include pulmonary oedema, persistent profound oliguria (< 0.5 ml/kg/h) despite fluid challenge and severe uncontrollable hypertension.

Sympathetic antagonists. In recent years there has been much interest in the use of *labetalol* for the control of hypertension associated with pre-eclampsia. Chronic use of oral labetalol and intravenous administration of labetalol to women with pre-eclampsia has been shown not to decrease interplacental blood flow, despite producing significant falls in blood pressure (Jouppila *et al.*, 1987). One difficulty with the use of labetalol in severe pre-eclampsia, however, is its variable efficacy. While in some reports a diastolic blood pressure of less than 100 mm Hg was easily achieved (Mabie *et al.*, 1987), in

others pressure control proved difficult (Ashe *et al.*, 1987). In the former study labetalol was administered as increasing boluses from 20 mg to 80 mg, while in the latter it was administered as a continuous infusion to a maximum of 160 mg/hour.

The use of non-specific β-blockers such as propanolol in pregnancy has been controversial, in particular because a reduction in birth weight and an increased incidence of small for gestational age infants has been attributed to the long-term antenatal prescription of propanolol (Lieberman *et al.*, 1978). Although one study (Sibai *et al.*, 1987) suggested that the use of labetalol was also associated with a reduction in birth weight, in general this agent seems less likely to produce such adverse effects.

Vasodilators (see also Chapter 4). *Hydralazine* is widely used in the treatment of pre-eclampsia, despite the observation that in many antenatal patients it causes significant fetal distress (Mabie *et al.*, 1987). Although its use is therefore not without hazard, the risks can be minimized by ensuring adequate hydration and careful dosing to achieve a diastolic blood pressure of approximately 100 mm Hg.

Sodium nitroprusside (SNP) is an extremely potent dilator of both the resistance and capacitance blood vessels and is administered by continuous infusion. Because of its rapid onset of action and short half-life, continuous intra-arterial blood pressure monitoring is essential. Experience with the use of SNP in the antenatal period is limited and there is concern that the capacity of the fetus to metabolize cyanide may be limited by relative immaturity of the hepatic enzyme systems. Nevertheless there have been a few case reports describing the use of SNP in severe pre-eclampsia complicated by pulmonary oedema. In the four cases reported by Stempel (1982), SNP produced a marked decline in PAOP that paralleled the decrease in MAP. Three of these patients had previously failed to respond to hydralazine. Cyanide was undetectable in blood samples obtained from one neonate and two mothers. When used carefully SNP is a safe and effective hypotensive agent in resistant or complicated cases of severe pre-eclampisa. Because of the precarious state of hydration in these patients the infusion should be started at a very low dose (e.g. 0.25 μg/kg/minute).

Glyceryl trinitrate (GTN) is also a suitable agent for controlling blood pressure in pre-eclampsia complicated by pulmonary oedema, although its efficacy may be limited in the well-hydrated patient. Like SNP, its rapid onset and short duration of action allows titration of a continuous infusion to achieve the desired blood pressure. Intra-arterial monitoring is required. Clinical reports of the use of GTN in severe pre-eclampsia have been limited to small studies (Cotton *et al.*, 1986).

As well as the fetal distress that can complicate

excessive iatrogenic reductions in blood pressure, there are specific concerns about the potential of vasodilators to exacerbate intracranial hypertension. Nevertheless in view of the possible role of NO deficiency in the aetiology of pre-eclampsia, both GTN and SNP, which are NO-donors, may have a limited, but important role in the more severe cases, especially those with pulmonary oedema.

Calcium channel blockers. These agents have a number of advantages as antihypertensive agents. They are easily administered in oral or sublingual form, and have a rapid onset of action with a duration of 3–5 hours. The ensuing reduction in MAP is proportional to the baseline blood pressure and serious hypotension is therefore rare. These agents also dilate the coronary vasculature and improve subendocardial myocardial perfusion. Enthusiasm for the use of calcium channel blockers in the antenatal period has, however, been tempered by animal studies demonstrating disproportionate reductions in uterine blood flow as well as theoretical concerns about their interaction with magnesium sulphate. This latter agent is favoured in some centres for seizure prophylaxis in pre-eclampsia (see later in this chapter), but is also a calcium antagonist. Currently the use of these agents is generally restricted to the treatment of hypertension in the postpartum period. *Sublingual nifedipine* may be prescribed in preference to intravenous hydralazine or labetalol (Fenakel *et al.*, 1991), usually in a dose of 10–20 mg three or four times daily.

Diuretics. In the past diuretics were widely prescribed to control the physiological oedema of pregnancy and, it was thought, thereby reduce the incidence of pre-eclampsia. It is now appreciated, however, that since the circulating volume is contracted in pre-eclampsia, diuretic therapy is contraindicated. Occasionally diuretic therapy is required for the treatment of specific complications such as pulmonary oedema, in which case the agent of choice is parenteral frusemide.

Prevention of seizures

Prophylactic *phenytoin* is routinely prescribed by some obstetricians to prevent seizures in severe pre-eclampsia (Slater *et al.*, 1987), although there are significant hazards associated with its use, of which hypotension is the most common. This appears to be related to the rate of intravenous infusion, which should not exceed 25 mg/minute. The ECG must be continuously monitored and the blood pressure measured frequently. The rate of infusion should be slowed if the systolic pressure falls below 110 mm Hg or bradyarrhythmias develop. The recommended loading dose is 15 mg/kg intravenously, a second dose of 500 mg should be given intravenously or orally 12 hours later, followed by a maintenance dose of 300 mg daily. This should be adjusted to maintain the blood level within the therapeutic range of 7–20 mg/l. It must also be remembered that newborn infants exposed to phenytoin may develop a bleeding tendency, which can be prevented by vitamin K administration at birth. Recurrence of convulsions has been reported despite achieving therapeutic levels of phenytoin (Tuffnel *et al.*, 1989).

Magnesium sulphate has retained its popularity in North America (Pritchard *et al.*, 1984) and South Africa (Richards *et al.*, 1986) despite the risk of toxicity leading to respiratory arrest. Some authors suggest that the dose can be titrated according to physical signs and that administration should be discontinued if there is oliguria or an absent patellar reflex. A typical regimen for the use of magnesium sulphate is provided in **Table 17.3**. The use of magnesium sulphate in obstetric practice remains controversial; it does not prevent convulsions in every case and has no effect on the abnormal electroencephalographic findings in eclampsia (Sibai *et al.*, 1984). Nevertheless a report from South Africa has suggested that phenytoin is not as effective an anticonvulsant in eclampsia as magnesium sulphate (Domisse, 1990).

Fluid balance

Currently treatment usually involves a combination of volume expansion and vasodilators. Judicious volume replacement has been shown to increase cardiac output and oxygen delivery, as well as reduce systemic vascular resistance (Cotton *et al.*, 1986), and vasodilation in the face of hypovolaemia may precipitate hypotension and fetal distress. On the other hand, severe pre-eclampsia may be complicated by cerebral oedema and cardiogenic or non-cardiogenic pulmonary oedema. In the more severe cases, central venous pressure (CVP) monitoring can be misleading as there may be significant disparity in the function of the left and right ventricles (Cotton *et al.*, 1985; Mabie *et al.*, 1989). Pulmonary artery catheterization is warranted in such cases and may provide useful information on oxygen transport variables. Severe pre-eclampsia is associated with abnormal tissue oxygen extraction (Belfort *et al.*, 1993).

COMPLICATIONS

Eclampsia (Moodley, 1990)

Should a patient have a seizure, the airway must be protected, oxygenation maintained and the seizure terminated with the intravenous administration of a benzodiazepine such as midazolam (1–2 mg) or diazepam (5–

Table 17.3   Guidelines for magnesium sulphate dosage in the management of pre-eclampsia and eclampsia

1   Give a loading dose of 4 g magnesium sulphate as a 20% solution (equivalent to 16.3 mmol Mg^{++}) intravenously at a rate of 1 g/min during eclamptic seizures or over 10–15 minutes for seizure prophylaxis

2   Start a continuous intravenous infusion of magnesium sulphate at the rate of 1–3 g/h (1–12 mmol/h) and continue the infusion for at least 24 h after delivery.

3   If convulsions persist after 15 mins give 2–4 g magnesium sulphate intravenously at a rate no faster than 1 g/min

4   Examine carefully every four hrs for the presence of limb reflexes, respiration rate of at least 16/min and urinary output of at least 30 ml/h. Measure serum magnesium concentrations if possible.

Normal range	0.75–1.25 (mmol/l)
Effective anticonvulsant	2–3.5 (mmol/l)
Reflexes disappear	5.00 (mmol/l)
Respiratory depression	7.50 (mmol/l)
Cardiac arrest	15.00 (mmol/l)

If reflexes are absent, respiration depressed, urinary output inadequate or if serum magnesium is within a dangerous range, discontinue magnesium sulphate infusion. In the event of cardiorespiratory arrest give 10–20 ml of 10% calcium gluconate intravenously slowly over 10 minutes in addition to advanced life support.

5   Magnesium sulphate may enhance the action of non-depolarizing muscle relaxants. Anaesthetists and paediatricians must be told that the drug is being used. The magnesium ion crosses the placenta and may cause the newborn to be flaccid.

---

10 mg) (see also Chapter 14). Sufficient anticonvulsant should be given to prevent further seizures while additional treatment is instituted. In many instances elective tracheal intubation and mechanical ventilation is indicated so that anticonvulsants can be administered freely without the risk of pulmonary aspiration and to control intracranial hypertension (Richards *et al.*, 1986). As well as the immediate control of convulsions it is important that raised blood pressure is treated promptly while avoiding reductions in cerebral blood flow (see Chapter 14). Many consider that the optimal MAP in obstetric patients with suspected cerebral oedema complicating severe pre-eclampsia/eclampsia is 80–100 mm Hg. In those who develop eclampsia, delivery of the baby is a priority.

Haemorrhage

A ruptured liver, intra-adrenal haemorrhage, life-threatening coagulopathy or rupture of a congenital intracerebral aneurysm are all possible life-threatening sequelae to pre-eclampsia.

Cerebral ischaemia

When associated with eclampsia, cerebral ischaemia is presumed to be secondary to vasospasm (Lewis *et al.*, 1988; Duncan *et al.*, 1989). The successful administration of nimodipine, a cerebral vasodilator which inhibits arterial contraction induced experimentally by

serotonin, to a moribund patient with eclampsia suggests that serotonin may be involved in the pathogenesis of this condition (Horn *et al.*, 1990).

Pulmonary aspiration

Pulmonary aspiration may complicate tracheal intubation, oversedation or convulsions. Adult respiratory distress syndrome (ARDS) is second only to intracerebral haemorrhage as the immediate cause of death in patients with hypertensive disorders of pregnancy (Sibai *et al.*, 1987) (see later in this chapter).

Acute renal failure

Acute renal failure is now rare, but may complicate the HELLP syndrome.

Differential diagnosis

Should the blood pressure not begin to fall within 24 hours of delivery other causes of hypertension such as phaeochromocytoma must be considered.

PREVENTION

The observation that pre-eclampsia is associated with increased thromboxane concentrations and low prostacyclin levels has provided the rationale for aspirin prophylaxis. Anecdotal reports were followed by two larger trials (Italian Study of Aspirin in Pregnancy, 1993; Sibai *et al.*, 1993), which failed to confirm efficacy, although both differed from earlier studies in that lower-risk women were recruited. Recently a large Collaborative Low-dose Aspirin Study in Pregnancy (CLASP) has shown that routine prophylactic low-dose aspirin (60 mg/day) is not effective in women at risk for pre-eclampsia or intrauterine growth retardation (CLASP Collaborative Group, 1994).

ADULT RESPIRATORY DISTRESS SYNDROME IN OBSTETRIC PATIENTS
(see Chapters 6 and 7)

In critically ill obstetric patients, ARDS may follow:

- amniotic fluid embolism;
- hypertensive disorders of pregnancy;
- haemorrhage;
- dead fetus syndrome;
- sepsis;
- inhalation of gastric contents;
- β-adrenergic agonist therapy with or without cortico-steroids for premature labour.

The incidence of ARDS complicating pregnancy appears to be increasing. This may be due partly to its more frequent recognition by pathologists and partly to patients surviving longer, thereby allowing time for the disease to become established.

Aspiration of gastric contents during anaesthesia

Although in the early Confidential Enquiries the proportion of deaths directly attributable to anaesthesia was small, their incidence has remained disappointingly constant, and complications related to anaesthesia are still one of the commonest causes of maternal death in the UK (Department of Health, 1994). This has been despite the introduction of epidural anaesthetic techniques and the widespread administration of antacids before delivery. These anaesthetic-related deaths are frequently a consequence of pneumonitis due to pulmonary aspiration of acidic gastric contents (Mendelson's syndrome) (Mendelson, 1946). The severity of aspiration pneumonitis depends on the acidity of the gastric contents as well as the volume aspirated (see Chapter 6).

PATHOGENESIS

In Mendelson's original series, women died from asphyxia, not from the aspiration pneumonitis that now carries his name. The increased lethality of this condition compared to Mendelson's original observations (Mendelson, 1946) may be due to the widespread practice of instituting intermittent positive pressure ventilation (IPPV) in such cases. This may only serve to disseminate inhaled gastric contents throughout the lung, thereby enlarging the acid burn to the alveolar–capillary membrane. Moreover, the free and liberal administration of crystalloid solutions, either as an adjunct to epidural analgesia or as a nutritional supplement during labour, combined with the routine administration of ergometrine or Syntometrine, both of which are pulmonary vasoconstrictors, may exacerbate oedema formation.

Aspiration pneumonitis is associated with hypoxia and hypovolaemia, which may precipitate splanchnic vasoconstriction, exacerbate generalized tissue hypoxia and initiate the release of inflammatory mediators. Patients are therefore at risk of developing primary multiple organ dysfunction syndrome (MODS), the systemic inflammatory response syndrome (SIRS) and eventually secondary MODS (see Chapter 4). The combination of a chemical burn to the alveolar–capillary membrane and a disseminated inflammatory response frequently leads to the development of ARDS.

MANAGEMENT

The management of pulmonary aspiration in obstetric patients should be the same as for the non-pregnant population. The airway must be secured and cleared of debris; this may require *bronchoscopy*, but broncho-alveolar lavage is not recommended. Appropriate *respiratory support* should be instituted (see Chapter 7), and in the most severe cases the use of *extracorporeal gas exchange* should be considered. *Steroid* administration is not thought to be of any benefit in aspiration pneumonitis. *Pulmonary artery catheterization* is often indicated to guide volume administration and haemodynamic support.

PREVENTION

Various studies have now discredited the particulate antacid magnesium trisilicate as effective prophylaxis against the consequences of aspirating gastric contents. A regimen involving the regular prescription of oral ranitidine (150 mg 6-hourly) together with the administration of 30 ml 0.3 M sodium citrate has been shown to be an effective means of controlling the acidity and volume of the gastric contents (Gillett *et al.*, 1984). Results from recent national surveys reveal that routine prophylaxis in the UK now generally consists of such a combination of H_2-receptor blockade (e.g. ranitidine) and a non-particulate antacid (e.g. 0.3 M sodium citrate) (Tordoff & Sweeney 1990; Grieff *et al.*, 1994).

Organizational changes prompted by the recommendations of the Confidential Enquiries have also meant that unsupervised junior staff no longer undertake anaesthesia for Caesarean section without adequate training and skilled assistance. The importance of correctly applied cricoid pressure and a rehearsed failed intubation drill have been emphasized repeatedly in successive reports.

Amniotic fluid embolism

Amniotic fluid embolism (AFE) is a rare, but catastrophic complication of pregnancy. Its incidence has been estimated at between 1/8000 and 1/80,000 deliveries.

RISK FACTORS

Risk factors for AFE include:

- increasing maternal age;
- the use of oxytocic agents to induce or augment labour;
- women of high parity;
- strong uterine contractions.

PATHOGENESIS

Conventionally, the cardiorespiratory complications of AFE were thought to be a consequence of acute right-sided heart failure secondary to severe pulmonary hypertension following occlusion of or vasospastic changes in the pulmonary vasculature. Recently, however, Clark (1990) has questioned this explanation. In contrast to observations in experimental models a review of published cases of AFE in humans has revealed only mild to moderate elevations in pulmonary artery pressure, variable increases in CVP, elevated PAOP and evidence of left ventricular dysfunction or failure (Clark *et al.*, 1985). Although the cause of the left ventricular failure remains obscure, it is the only significant haemodynamic abnormality that has been consistently documented in patients with AFE. To reconcile these experimental and clinical findings, Clark postulates a biphasic pattern of cardiorespiratory disturbance. The initial response of the pulmonary vasculature to the presence of amniotic fluid is perhaps vasospasm, which produces transient pulmonary hypertension and profound hypoxia. This initial period of hypoxia might account for the approximately 50% of patients who succumb to AFE within the first hour after the onset of symptoms. The transient nature of this initial haemody-

namic response could also account for the failure of subsequent invasive monitoring to document significant pulmonary hypertension. Those patients who survive this initial phase may experience a secondary phase of haemodynamic compromise, which involves left heart failure with right heart function returning to normal. While such a biphasic course is an attractive explanation it must be recognized that the existence of the initial phase of transient pulmonary vasospasm in humans is speculative.

The identification of fetal squames in the pulmonary vasculature is no longer considered pathognomonic for AFE (Plauche, 1983). Some fetal squames probably normally enter the venous circulation of pregnant women, raising the possibility that it is only *abnormal* amniotic fluid that causes the clinical syndrome of AFE. Intriguingly, metabolites of arachidonic acid can produce many of the haemodynamic and haematological effects found in patients with clinical AFE. Such metabolites, including the prostaglandins and leukotrienes, are present in amniotic fluid in increasing concentrations during labour (Karim & Devlin, 1967).

CLINICAL FEATURES (Steiner & Lushbaugh, 1941)

AFE presents as a sudden life-threatening collapse with *respiratory distress, cyanosis, hypotension* and *hypoxia*. This may progress rapidly to *refractory cardiorespiratory arrest*. Of those who survive the initial cardiovascular and respiratory insults 45% will develop *life-threatening coagulopathy* within the next four hours, which may be compounded by *uterine atony*. Almost three-quarters of those who survive the initial haemodynamic collapse will develop a secondary *non-cardiogenic pulmonary oedema* (Koegler *et al.*, 1994) due to an increased alveolar–capillary permeability. Patients surviving to receive invasive haemodynamic monitoring generally demonstrate left *ventricular dysfunction* or failure accompanied by moderate or severe elevations in PAOP and depressed left ventricular contractility (Vanmaele *et al.*, 1990). Superimposed *renal failure* worsens the prognosis.

DIAGNOSIS

There is no single clinical or laboratory finding that by itself can confirm or exclude AFE. The diagnosis must be made on the basis of clinical presentation and supportive laboratory studies. Fetal squames may be detected in samples of pulmonary capillary blood (Masson & Ruggieri, 1985) as well as at autopsy, when squamous cells or debris may be found in the pulmonary artery vasculature.

Laboratory abnormalities include *coagulopathy*

(decreased fibrinogen and elevated levels of fibrin split products, prolonged partial thromboplastin and prothrombin times) and *thrombocytopenia*. It must be emphasized that not all these coagulation abnormalities will be present in every case (Quinn & Barrett, 1993).

The *differential diagnosis* of AFE includes:

- septic shock;
- aspiration pneumonia;
- acute myocardial infarction;
- pulmonary thromboembolism;
- placental abruption.

History and examination should be supplemented with a 12-lead electrocardiogram (ECG) and chest radiograph. A right ventricular strain pattern on the ECG and perihilar infiltrates on the chest radiograph are suggestive, but not diagnostic. The onset of a haemorrhagic phase manifest by bleeding from venepuncture sites or surgical incisions is strongly suggestive of AFE in these circumstances.

MANAGEMENT

In addition to normal resuscitative measures, mechanical ventilation and the administration of pressor agents are central to the acute management of AFE. Management of the coagulopathy associated with AFE should include replacement of the circulating blood volume as well as administration of platelets and clotting factors as indicated (Quinn & Barrett, 1993). Some have speculated that cryoprecipitate may be particularly beneficial in AFE. It not only contains significant levels of fibrinogen and other factors, but also high concentrations of fibronectin. The latter facilitates clearance of cellular and particulate matter from the circulation by the reticuloendothelial system and might therefore improve outcome from AFE.

Recently a report of successful management of AFE syndrome with continuous haemofiltration (see Chapter 12) raises the possibility that this technique can effectively remove substances that might play an important role in the genesis of left ventricular and respiratory dysfunction (Weksler *et al.*, 1994).

PROGNOSIS

The overall mortality may be greater than 80%, and even in those patients who survive the initial cardiorespiratory events and subsequent multisystem organ dysfunction, the initial hypoxaemia may have caused irreversible damage to the maternal CNS, or even brain death.

ACUTE COAGULOPATHY IN PREGNANCY

Coagulation in pregnancy

Although blood loss after placental separation is controlled primarily by arterial constriction, the deposition of a fibrin mesh over the placental site is also important. In anticipation of this requirement, levels of Factor VII, VIII and X increase throughout pregnancy and the fibrinogen level at term is almost twice that in the nonpregnant state. Fibrin deposition occurs in the placental matrix and the walls of the spiral arteries. Systemic fibrinolytic activity is not, however, increased, tissue plasminogen activator is not found in the placenta (Letsky, 1989) and plasma fibrinolytic activity is reduced in mid and late pregnancy. Pregnancy is therefore associated with a procoagulant state.

Coagulation failure in pregnancy (Finley, 1989)

Endothelial damage unites the intravascular coagulation factors with their extravascular activators: the resultant fibrin formation is normally localized to the site of damage. If coagulation activators enter the circulation, however, uncontrolled fibrin deposition may lead to *disseminated intravascular coagulation* (DIC). Placental tissue is rich in thromboplastin, and amniotic fluid is a devastatingly effective activator of coagulation that can produce DIC of sudden onset and life-threatening severity. By comparison, slow release of thromboplastic substances into the circulation occurs in conditions such as missed abortion or mild pre-eclampsia. Some other causes of coagulopathy such as hypovolaemia and incompatible transfusion are not exclusive to pregnancy. Some conditions (such as placenta praevia, uterine rupture, vaginal or perineal tears) may be complicated by massive blood loss in which case the large volume transfusion (> 4–5 litres) may exacerbate any coagulopathy by haemodilution. Most authors do not now regard HELLP syndrome as a subvariant of DIC (Pousti *et al.*, 1994).

DIAGNOSIS OF COAGULATION FAILURE

Haemorrhage in the case of DIC may be localized to sites of tissue injury (venepunctures, intravenous and epidural cannula sites, uterus and perineum) or may be generalized with bruising, epistaxis, haematemesis and intracranial haemorrhage.

When coagulopathy is suspected, blood specimens should be taken for a 'DIC screen' (prothrombin time, partial thromboplastin time, fibrinogen and fibrin/fibrinogen degradation products), and sent to the haematology laboratory with samples for a full blood count and crossmatching. A fresh venepuncture should always be used for tests of coagulation.

TREATMENT OF COAGULATION FAILURE

General measures

Treatment priorities for the bleeding pregnant woman are the same as for the non-pregnant patient, always keeping in mind the normal physiological changes of pregnancy, including the increased tissue oxygen demands of the fetoplacental unit. *The best therapy for the fetus is rapid and effective resuscitation of the mother.*

Antepartum coagulopathy

DIC is always secondary to an underlying cause. If DIC is directly attributable to the gravid uterus as in pre-eclampsia, placental abruption or intrauterine death then evacuation of the uterus and delivery of the fetus may have to be considered.

Postpartum haemorrhage

Resuscitation of life-threatening postpartum bleeding must be accompanied by definitive measures to control haemorrhage. Such treatment may include infusing oxytocics and intramyometrial prostaglandins together with attempts at surgical control of the haemorrhage. Early hysterectomy or internal iliac artery ligation can be life-saving in extreme cases.

Specific management of DIC

If DIC is severe enough to cause bleeding or if there is coagulation failure due to massive haemorrhage, replacement of the depleted coagulation components will be necessary.

Fresh frozen plasma (FFP). One unit of FFP contains all the coagulation factors and fibrinogen of one donor unit of blood in approximately 180 ml. It does not contain platelets. Four units is standard therapy; in massive blood loss more will be required. FFP does not require crossmatch, but ABO compatibility is desirable to avoid transfusion of ABO antibodies. FFP is never indicated solely for volume replacement.

Platelet concentrates. One unit of platelet concentrate contains a minimum of 100×10^9 platelets in 50 ml plasma. The standard therapy is to transfuse five or six units. Platelet concentrates do not require crossmatch. They should be transfused as soon as they are received; their viability is greatly reduced by sedimentation and cooling. Platelets do not carry the Rhesus (D) antigen but, because of the possibility of red cell contamination of the concentrate, the administration of Rh(D)-positive platelets to a Rh(D)-negative obstetric patient should be followed by prophylactic injection of anti-D.

Cryoprecipitate. This blood product contains almost all the Factor VIII of one donor unit of blood in 100 ml of plasma and may be useful in the treatment of coagulation failure complicated by severe hypofibrinogenaemia. As with FFP, crycoprecipitate may contain red cells and when necessary should be followed by prophylactic anti-D therapy.

Blood product therapy should be given immediately and rapidly. The DIC screen and platelet count are then repeated to ascertain the response and the need for further therapy.

REFERENCES

Ashe RG, Moodley J, Richards AM & Philpott RH (1987) Comparison of labetalol and dihydralazine in hypertensive emergencies of pregnancy. *South African Medical Journal* **71**: 354-356.

Belfort MA, Anthony J, Saade GR *et al.* (1993) The oxygen consumption/oxygen delivery curve in severe preeclampsia: evidence for a fixed oxygen extraction state. *American Journal of Obstetrics and Gynecology* **163**: 1448-1455.

Clark SL (1990) New concepts of amniotic fluid embolism: a review. *Obstetrical and Gynaecological Survey* **45**: 360-368.

Clark SL, Montz JF & Phelan JP (1985) Hemodynamic alterations associated with amniotic fluid embolism: a reappraisal. *American Journal of Obstetrics and Gynecology* **151**: 617-621.

CLASP (Collaborative Low-dose Aspirin Study in Pregnancy) Collaborative Group (1994) CLASP: a randomised trial of low-dose aspirin for the prevention and treatment of pre-eclampsia among 9364 pregnant women. *Lancet* **343**: 619-629.

Collop NA & Sahn SA (1993) Critical illness in pregnancy. An analysis of 20 patients admitted to a medical intensive care unit. *Chest* **103**: 1548-1552.

Cotton DB, Jones MM, Longmire S, Dorman KF, Tessem J & Joyce TH 3rd (1986) Role of intravenous nitroglycerin in the treatment of severe pregnancy-induced hypertension complicated by pulmonary edema. *American Journal of Obstetrics* **154**: 91-93.

Cotton DB, Longmire S, Jones MM, Dorman KF, Tessem J & Joyce TH 3rd (1986) Cardiovascular alterations in severe pregnancy-induced hypertension: effects of intravenous nitroglycerin coupled with blood volume expansion. *American Journal of Obstetrics and Gynecology* **154**: 1053-1059.

Cotton DB, Gonik B, Dorman K & Harrist R (1985) Cardiovascular alterations in severe pregnancy-induced hypertension: relationship of central venous pressure to pulmonary capillary wedge pressure. *American Journal of Obstetrics and Gynecology* **151**: 762-764.

De Belder A, Lees C, Martin J, Moncada S & Campbell S (1995) Treatment of HELLP syndrome with nitric oxide donor. *Lancet* **345**: 124-125 (letter).

de Boer K, ten Cate JW, Sturk A, Borm JJJ & Treffers PE (1989) Enhanced thrombin generation in normal and hypertensive pregnancy. *American Journal of Obstetrics and Gynecology* **160**: 95-100.

Department of Health (1994) Report on Confidential Enquiries into Maternal Deaths in the United Kingdom 1988-1990. HMSO, London.

de Swiet M (1980) The cardiovascular system. In: Hytten F, Chamberlain G (eds), *Clinical Physiology in Obstetrics*. Oxford, Blackwell Scientific, pp. 3-42.

Dommisse J (1990) Phenytoin sodium and magnesium sulphate in the management of eclampsia. *British Journal of Obstetrics and Gynaecology* **97**: 104-109.

Duncan R, Hadley D, Bone I, Symonds EM, Worthington BS & Rubin PC (1989) Blindness in eclampsia: CT and MR imaging. *Journal of Neurology, Neurosurgery and Pyschiatry* **52**: 899-902.

Fenakel K, Fenakel G, Appelman Z et al. (1991) Nifedipine in the treatment of severe pre-eclampsia. *Obstetrics and Gynaecology* **77**: 331-337.

Finley BE (1989) Acute coagulopathy in pregnancy. *Medical Clinics of North America* **73**: 723-743.

Gillett GB, Watson JD & Langford RM (1984) Ranitidine and single-dose antacid therapy as prophylaxis against acid aspiration syndrome in obstetric practice. *Anaesthesia* **39**: 638-644.

Grieff JMC, Tordorff SG, Griffiths R & May AE (1994) Acid aspiration prophylaxis in 202 obstetric anaesthetic units in the UK. *International Journal of Obstetric Anaesthesia* **3**: 137-142.

Horn EH, Filshie M, Kerslake RW, Jaspan T, Worthington BS & Rubin PC (1990) Widespread cerebral ischaemia treated with nimodipine in a patient with eclampsia. *British Medical Journal* **301**: 794.

Italian Study of Aspirin in Pregnancy (1993) Low dose aspirin in prevention and treatment of intrauterine growth retardation and pregnancy-induced hypertension. *Lancet* **341**: 396- 400.

Jouppila P, Kirkinen P, Koivula A & Ylikorkala O (1986) Labetolol does not alter the placental and fetal blood flow or maternal prostanoids in pre-eclampsia. *British Journal of Obstetrics and Gynaecology* **93**: 543-547.

Karim SMM & Devlin J (1967) Prostaglandin content of amniotic fluid during pregnancy and labour. *Journal of Obstetrics and Gynaecology of the British Commonwealth* **74**: 230-234.

Kilpatrick SJ & Matthay MA (1992) Obstetric patients requiring critical care. A five-year review. *Chest* **101**: 1407-1412.

Koegler A, Sauder P, Marolf A & Jaegar A (1994) Amniotic fluid embolism: a case with non-cardiogenic pulmonary edema. *Intensive Care Medicine* **20**: 45-46.

Letsky EA (1989) Coagulation defects. In de Swiet M. (ed.) *Medical Disorders in Obstetric Practice*. Oxford, Blackwell Scientific Publications, 2nd edn., pp. 104-165.

Lewis LK, Hinshaw DB Jr, Will AD, Hasso AN & Thompson JR (1988) CT and angiographic correlation of severe neurologic disease in toxemia of pregnancy. *Neuroradiology* **30**: 59-64.

Lieberman BA, Stirrat GM, Cohen SL et al. (1978) The possible adverse effect of propanolol on the fetus in pregnancies complicated by severe hypertension. *British Journal of Obstetrics and Gynaecology* **85**: 678-683.

Mabie WC & Sibai BM (1990) Treatment in an obstetric intensive care unit. *American Journal of Obstetrics and Gynecology* **162**: 1-4.

Mabie WC, Gonzalez AR, Sibai BM & Amon E (1987) A comparative trial of labetolol and hydralazine in the acute management of severe hypertension complicating pregnancy. *Obstetrics and Gynecology* **70**: 328-333.

Mabie WC, Ratts TE & Sibai BM (1989) The central hemodynamics of severe preeclampsia. *American Journal of Obstetrics and Gynecology* **161**: 1443-1448.

Malee MP, Malee KM, Azuma SD, Taylor RN & Roberts JM (1992) Increases in plasma atrial natriuretic peptide concentration antedate clinical evidence of preeclampsia. *Journal of Clinical Endocrinology and Metabolism* **74**: 1095-1100.

Masson RG & Ruggieri J (1985) Pulmonary microvascular cytology: a new diagnostic application of the pulmonary artery catheter. *Chest* **88**: 908-914.

Mendelson CL (1946) The aspiration of stomach contents into lungs during obstetric anesthesia. *American Journal of Obstetrics and Gynecology* **52**: 191-205.

Moodley J (1990) Treatment of eclampsia. *British Journal of Obstetrics and Gynaecology* **97**: 99-101.

Plauche WC (1983) Amniotic fluid embolism. *American Journal of Obstetrics and Gynecology* **147**: 982-983.

Pousti TJ, Tominaga GT & Scannell G (1994) Help for the HELLP syndrome. *Intensive Care World* **11**: 62-64.

Pritchard JA, Cunningham FG & Pritchard SA (1984) The Parkland Memorial Hospital protocol for the treatment of eclampsia: evaluation of 245 cases. *American Journal of Obstetrics and Gynecology* **148**: 951-963.

Quinn A & Barrett T (1993) Delayed onset of coagulopathy following amniotic fluid embolism: two case reports. *International Journal of Obstetric Anaesthesia* **2**: 177-180.

Redman CWG (1988) Eclampsia still kills. *British Medical Journal* **296**: 1209-1210.

Redman CWG & Roberts JM (1993) Management of pre-eclampsia. *Lancet* **341**: 1451-1454.

Richards AM, Moodley J, Graham DI & Bullock MR (1986) Active management of the unconscious eclamptic patient. *British Journal of Obstetrics and Gynaecology* **93**: 554-562.

Roberts JM & Redman CWG (1993) Pre-eclampsia: more than pregnancy-induced hypertension. *Lancet* **341**: 1447-1451.

Sibai BM (1990) The HELLP syndrome (hemolysis, elevated liver enzymes, and low platelets): much ado about nothing? *American Journal of Obstetrics and Gynecology* **162**: 311-316.

Sibai BM, Spinnato JA, Watson DL, Lewis JA & Anderson GD (1984) Effect of magnesium sulphate on electroencephalographic findings in preeclampsia–eclampsia. *Obstetrics and Gynecology* **64**: 261-266.

Sibai BM, Gonzalez AR, Mabie WC & Moretti M (1987) A comparison of labetolol plus hospitalization versus hospitalization alone in the management of pre-eclampsia remote from term. *Obstetrics and Gynaecology* **70**: 323-327.

Sibai BM, Mabie WC, Harvey CJ & Gonzalez AR (1987) Pulmonary edema in severe pre-eclampsia–eclampsia: analysis of thirty-seven consecutive cases. *American Journal of Obstetrics and Gynecology* **156**: 1174-1179.

Sibai B, Caritis S, Phillips E *et al.* (1993) Prevention of pre-eclampsia: low-dose aspirin in nulliparous women: a double blind, placebo-controlled trial. *American Journal of Obstetrics and Gynecology* **167**: 286.

Slater RM, Wilcox FL, Smith WD *et al.* (1987) Phenytoin infusion in severe pre-eclampsia. *Lancet* **i**: 1417-1421.

Spargo BH, Lichtig C, Luger AM *et al.* (1976) The renal lesion in preeclampsia. In: Lindheimer MD, Katz AI, Zuspam FP eds. *Hypertension in Pregnancy*. New York, Wiley, pp. 129-137.

Steiner PE & Lushbaugh CC (1941) Maternal pulmonary embolism by amniotic fluid. *Journal of the American Medical Association* **117**: 1340-1345.

Stempel JE, O'Grady JP, Morton MJ & Johnson KA (1982) Use of sodium nitroprusside in complications of gestational hypertension. *Obstetrics and Gynecology* **60**: 533-538.

Tordoff SG & Sweeney BP (1990) Acid aspiration prophylaxis in 288 obstetric anaesthetic departments in the United Kingdom. *Anaesthesia* **45**: 776-780.

Tuffnell D, O'Donovan P, Lilford RJ, Prys-Davies A & Thornton JG (1989) Phenytoin in pre-eclampsia. *Lancet* **ii**: 273-274.

Vanmaele L, Noppen M, Vincken W, De Catte L & Huyghens L (1990) Transient left heart failure in amniotic fluid embolism. *Intensive Care Medicine* **16**: 269-271.

Wallenburg HCS (1988) Hemodynamics in hypertensive pregnancy. In: Rubin PC, (ed.) *Hypertension in Pregnancy. Handbook of Hypertension*, Vol 10. Amsterdam, Elsevier, pp. 66-101.

Weinstein L (1982) Syndrome of hemolysis, elevated liver enzymes and low platelet count: a severe consequence of hypertension in pregnancy. *American Journal of Obstetrics and Gynecology* **142**: 159-167.

Weksler N, Ovadia L, Stav A, Iuchtman M & Ribac L (1994) Continuous arteriovenous haemofiltration in the treatment of amniotic fluid embolism. *International Journal of Obstetric Anaesthesia* **3**: 1-5.

18 Poisoning

More than 100,000 people are admitted to hospital each year in the UK suffering from the effects of acute poisoning, accounting for over 10% of all medical admissions. Although only approximately 15% of poisoning victims require intensive observation and supportive care (with or without active treatment), management of such patients may account for up to one-third of admissions to a multidisciplinary intensive care unit, and in the USA acute self-poisoning accounts for 5-30% of admissions to medical intensive care units.

TYPES OF POISONING

Self-poisoning

The vast majority (about 95%) of adult cases of acute poisoning are self-administered. Most of these are manipulative or represent 'a cry for help' rather than a genuine attempt at suicide and there is often a history of previous similar episodes. The mean age of patients admitted to hospital with an overdose is approximately 25 years, with a female : male ratio of 1.3 : 1, whereas the mean age of successful suicide is about 50 years. In females the peak incidence is in those less than 25 years of age, whereas in males self-poisoning is commonest between the ages of 20 and 35 years.

Accidental poisoning

Accidental poisoning accounts for about 24,000 hospital admissions in England and Wales every year. It is most common in children between 1 and 5 years of age who ingest medicinal, domestic or cosmetic agents. In only about 15% of such cases presenting to a hospital does the child develop symptoms, and fatalities are unusual. Accidental poisoning may also be the result of industrial or agricultural mishaps.

Non-accidental poisoning

Non-accidental poisoning may be related to experimentation with drugs (usually in young adults) or may represent part of the syndrome of child abuse, in which

case poisoning is more often fatal than in accidental cases. Homicidal poisoning is rarely encountered in clinical practice.

Because the hospital mortality of acute poisoning is less than 1%, active measures to hasten the elimination of the poison (which are associated with a significant morbidity and, in some cases, mortality) can only be recommended in a few exceptional instances; indeed, the 'Scandinavian method' of elective supportive care was originally introduced because of the dangers associated with the use of analeptics in patients in barbiturate coma.

Above all else, therefore, the management of acute poisoning involves the application of the principles of *supportive care* detailed elsewhere in this book, including:

- maintenance and protection of the airway;
- respiratory support;
- expansion of the circulating volume;
- maintenance of fluid and electrolyte balance;
- correction of acid–base disturbances;
- occasionally the use of inotropes and/or vasopressors;
- provision of nutritional support;
- control of body temperature;
- skilled nursing care.

DIAGNOSIS AND ASSESSMENT

History

The diagnosis can usually be established from the history, often supported by circumstantial evidence. The quantity and nature of the substances taken must be determined. Currently self-poisoning episodes in the UK most commonly involve the ingestion of benzodiazepines, paracetamol, aspirin, or tricyclic antidepressants. In many cases a mixture of drugs will have been ingested, often including alcohol and a benzodiazepine. Inhalation of car exhaust fumes is the method favoured by men aged between 15 and 44 years. In most cases, a history can be obtained from the patient, although this is frequently misleading and about half will exaggerate or, less often, minimize the severity of poisoning (Wright, 1980). Sometimes patients refuse to divulge any information, while others are incoherent or unconscious. In all cases, therefore, the history should be corroborated by interviewing witnesses such as relatives, friends and ambulancemen, as well as by contacting the general practitioner when appropriate. Bottles, pills or other substances found on or about the patient may provide important clues as to the nature of the poisoning, although they can also be misleading (e.g. drugs may have been stored in incorrectly labelled bottles). Tablets can often be identified using the *Chemist and Druggist Directory*, and in some cases it may be appropriate to send a sample of the substance ingested to the laboratory for analysis. Clear documentation is essential.

Other important aspects of the initial enquiry include a history of previous psychiatric disorders and self-poisoning episodes, as well as evidence of complicating illnesses such as liver or renal disease, which might impair the patient's ability to handle poisons.

Examination

A detailed physical examination should be performed and should include a search for associated injuries (e.g. pressure necrosis) as well as medical conditions that might have precipitated the overdose (e.g. toxic psychosis) or be responsible for coma. When indicated, body temperature should be recorded with a low-reading rectal thermometer. An assessment of the patient's conscious level is particularly important; this should be repeated at regular intervals to follow progress and, in some cases, indicate the need for active intervention. A simple clinical grading of conscious level suitable for use in cases of acute poisoning is shown in **Table 18.1**.

Organic brain damage should be suspected when there is no improvement in the depth of coma within 24 hours, especially when the history of poisoning is dubious. Although the signs and symptoms may suggest intoxication with a specific poison there is in practice often little relationship between the drugs suspected on admission and those detected in the blood.

Investigations (Table 18.2)

When possible, samples of gastric contents (50 ml of vomit, aspirate or first portion of gastric lavage), blood (10 ml lithium–heparinized blood, 10 ml clotted sample, 2 ml of fluorided blood for ethanol assay) and urine (50 ml of the first sample voided after admission) should be obtained for laboratory identification of the poisons involved. Preferably these samples should be collected before the administration of medications, which might complicate toxicological analysis.

Since about 50% of those presenting to the accident and emergency department with coma of unknown cause are suffering from self-poisoning it is often advisable to perform a toxicological screen in all such cases. Automated devices for measuring blood levels of some of the common poisons are now available and can be positioned within, or close to, the intensive care unit. Meticulous maintenance and quality control is, however, essential, and purchase of such a device could only be recommended when the unit admits large numbers of poisoned patients. Assistance is always available from the local poisons information service.

Baseline determinations of haemoglobin concentration, blood sugar, urea and electrolyte levels and liver function tests should be performed in all cases. Blood gas analysis is also routine and may reveal hypercarbia due to respiratory depression or hypoxaemia related to pulmonary pathology such as infection, atelectasis, aspiration or oedema. A chest radiograph should also be obtained.

PRINCIPLES OF MANAGEMENT (Table 18.3)

Immediate management

It is worth reiterating that the majority of patients require only supportive treatment. This should include

---

Table 18.1 Clinical grading of conscious level in acute poisoning.

Grade 0	Fully conscious
Grade I	Drowsy, but responsive to verbal commands
Grade II	Unconscious, but responding to painful stimuli
Grade III	Unconscious, but responding only to maximal painful stimulus
Grade IV	Unconscious, not responding to pain

Table 18.2 Investigations in acute poisoning.

Toxicological analysis
    Gastric contents
    Blood
    Urine

Haemoglobin, white cell count

Blood sugar

Urea, creatinine and electrolytes

Liver function tests

Blood gas analysis

Chest radiograph

Table 18.3 Principles of management of acute poisoning.

Immediate management

Secure and protect airway
Respiratory support
Expand circulating volume
Occasionally inotropes and/or vasopressors
Treat arrhythmias
Pass nasogastric tube
Control seizures

Supportive care

Cardiovascular support
Respiratory support
Renal support
Prevent and treat neurological complications
Skilled nursing care
Physiotherapy

Stress ulcer prophylaxis
Enteral nutrition (rarely parenteral)
Antithrombotic prophylaxis

Control body temperature

Prevent further absorption of poison

Gastric aspiration and lavage
Activated charcoal
Induction of vomiting

Accelerated elimination of poison

Forced diuresis
Haemodialysis and/or haemoperfusion
Treat liver failure

Specific antidotes

immediate life-saving measures and prevention of complications such as hypotension, pulmonary aspiration, acid–base disturbances, fluid and electrolyte imbalances and hypothermia.

Airway

Patients with impaired cough and gag reflexes, as well as those with borderline airway protection who require gastric lavage, will require immediate tracheal intubation to secure their airway and prevent aspiration. All patients should be given supplemental oxygen.

Breathing

Mechanical ventilation should be instituted without delay in those with respiratory depression. Because hypoxia and hypercarbia can exacerbate intracranial hypertension and may cause or potentiate cardiac arrhythmias prompt treatment is essential. Some patients may have developed aspiration or hypostatic pneumonia before admission (see Chapter 6).

Circulation

Acutely poisoned patients are frequently hypotensive, predominantly as a result of peripheral vasodilatation. In most cases blood pressure can be restored by intravascular volume expansion, although occasionally vasopressors will be indicated, and in a few inotropic support may be required to counteract myocardial depression. In young, previously healthy patients invasive monitoring is rarely indicated.

Cardiac arrhythmias are common and may be due to hypoxia, hypercarbia, acid–base disturbances or electrolyte imbalance, as well as the direct effects of the toxin or drug (e.g. tricyclic antidepressants). A 12-lead electrocardiogram (ECG) should be obtained and the ECG should then be continuously monitored. When cardiac arrest does occur it is often resistant to attempts to restore sinus rhythm. It is therefore important to persist with cardiopulmonary resuscitation, especially since fixed dilated pupils may be attributable to the direct effects of the toxin.

Gastrointestinal

Gastric stasis is common in comatose patients and may be exacerbated by the effects of opiates or drugs with anticholinergic properties. A nasogastric tube should therefore be passed to decompress the stomach and reduce the risk of regurgitation.

Neurological

Seizures should be treated urgently with intravenous diazepam in the first instance (see Chapter 14).

Supportive care

As well as continued cardiovascular and respiratory support, subsequent management involves the institution of measures to prevent and treat complications. Intensive nursing care and physiotherapy are essential to prevent the complications of prolonged coma. It is important to document the presence or absence of neuropraxias, corneal abrasions and injury to pressure areas on admission to the intensive care unit.

Gastrointestinal

Stress ulcer prophylaxis should be instituted in the most seriously ill patients (see Chapter 10). Enteral nutrition should be established as soon as possible; if this is not possible parenteral nutrition given peripherally in the first instance should be considered (see Chapter 10).

Neurological

Neurological complications may include:

● coma;
● seizures (related to cerebral hypoxia, metabolic disturbances or the direct effects of the poison);
● cerebral oedema (due to severe hypoxia, cardiac arrest, profound hypotension, severe carbon monoxide (CO) poisoning);
● peripheral nerve injuries (due to prolonged pressure).

The possibility that neurological abnormalities are unrelated to poisoning should be considered when:

● the reduction in conscious level is out of proportion to the severity of poisoning;
● the conscious level fails to improve;
● there are lateralizing signs.

In such cases further investigations, including a cerebral computerized tomographic (CT) scan are warranted to exclude, for example, an intracranial haemorrhage.

Renal

Renal failure may be related to the direct effects of the toxin (e.g. in those poisoned with non-steroidal anti-inflammatory drugs (NSAIDs) or heavy metals), to prolonged hypotension or to sepsis/septic shock (e.g. in patients with pneumonia). *Rhabdomyolysis* is a common cause of renal failure in patients with poisoning and should be suspected in those who have been immobile for a prolonged period before admission, especially when pressure areas are seen to be discoloured with poor capillary refill. It may also be precipitated by prolonged seizures and extreme tissue hypoxia, such as may occur in severe CO poisoning.

A urinary catheter should be inserted in at-risk patients and measures instituted to reverse oliguria and prevent renal failure as outlined in Chapter 12. Those who progress to established renal failure will require artificial blood purification and fluid removal (see Chapter 12).

Liver

Liver failure should be treated as outlined in Chapter 13.

Temperature regulation (see Chapter 19)

Hypothermia is a common complication of prolonged coma outside hospital and is particularly likely in those poisoned with drugs that prevent vasoconstriction and shivering. Usually passive rewarming is sufficient, but occasionally active measures are warranted.

Hyperthermia may complicate intoxication with tricyclic antidepressants, cocaine, amphetamines or ecstasy, and is an important feature of the neuroleptic malignant syndrome. In severe cases, active cooling with sedation, muscle relaxation and mechanical ventilation with unheated gases may be required.

Prevention of further absorption of poison

GASTRIC ASPIRATION AND LAVAGE

When performed in seriously poisoned patients, gastric aspiration and lavage is associated with a considerable risk of complications, including:

● pulmonary aspiration;
● seizures;
● arrhythmias;
● perforation of the stomach.

It should therefore only be undertaken by experienced personnel with the facilities available to treat any complications, and then only if potentially dangerous amounts of a toxic substance have been ingested within about six hours of admission. This time limit can be extended up to 12 hours in cases of poisoning with agents that delay gastric emptying such as salicylates and tricyclic antidepressants. On the other hand, in those who have ingested agents that do not delay gastric emptying and are rapidly absorbed from the gastrointestinal tract (e.g. paracetamol), gastric aspiration and lavage may be ineffective, even when performed within 2–4 hours.

Gastric aspiration and lavage is effective for the majority of solid poisons, but it is debatable whether it should be performed when corrosive substances have been taken. Aspiration of kerosene or its derivatives can produce a particularly destructive form of lipoid pneumonia and the technique should be avoided in such cases.

PROCEDURE

Gastric aspiration and lavage should only be performed if the patient has adequate laryngeal and pharyngeal reflexes or has an endotracheal tube in place with the cuff inflated. The use of an intravenous anaesthetic agent and muscle relaxation to allow tracheal intubation of a semi-comatose patient is only justified when gastric lavage is clearly indicated; in the majority of cases, it is not. The semi-conscious patient should be positioned head down, lying on the left side. Facilities for pharyngeal suction must be immediately available. Foreign matter should be removed from the mouth, and pharynx before introducing a wide-bore tube into the mouth, which the patient is then persuaded to swallow (a large tube is less likely to enter the trachea and allows aspiration of particulate matter). The stomach contents are then aspirated and retained for analysis, following which lavage is performed with 250 ml warmed tap water. This procedure is repeated until the aspirate is clear of debris. Subsequently, the wide-bore tube is replaced by a Ryle's tube, which is aspirated hourly.

ACTIVATED CHARCOAL

Activated charcoal is a powerful non-specific adsorbent that not only irreversibly binds drugs within the gastrointestinal tract, thereby reducing absorption, but also reduces blood levels by creating a negative diffusion gradient between the gut lumen and blood—so called 'gastrointestinal dialysis' (Levy, 1982). Some therefore recommend administration of activated charcoal even when many hours have elapsed since ingestion, and repeated administration has been advocated as a cheap, safe and effective means of reducing drug levels. Others, however, consider that the efficacy of such treatment is relatively unproven and point out that pulmonary aspiration of activated charcoal can have serious consequences (Menzies *et al.*, 1988). There is also a risk of gastrointestinal obstruction and hypernatraemia from the sodium load. Moreover, the value of multiple doses of activated charcoal in acute salicylate poisoning is questionable (Kirshenbaum *et al.*, 1990) and they have not yet been shown to reduce morbidity and mortality. Comparative studies in human volunteers have, however, shown that activated charcoal is more effective than either induced emesis or gastric lavage in reducing drug absorption and on balance it seems to provide a relatively safe and effective means of limiting drug absorption when given soon after ingestion of specific poisons. Activated charcoal may also be effective when given repeatedly to selected cases. *Drugs that are well adsorbed to activated charcoal include*:

● benzodiazepines;

● barbiturates;
● anticonvulsants;
● theophylline;
● antidepressants.

Salicylates and paracetamol are only moderately well adsorbed. Current recommendations are that 50-100 g of activated charcoal should be given to adults who have taken a substantial overdose of a toxic substance no more than 2 hours previously. Severely poisoned adults should also be given 150-200 g via the nasogastric tube over 4-8 hours (Vale & Proudfoot, 1993).

INDUCTION OF VOMITING

Induction of vomiting should only be considered in fully conscious patients and in the knowledge that emesis precludes the subsequent administration of activated charcoal and oral antidotes. Because this technique is less traumatic than gastric lavage for conscious patients it is generally considered to be the preferred means of emptying the stomach in children. It is, however, contraindicated in those poisoned with corrosives, petroleum products or anti-emetics.

Ipecacuanha paediatric emetic draught BP can be administered in a dose of 10 ml in those 6-18 months old and 15 ml in those between 18 months and 5 years of age, followed by 200 ml water. This dose usually induces vomiting in 90-95% of patients within 20-30 minutes, but can be repeated once only if vomiting does not occur after 20-25 minutes. Recovery of stomach contents is, however, generally less than 50%, and there is little evidence that ipecacuanha prevents drug absorption or systemic toxicity (Vale *et al.*, 1986). The decision to induce emesis must be based on a clear history implicating a specific toxin, the estimated dose and the time of ingestion. Apomorphine should be avoided since it may induce protracted vomiting.

Accelerated elimination of poison

Active measures to increase the elimination of a poison are only indicated if the patient is seriously ill and deteriorating, if significant amounts of the poison can be removed and if this is likely to produce worthwhile improvement. In fact fewer than 5% of acutely poisoned patients merit such treatment and it is sensible to *first obtain the advice of a poisons centre*.

FORCED DIURESIS

Forced diuresis is based on the principle that an increase in urine volume will reduce the concentration difference between renal tubular and interstitial fluid, thereby minimizing reabsorption of the poison or its active metabolite(s). The technique is therefore only applicable to cases of poisoning in which either the drug itself or its active metabolites are excreted in the urine in significant amounts. Forced diuresis should only be considered when a toxic agent has been found in the blood in sufficient quantity to cause severe poisoning (Collee & Hanson, 1993). It is ineffective when the poison is strongly protein bound (e.g. tricyclic antidepressants, carbamazepine, phenytoin) and when its volume of distribution is large (e.g. tricyclic antidepressants, lithium, paracetamol). Urinary excretion can be further enhanced by altering the pH of the urine to increase the degree of ionization of the substance and reduce its lipid solubility. Therefore, in the case of weak acids (e.g. salicylates) the urine should be rendered alkaline, while for weak bases an acidic urine is required. Forced acid diuresis is very rarely indicated, but may be considered in severe chlorpromazine poisoning. Suitable regimens are shown in **Table 18.4**.

Forced diuresis is associated with a considerable risk of fluid overload and pulmonary oedema, especially in the elderly and those with renal impairment or heart disease. Cerebral oedema, as well as electrolyte and acid–base disturbances may also occur. It is therefore essential to ensure that a diuresis ensues and to monitor plasma and urinary electrolytes, as well as urine pH. The technique is probably best avoided in those at risk of fluid overload, but if it is considered essential, the volumes infused should be reduced appropriately. The use of mannitol is particularly liable to produce electrolyte disturbances, while acetazolamide can precipitate a metabolic acidosis and frusemide may compete for tubu-

lar secretion of salicylic acid. These diuretics should therefore be avoided, although frusemide may be required to treat pulmonary oedema.

HAEMODIALYSIS AND HAEMOPERFUSION (Cutler et al., 1987)

Haemodialysis and haemoperfusion are of dubious value, but are likely to be most effective when:

- the poison diffuses readily across the dialysis membrane or is avidly taken up by the adsorbent;
- the pharmacological effect of the toxin is closely related to blood levels;
- dialysis or haemoperfusion adds significantly to other routes of drug elimination.

On the other hand, drugs that are highly lipid-soluble and have a large volume of distribution are difficult to eliminate. There is also a danger that if the drug diffuses back into the intravascular compartment more slowly than the rate at which it is being removed, there may be a rebound increase in blood levels when the procedure is discontinued. Large molecules and poisons that are highly protein-bound cannot be cleared efficiently by haemodialysis and in such cases haemoperfusion is preferred.

Haemoperfusion/dialysis may be of value in the management of severe salicylate overdose and poisoning with death cap mushrooms (*Amanita phalloides*). Clearance of alcohol, ethanol, barbiturates, anticonvulsants, benzodiazepines, lithium, cardiac glycosides and many other less-commonly encountered poisons can certainly be enhanced with these techniques, but it is uncertain whether this reduces morbidity or mortality. Moreover, extracorporeal techniques are relatively complex and are associated with a significant risk of complications. Clearance of paracetamol, paraquat and tricyclic antidepressants is not significantly enhanced.

Haemodialysis or haemofiltration may also be considered in those with renal failure or refractory acid-base disturbances. It is occasionally indicated when a patient is deteriorating despite adequate supportive care as a result of poisoning with a dialysable substance. Peritoneal dialysis has no established role in the management of poisoning.

Specific antidotes

An antidote can be defined as any substance that can favourably influence the onset, severity or duration of the toxic effects of a poison (Collee & Hanson, 1993). Only a few specific antidotes are available and some may themselves have toxic effects. They may act by:

Table 18.4 Forced diuresis regimens.

Alkaline diuresis

500 ml sodium bicarbonate 1.26% or 1.4%
1 litre 5% dextrose
500 ml 0.9% saline + potassium chloride 20 mmol

This regimen should be administered for three successive hours.

(Some authorities recommend that this regimen should be repeated until the patient regains consciousness, or in salicylate overdose, until the blood level is reduced to less than 60 mg/100 ml)

Acid diuresis

500 ml 5% dextrose + 1.5 g ammonium chloride
500 ml 5% dextrose
500 ml 0.9% saline

This regimen should be administered at a rate of 1 litre/h and repeated four times over a four-hour period

competing for drug receptor sites (e.g. flumazenil, naloxone);

binding with the toxin to form less toxic chelates that are more easily excreted (e.g. digoxin-specific antibody fragments);

influencing metabolism of a poison to prevent or reduce the formation of harmful metabolites (e.g. acetylcysteine in paracetamol overdose).

The use of specific antagonists such as naloxone and flumazenil to reverse central nervous system (CNS) depression is controversial and is discussed later in this chapter. Analeptics should never be used.

MANAGEMENT OF SPECIFIC POISONS

Barbiturates

There has been a considerable reduction in the availability of these drugs, which should now only be prescribed as anticonvulsants, and as a result there has been a marked decrease in the incidence of barbiturate overdose.

CLINICAL FEATURES

Barbiturate overdose produces *generalized depression of the CNS*. The conscious level is reduced and this may progress to deep coma with flaccidity and hyporeflexia. The corneal reflex is often absent. The pupillary response to light is sluggish or absent and conjugate eye movement is lost. Unequal pupils suggest hypoxic cerebral damage and this possibility is supported by the presence of other focal neurological signs, which may sometimes be accompanied by seizures.

Profound cardiovascular depression may occur and is caused by a reduction in central vasomotor activity, a decrease in arteriolar tone and myocardial depression. Cardiac output and blood pressure are low, while central venous pressure (CVP) may be high (in those with myocardial failure) or low (in the presence of relative hypovolaemia). There may be a metabolic acidosis.

Respiratory depression causes hypoventilation with hypercarbia and hypoxaemia. The latter may be exacerbated by increased capillary permeability leading to the development of adult respiratory distress syndrome (ARDS) (see Chapter 6) and/or ventilation/perfusion mismatch (Sutherland *et al.*, 1977).

The reduction in muscle tone combined with cardiovascular depression causes *vascular stasis and tissue hypoxia*. Ischaemic muscle damage may lead to rhabdomyolysis, which may in the long term be followed by muscle calcification. Local hypoxia may also be re-

sponsible for the development of skin blisters, which are seen in approximately 5% of patients with barbiturate poisoning. Although these blisters often develop over pressure areas, they are not necessarily related to trauma and may occasionally complicate even a relatively trivial overdose.

Gastrointestinal motility is often depressed. It is thought that the fluctuations in conscious level that sometimes occur in barbiturate poisoning are due to the intermittent recovery of intestinal function leading to further absorption of the drug.

Hypothermia is a common complication of barbiturate overdose and is a result of impaired hypothalamic function, the reduction in muscle tone and vascular dilatation.

TREATMENT

The vast majority of those who reach hospital alive will survive with *aggressive supportive care*, provided they have not suffered irreversible cerebral damage. CVP monitoring and, in some cases, pulmonary artery catheterization, is required in seriously poisoned patients to guide intravenous volume replacement. Hypothermia must be prevented or treated (see Chapter 19).

Because prolonged coma may be complicated by pneumonia, some authorities recommend charcoal or resin haemoperfusion in those who are deeply unconscious and failing to improve following a massive overdose of a long-acting barbiturate. This technique is, however, most effective for medium- and short-acting agents and its value in the management of poisoning is disputed (Lorch & Garella, 1979). The possible benefits of a reduction in the duration of coma must be offset against the complications of the technique and it should be remembered that many patients will have taken a variety of toxins.

Tricyclic antidepressants

Tricyclic antidepressants are extensively prescribed for an 'at-risk' population of depressed patients. Furthermore, improvement in mood is often delayed for up to two weeks after the start of treatment. Consequently, acute poisoning with tricyclic antidepressants is common and the incidence is increasing.

CLINICAL FEATURES

The features of tricyclic antidepressant overdose are due to a mixture of *central excitation and depression* combined with *anticholinergic effects*. Although the conscious level may be decreased, coma is rare. Both pyramidal and extrapyramidal disturbances may occur and convulsions are common. Some patients hallucinate, and rapid distorted speech is characteristic. Respiration is frequently depressed. *Anticholinergic effects* are manifested as:

- widely dilated pupils;
- dry mouth;
- absent sweating;
- urine retention;
- paralytic ileus.

The combination of central depression and an inability to sweat impairs temperature regulation and may lead to *hyperthermia*. Examination may reveal hyperreflexia and extensor plantar responses. The diagnosis can be confirmed by detecting the drug in the urine.

The *cardiovascular effects* of tricyclic antidepressants are complex. Sinus tachycardia is common and both hyper- and hypotension may occur. Terminally, hypotension may become refractory, culminating in electromechanical dissociation (EMD). The ECG changes include a dose-related prolongation of the Q–T interval, widening of the QRS complex, AV block, and intraventricular conduction disturbances; right bundle branch block is characteristic. When the QRS complex is longer than 0.1 secs convulsions are likely, and when it is prolonged to more than 0.16 secs there is a considerable risk of ventricular arrhythmias (Boehnert & Lovejoy, 1985). Although in one case death occurred 5 days after the overdose (Masters, 1967), a review of 72 consecutive cases of tricyclic antidepressant overdose suggested that late unexpected complications are very rare and a 2-day period of intensive observation is probably sufficient (Stern *et al.*, 1985).

TREATMENT

Because stomach emptying may be delayed following an overdose of tricyclic antidepressants, *gastric aspiration and lavage* may be worthwhile up to 12 hours after ingestion. Active measures to hasten elimination of tricyclic antidepressants are, however, ineffective because these drugs are highly lipid-soluble, they are strongly protein-bound and only small amounts are excreted in the urine. Management is therefore supportive.

The ECG should be monitored continuously for 48–72 hours following a serious overdose. It has been recommended that all patients with respiratory depression, twitching or cardiac arrhythmias should be intubated and mechanically ventilated (Collee & Hanson, 1993). In this way hypercarbia and hypoxia, which may precipitate cardiac arrhythmias, and acidosis (respiratory or metabolic), which enhances cardiotoxicity, can be avoided. Also tracheal intubation secures the airway, thereby allowing the safe use of anticonvulsants such as benzodiazepines. Provided the patient is well oxygenated and the pH is maintained above 7.4 cardiac arrhythmias usually resolve. If hyperventilation alone fails to raise the pH above this level it has been suggested that small (50 mmol) doses of bicarbonate should be given.

If ventricular arrhythmias do occur, they may be resistant to conventional treatment, although some claim that they have experienced no difficulty in defibrillating such patients and that the subsequent infusion of lignocaine successfully prevents recurrence. A prophylactic intravenous infusion of lignocaine is also recommended for those with ventricular ectopics. Phenytoin may be useful since it can control both the ventricular arrhythmias and any accompanying convulsions, although it is a negative inotrope and as such could precipitate EMD.

Although it might seem logical to administer an anticholinesterase such as physostigmine, this is unwise in the acute phase since such treatment may precipitate seizures, bradycardia and cardiac failure. Similarly, administration of a β-blocker may cause extreme bradycardia and even asystole. Although a DC shock can be used when clearly indicated, there is a risk of precipitating asystole or EMD.

A few patients may be hypotensive in the absence of arrhythmias, but expansion of the circulating volume will usually restore the blood pressure. Inotropes should in general be avoided because of the danger of precipitating arrhythmias. If inotropic support is required, dobutamine is a suitable agent. Pulmonary artery catheterization should be avoided because of the risk of precipitating arrhythmias.

Cardiac toxicity generally resolves quite rapidly, within about 6 hours, and mechanical ventilation for convulsions is rarely required for more than 24 hours.

Extrapyramidal symptoms can be controlled with benztropine 1–2 mg intramuscularly or intravenously, while the agitation and convulsions that may occur during the recovery phase are best treated with intravenous diazepam.

Paracetamol

The incidence of poisoning with paracetamol has gradually increased over the last 20 years and this is now one of the commonest causes of fulminant hepatic failure (FHF) (see Chapter 13).

CLINICAL FEATURES

Patients who have taken a paracetamol overdose normally *remain fully conscious*. Clinical features may include pallor, perspiration, epigastric pain, nausea and vomiting. Occasionally, a massive paracetamol overdose may directly damage the myocardium and cause peripheral vasodilatation with *shock*. Metabolic acidosis may be severe. *Erythema, urticaria and mucosal lesions* are quite common. *Hyperglycaemia* may occur a few days after ingestion. Acute *haemolytic anaemia* may develop and produce *acute renal failure*.

These symptoms are not, however, a reliable indication of the severity of poisoning and there is a wide individual variability in tolerance to paracetamol, as well as susceptibility to *hepatotoxicity*. When liver damage does occur, the signs of hepatic failure are not usually apparent until 48 hours after the overdose. At this time, the patient may become jaundiced with an enlarged and tender liver. Liver function tests are most abnormal 3–5 days after ingestion. In severe, but non-fatal hepatotoxicity a cholestatic picture is usually seen, and in the most serious cases FHF develops about 3–7 days after ingestion.

MECHANISMS OF HEPATOTOXICITY

Paracetamol hepatotoxicity is due to a toxic metabolite, which is formed via an oxidative pathway dependent on cytochrome P450 and is normally scavenged by intracellular glutathione. Following an overdose, this mechanism may be overwhelmed and the highly reactive metabolite combines with sulphydryl groups of liver cell proteins, producing a centrilobular necrosis. Increased intracellular concentrations of calcium appear to play an important role in causing cellular injury.

Paracetamol-induced liver damage is likely to be more severe in patients exposed to hepatic enzyme-inducing agents such as barbiturates or alcohol. In patients with chronic alcoholism, however, increased susceptibility to paracetamol poisoning is probably related to decreased plasma and liver concentrations of glutathione, rather than enzyme induction.

INVESTIGATIONS

Plasma levels of paracetamol must be determined in any patient suspected of being poisoned with this agent and, when related to the time since ingestion, they correlate closely with the subsequent risk of liver damage. Therefore, in the absence of treatment, a level of more than 250 µg/ml at four hours or more than 100 µg/ml at 12 hours is usually hepatotoxic (Prescott *et al.*, 1976) (**Fig. 18.1**), while a level less than 100 µg/ml at four hours excludes the risk of liver damage. It is worth noting that large overdoses of paracetamol can triple its plasma half-life from 2.4 to 7.3 hours.

Laboratory investigations should include:

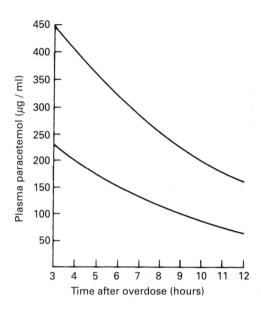

Fig. 18.1 Plasma paracetamol concentrations related to time since ingestion. Liver damage is likely to be severe above the upper line, severe to mild between the lines and clinically insignificant below the lower line. From Prescott *et al.* (1976), with permission.

- urea and electrolytes;
- coagulation studies;
- blood sugar level;
- liver function tests.

Blood glucose levels should be determined hourly.

TREATMENT

Gastric lavage is recommended if the patient is seen within 4 hours of ingestion, but the value of activated charcoal is unclear. Intravenous glucose should be administered to provide a total of 300 g daily. Renal replacement therapy may be required. Preventive treatment is based on the principle that by providing an alternative supply of sulphydryl groups, unstable precursors can be displaced from either glutathione or liver cell protein. A variety of agents have been recommended including cysteamine, methionine and *N*-acetylcysteine.

Cysteamine (2 g intravenously over 10 minutes, followed by three further 400 mg doses) is effective if given within 12 hours of ingestion, but can cause cutaneous vasodilatation, nausea, vomiting and drowsiness, which may last for up to 48 hours.

The side-effects of *oral methionine* are similar to those associated with cysteamine, but this agent (2.5 mg immediately followed by three further doses at four-hourly intervals) may be used in those who present within four hours of ingestion.

N-acetylcysteine, which repletes gluthathione stores is equally effective, but less toxic, and is now the treatment of choice. This agent should be given in a dose of 150 mg/kg intravenously over 15 minutes, followed by 50 mg/kg in 500 ml 5% dextrose over four hours and then 100 mg/kg in one litre of 5% dextrose over 16 hours.

Currently it is recommended that N-acetylcysteine is given to all patients who present within eight hours of ingesting more than 7 g of paracetamol and if the plasma concentration is above the lower line in **Fig. 18.1**. Treatment is still indicated at least as late as 24 hours after ingestion (Smilkstein *et al.*, 1988) and there is now evidence to suggest that acetylcysteine can improve outcome even when administered after the onset of paracetamol-induced FHF, possibly by improving oxygen delivery (D_{O_2}) and oxygen consumption ($\dot{V}_{O_2}$) and limiting the extent of vital organ dysfunction (Keays *et al.*, 1991) (see also Chapter 13). N-acetylcysteine is also a potent antioxidant and this may partly underlie its protective effect in paracetamol overdose. Very occasionally N-acetylcysteine may precipitate a histamine-mediated reaction.

Referral to a centre specializing in the management of paracetamol intoxication should be considered when:

- pH is less than 7.3 more than 24 hours after ingestion;
- prothrombin time is longer than 45 seconds at 48 hours, or longer than 50 seconds at 72 hours;
- creatinine concentration is increasing;
- there is rapid development of grade II encephalopathy.

Liver transplantation may be considered when:

- pH is less than 7.3;
- prothrombin time is longer than 100 seconds;
- serum creatinine is higher than 300 μmol/l;
- there is grade III or IV coma;

Salicylates

The increased use of paracetamol as a mild analgesic has resulted in some reduction in the incidence of salicylate poisoning. Nevertheless, it remains a relatively common cause of poisoning in children. Many readily available salicylate preparations do not mention that they contain aspirin. Oil of wintergreen, for example, contains methylsalicylate and is highly toxic.

MECHANISMS OF TOXICITY

Aspirin is normally deacetylated by plasma esterases and is eliminated by conjugation. Following intoxication, however, the conjugation pathway is saturated, free salicylate has to be eliminated via the kidneys and excretion is prolonged.

Aspirin uncouples oxidative phosphorylation, leading to increased metabolism of glucose and fats with a rise in $\dot{V}_{O_2}$ and carbon dioxide production. The respiratory centre is stimulated both directly and by the increased carbon dioxide production, thereby producing respiratory alkalosis. If salicylate levels are very high, however, respiratory depression may supervene. Blood levels of pyruvate, lactate and ketone bodies are increased and this, combined with the fact that aspirin is itself an organic acid, produces a metabolic acidosis.

CLINICAL FEATURES

The majority of patients present within six hours of ingestion and are conscious, alert and orientated, although some are *restless*, *irritable* and *confused*. *Hallucinations* may occur. Coma is rare and, in an adult, drowsiness indicates severe poisoning. Confusion and drowsiness are more frequently seen in children.

Other clinical features include:

- sweating;
- tinnitus and deafness;
- blurred vision;
- tachycardia;
- pyrexia;
- hyperventilation.

Initially there is a respiratory alkalosis, although in severe cases respiratory acidosis may occur as a terminal event, whilst in children a *metabolic acidosis* can develop rapidly and usually becomes the dominant abnormality.

Less commonly, patients poisoned with aspirin have *epigastric pain* and *vomiting* with *severe dehydration* and *oliguria*. Occasionally, they may develop acute renal failure. Gastrointestinal bleeding is uncommon, but may be related to *gastric erosions* and a *coagulopathy*. The latter is usually due to hypoprothrombinaemia, which can be corrected with fresh frozen plasma and vitamin K, but may also be due to thrombocytopenia, decreased production of factor VII or impaired platelet function.

In some cases, *pulmonary oedema* develops in association with an increase in capillary permeability, proteinuria and hypoproteinaemia. These patients may also be hypotensive and hypovolaemic; cautious administration of colloidal solutions has been recommended (Hormaechea *et al.*, 1979). Left ventricular failure may also occur secondary to cardiac arrhythmias, hypokalaemia or fluid overload.

Salicylate poisoning may also be associated with hypokalaemia, hyperglycaemia or hypoglycaemia; the latter may be particularly severe in children. Some patients develop an *encephalopathy* and *hyperthermia*.

INVESTIGATIONS

Investigations should include:

- blood gas and acid–base analysis;
- urea and electrolytes;
- coagulation studies;
- blood glucose.

In severe poisoning, protein and calcium levels should be determined and liver function tests should be performed.

The diagnosis should be confirmed, and the severity of poisoning assessed, by measuring *plasma salicylate levels*. This should be related to the time of ingestion, bearing in mind that absorption of aspirin continues for some time and peak levels may not be attained for up to eight hours. Therefore, a level of 300 mg/l may be significant 12 hours after ingestion, but is almost within the therapeutic range at 4–6 hours. Active treatment should be considered if the level is more than 500 mg/l within 12 hours of ingestion, and if it is over 300 mg/l beyond this time. In children, measures to hasten elimination are indicated when the level is more than 300 mg/l at 12 hours. Respiratory depression is a common mode of death when the plasma salicylate level exceeds 1000 mg/l.

TREATMENT

Gastric aspiration and lavage should be performed if the patient presents within 24 hours of ingestion. *Activated charcoal* should be administered in repeated doses via the nasogastric tube (although see comments earlier in this chapter).

When active treatment is indicated, it should be instituted immediately, since death can occur suddenly and unexpectedly. The clearance of salicylates is pH-dependent, increasing ten-fold when blood pH rises from 6.0 to 7.5, and excretion can therefore be enhanced by *forced alkaline diuresis* (see **Table 18.4**), which will also replace water and electrolyte losses and help to maintain blood sugar levels if 5% dextrose is used. Before promoting an alkaline diuresis, the intravascular volume must be replenished and any significant metabolic acidosis should be corrected. In selected cases, pulmonary artery catheterization may be indicated to guide volume replacement and avoid fluid overload. Other dangers of forced alkaline diuresis include hypernatraemia, hypokalaemia and metabolic acidosis.

Salicylate levels should be measured two hours after commencing a forced diuresis. If a moderate salicylate level has increased to within the dangerous range or if a severe level has failed to decrease, *haemodialysis* is indicated. If the salicylate level has fallen, however, treatment should be continued.

Opiates

Opiate poisoning is usually encountered in drug abusers who have taken an overdose, either intentionally or accidentally. Overdose may also occur with inexperienced users, when there has been a change in the purity of the supplied drug or when loss of tolerance has occurred during a period of abstinence. Drug couriers who swallow opiates in containers (e.g. a condom or plastic bag) may develop severe toxicity if the package leaks. An abdominal radiograph often reveals the package, which may require surgical removal. Occasionally, iatrogenic cases require admission to intensive care.

CLINICAL FEATURES

The triad of *coma, respiratory depression* (infrequent deep respirations) and *pinpoint pupils* (which are equal and reactive) is virtually diagnostic of opiate poisoning. *Cardiovascular depression* also occurs.

Physical examination may reveal *evidence of addiction* such as venepuncture scars, or the complications of intravenous drug abuse such as hepatitis and sepsis. Acute heroin intoxication can be complicated by *non-cardiogenic pulmonary oedema*, which may be related to hypoxia, hypersensitivity to the heroin or a contaminant, or to a direct toxic effect. Profound sedation may be associated with muscular compression which, especially when aggravated by hypoxia, acidosis and hypovolaemia, can precipitate *rhabdomyolysis*.

Death is usually due to respiratory depression, often combined with *pulmonary aspiration*.

TREATMENT

Coma and respiratory depression can be reversed by intravenous *naloxone* 0.1–0.8 mg intravenously or intramuscularly (in children 5–10 μg/kg). Because the half-life of naloxone is short (opiate reversal persists for only 15–30 minutes), repeated doses or an infusion are usually required. Naloxone can precipitate an acute withdrawal syndrome in addicts and may cause laryngeal spasm. In addition, a number of adverse reactions to naloxone have been described, including ventricular fibrillation, hypertension and pulmonary oedema. These are presumably related to disinhibition of the sympathetic nervous system. Caution is therefore required in those with known cardiovascular disease and in the authors' opinion it is safer to intubate the trachea and institute mechanical ventilation until the opiate effects have resolved spontaneously. Non-cardiogenic pulmonary oedema usually responds rapidly to intermittent positive pressure ventilation (IPPV) with positive end-expiratory pressure (PEEP).

Benzodiazepines

MECHANISMS

Many of the effects of benzodiazepines are mediated by occupation of specific receptor sites, thereby enhancing the effects of γ-aminobutyric acid (GABA), an inhibitory neurotransmitter.

CLINICAL FEATURES

When taken alone, benzodiazepines can produce *drowsiness, dizziness, ataxia* and *slurred speech*. More serious manifestations of overdose such as *coma* or *hypotension* are rarely seen and death due to isolated benzodiazepine poisoning, which is usually related to *respiratory depression* and *pulmonary aspiration*, is unusual. Many cases of self-poisoning, however, involve ingestion of a number of drugs, and benzodiazepines are included in as many as 40% of overdoses in the UK. Under these circumstances the clinical picture is often confusing and additive effects may aggravate or precipitate respiratory failure and hypotension.

Benzodiazepines are absorbed relatively slowly from the gastrointestinal tract and elimination of their active metabolites, as well as the parent compound, may take several days. In general, less than 5% of the ingested dose is recovered unchanged in the urine. Hospital stay may therefore be prolonged and the performance of skilled tasks (e.g. driving a car or operating machinery) can be impaired for weeks after apparent recovery from benzodiazepine poisoning.

TREATMENT

In general, management of benzodiazepine poisoning involves *supportive care* only. Although benzodiazepine antagonists (e.g. *flumazenil*) are now available that can effectively reverse coma in such cases (Ashton, 1985), their value is uncertain. It has been suggested that following isolated benzodiazepine overdose, they might speed recovery, reduce after-effects and shorten hospital stay, while in multiple self-poisoning they could reverse respiratory depression and facilitate diagnosis. Flumazenil can be given in aliquots of 0.1 mg to a total dose of 1.0 mg and has a rapid onset of action in less than a minute, with a maximal effect at five minutes. Because it has a relatively short half-life (54 minutes), repeated administration or a continuous infusion at 0.1–0.4 mg/h is usually required. Moreover, there is a danger of precipitating acute withdrawal symptoms. Convulsions may be produced, especially in epileptics and in the presence of proconvulsant agents such as tricyclic antidepressants, and rapid reversal may also precipitate

ventricular fibrillation. Many therefore now believe that flumazenil has no place in the management of benzodiazepine overdose (Collee & Hanson, 1993). Others, however, have shown flumazenil to be a safe aid to diagnosis in cases of multiple drug overdose and have claimed that this agent reduces the requirement for interventions such as gastric lavage, tracheal intubation, mechanical ventilation and CT scan of the brain (Höjer *et al.*, 1990).

Paraquat (Editorial, 1976)

Paraquat is a herbicide that is available commercially as a 20% solution (Gramoxone) and to the general public in the form of solid granules containing 2.5% paraquat and diquat (Weedol, Pathclear). Although measures instituted by the manufacturers have reduced the incidence of accidental poisoning with paraquat, this has been largely offset by an increase in the number of cases of deliberate overdose.

CLINICAL FEATURES

Paraquat is a *strong corrosive* that will burn the skin, tongue, mouth and oesophagus. This may not be apparent until 24–48 hours after ingestion when large white necrotic areas develop; these are often painless. If paraquat contaminates the eyes it will cause extreme irritation with ulceration of the conjunctivae and cornea. *Sweating, nausea* and *repeated vomiting* are usual, and in some cases the vomitus will contain gastric and oesophageal epithelial cells. *Tremor* and *convulsions* may occur.

Ingestion of large amounts of paraquat may be associated with *encephalopathy, myocarditis, liver damage, renal failure* and *haemorrhagic pulmonary oedema*. In such cases death usually occurs within 72 hours. When poisoning is less severe, evidence of myocardial, liver and renal dysfunction may be delayed for several days. Paraquat can, however, accumulate progressively in the lungs by an energy-dependent process (Rose *et al.*, 1974) even when plasma concentrations are relatively low. Subsequently, the alveolar epithelial lining is destroyed and this is followed by *progressive pulmonary fibrosis* culminating in hypoxaemic respiratory failure. Although this lung lesion may take 2–3 weeks to develop, it is irreversible and death is inevitable.

INVESTIGATIONS

The diagnosis of paraquat poisoning can be confirmed by examining the urine. Moreover, there is a good correlation between blood levels and the severity of poisoning.

TREATMENT

Gastric aspiration and lavage should be performed, followed by oral administration of *Fuller's earth*, 300 ml of a 30% suspension containing 30 g of Fuller's earth and 15 g of magnesium sulphate. This should be repeated after 2 and 4 hours. Fuller's earth is unpleasant to take and may have to be given via a nasogastric tube. These measures should be followed by aggressive supportive care since the hepatic lesion, renal failure and pulmonary oedema are all potentially reversible. Unduly high concentrations of oxygen should be avoided since this may accentuate the lung damage.

PROGNOSIS

An oral dose of approximately 2–3 g is likely to be fatal if untreated, and although as many as 90% of those who ingest Weedol survive, the mortality from poisoning with the concentrated solution is approximately 90%.

Cholinesterase inhibitors (organophosphorus compounds and carbamate insecticides)

MECHANISMS

Most of the organophosphorus compounds are highly lipid-soluble and are therefore well absorbed via all routes, including the skin. They also form very stable links with acetylcholinesterase. Recovery of anticholinergic activity is therefore delayed until sufficient quantities of enzyme have been manufactured. This may take days or even months. Carbamates, on the other hand, undergo spontaneous degradation and symptoms of poisoning with these substances last only 6–8 hours.

CLINICAL FEATURES

Poisoning with cholinesterase inhibitors causes:

- an increase in postganglionic parasympathetic nervous activity;
- muscle fasciculation followed by paralysis;
- central nervous stimulation followed by depression.

There is *anorexia, vomiting, abdominal colic* and *diarrhoea*. The patient is *restless* with *constricted pupils*; *coma* and *convulsions* may occur. Later, *respir-atory depression* supervenes with *paralysis of respiratory muscles, laryngobronchospasm*, increased *tracheobronchial secretions* and *excessive salivation*. Cardiovascular manifestations include *bradycardia* and *hypotension*.

TREATMENT

Immediate management must include measures to *prevent further exposure* to the poison, including the removal of contaminated clothing and thorough washing (initially with soap and water and then with ethanol). Those poisoned with an organophosphorus compound should receive *pralidoxime* (5 ml of a 20% solution) to break down the organophosphorus–cholinesterase complex. This should not be used in carbamate poisoning. *Atropine* should be administered in large doses for 2–3 days. Otherwise, treatment is *supportive* and may include mechanical ventilation.

Ethanol

CLINICAL FEATURES

Ethanol poisoning is usually simply related to overindulgence. In large quantities, ethanol can produce a deep, but short-lived *coma*, which may be complicated by *hypothermia* and, in a few cases, *hypoglycaemia*. Children may develop severe hypoglycaemia and a *metabolic acidosis*. The fatal dose is difficult to determine, but it is thought that in adults the equivalent of 600 ml pure ethanol consumed in less than 1 hour can be lethal.

TREATMENT

Treatment consists of *gastric aspiration and lavage* and, in severe cases, 200 g of *fructose* 40% infused over 30 minutes to correct hypoglycaemia and increase the rate of fall in blood alcohol levels. Some recommend *naloxone* administration to lighten coma.

Methanol

Acute methanol poisoning occurs most frequently in vagrants, although cases of accidental ingestion are occasionally encountered. Methanol is a constituent of antifreeze, paint removers and varnish and is produced in some home-made beverages. Methylated spirit, however, is composed largely of ethanol with only 5% methanol. Methanol is metabolized to formic acid and formaldehyde, both of which are extremely toxic.

CLINICAL FEATURES

The central effects of acute methanol intoxication may be delayed for 12–36 hours after ingestion at which time *nausea, vomiting, abdominal pain, headache* and *ataxia* can occur and may progress to *coma*. Often, there is a *profound metabolic acidosis* with Kussmaul respiration. If poisoning is severe (blood methanol > 500 mg/l, marked acidosis), the patient may develop an *acute optic nerve papillitis* with blurring of vision that can progress to blindness, dilatation of the pupils and papilloedema.

TREATMENT

Gastric aspiration and lavage should be performed if the patient is seen within four hours of ingestion and the *metabolic acidosis should be corrected*. Because *ethanol* competes with methanol for the enzyme alcohol dehydrogenase, administration of the former can limit the production of formic acid. *Haemodialysis* has been recommended if the patient fails to respond to these measures and has visual impairment, a severe metabolic acidosis or a blood methanol level greater than 1 g/l. There is no evidence, however, that dialysis is more effective than standard measures.

Cyanide

Cyanides are used industrially in electroplating and to clean or harden metals as well as in some chemical laboratories. Most cases of poisoning encountered in clinical practice are caused by ingestion or inhalation of sodium or potassium cyanide; free hydrocyanic acid (prussic acid) is almost instantaneously fatal if taken orally. The effects of inhaled prussic acid depend on the concentration of the vapour. The direct-acting vasodilator sodium nitroprusside is a complex cyanide that releases free hydrogen cyanide (HCN) *in vivo* and may produce related toxic effects when a gross overdose has been administered (see Chapter 4).

MECHANISMS

Cyanide produces its toxic effects by reacting with cytochrome oxidase, thereby inhibiting the final steps in oxidative phosphorylation.

CLINICAL FEATURES

If large quantities (1–2 g) are ingested, there is a rapid *loss of consciousness*, followed by *convulsions* and *death*. Lesser amounts produce *drowsiness, dizziness, breathlessness, confusion, nausea, vomiting* and *shock*. Coma and death may follow. *Severe lactic acidosis* and a *reduced* $C_{A-v}O_2$ are characteristic. Some are able to detect an odour of bitter almonds. Expired air resuscitation must *not* be given.

TREATMENT

When a patient is known to have ingested or inhaled cyanide, immediate treatment is imperative. A heparinized blood sample should be obtained for blood gas analysis and cyanide assay. General supportive measures including the administration of oxygen in high concentrations should be instituted and a specific antidote given. Immediately following massive exposure to cyanide (e.g. following an industrial accident) *intravenous dicobalt edetate* (CoEDTA) (300–600 mg over one minute, followed by a further 300 mg if the patient fails to improve) is the ideal antidote since it has a rapid action and although it is itself toxic, in the presence of HCN it forms a stable non-toxic complex. If the patient remains conscious some hours after assumed exposure to cyanide, CoEDTA should not be given since in the absence of HCN it is likely to produce an anaphylactic reaction, sometimes with severe laryngeal oedema. It may also precipitate atrial fibrillation, hypocalcaemia and hypomagnesaemia. Because CoEDTA can cause hypoglycaemia, it should be given in dextrose. Therefore, when some time has elapsed between ingestion and arrival in hospital or when there is doubt as to the nature of the poisoning, *sodium thiosulphate*, which converts cyanide to thiocyanate, is the antidote of choice. It should be given as a loading dose of 150 mg/kg intravenously followed by an infusion at a rate of 30–60 mg/kg/h.

Some consider that the administration of a *nitrite* (e.g. amyl nitrite or sodium nitrite) is a useful adjunct to thiosulphate in acute cyanide poisoning. These agents act by converting haemoglobin to methaemoglobin, the ferric iron of which then combines with HCN. Sodium nitrite (3%) should be given intravenously in divided 10 ml doses in order to convert approximately 25% of the haemoglobin to methaemoglobin; it is more effective than amyl nitrite. However, this clearly reduces the amount of haemoglobin available for oxygen transport and is particularly hazardous in children. In addition, nitrites can precipitate or exacerbate hypotension.

Iron

Iron tablets are most frequently prescribed to young women and they, or their children, therefore account for the majority of cases of poisoning.

CLINICAL FEATURES

Initially, most are asymptomatic, although a few develop an *acute gastritis* with abdominal pain, nausea, vomiting, haematemesis, melaena and *gastric perforation*. Some complain of a *metallic taste*. Those who are seriously poisoned become *hypovolaemic* and *shocked* 6-12 hours after ingestion. *Convulsions, coma, hepatic necrosis* and a *metabolic acidosis* may supervene approximately 24 hours later.

TREATMENT

Iron is slowly absorbed. *Gastric aspiration and lavage* should be performed and 10 g of *desferrioxamine*, which chelates iron, instilled into the stomach.

The severity of poisoning can be assessed by measuring the serum iron level, and if this is more than twice the upper limit of normal, 1-2 g of desferrioxamine should be administered intramuscularly and repeated 3-12 hours later. If the patient is shocked, this agent should be given intravenously (15 mg/kg/h up to a total dose of 80 mg/kg in 24 hours).

Digoxin

Digoxin has a narrow therapeutic index and is therefore particularly liable to produce life-threatening complications after accidental or deliberate overdose. Serious overdoses are frequently fatal, mortality being around 18% following ingestion of 15 mg digoxin and approximately 95% when more than 35 mg are taken. Digoxin may produce toxic effects when plasma levels exceed 2.5 μg/l, but serious problems are unusual at levels less than 10 μg/l. In general, however, plasma levels do not correlate closely with the severity of poisoning.

MECHANISMS

Digoxin overdose is associated with hyperkalaemia due to inhibition of Na^+/K^+ ATPase, the extent of the rise in plasma potassium being correlated with the clinical course.

CLINICAL FEATURES

Nausea and vomiting are constant features, while *diarrhoea* is less common. There may be *anorexia* and *abdominal pain*.

Cardiac toxicity may be associated with:

- bradycardia;
- varying degrees of atrioventricular block;
- supraventricular arrhythmias (with or without heart block);
- less commonly, ventricular arrhythmias including ventricular tachycardia/ventricular fibrillation.

Other features of toxicity may include extreme *fatigue, weakness* and *visual disturbances*, often with abnormal red–green colour perception. Some patients complain of *headaches, dizziness* and *abnormal dreams*.

MANAGEMENT

Gastric lavage, when indicated, should only be performed with extreme care because of the risk that increased vagal tone will precipitate cardiac arrest. Tissue stores of cardiac glycosides are large; measures to enhance their elimination such as forced diuresis, haemodialysis or haemoperfusion are therefore generally ineffective and the risks outweigh the benefits.

Bradycardia should be treated with atropine or transvenous pacing. Infusion of catecholamines should be avoided.

Hypokalaemia, which is most likely in those receiving chronic diuretic therapy, should be corrected.

Hyperkalaemia may be treated with intravenous dextrose and insulin (see Chapter 12), but inhibition of Na^+/K^+ ATPase may limit its efficacy.

The agents of choice for the treatment of *ventricular arrhythmias* are phenytoin and lignocaine. Quinidine and procainamide are less effective and may potentiate atrioventricular block. β-blockers should be avoided. The role of other anti-arrhythmic agents such as verapamil is unclear.

Severe digitalis intoxication should be treated with *digoxin-specific antibody fragments* (Fab) (Martiny *et al.*, 1988). These have a greater affinity for digoxin than does digoxin for its receptors, they do not fix complement and they are not susceptible to immune degradation. The antibody fragments easily pass into the interstitial spaces where they bind to molecules of digitalis glycoside, leading to an improvement in signs and symptoms within about 30 minutes. At this time plasma digoxin levels rise, although, because the drug is now bound, it is pharmacologically inactive. Plasma potassium levels fall. The digoxin–antibody complex is then eliminated via the kidneys. The plasma half-life after intravenous administration of Fab is 16-34 h in those with normal renal function. There is little experience of using Fab in renal failure and there is at least a theoretical danger that retained complex might be metabolized to release free digoxin with recurrence of toxicity.

Suggested indications for Fab treatment are:

- rising, uncontrollable potassium levels;

- life-threatening cardiac arrhythmias;
- serum digoxin concentration higher than 20 µg/l.

Following a test dose of 2 mg, a therapeutic amount is given diluted in 100 ml 5% dextrose over 15 minutes. The dose can be calculated from the quantity ingested in mg multiplied by a bioavailability factor of 0.8 for digoxin tablets and 1.0 for digoxin elixir, capsules or digitoxin. This should then be divided by 0.6 mg/vial to give the Fab dose in number of vials.

Although treatment with Fab has been associated with fever and renal dysfunction in some patients, it is not clear whether these complications were directly related to Fab administration. Similarly, the role of Fab therapy in precipitating heart failure in patients dependent on digoxin has not been precisely defined. There is a danger of hypersensitivity reactions or even anaphylaxis on re-exposure.

β-blocking drugs

β-blockers are extensively prescribed and readily available; poisoning with β-blockers is therefore relatively common.

CLINICAL FEATURES

Manifestations of profound ß-blockade include *lassitude, drowsiness, bradycardia* and *hypotension. Peripheral vasospasm* and *Raynaud's phenomenon* may occur. *Bronchospasm* may be precipitated, particularly in those with asthma or chronic obstructive pulmonary disease.

TREATMENT

Gastric aspiration and lavage should be performed if the patient is seen within four hours of ingestion. *Intravenous atropine*, 1–2 mg, and an *isoprenaline* infusion can be given in an attempt to counteract the bradycardia, although the latter is inefficient and very large doses may be required. Some recommend dopamine or dobutamine as alternatives to isoprenaline. Ideally, *cardiac pacing* should be instituted in those with extreme bradycardia. *Glucagon* is of unproven value, although its mechanism of action is thought not to involve the β-adrenoreceptor. Severe bronchospasm should be treated with *salbutamol*.

Phenothiazines

Although these major tranquillizers are often prescribed for the 'at-risk' population of patients with psychotic ill-

nesses, they are a relatively uncommon cause of self-poisoning.

CLINICAL FEATURES

Following an overdose, the patient becomes *drowsy* or *comatose* with *respiratory depression* and *hypotensive* with a *tachycardia. Arrhythmias* may occur and the ECG may show prolongation of the QT interval and flattening of the T waves. Sudden death is a possibility, probably as a result of torsades de pointes (see Chapter 8). Impaired hypothalamic function combined with cardiovascular depression makes the patient susceptible to *hypothermia. Extrapyramidal disturbances* such as oculogyric crises, dystonia and convulsions may also occur. Some may develop neuroleptic malignant syndrome (see Chapter 19).

TREATMENT

Methods to speed elimination are ineffective and treatment is therefore *supportive*. Plasma potassium should be maintained within the normal range and the pH should be kept above 7.4. Extrapyramidal disturbances can be treated with repeated intravenous administration of *benztropine mesylate*, 2 mg. Dystonia is generally relieved by *procyclidine*, 5–10 mg intravenously, while arrhythmias may respond to *physostigmine*. If hypotension requires specific treatment, an *α-stimulant* should be used.

Lithium intoxication

Toxicity may be precipitated by dehydration, concomitant administration of NSAIDs or diuretics and, because lithium is cleared via the kidney, renal failure.

CLINICAL FEATURES

Features of intoxication include:

- confusion;
- agitation;
- hypertonia;
- hyperreflexia;
- ataxia and tremor;
- convulsions;
- vomiting.

Patients may also develop *hyponatraemia, diabetes insipidus* and *renal failure*.

INVESTIGATIONS

In acute lithium poisoning the plasma level is usually higher than 5 mmol/l (therapeutic range 0.4–1.0 mmol/l).

TREATMENT

Management should include *gastric lavage* up to four hours after ingestion and *forced diuresis*. *Haemodialysis* is indicated in those with neurological symptoms, renal failure or both.

Cocaine (Cregler & Mark, 1986)

The recreational use of cocaine has increased dramatically over the last 10–15 years. It can be taken intravenously or by intranasal insufflation and can be smoked. 'Crack' (so-called because it crackles when burnt) is a more potent water-soluble alkaloid of cocaine that is suitable for smoking and is very rapidly absorbed. Abuse of 'crack' has now reached epidemic proportions.

MECHANISMS

Unlike other local anaesthetics, cocaine also impairs the presynaptic uptake of catecholamines and upregulates postsynaptic receptors. It also has other poorly understood actions within the central nervous system. When mixed with alcohol, cocaine may be metabolized in the liver to a longer lasting, more lethal metabolite (Randall, 1992). Street cocaine is frequently contaminated with adulterants such as amphetamines, LSD, quinine and heroin. Occasionally it is adulterated with strychnine, in which case it is known on the streets as 'death hit.'

CLINICAL FEATURES

The clinical features of cocaine intoxication are related to peripheral and central nervous system stimulation and include:

- euphoria (the desired effect);
- dysphoria;
- agitation, hyperactivity, confusion, headaches, aggression;
- delirium;
- paranoia;
- hallucinations;
- tremors, fasciculation, seizures;
- hyperthermia.

Increased peripheral sympathetic activity may cause *tachycardia, cardiac arrhythmias* and *hypertension* associated with marked *vasoconstriction*. Complications include myocardial infarction, dilated cardiomyopathy, cerebrovascular accidents, pulmonary toxicity?, rhabdomyolysis and maternal and fetal complications in pregnancy.

Myocardial infarction. This may occur in the absence of coronary artery disease and is probably related to increased myocardial oxygen requirements combined with a reduction in coronary flow. It is uncertain whether reduced coronary flow is a result of vasospasm, endothelial abnormalities or platelet aggregation. *Mesenteric ischaemia* and *bowel infarction* can also occur.

Dilated cardiomyopathy. This has recently been described and may be similar to catecholamine-induced cardiomyopathy. It generally improves with strict avoidance of further cocaine use. Myocarditis and aortic rupture have also been described.

Cerebrovascular accidents. Ischaemic or haemorrhagic strokes and transient ischaemic attacks can complicate cocaine abuse. Subarachnoid haemorrhage usually occurs in those with a pre-existing aneurysm or arteriovenous malformation and is probably related to episodes of hypertension. Recently subarachnoid haemorrhage has been described in the absence of pre-existing cerebrovascular disease and it has therefore been suggested that cocaine can cause a vasculitis. Some patients develop cerebral oedema.

Pulmonary toxicity. When taken intravenously, impurities will clearly be filtered by the lungs, but all forms of cocaine abuse can be associated with *noncardiogenic pulmonary oedema. Bronchiolitis obliterans* has also been reported. 'Crack lung' is characterized by bronchospasm, fever and transient pulmonary infiltrates. Because it is associated with elevated serum immunoglobulin E levels and eosinophilia it has been attributed to a hypersensitivity reaction. Those who smoke cocaine may perform a deep, prolonged and forceful Valsalva manoeuvre, which can be complicated by *subcutaneous emphysema, pneumomediastinum* and *pneumothorax*. Cocaine can also cause *pulmonary haemorrhage*.

Rhabdomyolysis. This can be particularly severe and may occur with or without renal failure (Steingrub *et al.*, 1989). It may be associated with *hyperthermia* and *disseminated intravascular coagulation* (DIC). Muscle damage may be due to overexertion, ischaemia or a direct toxic effect on the myocyte.

In pregnancy. Cocaine use has been associated with serious maternal and fetal complications including *abruptio placentae, spontaneous abortion* and *preterm labour.* It may also cause *placental ischaemia,* as well as *myocardial* or *cerebral infarction* in the fetus.

DIAGNOSIS AND INVESTIGATIONS

The clinical features of cocaine toxicity are similar to those of neuroleptic malignant syndrome (see Chapter 19), acute withdrawal from alcohol, sedatives or hypnotics, and an overdose of anticholinergics, hallucinogens or amphetamine.

Investigations should include:

- ECG;
- blood glucose;
- creatine phosphokinase (CPK) levels, urinary myoglobin;
- blood and urine cultures;
- in selected cases, cerebral CT scan and occasionally lumbar puncture;
- core temperature (should be measured frequently).

The metabolites of cocaine can be detected in the urine.

MANAGEMENT

The circulating volume should be expanded and adequate oxygenation ensured. Tracheal intubation and mechanical ventilation may be indicated in those with:

- extreme agitation ⎱ with danger
- deep coma ⎰ of aspiration
- seizures ⎱ difficult
- hyperthermia ⎰ to control.

Agitation should be controlled with intravenous *diazepam.* This will limit the severity of the cardiovascular disturbances as well as help prevent hyperthermia and acidosis. Diazepam is also indicated in those with *seizures.* More resistant cases will require a diazepam infusion, usually combined with tracheal intubation and mechanical ventilation. In general phenytoin is not a particularly effective anticonvulsant in those with cocaine toxicity and *barbiturates* are preferred. *Dantrolene* may have a place in the management of severe *hyperthermia* (core temperature > 41°C). Neuroleptic agents should be avoided.

Supraventricular tachyarrhythmias may not require specific treatment. There is some suggestion that lignocaine can aggravate cocaine toxicity and if *ventricular arrhythmias* persist despite treating the

hyperadrenergic state *bretylium* may be the best agent. Severe *hypertension* can be treated with an infusion of *sodium nitroprusside* or, possibly, *labetalol.* β-blockers should be avoided because there is a danger that the unopposed α-activity will precipitate extreme vasoconstriction, hypertension and a fall in cardiac output.

Myocardial ischaemia should be treated with nitrates and morphine. Surprisingly, calcium channel blockers have not proved useful and thrombolytic therapy is potentially dangerous.

Non-cardiogenic pulmonary oedema should be managed as outlined in Chapter 7, while steroids may be indicated in patients with bronchiolitis obliterans and 'crack lung'.

Amphetamines

Amphetamines are now rarely prescribed and episodes of poisoning are therefore usually related to illicit use of these drugs. Amphetamines can be injected, inhaled or taken orally.

CLINICAL FEATURES

In overdose, amphetamines produce:

- confusion;
- anxiety;
- restlessness;
- tremor;
- irritability.

The patient may be *hyperreflexic* with *dilated pupils.* An initial pallor is followed by *flushing, tachycardia* and *arrhythmias.*

TREATMENT

Treatment is *supportive* and includes sedation with a *benzodiazepine* or, if this fails, a *phenothiazine.* Although elimination of amphetamines can be enhanced by using a forced acid diuresis, this is rarely necessary.

MDA and MDMA (ecstasy)

3,4 methylene dioxyamphetamine (MDA) and 3–4 methylene dioxymethamphetamine (MDMA)—also known as *ecstasy*—are synthetic amphetamine derivatives with a mild amphetamine-like stimulant effect. They also induce a feeling of euphoria and increased sociability as well as enhance perception. Their hallucinogenic potential is, however, low (Henry, 1992). Side-effects include:

- loss of appetite, nausea;
- trismus and teeth grinding;
- muscle aches and stiffness;
- ataxia;
- sweating;
- tachycardia, hypertension;
- hyponatraemia and catatonic stupor (Maxwell *et al.*, 1993).

Afterwards there may be fatigue and insomnia.

Whereas in the USA ecstasy tends to be taken alone or at parties, in Britain it is used almost exclusively as a dance drug at 'rave' parties. The pharmacological effects of the drug can then be compounded by relentless drug-stimulated physical exertion in a hot environment with limited access to liquid refreshment. Under these circumstances acute severe complications may occur unpredictably and can include:

- hyperpyrexia;
- collapse, convulsions;
- rhabdomyolysis;
- DIC;
- acute renal failure.

This syndrome resembles malignant hyperpyrexia and heat stroke (see Chapter 19).

MANAGEMENT

Management is urgent and should include:

- control of convulsions;
- rapid rehydration;
- measurement of core temperature and possibly active cooling;
- cardiovascular and respiratory support;
- management of rhabdomyolysis, DIC and renal failure as described elsewhere.

Although some recommend administration of dantrolene, there is currently little evidence that this influences outcome (Watson *et al.*, 1993).

Monoamine oxidase inhibitors

Although an isolated overdose of these agents does not produce serious effects, severe toxicity may occur when they are taken in combination with foods containing precursors of biogenic amines or with drugs such as amphetamines and sympathomimetic amines.

CLINICAL FEATURES

Signs and symptoms of toxicity include:

- tachycardia;
- fluctuating blood pressure;
- warm peripheries;
- sweating;
- pyrexia;
- dilated pupils.

Muscle twitching may progress to diffuse *muscle spasm, trismus* and *opisthotonos*. As with amphetamine analogues, severe cases may be complicated by *rhabdomyolysis, DIC* and *renal failure*.

TREATMENT

Management is *supportive* combined with *cooling, sedation* and administration of *muscle relaxants* when core temperature is 39°C or more.

Corrosives

CLINICAL FEATURES

Acids and alkalis

Acids and alkalis are used for cleaning, both domestically and industrially, as well as being involved in chemical manufacturing processes. When swallowed, they can cause *extensive burns* of the mouth, tongue, pharynx, oesophagus and stomach. These are extremely painful and may lead to *perforation* of the oesophagus or stomach. Oedema of the epiglottis and larynx can produce severe *upper airway obstruction* necessitating endotracheal intubation. Systemic absorption produces profound *acid-base disturbances* and *shock*. Delayed deaths may be associated with necrosis and superimposed infection.

Long-term complications in survivors include *gastrointestinal scarring* and *stenosis*.

Phenolic compounds

Phenolic compounds are commonly found in antiseptics, disinfectants and preservatives. If swallowed, they cause blanching or erythema around the mouth and chin followed by *intense thirst, nausea, vomiting, diarrhoea* and *sweating*. Those who are severely poisoned may develop *abdominal pain, convulsions* and *coma*. *Acute renal failure* is common and *hepatic damage* may occur.

TREATMENT

Gastric lavage should probably be avoided because of the risk of aspiration, although some recommend it as a means of diluting the corrosive. Surgical intervention is required if there are signs of perforation. Otherwise, treatment is supportive and may include total parenteral nutrition.

Carbon monoxide (Meredith & Vale, 1988)

Since CO is no longer a constituent of domestic gas, the commonest sources of poisoning are motor vehicle exhaust fumes, incorrectly maintained and ventilated heating systems and smoke from fires (see Chapter 9). Approximately 1000 people die from CO poisoning in England and Wales every year and CO is the commonest cause of death from poisoning in children.

MECHANISMS

The affinity of CO for haemoglobin is some 200–250 times greater than that of oxygen, which it therefore displaces. It also shifts the oxyhaemoglobin dissociation curve to the left and may inhibit cellular respiration as a result of binding to other haem-containing proteins. Although CO only combines with cytochromes under hypoxic conditions, once binding occurs it is difficult to reverse with conventional oxygen therapy. The tissue effects may be the major cause of clinical toxicity and this may explain the discrepancy between clinical consequences and COHb levels. The net effect is tissue hypoxaemia, which in many cases is fatal.

CLINICAL FEATURES

The clinical course is directly related to the degree and duration of exposure. In general COHb levels less than 10% produce no symptoms whereas levels above 60% are associated with coma and a risk of cardiac arrest.

Repeated *chronic exposure* leads to fatigue, poor memory, impaired concentration, headaches, dizziness, visual disturbances, paraesthesiae, chest pain, abdominal pain and diarrhoea. Manifestations of *acute poisoning* include headaches, dizziness, hyperventilation, confusion, disorientation and, in severe cases, coma. Nausea, vomiting and faecal incontinence may also occur, as may hyperreflexia, convulsions and cardiac arrhythmias. Later, pulmonary oedema and respiratory depression may supervene, while extreme hypoxia may produce cerebral oedema, hyperpyrexia and myocardial ischaemia. Some patients develop rhabdomyolysis and renal failure.

The *pink discoloration of the skin* caused by the presence of large amounts of COHb is in practice uncommon, except in particularly severe poisoning. *Cyanosis* and *skin pallor* is more usual. *Skin blisters* may occur as a result of tissue hypoxia.

Late sequelae may include neuropsychiatric disturbances such as memory loss, impaired intellect and cerebellar damage, which may appear several weeks after exposure.

TREATMENT

Administration of oxygen in high concentrations, and IPPV if indicated, should be instituted immediately. The diagnosis may then be confirmed and progress monitored by estimating the percentage of COHb present in the blood. Arterial oxygen tension is usually normal. In severe poisoning, treatment for cerebral oedema should be instituted.

Hyperbaric oxygen

The elimination half-life of CO is reduced from 250 mins when breathing air to 59 mins when 100% oxygen is administered and to 22 mins when 100% oxygen is breathed at 2.2 atmospheric pressure. Treatment with hyperbaric oxygen can reduce the duration of coma and may decrease the incidence of delayed encephalopathy and long-term morbidity to less than 5%.

Suggested indications for hyperbaric oxygen therapy include (Collee & Hanson, 1993):

- conscious patient with COHb concentration higher than 20% (others suggest COHb > 40%);
- depressed conscious level, but able to maintain airway;
- recovery of consciousness after an initial COHb concentration higher than 40%.

Contraindications to hyperbaric oxygen are related to the practical difficulties of managing patients in single-person chambers and include:

- mechanical ventilation;
- inability to maintain an airway;
- hypovolaemic or inotrope dependent;
- cardiac arrhythmias potentially requiring urgent intervention;
- asthma.

Larger compression chambers in which medical attendants can also be pressurized are not widely available. Some consider that there is still a need for prospective trials to confirm the value of hyperbaric oxygen therapy in CO poisoning.

Mushroom poisoning

It has been claimed that early recognition of mushroom poisoning combined with aggressive treatment before liver failure has developed may be associated with mortality rates as low as 10–15% (Vesconi *et al.*, 1985). Over 90% of those who die as a result of fungal poisoning have eaten *A. phalloides*.

AMANITA PHALLOIDES (DEATH CAP)

Mechanisms

This fungus contains two toxins. The *phallotoxins* (heptapeptides) produce violent nausea, vomiting and diarrhoea, while the *amatoxins* (octapeptides) cause a fatal hepatorenal syndrome. The latter produce severe cellular damage by binding to the nuclear RNA polymerase B of eukaryotic cells, inhibiting enzyme activity and precipitating cell necrosis. In humans, amatoxins are specifically toxic to hepatocytes, intestinal epithelium and possibly the kidney.

Clinical features

Nearly all patients poisoned by *A. phalloides* first develop gastrointestinal symptoms some 6–18 hours after ingestion. There is *vomiting* and *abdominal pain*. *Diarrhoea* can be severe ('cholera like') leading to hypovolaemia, dehydration and hypokalaemia.

The *signs of hepatocellular necrosis* become evident about 36 hours after ingestion with elevated transaminase levels and, a little later, prolongation of the prothrombin time.

Treatment

The patient should be rehydrated and the circulating volume should be expanded.

Removal of circulating toxins by instituting a *forced diuresis* is the most effective, safest and cheapest immediate intervention.

Although other techniques such as haemodialysis, haemofiltration and haemoperfusion are effective, they should probably only be used when it proves impossible to produce a forced diuresis. *Activated charcoal* can be given to bind toxins within the gastrointestinal tract.

No specific *antidotes* are available although penicillin has been recommended. Its mechanism of action is unclear, but it may reduce hepatic uptake of amatoxins.

Fulminant hepatic failure (FHF) should be managed as outlined in Chapter 13. Liver transplantation has been performed in patients with FHF associated with mushroom poisoning.

OTHER RARE MUSHROOMS

Other rare mushrooms include:

- *Gyromitra*, the effects of which are similar to those produced by amatoxins except that it also produces neurological symptoms such as restlessness, stupor, dizziness, tremor, seizures, diplopia and nystagmus;
- *Orellanus*, which rarely causes initial gastrointestinal symptoms, and patients may develop renal failure 7–17 days after ingesting the mushrooms.

REFERENCES

Ashton CH (1985) Benzodiazepine overdose: are specific antagonists useful? *British Medical Journal* **290**: 805–806.

Boehnert MT & Lovejoy FH Jr (1985) Value of the QRS duration versus the serum drug level in predicting seizures and ventricular arrhythmias after an acute overdose of tricyclic antidepressants. *New England Journal of Medicine* **313**: 474–479.

Collee GG & Hanson GC (1993) The management of acute poisoning. *British Journal of Anaesthesia* **70**: 562–573.

Cregler LL & Mark H (1986) Medical complications of cocaine abuse. *New England Journal of Medicine* **317**: 1495–1500.

Cutler RE, Forland SC, Hammond PGStJ & Evans JR (1987) Extracorporeal removal of drugs and poisons by hemodialysis and hemoperfusion. *Annual Review of Pharmacology and Toxicology* **27**: 169–191.

Editorial (1976) Paraquat poisoning. *Lancet* **i**: 1057.

Henry JA (1992) Ecstasy and the dance of death. *British Medical Journal* **305**: 5–6.

Höjer J, Baehrendtz S, Matell G & Gustafsson LL (1990) Diagnostic utility of flumazenil in coma with suspected poisoning: a double-blind, randomised controlled study. *British Medical Journal* **301**: 1308–1311.

Hormaechea E, Carlson RW, Rogove H, *et al.* (1979) Hypovolemia, pulmonary edema and protein changes in severe salicylate poisoning. *American Journal of Medicine* **66**: 1046–1050.

Keays R, Harrison PM, Wendon JA, Forbes A, Gove C, Alexander GJM & Williams R (1991) Intravenous acetylcysteine in paracetamol-induced fulminant hepatic failure: a prospective controlled trial. *British Medical Journal* **303**: 1026–1029.

Kirshenbaum LA, Mathews SC, Sitar DS & Tenenbein M (1990) Does multiple-dose charcoal therapy enhance salicylate excretion? *Archives of Internal Medicine* **150**: 1281–1283.

Levy G (1982) Gastrointestinal clearance of drugs with activated charcoal. *New England Journal of Medicine* **307**: 676–678.

Lorch JA & Garella S (1979) Hemoperfusion to treat intoxications. *Annals of Internal Medicine* **91**: 301–304.

Martiny SS, Phelps SJ & Massey KL (1988) Treatment of severe digitalis intoxication with digoxin-specific antibody fragments: a clinical review. *Critical Care Medicine* **16**: 629-635.

Masters AB (1967) Delayed death in imipramine poisoning. *British Medical Journal* **iii**: 866-867.

Maxwell DL, Polkey MI & Henry JA (1993) Hyponatraemia and catatonic stupor after taking 'ecstasy'. *British Medical Journal* **307**: 1399.

Menzies DG, Busuttil A & Prescott LF (1988) Fatal pulmonary aspiration of oral activated charcoal. *British Medical Journal* **297**: 459-460.

Meredith T & Vale A (1988) Carbon monoxide poisoning. *British Medical Journal* **296**: 77-79.

Prescott LF, Sutherland GR, Park J, Smith IJ & Proudfoot AT (1976) Cysteamine, methionine and penicillamine in the treatment of paracetamol poisoning. *Lancet* **ii**: 109-113.

Randall T (1992) Cocaine, alcohol mix in body to form even longer lasting, more lethal drug. *Journal of the American Medical Association* **267**: 1043-1044.

Rose MS, Smith LL & Wyatt I (1974) Evidence for energy-dependent accumulation of paraquat into rat lung. *Nature* **252**: 314-315.

Smilkstein MJ, Knapp GL, Kulig KW & Rumack BH (1988) Efficacy of oral N-acetylcysteine in the treatment of acetaminophen overdose. Analysis of the national multicenter overdose (1976 to 1985). *New England Journal of Medicine* **319**: 1557-1562.

Steingrub JS, Sweet S & Teres D (1989) Crack-induced rhabdomyolysis. *Critical Care Medicine* **17**: 1073-1074.

Stern TA, O'Gara PT, Mulley AG, Singer DE & Thibault GE (1985) Complications after overdose with tricyclic antidepressants. *Critical Care Medicine* **13**: 672-674.

Sutherland GR, Park J & Proudfoot AT (1977) Ventilation and acid-base changes in deep coma due to barbiturate or tricyclic antidepressant poisoning. *Clinical Toxicology* **11**: 403-412.

Vale JA & Proudfoot AT (1993) How useful is activated charcoal? *British Medical Journal* **306**: 78-79.

Vale JA, Meredith TJ & Proudfoot AT (1986) Syrup of ipecacuanha: is it really useful? *British Medical Journal* **293**: 1321-1322.

Vesconi S, Langer M, Iapichino G, Constantino D, Busi C & Fiume L (1985) Therapy of cytotoxic mushroom intoxication. *Critical Care Medicine* **13**: 402-406.

Watson JD, Ferguson C, Hinds CJ, Skinner R & Coakley JH (1993) Exertional heat stroke induced by amphetamine analogues. Does dantrolene have a place? *Anaesthesia* **48**: 1057-1060.

Wright N (1980) An assessment of the unreliability of the history given by self-poisoned patients. *Clinical Toxicology* **16**: 381-384.

19 Disturbances of Body Temperature

ACCIDENTAL HYPOTHERMIA

Causes

Three types of cold injury may be encountered.

- *Frostbite* is due to freezing of tissue with intracellular ice crystal formation and microvascular occlusion. It can be classified into first, second, third and fourth degree according to the depth of the injury.
- *Non-freezing cold injury* to the extremities is due to microvascular endothelial damage, stasis and vascular occlusion. With ambient temperature above freezing, prolonged exposure over several days leads to 'trench foot'. Although the entire foot may appear black, deep tissue destruction may not be present.
- *Hypothermia* is defined as a core temperature below 35°C.

Accidental hypothermia may follow exposure to low environmental temperatures or immersion in cold water and is frequently associated with impaired temperature regulation. Factors predisposing to exposure hypothermia include inadequate or wet clothing, strong winds, contact with snow and strenuous exercise. Paradoxically, it is more common in relatively temperate regions where the dangers of, for example, hill walking in winter are often underestimated and preventive measures are consequently inadequate. The incidence of immersion hypothermia is rising, probably because of the widespread use of life-jackets, which support the head above water and prevent drowning (Golden & Rivers, 1975), as well as the increasing popularity of water sports. The rate of heat loss in water is approximately 25 times greater than that in air at the same temperature and this is accelerated by the increase in cutaneous blood flow that accompanies exertion (e.g. swimming) as well as a redistribution of the warmed water layer surrounding the body. Subcutaneous fat provides insulation and obese subjects can generally survive longer periods of immersion; even non-waterproof conventional clothing is protective.

Diseases in which the metabolic rate is reduced (e.g. *myxoedema*, *hypopituitarism* and *malnutrition*) limit the ability to maintain body temperature by increasing heat production. Similarly, patients with *spinal cord lesions* are unable to produce thermal energy by increasing muscular activity, and this is exacerbated by an inability to adjust skin blood flow (see Chapter 9). *Hypothalamic lesions* can impair thermoregulation and patients in coma (e.g. due to a cerebrovascular accident, alcohol abuse or self-poisoning) are frequently hypothermic. Furthermore, *alcohol* and many *sedative drugs*, especially the barbiturates, increase heat loss by producing cutaneous vasodilatation. The *elderly* are particularly vulnerable to cold because of inactivity, impaired shivering, low metabolic rate, malnutrition, reduced subcutaneous fat, decreased vasoconstriction in response to cold and poor social conditions (Editorial, 1977).

Clinical manifestations and pathophysiology

The clinical manifestations of hypothermia at a particular body temperature are variable and probably depend on the rate of cooling and the duration of hypothermia. Nevertheless, if the core temperature is greater than 33°C, physiological changes are generally minimal and thermoregulatory mechanisms remain intact. At temperatures between 33°C and 30°C there is progressive physiological dysfunction, while cooling to below 30°C produces severe cardiorespiratory and neurological abnormalities with failure of thermoregulation. Body temperatures of less than 27–28°C can mimic death, and extreme hypothermia (< 24–26°C) is usually incompatible with life, although some remarkable cases of survival under these circumstances have been reported (see Chapter 9).

METABOLIC RESPONSES

Initially, metabolic rate increases and the victim shivers in an attempt to maintain body temperature. If this is unsuccessful, thermoregulation eventually fails and oxygen consumption ($\dot{V}_{O_2}$) falls (e.g. $\dot{V}_{O_2}$ may be reduced to about 80 ml/min/m² at a core temperature of 32°C)

(Harari *et al.*, 1975). As would be expected, the reduction in metabolic rate is greater in those with myxoedema coma.

NEUROLOGICAL MANIFESTATIONS

The severity of the neurological disturbance depends on the rate of cooling. In general, cerebral metabolism is depressed and this minimizes cerebral damage during episodes of ischaemia or hypoxia. At core temperatures below 33°C, the patient is dysarthric and cerebration is slowed. Conscious level falls progressively until at 30°C the victim is usually stuporous and hypertonic with infrequent voluntary movements. Tendon reflexes are slowed, with prolonged contraction and relaxation phases. At core temperatures below 27°C, patients are usually comatose and hypertonic with absent tendon and plantar reflexes. The pupils do not react to light and voluntary movements are absent.

CARDIOVASCULAR CHANGES

At first, cardiac output rises to satisfy the increased metabolic demands, but subsequently the cardiovascular system is depressed in proportion to the fall in body temperature. Progressive bradycardia, probably due to a direct effect of cold on the sinus node (30–40 beats/min at 28–29°C, 10 beats/min at 25–26°C), produces a dramatic fall in cardiac output, despite a normal or increased stroke volume. Initially, blood pressure is maintained by vasoconstriction and an increase in viscosity, but hypotension usually supervenes at temperatures below 30°C. In addition, many hypothermic patients are hypovolaemic (Harari *et al.*, 1975) and vasodilatation induced by rewarming can precipitate serious hypotension. Blood pressure may also fall when the increase in viscosity is reversed by intravenous fluid administration. There is some evidence that myocardial performance can be impaired following prolonged exposure to cold (Harari *et al.*, 1975).

Although sinus rhythm is maintained during moderate hypothermia, atrial flutter or fibrillation, sometimes with ventricular premature contraction, often supervenes in the more serious cases. With more profound falls in body temperature, an idioventricular rhythm is common and atrial activity may completely disappear. There is a risk of ventricular fibrillation (VF) when core temperature falls below 30°C and this may be precipitated by hypoxia, hypotension or stimulating procedures such as endotracheal intubation. At core temperatures of less than 28°C, there is a pronounced tendency to develop VF.

The electrocardiogram (ECG) in hypothermia shows evidence of reduced conductivity with prolongation of

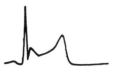

Fig. 19.1 The electocardiogram in accidental hypothermia. Lead V5 showing 'J' wave and ST segment changes.

the PR and QT intervals, as well as widening of the QRS complex. The ST segment is generally depressed or concave, but is sometimes elevated. Classically, a 'J' wave is seen at the junction of the QRS and ST segments (**Fig. 19.1**) and this finding is almost constant at temperatures below 31°C.

RESPIRATORY CHANGES

Hypothermia reduces the ventilatory response to hypoxaemia and hypercarbia, and tidal volume and respiratory rate fall progressively. This reduction in minute volume is, however, accompanied by a fall in both $\dot{V}O_2$ and carbon dioxide production. The arterial carbon dioxide tension (P_aCO_2) corrected to body temperature may therefore be low, normal or high depending on the balance between the reduction in alveolar ventilation and the fall in carbon dioxide production. On the other hand, hypothermic patients are consistently hypoxaemic (when arterial oxygen tension is corrected to body temperature), with an increased $P_{A-a}O_2$, largely due to ventilation perfusion (V/Q) mismatch. Although the consequences of a reduction in arterial oxygen tension (P_aO_2) are minimized by the fall in $\dot{V}O_2$, and are generally well tolerated, a metabolic acidosis is common. Moreover, significant tissue hypoxia can develop when the metabolic rate rises during rapid rewarming or shivering, and restoration of blood flow to previously ischaemic areas washes accumulated acid into the general circulation. This metabolic acidosis is exacerbated by impaired hepatic clearance of lactic acid and a reduction in the capacity of the kidneys to excrete hydrogen ions.

Bronchopneumonia is a relatively common complication of hypothermia; both its incidence and severity are related to the duration and the degree of hypothermia.

RENAL DYSFUNCTION

Hypothermia is associated with a diuresis and haemoconcentration, despite a reduction in renal blood flow. This polyuria may be related to a central shift of the blood volume as well as impaired tubular function due to inhibition of enzyme systems and a reduced responsiveness to antidiuretic hormone (ADH). Hypothermic patients therefore produce dilute, eventually almost iso-osmotic urine, with a reduced creatinine clearance, an elevated blood urea and increased sodium excretion. Potassium is retained, but this seldom causes significant alterations in plasma levels.

A few patients develop established acute renal failure and require dialysis. This is unlikely to be the result of hypothermia alone and is probably related to associated abnormalities such as hypoxia, hypotension and hypovolaemia.

OTHER ABNORMALITIES

Serum amylase levels are often raised in hypothermia, and this probably reflects a mild acute pancreatitis. Occasionally, this pancreatitis contributes to the development, sometimes delayed, of diabetic ketoacidosis (MacLean et al., 1973).

Initially, glucose is released from liver glycogen and its use is increased. Later, glucose uptake decreases, possibly because of insulin resistance or inactivation of hexokinase, and hyperglycaemia is exacerbated by elevated cortisol levels.

Thrombocytopenia and various coagulation abnormalities have been described, but these are of doubtful clinical significance.

Management

MONITORING

The diagnosis can be established using a *low-reading rectal thermometer*. Subsequently, body temperature can be monitored using a rectal probe. This must be inserted at least 10 cm beyond the anal sphincter and will record a temperature 0.25-0.5°C below that of blood. An oesophageal probe may more closely reflect the temperature of the blood and the myocardium.

Blood pressure, central venous pressure (CVP), the ECG and urine output should also be monitored in all cases. Insertion of a pulmonary artery catheter is generally not recommended since passage of the catheter may precipitate ventricular fibrillation. Urea and electrolytes and blood sugar concentrations should be measured frequently.

Determination of blood gas tensions is complicated by the influence of alterations in body temperature on the position of the dissociation curve. Measurements are made at 37°C and if corrected, for example, to a body temperature of 25°C, a P_aO_2 of 13.3 kPa (100 mm Hg) and a P_aCO_2 of 5.3 kPa (40 mm Hg) become 6.7 and 3 kPa (50 and 22.5 mm Hg) respectively. Changes in temperature also affect pH measurements; a fall of 1°C increases pH by 0.0147 units.

SUPPORTIVE TREATMENT

Patients who are profoundly hypothermic may survive despite apparently being dead on admission. Moreover, survival has been reported even following prolonged cardiac arrest or VF. Attempts at resuscitation should therefore continue until rewarming has been achieved or until it is clear that the situation is hopeless. In all cases, underlying diseases must also be treated.

Hypoxaemia must be corrected by securing the *airway* and administering *oxygen*; this is particularly important during rewarming when oxygen requirements increase. A few patients will require *controlled ventilation*. To avoid extreme hypocarbia, which can exacerbate peripheral vasoconstriction and may precipitate VF, the minute volume must be adjusted to match the reduced carbon dioxide production.

Intravenous *fluid replacement* should be started with 5% or 10% dextrose, combined with sodium bicarbonate as required to correct significant metabolic acidosis. *Expansion of the circulating volume* is essential during rewarming and this can be achieved using a colloidal solution. Subsequent intravenous fluid administration should be guided by frequent estimation of urea, electrolytes and blood sugar levels, and haematocrit.

Occasionally, hypothermic patients develop cardiac failure during rewarming, with an elevated CVP, persistent hypotension, oliguria and acidosis. This may require the administration of an *inotropic agent*, although there is a considerable risk of inducing arrhythmias. The heart rate normally increases progressively as body temperature rises and definitive treatment of the bradycardia is not indicated. Intracardiac pacing is generally ineffective and can be harmful. Patients in VF will require direct current *defibrillation*. Although successful defibrillation has been reported at temperatures as low as 24°C (Siebke et al., 1975), in general restoration of an effective cardiac rhythm is unlikely until core temperature has reached 28-30°C.

Steroids are of no value in hypothermia, and antimicrobial therapy should be reserved for those with established infection.

REWARMING

The risk of complications such as myocardial failure, bronchopneumonia and neurological dysfunction increases the longer hypothermia persists. Furthermore, spontaneous rewarming takes place more slowly following prolonged hypothermia.

Spontaneous rewarming is the rule in patients whose body temperature is greater than 33°C, and may be possible in a few with core temperatures as low as 26-27°C. Passive rewarming is also preferred by some for elderly patients with prolonged hypothermia and underlying disease (e.g. myxoedema). The patient should be moved to a warm room (25–30°C) with warm blankets and clothing. It is also important to insulate the patient's head since scalp vessels do not constrict in response to cold and considerable heat can be lost from this region. Reported rewarming rates range from 0.1–3.7°C/hour.

In other patients, particularly those with impaired thermoregulation and an inability to shiver, *active measures* are required to restore body temperature. This can be achieved with *surface heat* using hot water bottles, heat cradles, heated mattresses or electric blankets. This method is usually suitable for young patients with moderate hypothermia (28–30°C) of short duration and for elderly patients who fail to respond to passive rewarming. Warming rates vary from 1–4°C/hour. Surface rewarming can, however, produce abrupt vasodilatation and hypotension ('*rewarming shock*'), while reperfusion of cold ischaemic regions can cause a fall in central body temperature of as much as 3–4°C ('*after-drop*') as well as exacerbate metabolic acidosis. In addition, this technique is relatively inefficient and may cause skin burns. *Hot baths* (at 40–45°C), with the limbs out of the water to avoid after-drop and minimize hypotension, are suitable for fit young adults, particularly following a short period of immersion in cold water, but should not be used in the elderly. Warming rates range from 5–7°C/hour. With this method, active rewarming should be discontinued when the core temperature reaches 33°C.

Theoretically, *central rewarming*, which warms the 'core' before the 'shell', should avoid some of the dangers of surface heating as well as ensure that the myocardium warms early and is able to respond to the increasing metabolic demands. Moreover, it is the only practicable method in those with cardiac arrest.

Central rewarming at a rate of up to 15°C/hour can be achieved using an *extracorporeal circulation* via a femoral artery and vein. This method is relatively complex and its use should be restricted to those with severe hypothermia (< 28°C) complicated by myocardial failure or cardiac arrest. Some use *venovenous bypass* to actively warm those whose core temperature is below 31°C and who are not warming steadily (> 1°C/hour) with non-invasive methods. *Peritoneal lavage* with warm fluid is less efficient, but may be useful in self-poisoning since it can also hasten drug elimination.

Intravenous administration of warm fluids and ventilation with warmed humidified gases are inadequate when used alone, but are useful adjuncts to other measures. Indeed, the optimal approach in an individual patient is often to use a carefully selected combination of the available techniques.

Prognosis

The overall mortality of accidental hypothermia may approach 60%, being as high as 75% in patients with an underlying primary disease and as low as 6% in those with hypothermia alone. Hypothermia associated with poisoning has a good prognosis.

HYPERTHERMIA

Although still uncommon, the incidence of severe hyperthermia has recently increased, due principally to the popularity of long-distance running events and the increased availability and use of amphetamine-like drugs such as 'Ecstasy' at night-clubs, raves and parties (see Chapter 18).

Definitions

Hyperthermia is defined as a core body temperature above normal, and *severe hyperthermia* or *heat stroke* as a core temperature of 40.5°C or higher sustained for at least 1 hour (Rosenberg *et al.*, 1986). Mild hyperthermia includes the syndromes of *heat cramps* and *heat exhaustion*, while severe hyperthermia encompasses the more serious *heat stroke*, *malignant hyperthermia* and *neuroleptic malignant syndrome*. For the purposes of this chapter, fever due to infection is excluded from this definition.

Causes (Table 19.1)

Heat cramps occur in heavily exercised muscles, usually the calves, during unaccustomed exercise when the environmental temperature is high. They are caused by a combination of dehydration and sodium loss and are therefore more common in those who sweat profusely and when lost fluids are replaced with water without added salts.

Most cases of *severe hyperthermia* are caused by a combination of exogenous and endogenous factors that results in an excessive heat load, impaired heat dissipation or a combination of both. A large number of predisposing factors have been identified (**Table 19.2**). Many cases follow extreme exertion such as long-distance running, training in the armed forces or prolonged dancing in association with drug abuse, and the incidence is higher when ambient temperature and humidity are high.

Drug toxicity is frequently implicated. Severe hyperthermia has, for example, been described following the use of many 'recreational drugs', although it is not always certain whether this is related to idiosyncratic

Table 19.1 Causes of hyperthermia.
Increased heat production
Increased muscular activity
Exercise
Seizures
Agitation
Rigidity
Uncoupling of oxidative phosphorylation
Salicylates
Stimulation of hepatic metabolism
Sympathomimetics
Alterations in brain chemistry
Reduced heat dissipation
Behavioural dysfunction
High ambient temperature and humidity
Pre-existing disease
Drug-related
Specific syndromes
Malignant hyperthermia
Neuroleptic malignant syndrome

Table 19.2 Predisposing factors to hyperthermia.
Pre-existing disease
Cardiovascular disease
Endocrine disease
Autonomic dysfunction
Dehydration
Fever
Delirium tremens
Psychosis
Neonates/elderly
Malignant hyperthermia
Parkinsonism
Drugs
Anticholinergics
Phenothiazines
Tricyclic antidepressants
Monoamine oxidase inhibitors (MAOIs)
β-blockers
α-blockers
α-agonists
Sympathomimetics
Hallucinogens
Salicylates
Diuretics
Alcohol
Behaviour
Overexertion
Inappropriate clothing
Poor fluid intake
Poor acclimatization

reactions, overdose or a genetic predisposition to exertional heat stroke (Hopkins *et al.*, 1991), or is simply a result of unremitting drug-stimulated exercise in hot and humid conditions with inappropriate clothing and inadequate hydration. Responsible drugs may include:

- amphetamines and amphetamine derivatives;
- cocaine;
- lysergic acid diethylamide (LSD);
- mescaline;
- phencyclidine.

Drugs that reduce sweating such as the tricyclic antidepressants, atropine and antihistamines, as well as those that uncouple oxidative phosphorylation such as the salicylates have also been implicated in precipitating hyperthermia. Sympathomimetic agents increase heat production by stimulating hepatic metabolism of glucose and fat, while α-agonists such as phenylephrine and some appetite suppressants, as well as amphetamine and its derivatives, cocaine, PCP ('angel dust') and ketamine ('special K'), cause cutaneous vasoconstriction with reduced heat loss. Drugs that cause seizures or rigidity such as tricyclic antidepressants or monoamine oxidase inhibitors (MAOIs) may also increase heat production. Malignant hyperthermia and neuroleptic

malignant syndrome are distinct syndromes related to the administration of specific drugs (see later in this chapter).

Increased *centrally mediated thermogenesis* may be due to dopamine hyperactivity (which also causes extrapyramidal rigidity) and excess serotoninergic activity. This is an additional mechanism for hyperthermia associated with amphetamine derivatives, MAOIs and the antidepressant fluoxetine.

Failure to adapt to environmental conditions often contributes to the development of hyperthermia. For example, the mentally ill, small babies, the elderly or infirm and soldiers in training may fail to remove excess clothing or move to a cooler place. Ingestion of alcohol or drugs may also prevent appropriate responses to hot and humid environments.

The ability to increase cardiac output and therefore cutaneous bloodflow is also crucial to the dissipation of heat and may be impaired in the elderly, those with pre-existing cardiac disease and by dehydration. Additionally exercise diverts blood to muscles, thereby further reducing cutaneous blood flow.

Pathophysiology

When temperature regulation fails and core temperature exceeds 42°C, oxidative phosphorylation is uncoupled and enzymes cease to function. Simultaneously energy stores are depleted, membrane permeability increases and there is influx of sodium into the cells. ATP is depleted by increased membrane depolarization and neurotransmitter activity leading to further heat production. Therefore as temperature control fails, hyperthermia is accelerated, proteins denature and there is widespread damage to vital organs. Tissues most at risk include vascular endothelium, nervous tissue and hepatocytes. In severe cases there may be coma, liver failure, renal failure, adult respiratory distress syndrome (ARDS), rhabdomyolysis and disseminated intravascular coagulation (DIC).

History and clinical features

Usually it is not possible to obtain an adequate history from the patient, and family, friends or bystanders may be unable or reluctant to provide information, especially if drug abuse is involved. It is important to establish whether the patient has been exposed to excessive heat loads and whether drug abuse, medications or intercurrent illness are implicated.

Heat exhaustion is characterized by:

- headache;
- malaise;
- dizziness;
- nausea and vomiting;
- body temperature higher than 37°C, but less than 39°C;
- normal mental function.

Traditionally *severe hyperthermia* or heat stroke has been divided into *classical heat stroke*, which is seen in those with compromised homeostatic mechanisms when ambient temperature is high and *exertional heat stroke*, which occurs in young previously healthy people, usually in association with extreme physical exertion. Classical heat stroke has a slower onset and is often associated with an absence of sweating, whereas exertional heat stroke has a rapid onset and sweating may be profuse.

The core temperature (measured using a rectal or oesophageal probe) will be high (> 40.5°C), although the patient may already have begun to cool by the time of presentation and may feel deceptively cool as a result of cutaneous vasoconstriction.

The patient's mental state is invariably altered and *neurological changes* are the hallmark of severe hyperthermia. These may include:

- confusion/irritational behaviour;
- seizures;
- abnormal posturing;
- ataxia;
- syncope;
- focal neurological signs;
- coma.

The muscles are likely to be flaccid in those with exertional or environmental hyperthermia, but may be rigid or dystonic in patients with drug-induced hyperthermia. Most of these neurological symptoms and signs resolve, provided treatment is not delayed. Nevertheless long-term sequelae do occur and may include cerebellar ataxia, paresis and personality changes.

Muscle damage and *rhabdomyolysis* are common, particularly when hyperthermia is secondary to drug abuse and/or unremitting exertion. Muscles are swollen and painful, creatine kinase levels are grossly elevated and there is myoglobinuria.

The *cardiovascular system* is usually hyperdynamic, with tachycardia, normotension with a wide pulse pressure or hypotension associated with hypovolaemia. Early cutaneous vasodilatation may be followed later by peripheral vasoconstriction. Eventually cardiac failure may supervene with a normal or high peripheral vascular resistance. It is worth noting that myocardial contractility is impaired when body temperature exceeds 40°C.

Hyperthermic patients are often *tachypnoeic* and their appearance has been likened to that of a 'panting' dog. Later *pulmonary oedema* may develop. This may be the result of fluid overload, perhaps exacerbated by central redistribution of the circulating volume during cooling and myocardial dysfunction. Alternatively pulmonary endothelial injury may lead to the development of ARDS.

DIC is a common and sinister complication of hyperthermia. It is probably related to activation of the clotting cascade by endothelial damage and heat-induced denaturation of clotting factors.

Acute renal failure is also a common complication of severe hyperthermia and may be related to hypovolaemia, hypotension, direct thermal injury, rhabdomyolysis and haemolysis. Similarly *liver dysfunction* is almost universal and may be due to impaired perfusion, hypoxia or direct thermal injury. Liver failure will exacerbate the coagulopathy.

The combination of extreme exertion, muscle rigidity, seizures and circulatory insufficiency may precipitate *lactic acidosis*, while hypermetabolism and respiratory failure may be complicated by *respiratory acidosis*.

Electrolyte disturbances include hypernatraemia and hypokalaemia, which may be followed later by dangerous hyperkalaemia secondary to rhabdomyolysis and acute renal failure. Hypocalcaemia is common, but rarely requires intervention.

Differential diagnosis

The most important differential diagnosis in a patient with the combination of fever and neurological signs is *meningoencephalitis*. If there are signs of meningeal irritation and the history is unclear, appropriate antibiotics should be administered until the diagnosis is clarified by lumbar puncture and, when indicated, CT scan. *Sepsis* may also cause fever and altered mental status. It is particularly important to enquire about foreign travel and the possibility of malaria or other tropical diseases. *Prolonged status epilepticus* or other disorders in which muscle tone is markedly increased such as *discontinuation of anti-Parkinsonian treatment*, as well as some *psychoses*, can also present as hyperthermia.

Occasionally *cerebrovascular thrombosis or haemorrhage* involving the hypothalamus or *endocrine disorders* such as thyroid storm or phaeochromocytoma may present with severe hyperthermia and altered mental state.

Investigations

Investigations should include:

- full blood count (thrombocytopenia in DIC; elevated white cell count in hyperthermia, but may also indicate infection);
- coagulation screen (coagulopathy may develop rapidly);
- liver function tests;
- creatine kinase;
- urea and electrolytes, blood glucose;
- blood gas and acid–base analysis;
- electrocardiogram;
- chest radiograph;
- CT scan;
- lumbar puncture.

Treatment

Rapid institution of treatment aimed at rapidly cooling the patient while maintaining oxygen delivery increases the chances of a successful outcome. Depending on the cause of hyperthermia, specific therapy may be indicated. Subsequent treatment involves supporting vital organ function.

PREHOSPITAL MANAGEMENT

The victim should be moved immediately to a cooler environment and their clothing removed. Cooling should be achieved by whatever means are available (e.g. the patient can be sprayed or splashed with water and evaporation encouraged by opening windows or doors, using a fan or even the down-draught from helicopter blades). Ice packs, when available, should be applied to the neck, axillae or groins. If possible oxygen should be given and an intravenous infusion of crystalloid established.

MANAGEMENT IN HOSPITAL

Cooling

Aggressive measures to cool the patient should be started as soon as the diagnosis has been established. Immersion in ice-cold water is impractical and its efficacy is limited by cutaneous vasoconstriction, which diminishes the capacity for heat loss. The most effective methods combine evaporation and convection, most simply by splashing or sponging the patient with tepid (not cold) water and exposing them to a continuous current of air (e.g. using a fan). The Mecca body cooling technique is unsurpassed as a means of reducing body temperature in heat stroke victims. It involves spraying the naked victim with lukewarm, atomized water (at 15°C) while warm air (at 40–50°C) is blown over the body and the skin temperature is maintained above 30°C to encourage cutaneous vasodilatation (Weiner & Khogali, 1980). As well as administering cold humidified oxygen and cold intravenous fluids, which contribute minimally to heat loss, iced gastric lavage is a relatively simple procedure that has been used in combination with evaporative techniques.

If these measures fail to reduce core temperature to below 40°C within about 30 minutes then additional measures such as iced peritoneal lavage (instillation of 2 litres of iced 0.9% saline into the peritoneal cavity, which is drained after 30 minutes) or, rarely, extracorporeal cooling may be used.

Drug therapy

Dantrolene is a direct-acting muscle relaxant that inhibits the release of calcium from the sarcoplasmic reticulum. It reduces heat production by preventing muscle contraction. Dantrolene reverses the clinical features of malignant hyperthermia (Kolb *et al.*, 1982) and can prevent it when given prophylactically to susceptible patients undergoing general anaesthesia. Dantrolene is also probably useful in neuroleptic malignant syndrome, but it seems to be of no benefit in heat stroke (Bouchama *et al.*, 1991) and there is little evidence to support its use in severe hyperthermia associated with the use of amphetamine analogues (see Chapter 18).

Serotonin antagonists such as ketanserin may be useful in the treatment of drug-induced hyperthermia due to agents such as fluoxitene, MAOIs and some amphetamine derivatives whose hyperthermic activity may be partially attributable to increased serotonin levels.

Calcium antagonists such as nimodipine may also inhibit calcium-dependent release of serotonin from storage vesicles (Azmitia *et al.*, 1990).

Drugs that *increase dopaminergic activity* such as bromocriptine, amantidine and Levodopa and *anticholinergics* such as benztropine may be useful in neuroleptic malignant syndrome, although there is no clear evidence for their efficacy.

In some cases the muscle relaxant properties of *diazepam* may be useful.

Supportive measures

In severe cases supportive measures may include:

- tracheal intubation and mechanical ventilation, which can be combined with neuromuscular blockade to reduce muscular activity and heat production;
- expansion of the circulating volume (guided by CVP and/or pulmonary artery occlusion pressure (PAOP) monitoring as indicated);
- inotropic support, though this is rarely required (avoid α agonists, which may cause cutaneous vasoconstriction and impair heat loss);
- management of pulmonary oedema and/or ARDS (see Chapter 7).
- management of rhabdomyolysis (see Chapter 12);
- prevention of agitation and seizures (which increase heat production) with prophylactic phenytoin and diazepam as indicated;
- early haemofiltration for severe rhabdomyolysis and/or renal failure (see Chapter 12);
- administration of blood and blood products as indicated to treat coagulopathy;
- supportive measures for liver impairment (see Chapter 13).

Prognosis

Morbidity and mortality are directly related to the peak temperature and the duration of hyperthermia. Prolonged coma and DIC are associated with a poor prognosis. Mortality seems to be reduced if patients are rapidly cooled during the first hour of treatment and survival is possible even when core temperature exceeds 42°C (Logan *et al.*, 1993).

Malignant hyperpyrexia

Malignant hyperpyrexia (MH) is a rare inherited disorder of muscle that predisposes individuals to develop a hypermetabolic state when exposed to certain 'triggering' agents such as suxamethonium and a variety of anaesthetic agents. The incidence is thought to be around 1/62,000 anaesthetics involving recognized triggering agents.

PATHOGENESIS

It appears that MH is precipitated when exposure of a susceptible individual to a 'triggering' agent leads to a sudden increase in intracellular calcium concentrations, probably as a result of impaired uptake of calcium by the sarcoplasmic reticulum or inappropriate release of calcium from intracellular stores. The increase in intracellular calcium concentration accelerates hydrolysis of ATP, induces muscle rigidity and uncouples oxidative phosphorylation. These changes induce a hypermetabolic state with increased heat production, impaired active transport mechanisms and eventual depletion of ATP.

Responsible agents include:

- succinylcholine;
- inhalational anaesthetic agents (except nitrous oxide);
- amide local anaesthetics;
- caffeine;
- halogenated radiographic contrast media (rarely);
- phenothiazines (increase intracellular calcium).

Ketamine is probably safe, but is best avoided because the hypertension and tachycardia that usually accompanies its use might confuse management of a susceptible patient. The condition may also be triggered by strenuous exercise or massive muscle injury, especially in hot and humid conditions, as well as by emotional stress.

CLINICAL FEATURES

Susceptibility to MH is associated with subclinical and clinical myopathies such as Duchenne muscular dystrophy. There may be a history of previous episodes, unexplained perioperative fever or an aborted anaesthetic. MH often presents insidiously in a patient undergoing general anaesthesia. The earliest reliable indication is usually *increased carbon dioxide production*, which may be detected as a rise in the end-tidal carbon dioxide concentration in mechanically ventilated patients or as an increase in minute ventilation in those breathing spontaneously. Unusual and rapid exhaustion of the carbon dioxide absorbent may also be recognized. *Muscle rigidity* is often first noted in the jaw muscles, but later becomes generalized, although the specificity of masseter spasm as a sign of MH has been questioned. Tachycardia, arrhythmias and hypertension may be followed later by hypotension as cardiac function deteriorates. As the hypermetabolic state progresses *body temperature increases*, although this is usually a late sign, and the rate of temperature rise is variable (from 1°C/hour to 1°C every 5 minutes). The onset of fever is also influenced by the precipitating agent (e.g. the combination of suxamethonium and halothane produces an earlier and more rapid rise in body temperature). Cyanotic mottling of the skin, especially over the head, neck and upper chest may also be noted.

As the condition progresses patients may develop:

- pulmonary oedema and cardiac failure;
- DIC;
- rhabdomyolysis;
- haemolysis;
- neurological damage;
- acute renal failure;
- lactic acidosis;
- early hyperkalaemia followed by prolonged hypokalaemia;
- changes in serum calcium, phosphorus and magnesium levels.

INVESTIGATIONS AND MONITORING

Investigations may include:

- blood gas and acid–base analysis;
- plasma electrolytes, urea and glucose;
- creatine kinase;
- liver enzymes;
- coagulation screen and platelet count;
- tests for haemolysis;
- blood lactate.

Body temperature, end-tidal carbon dioxide, ECG, blood pressure, CVP and urine output should be continuously monitored.

Investigation of susceptibility to MH involves testing contractile responses to halothane, caffeine, or a combination of the two in a fresh viable muscle biopsy obtained from the patient. Testing is performed in a limited number of specialist centres and the results can be inconsistent.

TREATMENT

The treatment of MH is as follows:

- terminate anaesthesia and surgery as soon as possible;
- hyperventilate with oxygen, preferably through a vapour-free circuit;
- if surgery cannot be concluded immediately, use narcotics and non-depolarizing muscle relaxants;
- administer dantrolene 1 mg/kg intravenously every 5 minutes to a total dose of 10 mg/kg;
- correct acidosis;
- control potassium;
- institute measures to cool the patient (see above);
- give mannitol and frusemide to promote a diuresis;
- control arrhythmias;
- minimize movement and handling of the patient since this may precipitate ventricular arrhythmias.

Drugs such as barbiturates, narcotics and antipyretics are probably of little value. Steroids have been recommended, but their role is unclear. Chlorpromazine may help to promote heat loss by reversing peripheral vasoconstriction and inhibiting shivering.

Drugs that must be avoided at all costs during an episode of MH include amide local anaesthetics, cardiac glycosides, belladonna alkaloids, vasopressors and calcium chloride.

PROGNOSIS

In the 1960s the mortality from MH was around 80%, but improved treatment, earlier detection and increased recognition and understanding of the syndrome has reduced the mortality to less than 10%.

Neuroleptic malignant syndrome

Neuroleptic malignant syndrome (NMS) is a potentially fatal idiosyncratic response to neuroleptic drugs including the phenothiazines, butyrophenones, thioxanthenes and other major tranquillizers such as lithium. It has also occurred after withdrawal of anti-Parkinsonian drugs and metoclopramide. The estimated incidence is 0.5–1.0% of those taking neuroleptics and in susceptible patients the syndrome may be triggered by factors such as exhaustion, dehydration and organic brain disease. It affects people of all ages, but is commoner in males and in those less than 40 years of age.

PATHOGENESIS

NMS is thought to be precipitated by blockade of dopamine receptors in the basal ganglia and hypothalamus. Hyperthermia is probably related to impaired temperature regulation and sustained muscle contraction.

CLINICAL FEATURES

Frequently the syndrome occurs within 2 weeks of instituting treatment or when the dosage is increased; symptoms usually progress rapidly over 2-3 days. Characteristic features include:

- hyperthermia;
- muscle rigidity and tremors;
- akinesia;
- impaired consciousness and confusion;
- autonomic dysfunction with tachycardia, labile blood pressure and sweating;
- tachypnoea;
- dysarthria and sialorrhoea;
- urinary retention/incontinence.

Investigations may reveal a leucocytosis, abnormal liver function tests (increased transaminases), a raised creatinine kinase, myoglobinuria and metabolic acidosis.
The *differential diagnosis* includes:

- MH;
- Parkinson's disease;
- catatonia;
- heat stroke;
- central cholinergic syndrome;
- drug interactions with MAOIs;
- sepsis;
- tetanus;
- meningoencephalitis.

Admission to intensive care may be precipitated by cardiac arrest (e.g. due to myocardial infarction or pulmonary embolism), respiratory failure (pulmonary oedema, aspiration pneumonitis), seizures or acute renal failure (related to dehydration and/or myoglobinuria).

TREATMENT

The offending drug should be withdrawn and supportive therapy instituted. This should include:

- cooling;
- rehydration;
- measures to prevent acute renal failure;
- cardiovascular support;
- mechanical ventilation if indicated.

Specific treatment is intended to alter the balance between dopaminergic and cholinergic activity in the basal ganglia as well as to provide muscle relaxation. Suggested pharmacological interventions include:

- Levodopa orally;
- bromocriptine (can be used with dantrolene);
- amantidine;
- benztropine;
- dantrolene (can be combined with dopaminergic agents);
- other muscle relaxants such as diazepam and non-depolarizing agents.

REFERENCES

Azmitia EC, Murphy RB & Whitaker-Azmitia PM (1990) MDMA (Ecstasy) effects on cultured serotonergic neurons: evidence of Ca$^{2(+)}$ dependent toxicity linked to release. *Brain Research* **510**: 97-103.

Bouchama A, Cafege A, Devol EB, Labdi O, el-Assil K & Seraj M (1991) Ineffectiveness of dantrolene sodium in the treatment of heatstroke. *Critical Care Medicine* **19**: 176-180.

Editorial (1977) The old in the cold. *British Medical Journal* **i**: 336.

Golden FStC & Rivers JF (1975) The immersion incident. *Anaesthesia* **30**: 364-373.

Harari A, Regnier B, Rapin M, Lemaire F & Le Gall JR (1975) Haemodynamic study of prolonged deep accidental hypothermia. *European Journal of Intensive Care Medicine* **1**: 65-70.

Hopkins PM, Ellis FR & Halsall PJ (1991) Evidence for related myopathies in exertional heat stroke and malignant hyperthermia. *Lancet* **338**: 1491-1492.

Kolb ME, Horne ML & Martz R (1982) Dantrolene in human malignant hyperthermia: *Anaesthesiology* **56**: 254-262.

Logan AS, St. C, Stickle B, O'Keefe N & Hewitson H (1993) Survival following 'Ecstasy' ingestion with a peak temperature of 42°C. *Anaesthesia* **48**: 1017-1018.

MacLean D, Murison J & Griffiths PD (1973) Acute pancreatitis and diabetic ketoacidosis in accidental hypothermia and hyperthermic myxoedema. *British Medical Journal* **4**: 757-761.

Rosenberg J, Pentel P, Pond S, Benowitz M & Olson K (1986) Hyperthermia associated with drug intoxication. *Critical Care Medicine* **14**: 964-969.

Siebke H, Rod T, Breivik H & Lind B (1975) Survival after 40 minutes: submersion without cerebral sequelae. *Lancet* **i**: 1275-1277.

Weiner JS & Khogali M (1980) A physiological body-cooling unit for treatment of heat stroke. *Lancet* **ii**: 507-509.

20 Transporting the Critically Ill

Critically ill patients may have to be transported to hospital from the site of illness or injury (*primary transport*) or be transferred from one hospital to another for specialist investigations and treatment (*secondary transport*); sometimes transfer is necessary because of a shortage of staffed intensive care beds. Seriously ill patients may also have to be moved within the hospital (e.g. to the operating theatre for surgical procedures or for investigations such as CT scanning or angiography).

Moving critically ill patients is potentially extremely dangerous, especially when they are receiving intensive haemodynamic and respiratory support and when unqualified or inexperienced staff are involved (Bion *et al.*, 1988). Not only is there a considerable risk of mishaps such as accidental extubation, loss of intravascular access and discontinuation of vasoactive or sedative agents, but seriously ill patients are intolerant of lifting, tipping, abrupt movements, vibration and acceleration/deceleration. Transfer is often associated with a significant deterioration in oxygenation, while accelerational forces and vertical movements can precipitate cardiovascular instability, especially in those who are volume depleted or vasodilated due to sepsis, sedation or drugs. The mechanisms underlying the reduction in cardiac output that often occurs under these circumstances have not been fully explained, but both venous pooling and vagally mediated responses via the eighth nerve are possibilities. Transfer may also cause significant changes in intracranial pressure. Accelerational forces in the longitudinal plane, for example, will alter the pressure in central veins, intracranial sinuses and cerebrospinal fluid. Placing patients in the head-down position (e.g. when they are being loaded into an ambulance) may also exacerbate intracranial hypertension. Physical difficulties such as narrow corridors, small lifts and cramped vehicles, as well as poor weather conditions, may also be encountered. Table 20.1 shows a summary check-list.

PRIMARY TRANSPORT

Most often, primary transport of critically ill patients is required for the victims of cardiorespiratory collapse or major trauma, including severe head injuries, and may involve extrication of trapped individuals, handling of mass casualties and evacuation from isolated locations.

Composition of the pre-hospital team

In many countries primary transport is normally performed by medical technicians trained in simple first aid or by paramedics; the latter may be trained to provide basic life support (BLS) only or to administer advanced life support (ALS). Some have questioned whether the additional skills of medically qualified personnel can be used to advantage in the pre-hospital environment, although others are convinced that the inclusion of a doctor in the emergency team is valuable, and it has been claimed that the survival of patients with blunt trauma is improved when they are attended by flight crews that include a physician (Baxt & Moody, 1987). Those who advocate including a physician in the team argue that although ambulancemen with advanced training may be competent to perform the commonly required practical procedures, the particular skills of a doctor are invaluable for diagnosis, assessing the severity of the injury, deciding priorities and triage. There are also reservations about those without medical knowledge using advanced resuscitation techniques unsupervised.

It is claimed that a number of other benefits may arise from specialist medical involvement in pre-hospital care. For example it becomes unnecessary to dispatch relatively inexperienced doctors in training, unsupervised, to the scene of an incident, and hospitals are not deprived of doctors when patients require transfer. Also the training of doctors in emergency medicine at the roadside is improved and experienced doctors are immediately available to respond to major disasters. Certainly the French have insisted that doctors should play a central role in the control and provision of pre-hospital emergency care and to this end have created an emergency medical assistance service—Service d'Aide Médicale Urgente (SAMU)—which each département is now legally required to provide. Every SAMU has a control room, offices and a garage for the rescue vehicles. The control room acts as a centre for the reception of medical emergency calls and is under the control of a full-time 'chef de service'. The main functions of the SAMU are:

Table 20.1 Transporting critically ill patients—a checklist.

Administration

Establish effective communication between transferring and receiving hospitals and ambulance authority

Notify and explain reasons for transfer to relatives

For the conscious patient, explain the reasons for the transfer

Collect together patient records to accompany patient

Ensure appropriately experienced and qualified staff accompany patient

Select most appropriate mode of transport—surface ambulance, air transport—(fixed wing, helicopter), sea

Preparation of Patient

Optimize patient's condition
   Circulating volume
   Haemodynamic support
   Respiratory support
   Appropriate monitoring
   Appraise need for sedation, analgesia and muscle relaxants
   Rarely need surgery before transfer

Underwater seal drains—do not clamp or lift above patient

Nutritional support—if this is discontinued, beware of hypoglycaemia

Maintain body temperature

Investigations
   Radiographs to confirm position of endotracheal tube, intravascular cannulae and chest drains

Equipment

Provision of respiratory support and monitoring

   Gas supply—oxygen ± air
      Cylinders
      Portable liquid oxygen containers
      Air compressor
   Mechanical ventilation
      Portable ventilator
      Heat and moisture exchanger
      Suction apparatus
   Monitoring
      Airway pressure gauge
      Wright's respirometer
      Pulse oximeter
      (Capnography)
Provision of cardiovascular monitoring and support
   Fluid administration—infusion pump
   Vasoactive agents and inotropes—syringe pump
   Portable defibrillator
   Continuous ECG monitoring
   Continuous direct intra-arterial pressure monitoring
   (Pulmonary artery pressures)
   (Intracranial pressure)
   (Cardiac output)
   (Intra-aortic balloon pump)
   (Continuous haemofiltration)

- centralization of emergency medical calls;
- organization of the appropriate response;
- ensuring that medical assistance arrives rapidly;
- continuous radio link with the hospital during initial medical care;

- preparation of hospital reception;
- organization of interhospital and intrahosptial transports;
- promotion of research and teaching in emergency and disaster medicine for medical, nursing and paramedical personnel.

In other countries separate accident, coronary and obstetric 'flying squads' have been used to provide expert medical assistance at the scene, but in general their value has been difficult to establish and, at least in the UK, they are few in number. Most large hospitals do, however, have major accident protocols, which include the provision of suitably experienced and qualified medical and nursing staff at the scene of the incident. To ensure the appropriate level of response, it is essential to establish good communications and to ensure that the response is supervised and coordinated by a senior physician in the receiving hospital's emergency department.

Conduct of primary transport

It is important to take measures to secure the safety of personnel involved in pre-hospital care including the provision of safe transport, as well as issuing protective, clearly visible, dress and headgear with clear identification. Environmental safety measures such as controlling fires and protection from oncoming traffic are also important.

There are two broad approaches to the primary transport of seriously ill patients.

- 'Scoop and run' is intended to avoid wasting valuable time while inadequately trained personnel attempt complex life-saving measures.
- The alternative approach of 'field stabilization' is based on the premise that prior resuscitation may reduce morbidity and mortality, mainly by decreasing the risks of deterioration during transport, especially when journey times are long.

In practice the most appropriate approach in an individual patient is determined by the anticipated journey time and the nature of the illness or injury. Therefore when the patient is close to a hospital in an urban environment, immediate transfer is often preferable, whereas when longer distances are involved, the patient should be fully resuscitated before being moved. Patients with penetrating thoracic injuries involving the myocardium are best taken immediately to the nearest major hospital with only the minimum of pre-hospital care, whereas endotracheal intubation is clearly indicated for many head injuries before transfer.

All patients should receive *supplemental oxygen* to an *unobstructed airway* and most will benefit from establishing venous access and *expansion of their circulating volume* before transfer. *Stabilization of the cervical spine* is quick and of proven value whereas application of military antishock trousers (MAST) takes time and is of uncertain benefit except in a few clearly defined circumstances (see Chapter 4). *Pleural drainage*, when indicated, is most easily established via the second intercostal space in the mid-clavicular line where it can be easily observed with the patient on a stretcher. A *Heimlich valve* connected to a simple wound drainage bag can be useful under these circumstances. Appropriate intravenous, gaseous or regional *analgesia* should usually be given, and gross angulated *fractures* with vascular compression should be corrected and splinted. Objects impaling the trunk should not be removed.

Benefits of pre-hospital emergency treatment

The provision of pre-hospital emergency medical services is of proven value for victims of a cardiac arrest provided that cardiopulmonary resuscitation is initiated by a bystander, the paramedics arrive at the scene within a few minutes and the patient is rapidly transferred to hospital for definitive care. The benefits for trauma victims are less clear, except when a coordinated approach from primary transport to specialized trauma centres is established.

SECONDARY TRANSPORT

Considerably fewer seriously ill patients require secondary transport, although in the UK it is thought that at least 10,000 critically ill patients require interhospital transfer each year. The increasing tendency to concentrate specialist services such as neurosurgery, plastic surgery, cardiothoracic surgery, nephrology and intensive care in regional centres is likely to increase the demand for secondary transfer of the most seriously ill patients.

Principles of safe secondary transport
(see **Table 20.1**)

OPTIMIZE PATIENT'S CONDITION BEFORE TRANSFER

A detailed systems-based assessment of the patient's condition should be performed before instituting measures to prepare the patient for transfer. Most will require optimization of their circulating volume, as well as institution of mechanical ventilation and appropriate

monitoring if these are not already in progress. It is important to ensure adequate sedation, analgesia and, when indicated, muscle relaxation before moving the patient. A few may need surgery before transfer (e.g. to evacuate an acute intracranial haematoma). Investigations may include radiographs to confirm the positions of the endotracheal tube, intravascular cannulae and chest drains. Underwater seal drains should not be clamped or lifted above the patient during transfer. It is important to appreciate that abrupt cessation of glucose administration (e.g. if parenteral nutrition is discontinued) may precipitate dangerous hypoglycaemia. Measures should be taken to maintain body temperature. If the patient is conscious the proposed transfer and all that is entailed should be explained to them.

Although in general the patient's condition improves after initial resuscitation and with careful medical care does not usually deteriorate further during transport (Bion *et al.*, 1985), the more widespread use of invasive monitoring, and in particular pulmonary artery catheterization, has clearly demonstrated that transport can sometimes adversely affect even those patients who have been adequately resuscitated. Nevertheless mortality rates during transfer are in practice remarkably low (< 1%).

MAINTAIN A HIGH STANDARD OF CARE DURING TRANSFER

Medically qualified personnel are nearly always involved in secondary transport, although in certain circumstances (e.g. patients with impending cardiac crises who are not mechanically ventilated) transfer by paramedics may be appropriate. In some countries (e.g. North America, Australia and France) comprehensive transport systems have been developed, but in the UK the provision of facilities for secondary transfer is poor. In 1987, for example, 65% of intensive care units did not have access to a dedicated ambulance and 80% lacked a specialized trolley on which to base a mobile intensive care unit (MICU) (Wright *et al.*, 1988). Moreover medical care during transfer is often deficient. In a series of 50 mainly postoperative patients, for example, seven developed life-threatening complications including obstruction of an endotracheal tube, respiratory arrest, unrecognized disconnection of arterial and central venous cannulae and severe hypotension (Bion *et al.*, 1988). This study also suggested that patients under the care of experienced anaesthetists deteriorated less during transport than those supervised by other medical specialties (Bion *et al.*, 1988). It is therefore recommended that an anaesthetist with intensive care training who is not prone to motion sickness, does not have ear or sinus problems and has no difficulty working in a confined space, should accompany the patient. The use of specialized 'retrieval teams' by major centres has considerable advantages.

COMMUNICATION AND COOPERATION

Communication and cooperation between the transferring and receiving hospitals as well as the ambulance authority is fundamental to the success of secondary transport. Changes in the patient's condition and their response to treatment during transfer should be recorded and this, together with a written summary of the patient's history and initial treatment, must be handed over to the receiving staff.

MODES OF TRANSPORT

Selection of the most appropriate mode of transport requires consideration of the following:

- the patient's diagnosis and the possible effects of transport on their condition;
- the degree of any instability;
- the urgency of the transfer;
- the level of medical care the patient is receiving;
- the level of medical care the patient requires;
- the distance and duration of the journey;
- the methods of transport available.

Surface ambulances

Surface ambulances are probably the most practical and efficient means of transport within urban areas and for journeys not exceeding 25–30 miles. Despite recent improvements in the design of standard ambulances, however, unmodified, multipurpose vehicles are not ideal for transferring critically ill patients. On the other hand, purpose-built MICUs or 'critical care ambulances' are expensive and inflexible.

The advantages of surface ambulances include:

- door to door service;
- no requirement for landing zone or runway;
- little or no restrictions due to weather;
- in an emergency the vehicle can be stopped to facilitate performance of procedures;
- can divert to the nearest hospital if the patient deteriorates or supplies are exhausted;
- relative ease of personnel training.

The main disadvantages of surface transport include:

- long journey times, especially when there is traffic congestion, poor road conditions, inclement weather or road works;

- the uncomfortable rough ride, 'sway and bounce,' vibration, repetitive acceleration and/or deceleration;
- motion sickness;
- limited accessibility, poor lighting and limited power;
- difficulty gaining access to remote or restricted areas;
- potential breakdown in communications on long journeys.

Air transport

The main advantage of air transport is the shorter journey time; it is therefore used more frequently in North America and Australia where patients often have to be transported over long distances. Air transport may also be used to achieve rapid delivery of paramedics and doctors to the scene of the incident. Elective movement of patients between hospitals by air may also be preferred because of the reduction in journey times. Secondary transportation of trauma victims by air following stabilization at the receiving hospital can be performed safely and many consider this to be an important aspect of regionalized trauma care. Some authors (Moylan et al., 1988) have demonstrated improved survival of trauma victims transported by air rather than surface ambulance, although the efficacy of air transport probably depends on local geography since in an urban setting the use of a helicopter appeared to offer no advantage compared to a sophisticated paramedic-based system of pre-hospital care (Schiller et al., 1988).

DANGERS OF AIR TRANSPORTATION

Reduction in atmospheric pressure

Even in 'pressurized' aircraft the cabin pressure is equivalent to an altitude of 2000–2500 m (i.e. about 75 kPa) and this is associated with a fall in the atmospheric partial pressure of oxygen. There is therefore a danger of precipitating *hypoxia* in those breathing room air, although critically ill patients will, of course, be receiving supplemental oxygen.

The reduction in atmospheric pressure may also be associated with *expansion of closed cavities*. Pneumothoraces, for example, may enlarge and it is important to ensure that chest drains are patent and correctly positioned; in some cases prophylactic drainage may be indicated. There may also be damage to the middle ear if the eustachian tube is obstructed (e.g. in those with upper respiratory tract infections, sinusitis, ear infections or allergy), while expansion of air trapped in abscesses or behind crowns may cause toothache. Expansion of gas in the gastrointestinal tract may be associated with discomfort, nausea, vomiting and shortness of breath. In extreme cases, venous return may be compromised and, if pain is severe, the vasovagal response may cause hypotension and synope. The cuff on the endotracheal tube may also expand and if the intracuff pressure exceeds about 25 mm Hg it may be wise to remove excess air; during descent the cuff may deflate and a leak can develop around the tube. The air in MASTs may also expand causing worsening regional compression, while limbs encased in plaster of Paris can swell and may have to be released using plaster shears. Expansion of the air in intravenous fluid containers may increase the rate of transfusion. Finally, gas emboli in those with decompression sickness can also expand.

The effect of air space expansion at altitude (e.g. in those with gut distension, blocked sinuses or intracranial air) can be minimized by administering 100% oxygen to denitrogenate the patient before and during the flight. Patients with bowel obstruction and those who have recently undergone abdominal surgery must have a patent nasogastric tube in place before transport.

Effects of turbulence

Apart from precipitating *nausea and vomiting* with a risk of aspiration, turbulence may have adverse effects on *unstable spinal fractures* and on an *irritable myocardium*.

Temperature and humidity

Cabin temperature tends to fall at altitude and this may lead to an *increased metabolic rate* and oxygen demand. The reduction in humidity can cause *dehydration* in both the patient and the crew.

Noise

Noise hampers communication, renders audible alarms useless and makes it difficult or impossible to use a stethoscope. It may also cause discomfort, headache, fatigue, nausea, visual disturbances, vertigo, temporary or permanent ear damage and poor performance of tasks. The use of ear plugs, headsets and helmets ameliorates the effects of noise.

Vibration

Vibration causes a slight increase in metabolic rate. Low-frequency vibration may lead to fatigue, shortness of breath, motion sickness, blurred vision and chest or abdominal pain. Vibration may also interfere with thermoregulation by causing vasoconstriction and a reduced ability to perspire.

Gravitational forces

Gravitational forces occur during ascent and descent as well as during changes in speed or direction (see elsewhere in this chapter).

Fluid losses

As barometric pressure falls, fluid may extravasate from the intravascular to the interstitial space causing oedema, tachycardia and hypotension, as well as exacerbating the effects of dehydration.

Effects in those with penetrating eye injuries

Vomiting, coughing, straining and hypoxia may lead to expulsion of vitreous and other intraocular contents. Expansion of entrapped air may lead to discharge of the globe. Recommended preventive measures have included eye binding, sitting the patient up, the administration of 100% oxygen and anti-emetics.

Problems caused by altitude may also be occasionally encountered when transporting by road over mountainous terrain.

HELICOPTERS

When compared to surface transport, helicopters reduce journey times by between one-third and one-half, they cause less road disruption and they facilitate patient management during a long transfer. They are also able to land close to an incident and gain access to difficult locations. Helicopters have been shown to be a practical means of transporting critically ill patients between hospitals (Kee *et al.*, 1992). Although vibration and motion sickness can cause difficulties, transfer by helicopter may be less deleterious to critically ill patients than other forms of transport because:

- acceleration/deceleration can be achieved more smoothly than in a land vehicle;
- a helicopter only accelerates at the beginning of transfer, following which a steady speed can be maintained throughout the flight;
- there is less vibration;
- if patients are flown 'feet first' they will be tilted slightly head-up during acceleration and slightly head-down during deceleration—this may minimize the changes in cardiovascular function and intracranial pressure normally seen during transport (Kee *et al.*, 1992);
- helicopters typically fly at below 2000 feet, thereby

avoiding the problems associated with depressurization;

- the likelihood of an accident is less than with ground transport.

The disadvantages of helicopters include the requirement for a helipad or unobstructed landing zone, space and weight limitations, and the noise, which may interfere with monitoring, especially audible warning devices. Communication difficulties are overcome relatively easily by wearing headsets. Finally, helicopters need a minimum visibility to fly, although most other weather conditions are not usually a problem. They are generally more expensive than ground transport.

FIXED-WING AIRCRAFT

Fixed-wing aircraft can be used for more rapid transport over longer distances. There is usually more space and the patient can often be positioned transversely to minimize the effect of acceleration/deceleration. Fixed-wing aircraft can fly above or around inclement weather. They can, of course, only operate from landing strips, and therefore intermediary transport is normally required.

Transport by sea

It is sometimes necessary to treat severely injured divers in a compression chamber on the surface at the scene of the accident. In some circumstances the patient may subsequently be transferred under pressure. More often the patient is treated and resuscitated before being rapidly evacuated to a specialist facility onshore.

EQUIPMENT FOR TRANSPORT

MICUs consist of a dedicated, purpose-built vehicle and trolley equipped to provide respiratory support and continuous monitoring. Alternatively trolleys can be designed to fit into conventional ambulances. They should be robust but light, stable but manoeuvrable and fit easily into lifts. They must be fully equipped with their own supply of power and gas so that they can provide patient support independently. All equipment must be securely mounted while in transit.

Provision of respiratory support

GAS SUPPLY

The gas supply can be from *cylinders*, which are relatively heavy and cumbersome, require reducing valves

and flow gauges, and cannot be refilled on-site, or *portable liquid oxygen containers*, which have a built-in flow meter, connect directly to the equipment or a face mask and overcome the problem of safety and weight in aircraft. Flexible pipe line extensions can be used to connect to wall supplies in hospitals and to larger cylinders in ambulances. Accurate low-flow oxygen delivery is also required for those breathing spontaneously. Gas-powered ventilators will entrain air, but have a limited selection of inspired oxygen concentrations, whereas minute volume dividers will require a source of diluent gas (either air or nitrous oxide) as well as a supply of oxygen. Compressed air is best provided by a compressor to avoid the difficulties associated with cylinders. An audible alarm must be used to warn of failure of the oxygen supply or the accidental delivery of a hypoxic mixture of gases, bearing in mind the limitations of an audible alarm in a noisy transport vehicle.

MECHANICAL VENTILATION

Manual ventilation with self-inflating bags may be associated with inadequate ventilation, carbon dioxide retention and hypoxaemia. Mechanical ventilation is therefore preferred and it should be possible to apply a positive end-expiratory pressure when necessary. The expired tidal volume can be measured using a *Wright's respirometer* (see Chapter 5) and an *airway pressure gauge* is vital to provide a warning of disconnection. *Capnography* tends to be unreliable during transport, although it is the only continuous method of ensuring that the endotracheal tube has not been displaced. It also provides a visual disconnect alarm and can be helpful in detecting catastrophic reductions in cardiac output. To fulfil these roles, the chosen capnograph must have a continuous graphic display. *Pulse oximeters* are an invaluable means of continuously monitoring oxygenation.

Humidification of inspired gases is best achieved using a heat and moisture exchanger. Electrically operated *suction apparatus* can be used in ambulances and aircraft, but manual or Venturi devices are preferred when transporting patients on trolleys.

Provision of cardiovascular monitoring and support

During transport fluid is most accurately and reliably administered using an infusion pump. Syringe pumps, which are cheaper, smaller and use less power, may be preferred for administering vasoactive agents and other drugs.

Clinical assessment of cardiovascular function is extremely difficult during transport and it is therefore essential to establish reliable accurate continuous monitoring of important haemodynamic variables using a lightweight battery-powered monitor. Devices are now available with excellent screen quality that allow continuous monitoring of two pressures, ECG, two temperatures, pulse oximetry, non-invasive blood pressure and even cardiac output. *Continuous ECG monitoring* will detect arrhythmias and alterations in heart rate, and may indicate the development of myocardial ischaemia or biochemical abnormalities such as hyperkalaemia. Indirect measurement of blood pressure by palpation is difficult and unreliable during transport because of artefact and interference. Direct *intra-arterial pressure monitoring* is therefore preferred, and in some cases central venous pressure, intracranial pressure or, occasionally, pulmonary artery pressures should also be continuously displayed. Because continuous flush systems are relatively bulky, intermittent manual flushing can be used as an alternative. A less satisfactory, but clinically acceptable, system is to use a heparin–saline-filled line connected to the air in an aneroid pressure-monitoring device to measure mean arterial pressure (Runcie *et al.*, 1990).

A modern portable external *defibrillator*, which may also display and print the ECG as well as act as an external pacemaker, should be carried on all transport trolleys and in ambulances. Some trolleys and ambulances are designed to enable intra-aortic balloon counterpulsation to continue during transfer and, in some cases, especially when journey times are long, continuous arteriovenous haemodiafiltration may be continued.

TRANSPORT WITHIN THE HOSPITAL

Intrahospital transport may in some instances be more hazardous than out of hospital transfers; also patients may be outside a critical care area (e.g. in the CT scanner) for long periods of time.

Even for these relatively short journeys, adequate resuscitation and preparation before moving the patient, the provision of comprehensive continuous monitoring and meticulous care by skilled medical and nursing staff during transfer are essential. Transfer within the hospital may be associated with various complications including hypotension, hypertension, cardiac arrhythmias, airway obstruction and cardiac arrest (Link *et al.*, 1990), and is further complicated if the patient is emerging from anaesthesia on return from the operating theatre. It is important to move at a time and along a route likely to be associated with the least delay, and it is sensible to delegate a team member to commandeer lifts and clear corridors.

TRANSPORT OVER LONG DISTANCES

Transport over long distances poses special problems, especially when international travel is involved. In most cases the patient should not be moved until the acute illness has resolved. Transfer can then be by private aeromedical transport organization, military aircraft, chartered executive jet or commercial airliner, preferably non-stop. Arrangements can be complex, and good liaison is essential. It is important that sufficient staff are employed to allow them to work conventional 8–12 hour shifts. In a commercial jet aircraft up to 15 seats may be required for a complex case—6–8 for the stretcher, two for the equipment, two for medical gases and one for each team member. A spare ventilator, preferably able to operate using room air, and twice the anticipated gas supplies should be carried. On these long flights waste disposal becomes an important consideration.

REFERENCES

Baxt WG & Moody P (1987) The impact of a physician as part of the aeromedical prehospital team in patients with blunt trauma. *Journal of the American Medical Association* **257**: 3246–3250.

Bion JF, Edlin SA, Ramsay G, McCabe S & Ledingham IMcA (1985) Validation of a prognostic score in critically ill patients undergoing transport. *British Medical Journal* **291**: 432–434.

Bion JF, Wilson IH & Taylor PA (1988) Transporting critically ill patients by ambulance: audit by sickness scoring. *British Medical Journal* **296**: 170.

Kee SS, Ramage CMH, Mendel P & Bristow ASE (1992) Interhospital transfers by helicopter: the first 50 patients of the Carelight project. *Journal of the Royal Society of Medicine* **85**: 29–31.

Link J, Krause H, Wagner W & Papadopoulous G (1990) Intra-

hospital transport of critically ill patients. *Critical Care Medicine* **18**: 1427–1429.

Moylan JA, Fitzpatrick KT, Beyer AJ III & Georgiade GS (1988) Factors improving survival in multisystem trauma patients. *Annals of Surgery* **207**: 679–685.

Runcie CJ, Reeve W, Reidy J & Dougall JR (1990) A comparison of measurements of blood pressure, heart-rate and oxygenation during inter-hospital transport of the critically ill. *Intensive Care Medicine* **16**: 317–322.

Schiller WR, Knox R, Zinnecker H *et al.* (1988) Effect of helicopter transport of trauma victims on survival in an urban trauma center. *Journal of Trauma* **28**: 1127–1134.

Wright IH, McDonald JC, Rogers PN & Ledingham IMcA (1988) Provision of facilities for secondary transport of seriously ill patients in the United Kingdom. *British Medical Journal* **296**: 543–545.

INDEX